Portal Hypertension

CLINICAL GASTROENTEROLOGY

George Y. Wu, SERIES EDITOR

PORTAL HYPERTENSION

PATHOBIOLOGY, EVALUATION, AND TREATMENT

Edited by

ARUN J. SANYAL, MBBS, MD

Division of Gastroenterology,
Virginia Commonwealth Medical Center, Richmond, VA

VIJAY H. SHAH, MD

GI Research Unit, Mayo Clinic, Rochester, MN

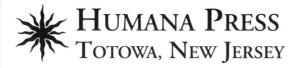

HUMANA PRESS
TOTOWA, NEW JERSEY

© 2005 Humana Press Inc.
999 Riverview Drive, Suite 208
Totowa, New Jersey 07512
humanapress.com

For additional copies, pricing for bulk purchases, and/or information about other Humana titles, contact Humana at the above address or at any of the following numbers: Tel: 973-256-1699; Fax: 973-256-8341; E-mail: orders@humanapr.com or visit our Website at humanapress.com

This publication is printed on acid-free paper.∞
ANSI Z39.48-1984 (American National Standards Institute)
Permanence of Paper for Printed Library Materials.

Cover Illustration: *Foreground*—Figure 3, Chapter 18, and *background*—Figure 1, Chapter 18, by Charmaine A. Stewart and Patrick S. Kamath.

Cover design by Patricia F. Cleary.

Printed in the United States of America.   10 9 8 7 6 5 4 3 2 1

Library of Congress Cataloging-in-Publication Data
Portal hypertension : pathobiology, evaluation, and treatment / edited by Arun J. Sanyal and Vijay H. Shah.
          p. ; cm. — (Clinical gastroenterology)
     Includes bibliographical references and index.
     ISBN 1-58829-386-6 (alk. paper) e-ISBN 1-59259-885-4
     1. Portal hypertension.   I. Sanyal, Arun J. II. Shah, Vijay H. III. Series.
     [DNLM: 1. Hypertension, Portal.   WI 720 P8423 2005]
 RC848.P6P678 2005
  616.3'62—dc22   2004016771

PREFACE

The past several years have seen a logarithmic increase in progress in the field of portal hypertension, both in clinical management as well as in pathobiology. For example, the implementation of beta-blockers in the primary and secondary prophylaxis of variceal hemorrhage and the establishment of endoscopic variceal band ligation in the management of acute variceal hemorrhage have become mainstays of clinical management of patients with portal hypertension. From a scientific standpoint, discoveries such as the elucidation of the hepatic stellate cell as a contractile sinusoidal effector cell and the understanding of nitric oxide as a key mediator of vascular responses have provided a cellular framework for the pathogenesis of portal hypertension. However, these discoveries and treatment advances are just the tip of the iceberg, with new therapies and pathogenic principles coming under scrutiny and likely to reach fruition in the years to come.

In this spirit, we hope that *Portal Hypertension: Pathobiology, Evaluation, and Treatment* will provide useful information for individuals actively engaged in the investigative aspects of portal hypertension, as well as clinicians who care for patients with portal hypertension throughout the world. The goal of this text is to provide scientific updates from leading portal hypertension researchers on key topics relating to the clinical and basic investigation of portal hypertension, as well as to provide input from leading portal hypertension clinicians regarding the revaluation and management of specific clinical circumstances relating to portal hypertension. We have garnered contributions from experts throughout the world, consistent with the global contributions that have been made in the field of portal hypertension.

We hope that the readership finds *Portal Hypertension: Pathobiology, Evaluation, and Treatment* useful as a reference as well as enjoyable as a cover-to-cover read!

Arun J. Sanyal, MBBS, MD
Vijay H. Shah, MD

CONTENTS

Part V: Evaluation and Treatment in Special Circumstances of Portal Hypertension

COLOR PLATES

CONTRIBUTORS

JUAN G. ABRALDES, MD • *Liver Unit, Institut de Malalties Digestives, Institut d'Investigacio Biomedica August Pi Sunyer, University of Barcelona, Barcelona, Spain*

MARIA H. ALONSO, MD • *Department of Surgery, University of Cincinnati, Cincinnati Children's Hospital Medical Center, Cincinnati, OH*

MEENA B. BANSAL, MD • *Division of Liver Diseases, Mount Sinai School of Medicine, New York, NY*

JAIME BOSCH, MD • *Liver Unit, Institut de Malaties Digestives, Institut d'Investigacio Biomedica August Pi Sunyer, University of Barcelona, Barcelona, Spain*

THOMAS D. BOYER, MD • *Liver Research Institute, University of Arizona, Tuscon, AZ*

ANDRÉS CÁRDENAS, MD, MMSc • *Division of Gastroenterology and Hepatology, Harvard Medical School, Beth Israel Deaconess Medical Center, Boston, MA; Liver Unit, Institut de Malalties Digestives, Institut d'Investigacio Biomedica August Pi Sunyer, University of Barcelona, Barcelona, Spain*

JOHN P. CELLO, MD • *Department of Medicine, School of Medicine, University of California, San Francisco, CA*

ROBERTO DE FRANCHIS, MD • *Gastroenterology and Gastrointestinal Endoscopy Service, Department of Internal Medicine, IRCCS Ospedale Policlinico, University of Milan, Milan, Italy*

ÀNGELS ESCORSELL, MD • *Liver Unit, Institut de Malalties Digestives, Institut d'Investigacio Biomedica August Pi Sunyer, Barcelona, Spain*

MICHAEL B. FALLON, MD • *Liver Center, University of Alabama at Birmingham, Birmingham, AL*

SCOTT L. FRIEDMAN, MD • *Division of Liver Diseases, Mount Sinai School of Medicine, New York, NY*

GUADALUPE GARCIA-TSAO, MD • *Section of Digestive Diseases, Yale University School of Medicine, Connecticut VA Healthcare System, New Haven, CT*

PERE GINÈS, MD • *Liver Unit, Institut de Malalties Digestives, University of Barcelona, Barcelona, Spain*

NORMAN D. GRACE, MD • *Gastroenterology Division, Brigham and Women's Hospital, Boston, MA and Faulkner Hospital, Jamaica Plain, MA*

ROBERTO J. GROSZMANN, MD • *Hepatic Hemodynamic Laboratory, Yale Liver Center, West Haven, CT*

PETER C. HAYES, MD, PhD • *Department of Hepatology and Radiology, Royal Infirmary, Edinburgh, UK*

J. MICHAEL HENDERSON, MD • *Department of General Surgery, The Cleveland Clinic Foundation, Cleveland, OH*

PIERRE-MICHEL HUET, MD, PhD • *Hopital l'Archet, Centre Hospitalier Universitaire, Nice, France*

RAJIV JALAN, MBBS, MD • *Institute of Hepatology, Royal Free and University College Medical School, London, UK*

WLADIMIRO JIMÉNEZ, PhD • *Hormonal Laboratory, University Hospital Clinic, University of Barcelona, Barcelona, Spain*

PATRICK S. KAMATH, MD • *Division of Gastroenterology, Mayo Clinic and Medical School, Rochester, MN*

SAKIB KARIM KHALID, MD • *Section of Digestive Diseases, Yale University School of Medicine, Connecticut VA Healthcare System, New Haven, CT*

W. RAY KIM, MD, MBA • *Mayo Clinic and Foundation, Rochester, MN*

MICHAEL J. KROWKA, MD • *Divisions of Pulmonary and Critical Care and of Gastroenterology and Hepatology, Mayo Clinic, Rochester, MN*

W. WAYNE LAUTT • *Department of Pharmacology and Therapeutics, University of Manitoba, Winnipeg, Manitoba, Canada*

DIDIER LEBREC, MD • *Laboratoire d'Hemodynamique Splanchnique et de Biologie Vasculaire, Hopital Beaujon, Clichy, France*

ZHI MING • *Department of Pharmacology and Therapeutics, University of Manitoba, Winnipeg, Manitoba, Canada*

MANUEL MORALES-RUIZ • *Hormonal Laboratory, University Hospital Clinic, University of Barcelona, Barcelona, Spain*

RICHARD MOREAU, MD • *Laboratoire d'Hemodynamique Splanchnique et de Biologie Vasculaire, Hopital Beaujon, Clichy, France*

ROSA MARIA MORILLAS, MD • *Liver Unit, Department of Gastroenterology, Hospital Universitari Germans Trias I Pujol, Barcelona, Spain*

KEVIN MOORE, MBBS, PhD • *Centre for Hepatology, Royal Free and University College Medical School, University College London, London, UK*

MASSIMO PINZANI, MD, PhD • *Laboratorio di Epatologia, Dipartimento di Medicina Interna, Universita di Firenze, Firenze, Italy*

RAMON PLANAS, MD • *Liver Unit, Department of Gastroenterology, Hospital Universitari Germans Trias I Pujol, Barcelona, Spain*

G. POMIER-LAYRARGUES, MD • *Andre-Viallet Clinical Research Centre, Hopital Saint-Luc, Montreal, Canada*

DORIS N. REDHEAD • *Department of Hepatology and Radiology, Royal Infirmary, Edinburgh, UK*

JUERG REICHEN, MD • *Department of Clinical Pharmacology, University of Berne, Berne, Switzerland*

ADRIAN REUBEN, MBBS, FRCP • *Division of Gastroenterology and Hepatology, Medical University of South Carolina, Charleston, SC*

DON C. ROCKEY, MD • *Liver Center, Duke University Medical Center, Durham, NC*

FREDERICK C. RYCKMAN, MD • *Department of Surgery, University of Cincinnati, Cincinnati Children's Hospital Medical Center, Cincinnati, OH*

BIMALJIT SANDHU, MD • *Division of Gastroenterology, Hepatology, and Nutrition, Virginia Commonwealth University, Richmond, VA*

ARUN J. SANYAL, MBBS, MD • *Division of Gastroenterology, Hepatology, and Nutrition, Virginia Commonwealth University, Richmond, VA*

SHIV K. SARIN, MD • *Department of Gastroenterology, University of Delhi, GB Pant Hospital, New Delhi, India*

VIJAY H. SHAH, MD • *GI Research Unit, Mayo Clinic, Rochester, MN*

CHARMAINE A. STEWART, MD • *Division of Gastroenterology, Mayo Clinic, Rochester, MN*

KAREN L. SWANSON, DO • *Division of Pulmonary and Critical Care, Mayo Clinic, Rochester, MN*

JAYANT A. TALWALKAR, MD, MPH • *Mayo Clinic and Foundation, Rochester, MN*

GREG TIAO, MD • *Department of Surgery, University of Cincinnati, Cincinnati Children's Hospital Medical Center, Cincinnati, OH*

RICHARD S. TILSON, MD • *Gastroenterology Division, Brigham and Women's Hospital, Boston, MA*

DHIRAJ TRIPATHI • *Department of Hepatology and Radiology, Royal Infirmary, Edinburgh, UK*

HUGO E. VARGAS, MD • *Division of Transplantation Medicine, Mayo Clinic, Scottsdale, AZ*

FRANCESCO VIZZUTTI, MD • *Laboratorio di Epatologia, Dipartimento di Medicina Interna, Universita di Firenze, Firenze, Italy*

MANAV WADHAWAN, MD • *Department of Gastroenterology, University of Delhi, GB Pant Hospital, New Delhi, India*

FLORENCE WONG, MD • *Division of Gastroenterology, University of Toronto, Toronto General Hospital, Ontario, Canada*

I HISTORICAL PERSPECTIVE

1

Portal Hypertension

A History

Adrian Reuben, MBBS, FRCP
and Roberto J. Groszmann, MD

CONTENTS

REFERENCES

The term *portal hypertension* or, more strictly, *portal venous hypertension*, refers explicitly to a pathologic elevation of pressure in the veins that carry blood from the splanchnic organs (including the spleen) to the liver. Implicit in the working definition of portal hypertension is the necessary condition that the rise in portal pressure is not simply a consequence of an increase in systemic venous pressure, as might occur with congestive heart failure for example, but is intrinsically part of an increase in the pressure gradient between the portal venous inflow to the liver and its hepatic venous outflow. Increased pressure in the hepatic veins from any cause, such as hepatic vein thrombosis, a suprahepatic inferior vena cava web, right heart dysfunction, constrictive pericarditis, or any other comparable anatomic and/or functional lesion, elevates portal pressure above its normal baseline value and can cause splenomegaly and ascites. Notwithstanding, without secondary structural changes in the liver, however subtle, portal pressure elevation that is solely caused by impaired hepatic venous drainage does not lead to the formation of esophagogastric varices and the other pathophysiologic complications of an increased portal–systemic pressure gradient that are discussed in detail in this book. It is now self-evident that in health splanchnic blood percolates from the portal vein through low-resistance intrahepatic vascular channels (sinusoids) to the hepatic veins— but this was not always conventional wisdom. Ideas about the splanchnic and hepatic vascular architecture and blood flow have evolved over millennia *(1)*, as have concepts of the nature of portal hypertension *(2)*, although the time frame for the latter is only a couple of hundred years at most.

Recognition that the liver is a highly vascular organ dates back more than 30,000 yr to Paleolithic times, as shown by the remarkable cave art of prehistoric hunters found at Lascaux in Southern France *(3)* and at other sites. The ancient Egyptians also must have noticed the bloody content of the livers that they so carefully preserved for the next world, along with other vital organs of their departed nobility and deceased privileged

From: *Clinical Gastroenterology: Portal Hypertension*
Edited by: A. J. Sanyal and V. H. Shah © Humana Press Inc., Totowa, NJ

classes. Conversance with the vascularity of the liver was also common among people of antiquity in the Mediterranean basin and the Near East, who practised the now lost art of *haruspicy* or divination of the future by scrutinizing livers from sacrificed animals. Egyptian physicians, however, were the first to record a description of the hepatic vasculature that they thought consisted of four veins *(4)* but, like Diogenes, Hippocrates, and Aristotle in the 4th and 5th centuries BCE in Greece, and Galen in 2nd century CE Rome, they got it wrong. Aristotle was confused about the portal vein, for he thought that the vena cava supplied blood to the liver from above and that the liver and spleen were connected by veins to the right and left arms, respectively *(5)*, permitting targeted phlebotomy for the ill *humors* of those organs. For Galen and his contemporaries and followers, in contrast, the liver was the *"fons venarum,"* the source of the major veins of the body and the *"sanguifactionis officina,"* or the "factory of the blood," the site of sanguification. Galen did recognize that veins from the mesentery entered the *"porta hepatis"* or gateway of the liver on its concave side *(6)*, in his belief bringing digested food from the intestines to be converted into blood in the liver by *"(con)coction"* (*pepsis*), with separation of light, yellow bile that is excreted by way of the bile ducts and gallbladder and heavy, black bile that passes via the spleen to the stomach; the residue remained in the intestine to be voided. Galen reported the insightful view of Erasistratus of Chios, an Alexandrian scientist of the 2nd century BCE, who reasoned that there must be a labyrinthine system of channels in the liver connecting the portal vein to the vena cava *(7)*, to allow the blood to pass through. In many respects, Galen was a bitter critic of his Alexandrian predecessor *(8)*, who flourished 400 yr earlier *(9)* and who, with his contemporary Herophilus of Chalcedon *(10)*, founded the Alexandrian school of anatomy that was based on dissecting human corpses. Galen disapproved of Erasistratus's materialism and his dependence on morphology as the only indication of an organ's function.

After the fall of Rome in 476 CE, and with it the decline of Greco-Roman civilization and learning, there were no advances in understanding the anatomy and function of the liver, nor indeed anatomy in general, until the Renaissance dawned one thousand years later. Throughout the Dark Ages, from the 5th to the 10th century CE, and even in the latter half of the Middle Ages, the views and schemes of Aristotle and Galen were preserved in the East in the Byzantine Empire and in the Arabic (Islamic) culture. In the West, with its religious preoccupation with death and salvation, the soul was more important than the body in which clerics and philosophers sought its haven. The graphic demonstrations of bodily structures by Leonardo da Vinci in the 15th century *(11)* and Andreas Vesalius in the 16th century *(12)* exemplified the revival of interest in anatomy but it was not until William Harvey's publication in 1628 of his discovery of the circulation of the blood *(13)* that the Galenic perspective of the vasculature of the liver was seriously challenged. Harvey reasoned that if blood could pass through a dense organ like the liver, from the portal vein to the vena cava, seemingly without any local propulsive force, then blood could surely flow through the delicate spongy lungs driven by the contractions of the heart's right ventricle. Yet it took a mere 1900 yr before Erasistratus's hypothesis of transhepatic blood flow was conclusively proved empirically by Francis Glisson (1597–1677) *(14)*, then Regius Professor of Physic at Cambridge, cofounder of the Royal Society, and one-time President of the Royal College of Physicians of London. Using an ox bladder attached to a syphon, such as was used in those days to administer enemas, Glisson injected "warm water, coloured with a little milk" into the portal vein of a fresh human cadaver, and found that the liver blanched when all the blood in it was expelled. With this demonstration, Glisson not only vindicated Erasistratus and his theory of intrahepatic vascular channels, but he also provided direct proof for Harvey's assertion that blood flows through the lungs, because the milky contrast passed sequentially through the right heart, the lungs, and the left heart into the systemic arterial circulation.

The structural proof of Harvey's theory and of Glisson's functional demonstration of a connection between arteries and veins—and, in the case of the liver, of a low-resistance pathway between portal and hepatic veins—was made possible by Marcello Malpighi's landmark microscopic identification of capillaries that he first saw in the lung of a living frog *(15)*. Following the discovery by Wepfer, in the latter half of the 17th century, of lobules or *acini* in the liver of the pig *(16)*, a finding confirmed by Malpighi in many other species *(17)*, one would have expected that the fundamental anatomic hepatic unit would have been well authenticated and universally agreed upon by now, but it has not *(1)*. Kiernan, using only a hand lens and a quicksilver injection technique, distinguished triangular spaces containing minute branches of the hepatic artery, portal vein, and bile duct, in other words portal tracts or triads, at the periphery of classic hexagonal lobules *(18)*. Elias, using elegant three-dimensional (3D) microscopic reconstructions *(19)*, confirmed Hering's original layout of one-cell-thick hepatocyte plates separating and bordering vascular spaces *(20)*, which many authors continued to call capillaries. Later, Minot *(21)* distinguished the smallest blood vessels in the liver by the term "*capilliform sinusoids*" (later, plain sinusoids) because of their unique endothelial structure and associated perisinusoidal cells, an arrangement that was later fully elucidated and is well recognized today. It has yet to be settled whether the once popular *acinus* of Rappaport *(22)* or the more current hepatic microcirculatory unit of Ekataksin *(23)*, or some other model, will be universally accepted as the ultimate morphofunctional unit of the liver. Irrespective, in health, the sinusoidal system that connects portal and hepatic veins, which Malpighi originally identified *(17)*, constitutes a low-resistance vascular pathway. It follows that any derangement of sinusoidal structure or venous drainage that is likely to increase resistance to blood flow through the liver may thereby initiate portal hypertension.

The major complications of portal hypertension, notably ascites and to a lesser extent variceal hemorrhage, were recognized long before their pathogenesis was understood. Ascites is mentioned in the most ancient of medical texts, i.e., the papyrus Ebers of Ancient Egypt *(25)* and the Ayurveda of the Hindu tradition *(26)*, both dating from as early as 1500–1600 BCE and both offering remedies for accumulation of abdominal fluid that the Hindus call *Jalodara (26)*. In Central America, at about the same time, the Ancient Mayans knew of the association between tense ascites and umbilical herniation, which they vividly depicted in the clay figurines of the time. The term ascites first appeared in English in the late 14th century as *aschytes*, and was taken from the Greek word for dropsy "*askiTes*" (ασκϊτηξ), itself derived from "*askos*" (ασκοξ), an ancient Greek word for a leather bag or sheepskin that was used for carrying water, wine, oil, and so on. Whereas the Old Testament blamed ascites on adultery *(27)*, Hippocrates knew of its seepage from the liver and its poor prognosis *(28)*. Erasistratus almost solved the pathogenesis of ascites when he argued that "the water cannot accumulate... in any other way than from narrowness of the blood vessels going through the liver," *(29)* which, as usual, invited scorn from his nemesis Galen. In contrast to the ample documentation available of the history of ascites and its treatment through the ages *(29–31)*, relatively little has been written before the modern era about varices and variceal hemorrhage in patients with cirrhosis or portal vein occlusion.

In patients with portal hypertension, esophagogastric varices were undoubtedly common but their discovery in life would have been almost impossible before the advent of radiology and endoscopy. Even in death from variceal hemorrhage, collapsed luminal varices are difficult to identify at autopsy. Bleeding from esophageal varices was described with certainty in France *(32)* and America *(33)* in the mid-19th century, and a little later by Osler *(34)*. Yet, in 1860, Friedrich Theodor von Frerichs, who is widely regarded as the founder of modern hepatology, considered variceal bleeding to be a rare complication of cirrhosis and hemorrhoids to be infrequent *(35)*, even though he and others *(35–37)* ably demonstrated, by injection opacification, an extensive portal collateral circulation in cirrhosis, including the legendary *caput Medusæ (35)* and congestive splenomegaly *(35)*.

If we ignore the hypothesis proposed by the German physician and chemist Georg E. Stahl (1660–1734) that congestion of the portal vein, so-called *abdominal plethora*, is responsible for most if not all chronic illness *(38)*, then the concept of portal hypertension can be considered to have been introduced at the turn of the 20th century by Gilbert and Villaret in Paris, who also coined the term that we use today *(39)*. Gilbert and Weil had shown previously that pressure in ascitic fluid was high in patients with cirrhosis *(40)*, in which setting they inferred that portal venous pressure must be high too *(39)*. However, the next obvious deduction was not made, namely, that the cirrhotic liver must be responsible in some way for portal pressure elevation and its many consequences, including splenomegaly. What followed instead was the classic error of confusing cause with effect, as the enlarged spleen was thought to be the cause and not the result of the portal pressure elevation. This conclusion was based on the faulty reasoning of the renowned Florentine physician and pathologist Guido Banti *(41)*, whose erroneous hypothesis was not accepted by his colleagues in Europe but was supported for the longest while by none other than the most respected physician of the day in Britain and America, William Osler *(42,43)*. Banti reasoned that in patients with splenomegaly, anemia, and leukopenia [so-called splenic anemia *(44)* or Banti's disease], the spleen was damaged by a toxin *(45)* and, in turn, the *splenopathy* injured the liver and caused cirrhosis in a syndrome he labeled *hepatosplenopathy (46)* (later called Banti's syndrome). Osler later withdrew his support for the notion that a primary splenic disorder causes portal hypertension but not before surgeons, from Harvey Cushing to William Mayo, removed the offending spleens with gusto, despite recurrent hemorrhage and late mortality *(41)*. Other surgeons performed omentopexy, producing decompressing portosystemic collaterals by sewing the omentum to the peritoneum *(47)*. Despite its obvious shortcomings, Banti's theory held sway from the 1880s to the 1950s, until the weight of evidence from pathologic, radiologic, hemodynamic, and surgical shunt studies laid to rest the legend of hepatosplenopathy *(41,48–53)*.

The rejection of Banti's hepatosplenopathy hypothesis cleared the way for less enigmatic solutions to the pathogenesis of portal hypertension. Plausible, testable mechanistic explanations were lacking for the perplexing association between cirrhosis and esophagogastric varices *(54)*, as were more rational treatments than splenic amputation. To answer these needs, one of the arguably most significant contributions came from the extensive anatomic, pathologic, and liver-perfusion studies reported by a young New Zealander trainee in pathology and surgery at the Mayo Clinic, Archibald McIndoe *(55)*. McIndoe— who later found fame in Great Britain, during World War II and its aftermath, for his innovative plastic and reconstructive surgery on severely burned and injured airmen, other service personnel, and civilians—concluded from the results of his experiments that portal hypertension was a result of vascular obstruction in the cirrhotic liver *(55)*. Banti's "forward flow hypothesis" was thus replaced by McIndoe's "backflow" phenomenon. McIndoe also suggested that portal hypertension could be ameliorated by the use of the portocaval fistula devised by the Russian surgeon, bureaucrat, and engineer, Nicolai Vladimirovich Eck, working in St. Petersburg 50 yr earlier *(56)*. Whipple, Rousselot, Blakemore, Sengstaken, and many other surgeons at Columbia University in New York City and elsewhere pioneered a mainly surgical approach to decompression of the portal venous system *(41)*, which will be discussed and updated later by Dr. Michael Henderson (Chapter 16) as will nonsurgical shunts, the radiologic counterparts, by Dr. Rajiv Jalan (Chapter 17).

The abandonment of Banti's hypothesis does not mean that forward flow is discredited as a contributory factor in portal hypertension. Patients with advanced liver disease have long been recognized to exhibit the physical signs of a hyperdynamic circulation *(57,58)*. Whereas many possible mechanisms have been proposed for the hyperdynamic circulatory state seen in cirrhosis and portal hypertension *(59)*, central to the syndrome is arterial vasodilatation in both the splanchnic and peripheral vascular beds *(60–62)*, which will be analyzed and explained by Dr. Didier Lebrec (Chapter 4). Despite normalization of resistance to portal blood flow as a result of portal–systemic collateralization, elevated portal pressure is not abolished but persists, now being maintained largely by the hyperdynamic increase in portal blood flow. Thus, the hyperdynamic portal inflow and not only the resistance provides the impetus for preserving an elevated portal venous pressure. In other words, the backflow phenomenon gives way to and/or is augmented by forward flow, as shown well in experimental animal models *(60,63)*.

Parenthetically, one must concede that Banti's ghost still stalks from time to time, especially but not exclusively in the case of patients with hematological causes of splenomegaly who also have portal hypertension and varices *(64)*. Hematologists and others have argued that the increased blood flow from a grossly enlarged spleen meaningfully contributes to, or can even cause, portal pressure elevation, in much the same way as the hyperdynamic circulation of cirrhosis does and can occur in the extreme case of splenic arteriovenous fistula *(65)*. This argument is often used to justify splenectomy, which can be hazardous by causing portal and/or mesenteric thrombosis *(66–69)*, possibly because of the thrombogenic effect of a temporary slowing of portal blood flow *(70)*, in the presence of vessel wall injury and thrombocytosis. In cirrhotic patients undergoing distal splenorenal shunt surgery there appears to be no correlation between spleen size and estimated sinusoidal pressure, and direct measurement intraoperatively shows no reduction of portal pressure with splenic vein clamping *(71)*. In patients with certain hemologic disorders, portal hypertension is either the result of a subtle change in sinusoidal structure *(72)*, hepatic fibrosis *(73)*, or portal vein lesions with the secondary development of other liver lesions such as nodular regenerative hyperplasia *(72)*. Whether laparoscopic splenectomy *(74)*, which is being used increasingly in cirrhotic patients to alleviate thrombocytopenia *(75)*, will prove less hazardous than open splenectomy remains to be seen as portal thrombosis has already been reported in patients with splenomegaly who undergo laparoscopic splenectomy *(75)*.

The final stop in this historical romp through portal hypertension is to review the introduction of portal pressure measurements in humans, for investigational and clinical purposes. Portal pressure had been measured directly intraoperatively since the 1930s at least *(52,77)*. The introduction of hepatic vein catheterization in 1944 for blood sampling *(78)* was preparatory to the earliest efforts at hepatic venous pressure measurement and sinusoidal pressure estimation by Friedman and Weiner *(79)* and Myers and Taylor *(80)* in

1951, and Paton et al. in 1953 *(81)* using an occlusion (wedged) technique, which was preferred to both abdominal wall vein *(82)* and splenic pulp *(83)* puncture. While the precise role of wedged hepatic venous pressure measurements in routine clinical practice is still being debated *(84)*, the importance of making the measurements correctly cannot be overemphasized *(85)* lest the technique fall into disrepute because of inadequate performance.

In this introductory chapter, we have shown that the history of the discovery and investigation of the hepatic vasculature and portal hypertension is a colorful and illustrious one in hepatology and in medicine in general. The remainder of this volume will build on this historical account by providing explanations of the pathophysiology of portal hypertension and its complications, clinically and experimentally, with data ranging from studies in conscious humans to minutiae at the cellular and molecular levels, and embracing the most modern and rational approaches to therapy. The Ancient Egyptians, Mayans, Hindus, Greeks, Romans, and others will surely applaud our progress with the organ once considered to be the "seat of the soul."

REFERENCES

1. Reuben A. Now you see it, now you don't. Hepatology 2003;38:781–784.
2. Reuben A. The way to a man's heart is through his liver. Hepatology 2003;37:1500–1502.
3. Glyn D. Lascaux and Carnac. Butterworth, London, 1965.
4. Bryan CP. The papyrus Ebers (translated from the German version). D. Appleton, New York, 1931, pp. 126,127.
5. Harris CRS. The Heart and Vascular System in Ancient Greek Medicine; from Alcmæn to Galen. Clarendon, Oxford, UK, 1973.
6. Singer C. Galen on Anatomical Procedures. Translation of Surviving Books with Introduction and Notes. Oxford Univ Press, London, UK, 1956.
7. Brock AJ. Galen on the Natural Faculties (translated from the Greek). Loeb Classical Library, London, 1928.
8. Bradley SE. In: Fishman AP, Richards DW, eds. Circulation of the Blood: Men and Ideas. Oxford Univ Press, New York, 1964, Ch X. The Splanchnic Circulation.
9. Dobson JF. Erasistratus. Proc Roy Soc Med 1927;20:825–832.
10. Dobson JF. Herophilus of Alexandria. Proc Roy Soc Med 1925;18:19–32.
11. Da Vinci L. Quardeni di'anatomia. Volume 1. Tredici Fogli della Royal Library di Windsor. Respirazione Cuore, Viscera addominali–Christiana, Dybwad. 1911.
12. Vesalius A. De humani corporis fabrica. Basileae, ex office. J. Oporini 1543.
13. Harvey W. Exercitatio Anatomica de Motu Cordis et Sanguinis in Animalibus. W. Fitzer, Frankfurt, Germany, 1628.
14. Glisson F. Anatomia Hepatis. O. Pullein, London, 1654.
15. Malpighi M. De viscerum structura excercitatio anatomica. London, 1666.
16. Wepfer JJ. De Dubiis Anatomicis. Epistola ad Jacob Henricum Paulli. In: Paulli JH, ed. Anatomiae Bilsianae Anatome Occupata Imprimis Circa Vasa Mesereraica et Labyrinthum in Ductu Orifero, 93–100. Simonem Paulli: Argentorati, 1665.
17. Malpighi M. Discours anatomiques sur la structure des visceres sçavioir due foye, du cerveau, des reins, de la ratte, du polype du coeur et de poulmons. 2nd ed, Paris, D'Houry, 1687.
18. Kiernan F. The anatomy and physiology of the livers. Philos Trans R. Soc Lond B Biol Sci 1833;123: 711–770.
19. Elias H. A re-examination of the structure of the mammalian liver. 1. Parenchymal architecture. Am J Anat 1949;84:311–334.
20. Hering E. The liver. In: Stricker S, ed. Manual of Human and Comparative Histology. Translated by H. Power, Volume 2. New Sydenham Society, London, 1870–1873, pp. 1–33.
21. Minot CS. On a hitherto unrecognized form of blood circulation without capillaries in organs of vertebrata. Proc Boston Soc Natl Hist 1901;29:185–215.

22. Rappaport AM. The microcirculatory unit. Microvasc Res 1973;6:212–228.
23. Ekataksin W, Zou Z, Wake K, et al. The hepatic microcirculatory sub units: an over-three-century-long search for the missing link between an exocrine unit and an endocrine unit in mammalian liver lobules. In: Motta PM, ed. Recent Advances in Microscopy of Cells, Tissues and Organs. Rome, Italy, Antonio Delfino Editore, 1997, pp. 407–412.
24. McCuskey RS. The hepatic microvascular system. In: Arias IM, Boyer JL, Fausto N, et al., eds. The Liver: Biology and Pathobiology. 3rd ed. Raven, New York, 1994, Chapter 57.
25. Bryan CP. The papyrus Ebers (translated from the German version). D. Appleton, New York, 1931, pp. 135–136.
26. Majumdar A, ed. Jalodara. In: Hand Book of Domestic Medicine and Common Ayurvedic Remedies. Documentation and Publication Division. Central Council for Research in Ayurveda and Siddha. New Delhi, 1999, pp. 88–89.
27. Old Testament. Numbers 5:22.
28. Sprengell C. The aphorisms of Hippocrates, and the sentences of Celsus; with explanations and references to the most considerable writers in physick and physiology, both ancient and modern. To which are added, aphorisms upon several distempers, not well distinguished by the ancients. The second edition, corrected and very much enlarged. London, Wilkin J, Bonwich J, Birt S, Ward T, Wicksteed E. 1735. Special Limited Edition containing excerpts from the Aphorisms of Hippocrates. Presented as a service to medicine by Lederle Laboratories from the Collection of the Yale Univ Med Hist Libr. Classics in Med Lit by DevCom, Inc. Wayne, NJ, DevCom, Inc., 1987.
29. Dawson AM. Historical notes on ascites. Gastroenterology 1960;39:790,791.
30. Runyon BA. Historical aspects of treatment of patients with cirrhosis and ascites. Seminars Liver Disease 1997;17:163–173.
31. Reuben A. Out came copious water. Hepatology 2002;36:261–264.
32. LeDiberdier and Fauvel. De l' hématémèse due à des varices de l' oesophage, à propos de deux observations. Rec Trav Soc Méd (Paris) 1857–1858;1:257–284.
33. Power W. Contributions to pathology. Maryland Med Surg J 1840;1:306–318.
34. Osler W. Cirrhosis of the liver: fatal hemorrhage from esophageal varix. Trans Pathol Soc Philadelphia 1887;13:276,277.
35. von Frerichs FT. A clinical treatise on diseases of the liver. Translated by Murchison C. Volume 2, Chapter III. Inflammation of the liver. Its various forms and consequenes. Wm. Wood, New York, 1879, p. 81.
36. Retzius MG. Bemerkungen über Anastomsen zwischen der Pfortader und der untern Hohlader ausserhalb der Leber. Z Physiol 1835;5:105–106.
37. Sappey C. Récherches sur quelques veines portes accessoires. Mém Compt Rend Soc Biol 1859;11: 3–13.
38. Stahl GE. De vena Portæ, porta malorum hypochondriaco–splenectico-sufferativo, hysterico-colico hemorrhoidariorum. Halle 1698.
39. Gilbert A, Villaret M. Contribution à l'étude du syndrome d' hypertension portale: cytologie des liquides d' ascite dans les cirrhoses. Compt Rend Soc Biol 1906;60:820–823.
40. Gilbert A, Weil E. Sur la tension des liquides ascitiques. Compt Rend Soc Biol 1899;51:511–514.
41. Grannis FW. Guido Banti's hypothesis and its impact on the understanding and treatment of portal hypertension. Mayo Clin Proc 1975;50:41–48.
42. Osler W. On splenic anemia. Am J Med Sci 1900;119:54–73 and 1902;124:751–800.
43. Osler W, McCrae T. Modern Medicine: Its Theory and Practice. Vol. 1 and 2, Third edition. Leo and Febiger, Philadelphia, 1925.
44. Gretsel K. Eine Fall von Anaemia splenica bei einem Kinde. Berl Klin Wocheuschr 1886;3:212–214.
45. Banti G. Dell' anemia splenica. Arch Scuola Anat Pat Firenze 1883;124:53–122.
46. Banti G. La splenomegalia con cirosi del fegato. Lo Sperimentale Firenze 1894;48:407–432 and 48: 447–452 (translated in Medical Classics 1937;1:907–912).
47. White S. Discussion on the surgical treatment of ascites secondary to vascular cirrhosis of the liver. Br Med J 1906;2:1287–1296.
48. Dock G, Warthin AS. A clinical and pathological study of five cases of splenic anemia, with early and late stages of cirrhosis. Am J Med Sci 1904;127:24–55.

49. Herrick FC. An experimental study into the cause of the increased pressure in portal cirrhosis. J Exper Med 1907;9:93–104.

50. Klemperer P. Cavernous transformation of the portal vein: its relation to Banti's disease. Arch Pathol 1928;6:353–377.

51. Larrabee RC. Chronic congestive splenomegaly and its relationship to Banti's disease. Am J Med Sci 1934;188:745–760.

52. Thompson WP, Caughey JL, Whipple AO, Rousselot LM. Splenic vein pressure in congestive splenomegaly (Banti's syndrome). J Clin Invest 1937;16:571–572.

53. Thompson WP. The pathogenesis of Banti's disease. Ann Intern Med 1940;14:255–262.

54. Preble RB. Conclusions based on sixty cases of fatal gastrointestinal hemorrhage due to cirrhosis of the liver. Am J Med Sci 1900;119:263–280.

55. McIndoe AH. Vascular lesions of portal cirrhosis. Arch Pathol 1928;5:23–40.

56. Eck NV. K. voprosu o perevyazkie vorotnois veni: predvaritelnoye. Soobshtshjenye. Voen Med J (St. Petersburg) 1877;130:1,2.

57. Kowalski HJ, Abelman WH. The cardiac output at rest in Laennec's cirrhosis. J Clin Invest 1953;32:1025–1033.

58. Murray JF, Dawson AM, Sherlock S. Circulatory changes in chronic liver disease. Am J Med 1958;24:358–367.

59. Abelman WH. Hyperdynamic circulation in cirrhosis: a historical perspective. Hepatology 1994;20:1356–1358.

60. Vorobioff J, Bredfeldt JE, Groszmann RJ. Hyperdynamic circulation in portal-hypertensive rat model: a primary factor for maintenance of chronic portal hypertension Am J Physiol 1983;244:G52–G57.

61. Schrier RW, Arroyo V, Bernardi M, et al. Peripheral arterial vasodilatation hypothesis: a proposal for the initiation of renal sodium and water retention in cirrhosis. Hepatology 1988;8:1151–1157.

62. Groszmann RJ. Hyperdynamic circulation of liver disease 40 years later: pathophysiology and clinical consequences. Hepatology 1994;20:1359–1363.

63. Blancher L, Lebrec D. Changes in splanchnic blood flow in portal hypertensive rats. Eur J Clin Invest 1982;12:327–330.

64. Lukie BE, Card RT. Portal hypertension complicating myelofibrosis: reversal following splenectomy. Can Med Ass J 1977;117:771–772.

65. Murray MJ, Thal AP, Greenspan R. Splenic arteriovenous fistula as a cause of portal hypertension. Am J Med 1960;29:849–856.

66. Rossi P, Passariello R, Simonetti G. Portal thrombosis: high incidence following splenectomy for portal hypertension. Gastrointest Radiol 1976;1:225–227.

67. Broe PJ, Conley CL, Cameron JL. Thrombosis of the portal vein following splenectomy for myeloid metaplasia. Surg Gynecol Obstet 1981;152:488–492.

68. Eguchi A, Hashizume M, Kitano S, et al. High rate of portal thrombosis after splenectomy in patients with esophageal varices and idiopathic portal hypertension. Arch Surg 1991;126:752–755.

69. Winslow ER, Brunt LM, Drebin JA, Soper NJ, Klingensmith ME. Portal vein thrombosis after splenectomy. Am J Surg 2002;184:631–635.

70. Nakamura T, Moriyasu F, Ban N, et al. Hemodynamic analysis of postsplenectomy portal thrombosis using ultrasonic Doppler duplex system. Am J Gastroenterol 1987;82:1212–1216.

71. Gusberg RJ, Peterec SM, Sumpio BE, Meier GH. Splenomegaly and variceal bleeding–hemodynamic basis and treatment implication. Hepatogastroenterology 1994;41:573–577.

72. Wanless IR, Petersen P, Das A, et al. Hepatic vascular disease and portal hypertension in polycythemia vera and agnogenic myeloid metaplasia: a clinicopathological study of 145 patients examined at autopsy. Hepatology 1990;12:1166–1174.

73. Lafon ME, Bioulac-Sage P, Balabaud C. Hepatic fibrosis with idiopathic thrombocytopenic purpura. Liver 1988;8:24–27.

74. Hashizume M, Tanoue K, Akahoshi T, et al. Laparoscopic splenectomy: The latest modern technique. Hepatogastroenterology 1999;46:820–824.

75. Kerchev KW, Carbonell AM, Heniford BT, et al. Laparoscopic splenectomy reverses thrombocytopenia in patients with hepatitis C cirrhosis and portal hypertension. J Gastrointestinal Surg 2004;8:120–126.

76. Sok J, Su W, Hopkins MA. Portal vein thrombosis following laparoscopic splenectomy for beta-thalassemia: a case study. Surg Endosc 2001;15:1489.

77. Rousselot LM. The role of congestion (portal hypertension) in so-called Banti's syndrome: a clinical and pathological study of thirty-one cases with late results following splenectomy. J Am Med Assoc 1936;107:1788–1793.
78. Warren JV, Brannon ES. A method of obtaining blood samples directly from the hepatic vein in man. Proc Soc Exp 1944;55:144–146.
79. Friedman EW, Weisner RS. Estimation of hepatic sinusoid pressure by means of venous catheter and estimation of portal pressure by hepatic vein catheterization. Am J Physiol 1951;165:527–531.
80. Myers JD, Taylor WJ. An estimation of portal venous pressure by occlusive catheterization of a hepatic venule. J Clin Invest 1951;30:662,663.
81. Paton A, Reynolds TB, Sherlock S. Assessment of portal venous hypertension by catheterization of hepatic vein. Lancet 1953;1:918–921.
82. Davidson CS, Gibbons TB, Falloon WW. Systemic and portal venous pressures in cirrhosis of the liver. J Lab Clin Med 1950;35:181–187.
83. Atkinson M, Sherlock S. Intrasplenic pressure as an index of portal venous pressure. Lancet 1954;1: 1325–1327.
84. Huet P-M, Pomier-Layrargues G. The hepatic venous pressure gradient: "Remixed and Revisited." Hepatology 2004;39:295–298.
85. Groszmann RJ, Wongcharatrawee S. The hepatic venous pressure gradient: Anything worth doing should be done right. Hepatology 2004;39:280–282.

II PATHOBIOLOGY AND EXPERIMENTAL PROGRESS IN PORTAL HYPERTENSION

2

Anatomy and Vascular Biology of the Cells in the Portal Circulation

*Massimo Pinzani, MD, PhD
and Francesco Vizzutti, MD*

CONTENTS

INTRODUCTION
ANATOMIC CONSIDERATIONS OF THE NORMAL PORTAL CIRCULATION
BIOLOGY OF PORTAL CELLS INCLUDING SINUSOIDAL ENDOTHELIAL
  CELLS AND HSCs
MAJOR SIGNALING PATHWAYS RELEVANT TO ENDOTHELIAL–SMOOTH
  MUSCLE CELL INTERACTIONS
REFERENCES

INTRODUCTION

Portal hypertension occurring during the natural course of liver cirrhosis is a consequence of the increased intrahepatic resistance to portal flow. For a long time, this phenomenon has been ascribed only to the profound changes of liver tissue angioarchitecture consequent to the progression of the fibrogenic process. However, studies performed during the last decade have demonstrated that there is also an increased vascular tone that could be modulated to a certain extent by pharmacological agents. The aim of this chapter is to provide general information on the anatomy of the portal systems and on the regulation of vascular tone in this specific vascular district and in the splanchnic circulation. Information about the collateral circulation that becomes relevant in the case of portal hypertension is also provided.

In addition, because of the many studies performed in animal models and isolated and cultured hepatic cell, attention will be paid to the biology of these cells and to the relative pathophysiological implications. In particular, hepatic stellate cells, now regarded as liver-specific pericytes, are likely to play an important role in the progression of portal hypertension because of their active role in the deposition of fibrillar extracellular matrix and of their contractile properties. In this context, several vasoconstricting agonists, whose expression is increased in fibrotic liver, may play a role in inducing contraction

From: *Clinical Gastroenterology: Portal Hypertension*
Edited by: A. J. Sanyal and V. H. Shah © Humana Press Inc., Totowa, NJ

of hepatic stellate cells as well as of other resident cells characterized by contractile ability. The features of different vasoactive agents will be analyzed and their potential involvement in physiological and pathological conditions thoroughly discussed.

ANATOMIC CONSIDERATIONS OF THE NORMAL PORTAL CIRCULATION

A portal venous system is defined as one beginning and ending in capillaries. The name "portal vein" derives from the notion that it is the gate into which the splanchnic circulatory system is connected to the liver (*porta* = gate). The name portal vein is applied to the venous system that originates in the capillaries of the intestine and terminates in the hepatic sinusoids. Nutrients absorbed from the gastrointestinal tract, in addition to hormones such as glucagons and insulin released by the pancreas, are directly delivered to the liver in high concentrations.

Embryology of the Portal System

The portal venous system originates from the two vitelline and the two umbilical veins. The vitelline veins, which drain blood from the yolk sac, intercommunicate in the septum trasversum, at which point the liver sinusoids and lobules develop. The extrahepatic portal system develops primarily from the left vitelline vein (which is later joined by the splenic vein to form the portal vein), whereas the intrahepatic portal circulation originates from the umbilical veins. In addition, the left umbilical vein communicates with the venous sinus connecting with the inferior vena cava, thus allowing a large quantity of blood to bypass the liver in the fetal circulation. Soon after birth, the umbilical vein is obliterated and the normal adult circulation is established. Despite this complexity in the development of the portal system, only very few congenital anomalies of the portal venous system are observed.

Gross Anatomy of the Portal System

The portal vein is a vessel collecting the venous blood of the abdominal part of the alimentary tract, spleen, pancreas, and gallbladder to the liver. The portal vein begins at the level of the second lumbar vertebra, just behind the neck of the pancreas as an upward continuation of the superior mesenteric vein after this vessel has been joined by the splenic vein. The superior mesenteric vein (0.78 cm in diameter) is primarily formed by all the veins draining the small bowel, with significant further contributions of the ileocolic, right colic, and middle colic veins. It runs in the root of the mesentery, in front of the third portion of the duodenum to merge with the splenic vein. The splenic vein (0.94 cm in diameter) originates with five to six branches that return the blood from the spleen and unite to form a single nontortuous vessel at the splenic hilum and join near the tail of the pancreas with the short gastric vessels to form the main splenic vein. This vein proceeds transversally, close to the hilum of the left kidney, in the body and head of the pancreas, receiving numerous tributaries from this latter portion of the pancreas. The left gastroepiploic vein joins the splenic vein near the spleen, and the inferior mesenteric vein (0.24 cm diameter), collecting blood from the left part of the colon and rectum, usually enters its middle third. Occasionally (one-third of subjects) the inferior mesenteric vein enters directly into the superior mesenteric vein or at its junction with the splenic vein. On its way to the porta hepatis, the portal vein trunk receives (in some variants) the superior pancreaticoduodenal vein (with right gastroepiploic vein) and the right gastric (pyloric) veins. The left gastric (coronary) vein joins the portal vein at its origin 50% of the time, and it joins the splenic instead of the portal vein in the other 50% of subjects. Coronary vein runs upward along the lesser curvature of the stomach, where it receives some esophageal veins.

The portal system carries all the blood from the alimentary tract to the liver and, thus, in the normal subject all of the above-named veins have blood flow directed toward the liver. The segment of the portal vein after the last afferent branch runs in the hepatoduodenal ligaments (the free edge of the lesser omentum) in a plane dorsal to the bile ducts and the hepatic artery. This segment extends for approx 6–8 cm before entering the liver and it is 1–1.2 cm in diameter. The portal vein is not provided with valves, so the pressure is transmitted freely back to the afferent branches. The portal vein pressure normally ranges between 5 and 10 mmHg (depending on the method of measurement). Normal fasting hepatic blood flow is approx 1500 mL/min. The best available estimates in humans indicate that about two-thirds of the total hepatic blood flow and about one-half of the oxygen consumption are supplied by the portal vein, whereas the remainder is supplied by the hepatic artery. This dual hepatic blood supply makes the liver rather resistant to hypoxia. Accordingly, ligation of the portal vein does not cause hepatocellular necrosis. Similarly, accidental ligation of the hepatic artery or its major branches does not necessarily lead to hepatic failure. The portal trunk divides into two lobar veins before entering the portal fissure. The right lobar branch, short and thick, then receives the cystic vein. The left lobar vein is longer than the right and consists of a transverse and an umbilical part. The latter is the remainder of the umbilical parts. The recanalized umbilical or paraumbilical veins arise from the umbilical portion of the left portal vein and pass through the round ligament to the anterior abdominal wall, where they may become evident, in the presence of portal hypertension, in the umbilical varices.

According to the distribution of major portal vein branches, so-called segmental branches, the liver can be divided into functional segments. Each segment depends on its major vessel for blood supply. The right branch of the portal vein is usually less than 3 cm long and runs more vertically. It divides into anterior and posterior branches, which supply the anterior and posterior parts of the right lobe. Each of these vessels divides again into superior and inferior branches. The left lobar vein gives branches to the quadrate lobe and to the caudate lobe, before entering the parenchyma at the left end of the porta hepatis. A separate branch may arise near the bifurcation to supply the caudate lobe. The vein is then joined by the obliterated umbilical vein as it turns medially. The terminal part of the vessel continues into segment IV, which it supplies with ascending and descending branches. In addition to the main portal vein and its branches, the liver receives other veins from the splanchnic circulation, the so-called parabiliary venous system of Couinaud. This highly variable plexus includes several veins that arise from the pancreaticoduodenal or pyloric veins and drain into the portal vein or directly into hepatic segments, especially segment IV. This plexus provides examples of the metabolic effects of proximity to an insulin source. Veins arising from the pancreatic region would carry blood with high insulin levels and pyloric veins would carry low-insulin blood. The anatomy of these veins could explain some examples of focal fatty liver and focal fatty sparing, in fact, insulin determines the ability of the liver to accumulate triglycerides (1).

The other vessel supplying the liver is the hepatic artery. About one-third of the total hepatic blood flow is supplied by the hepatic artery. The common hepatic artery is the second major branch of the celiac axis. It runs to the right along the upper border of the pancreas in the context of the right gastropancreatic fold, which conducts the artery to the medial border of the hepatoduodenal part of the lesser omentum. It ascends in front of the portal vein in 91% of subjects and to the left of and behind the bile duct in 64% of cases. It divides into the left and the right hepatic arteries to supply the corresponding hemilivers. Although the left and right hepatic arteries are end-arteries, they often anastomose within the hilar tissue *(2)*. The right and left hepatic arteries each divide into two arteries that supply the right anterior and posterior sections and the left medial lateral sections, respectively. Another branch, the middle hepatic artery, arises from the left or right hepatic artery and supplies the quadrate lobe. The cystic artery arises from the right hepatic artery in the upper part of the Calot triangle (formed by the cystic duct, common hepatic duct, and inferior surface of liver) *(3)*.

Portal Collateral Circulation

The portal system has numerous collaterals that interconnect with the systemic circulation. When portal pressure rises above 10 mmHg potential portosystemic collaterals may develop. Formation of collaterals is a complex process involving the opening, dilation, and hypertrophy of preexisting vascular channels. It is possible that active neoangiogenesis is involved in the formation collateral vessels *(4)*. The sites for the development of portal collateral vessels are those areas where veins draining into the portal system are in immediate juxtaposition to veins draining into the superior or inferior vena cava. Collaterals vessels could be classified into tree embryological groups: (1) junction of absorp-tive and protective epithelium (gastroesophageal and hemorrhoidal plexuses); (2) obliterated fetal circulation (umbilical or paraumbilical veins in round and falciform ligaments); and (3) organs derived from the gastrointestinal tract that became retroperitoneal or adhere to the abdominal wall because of pathologic process (portorenal plexus, veins of Retzius, surgical stomata, and other interventions connecting portal bed with the ascending lumbar azygos, renal, and adrenal veins).

The most important sites for the development of portosystemic collateral vessels are: (1) esophageal submucosal veins, supplied by the left gastric vein and draining into the superior vena cava through the azygos vein; (2) paraumbilical veins, although normally nonfunctional, can serve as an anastomosis between the umbilical part of the left portal vein and the hepigastric veins of the anterior abdominal wall that drain into the superior or inferior vena cava, and in special circumstances may form caput medusae at the umbilicus (Cruveilhier–Baumgarten syndrome); (3) rectal submucosal veins, supplied by the inferior mesenteric vein through the superior rectal vein and draining into the internal iliac veins through the middle rectal vein; (4) splenorenal shunts, in this case venous blood may be carried to left renal vein, either directly or by way of the diaphragmatic, pancreatic, or gastric veins; (5) short gastric veins communicate with the esophageal plexus. Moreover, within the cirrhotic liver, there is significant collateral flow in small veins that connect branches of the portal and hepatic veins *(5)*.

The Gastroesophageal Junction

The normal venous anatomy of the gastroesophageal junction and of the lower esophagus is particularly relevant to this introductory chapter. Studies of Vianna et al. documented four distinct zones of esophageal venous drainage (from distal to proximal): (1) the gastric zone, which extends for 2–3 cm just below the gastroesophageal junction. This is the junctional zone between the stomach and lower oesophagus. Veins from this zone drain into the short gastric and left gastric veins. (2) The palisade zone extends 2–3 cm superiorly from the gastric zone into the lower esophagus and represent the watershed between the portal and systemic circulation. (3) The perforating or transitional zone extends approx 2 cm further up the esophagus above the palisade zone. Here, the organized longitudinal structure is lost, with veins looping and forming a network. The main feature of this zone is represented by the presence of perforating veins through the muscle wall of the esophagus linking the submucosal and paraesophageal venous plexuses that are tributaries of the azygos venous system. These perforating veins run circumferentially around the esophageal wall. In portal hypertensive patients, dilated perforating veins become incompetent and allow retrograde blood flow from the paraesophageal to the submucosal veins. This associated with the turbulent flow caused by pressure changes as a result of the respiratory movements, coughing and stretching may contribute to formation and dilation of varices. (4) The truncal zone is 8–10 cm long and is characterized by four of five longitudinal veins in the lamina propria. In this zone, perforating veins penetrate from the submucosa at irregular intervals to the external esophageal venous plexus.

In summary, venous drainage from the gastric fundus and the lesser curvature is directed inferiorly to the portal vein. In the palisade zone, there is to/from flow that is probably respiration dependent. The perforating veins connect the intrinsic and extrinsic esophageal plexuses. Flow in the truncal zone is inferior to the perforating zone. In conclusion, the perforating, transitional zone is the "critical area" for variceal rupture. Indeed, varices tend to be bigger and to form "nodules" at the distal end of the esophagus, at the level of the perforating veins *(6)*.

Structure and Function of the Splanchnic Vasculature

The splanchnic circulation consists of those vascular beds perfused by the celiac, superior and inferior mesenteric arteries, and the portal vein. The organs perfused by the splanchnic vasculature receive about 25% of cardiac output and account for about 30% of total body oxygen consumption under resting conditions. Functional and/or structural changes in arterioles, capillaries, and venules can initiate or perpetuate an elevated portal pressure (e.g., dilation of arterioles, passive occlusion of capillaries, and active constriction of hepatic venules). The structural and functional characteristics of the microvasculature of the stomach and small and large intestine are very different from those of the liver. First, splanchnic capillaries are much less porous than the hepatic sinusoids and have a well-defined basement membrane. Although most splanchnic capillaries are fenestrated, the estimated pore size, 3.7 to 12 nm in radius, is between 50 and 100 times lower than that of the hepatic sinusoids. A very little amount of the total protein oncotic pressure may pass across a splanchnic capillary membrane; consequently, any increase in filtration in the splanchnic capillaries is quickly counterbalanced by an increase in the oncotic pressure difference between capillary lumen and interstitial space. In addition, there is evidence that the intestinal microvasculature autoregulates the capillary pressure and capillary filtration coefficient. There are significant differences between the intestinal and hepatic interstitium in terms of compliance; in fact, considerable interstitial fluid can accumulate without causing any major changes in interstitial pressure. Moreover, the intestines have a very efficient lymphatic system to remove interstitial edema. In normal conditions, approx 20% of the fluid absorbed by the small intestine is carried out to the general circulation by the lymphatics *(7)*.

Under basal conditions, splanchnic arterioles are partially constricted, and have the capacity to either further constrict or dilate. This arteriolar smooth muscle tone is the sum of multiple factors that tend to either relax or constrict vascular smooth muscle. A variety of metabolic end-products (e.g., adenosine), some endothelium-derived substances (e.g., nitric oxide), and certain neurotransmitters (e.g., acetylcholine) are known to relax arteriolar smooth muscle and produce vasodilation. Important vasoconstrictors influences on splanchnic arterioles include some circulating agents (e.g., angiotensin II), certain endothelium-derived substances (e.g., endothelin), and some neurotransmitters (norepinephrine). These factors can alter the contractile state of arteriolar smooth muscle either by acting directly on vascular smooth muscle (e.g., metabolic mediators) or by stimulating endothelial cells to release vasoactive agents that act on the underlying adjacent vascular smooth muscle (e.g., acetylcholine). Hypoxia, in terms of reduced oxygen delivery or increased oxygen demand, can lead to changes in arteriolar tone and consequent changes in blood flow. This effect appears to be mediated by terminal products of oxidative metabolism, such as adenosine, and tissue oxygen tension (pO_2) and appear to be one of the principal mechanisms of postprandial hyperemia. In fact, when tissue pO_2 falls or extracellular adenosine concentration rises, arterioles dilate. Normally, splanchnic arterioles are exquisitely sensitive to acute changes in intravascular pressure. Vascular smooth muscle of splanchnic arterioles contracts intensely in response to stretch (inducing a sudden elevation in portal pressure). The intense dilation of arterioles observed in chronic portal hypertension likely reflects the accumulation of vasodilators [e.g., increased nitric oxide (NO) production, increased blood levels of glucagons] that overcome intrinsic myogenic vasoconstrictor factors *(8)*.

Norepinephrine, angiotensin II, and vasopressin are estimated to account for more than two-thirds of basal splanchnic vascular tone. Norepinephrine generally elicits a profound, yet transient, reduction in splanchnic blood flow. Increased tissue levels of adenosine during vasoconstriction-mediated arterioles escape from norepinephrine-mediated vasoconstriction. On the contrary, vasopressin and angiotensin II cause a sustained reduction in splanchnic blood flow. Glucagon attenuates the splanchnic vasoconstrictive response induced by catecholamines, vasopressin, and angiotensin II through a downregulation of receptors and/or postreceptor mechanisms such as impairment of second-messenger activation in splanchnic vascular smooth muscle. A wide variety of hormones and peptides produced within the alimentary tract are capable of altering splanchnic blood flow when infused into arterial blood. Somatostatin and neuropeptide-Y are locally produced peptides that exert potent vasoconstrictor actions. Vasoactive intestinal polypeptide, substance P, cholecystokinin, and gastrin are examples of gastrointestinal peptides that dilate splanchnic arterioles and increase blood flow.

Splanchnic organs exhibit an intrinsic ability to regulate local blood flow by modulating the tone of arterioles. Two examples of intrinsic vasoregulation are pressure-flow autoregulation and functional (postprandial) hyperemia. Pressure-flow autoregulation is the ability of an organ to maintain its constant blood flow when arterial pressure is reduced. This regulatory mechanism depends on metabolic or myogenic-mediated dilation of arterioles at lower intravascular pressures. However, pressure-flow autoregulation of splanchnic organs is not as potent and precise as in other vascular beds such as the heart, the brain, and the kidneys. Nevertheless, this autoregulation is improved in the postprandial phase (increased metabolic demand), when arterioles become more sensible to reductions in arterial pressure. Postprandial hyperemia has recently received much attention as a potential cause of rapid elevation in splanchnic blood flow and portal pressure that may lead to variceal formation, dilation, and explosion *(9,10)*. Splanchnic vasodilation and hyperemia is caused by the interaction of intrinsic (change in arteriolar transmural pressure and/or increase in vasodilator tissue metabolites) or extrinsic mechanisms (autonomic nervous system especially noncholinergic vagal reflexes) and the effect of nitric oxide, gastrointestinal hormones and peptides (gastrin, cholecystokinin and glucagons), autacoids (histamine, serotonin), osmolality, and prostaglandins. The relative contribution of these different factors is influenced by the composition of the meal (i.e., long-chain fatty acids appear to be the most potent stimulus) and the preprandial metabolic status of the affected organ.

Nerves

The liver is predominantly innervated by two plexuses, the anterior and the posterior, which communicate with each other. The anterior plexus surrounds the hepatic artery and is made up of fibers from the celiac ganglia and anterior vagus nerve. The posterior plexus surrounds the portal vein and bile duct and is formed from branches of the right celiac ganglia and posterior vagus. The vast majority of nerve fibers terminate in plexuses in the adventitia around hepatic arterioles and venules. Small fibers from these plexuses then end on smooth muscle cells in the media of these vessels. Within the liver cell plate, the majority of nerve fibers are observed in periportal regions. Some of the nerve fibers terminate on endothelial cells in the smallest hepatic arterioles, near the space of Disse, on Kupffer cells, and on hepatic stellate cells (HSC).

Hepatic innervation can be distinguished in extrinsic and intrinsic. The extrinsic innervation of the liver is constituted by: (1) efferent sympathetic nerve fibers and parasympathetic nerve fibers; these play a role in regulating the metabolic load of hepatocytes, hemodynamic and biliary motility; (2) afferent fibers, which are thought to be involved in osmo- and chemoreception. At the hilus, amyelinic fibers from the anterior and posterior plexuses enter the liver mainly around the hepatic artery. The intrinsic innervation is composed of fibers (mostly adrenergic, but also cholinergic and peptidergic) mainly associated with vascular and biliary structures in the portal spaces *(11)*. Certain fibers enter liver lobule where they form a network around hepatocytes and extend into the sinusoidal wall, sometimes reaching the centrilobular vein. Some neuropeptides have been identified, such as vasointestinal peptide, neuropeptide Y, substance P, glucagon, and calcitonin gene-related peptide. Stimulation of sympathetic fibers causes an increase in vascular resistance and a decrease in hepatic blood volume.

The Hepatic Portal Tree

Segmental branches of the portal vein split dichotomously into equal sized branches, constituting a tree of conducting vessels that terminate in venules having an inner diameter of about 400 μm. Each branch of the afferent vessels is essential for proper function because it supplies blood to a specific area. There are few, if any, anastomoses that could provide collateral circulation if a major branch is impaired. In other words, the first portion of the portal system is merely conductive up to the branching into preterminal portal venules with an inner diameter of 80–40 μm. This latter portion appears to be the main site of the constrictive response of the portal tree to various constrictive stimuli and, as such, the main mechanism for controlling blood distribution within the liver. Further downstream, the so-called terminal portal venules are endothelial tubes surrounded by a thin layer of smooth muscle. These structures do not contract and splits into septal, perilobular, and lobular branches that supply directly blood to sinusoids via inlet venules and give a constant but sluggish blood flow *(12)*. At this last level, a sphincter mechanism is created by the nuclei of endothelial cells residing at origin of sinusoids. The branching of the distribution portion of portal tree is paralleled by the arterial and lymphatic components of the portal tract *(13)*.

Arterial Supply

Arterial supply, which normally represents from 25% to 30% of the hepatic blood flow, satisfies the oxygen demands of the stromal and parenchymal compartments of the liver. The arteries form a peribiliary plexus that surrounds and nourishes small bile ducts. Intrahepatic arteries are thick-walled and become smaller as the arteries branch. Terminal branches contain only endothelium surrounded by a thin adventitia. Entry of arterial blood into sinusoids takes place at different levels, mainly zone 1 and 2 of the acinus. Additional entrances in zone 3 have also been postulated. Drainage of the plexus is both directly in sinusoids and into small branches of the portal veins *(14)*. In physiological conditions, the arterial flow varies inversely with portal vein flow, and compensates for the eventual shortage of portal perfusion *(15,16)*. The hepatic artery provides a pulsatile but small-volume flow that appears to enhance sinusoidal flow, especially in periods of reactive arterial flow, such as the postprandial hyperemia. The proportion of arterial perfusion rises in portal hypertension irrespective of the etiology and reflects a deterioration of liver conditions *(17)*.

The Functional Unit of the Liver—Rappaport's Acinus

Rappaport's acinus is a parenchymal mass lying between two centrilobular veins. Its axis is a small radicle of the portal triad containing a terminal portal vein (diameter <40 µm), a hepatic arteriole (diameter >15 µm), nerves, lymph vessels, and bile ducts or cholangioles. This axis, seldom seen by light microscopy, corresponds to the connective tissue septa. Blood drain into centrilobular veins (diameter <65 µm) from the terminal branch of the portal vein. In sinusoids, flow is unidirectional, from periportal to centrilobular hepatocytes. The concept of functional heterogeneity has been based on this organization. The acinus is arbitrarily divided into three zones; (zone 1) periportal; (zone 2) mediolobular; (zone 3) centrolobular *(18)*. In Rappaport's acinus, blood flows unidirectionally from zone 1 to zone 3. This is because of: (1) the presence of sinusoidal inlet and outlet sphincters composed of sinusoidal lining cells bulging into the lumen; (2) transient leucocyte plugging; (3) variations in the morphology of sinusoids in the different zones; and (4) the contribution of arterial flow at the beginning of the sinusoidal structures *(19)*.

Sinusoids

Between the genuinely interdigitating networks of afferent and efferent vessels, there is a space filled with plates and columns of hepatocytes, among which a complex network of sinusoids is found. In other words, the hepatic sinusoids can be seen as conduits connecting the terminal portal venule and terminal hepatic arteriole with the hepatic venules. The length of a human sinusoid varies between 223 and 477 µm. The average velocity of erythrocyte flow in sinusoids ranges between 270 and 410 µm/s. Average blood pressure has been measured to be about 4.8 mmHg in terminal portal branches, 30–35 mmHg in arterial blood, and 1.7 mmHg in collecting vessels *(20)*. The huge cross-sectional area of the sinusoids is responsible for the normally low transsinusoidal vessel resistance, pressure gradient, and flow velocity. It is estimated that 80% of the sinusoidal profile would have to be obliterated to cause portal pressure to rise *(21)*. This portion of the liver circulation is unique in comparison to most other capillary beds. Its endothelial lining is made up of flat, lobulated, fenestrated cells, which overlap loosely without being attached to one another, i.e., intercellular junctions are absent. In contrast with other capillaries, hepatic sinusoids are not provided with a basal membrane. The presence of elements of the cytoskeleton in these fenestrations have raised the issue of whether fenestrations may contract and to what extent this may influence the passage of solutes into the space of Disse. This is a space located between the sinusoidal domain of the hepatocyte plasma membrane and the endothelial cells forming the walls of the hepatic sinusoids.

This space, which is not normally discernible in biopsy material by standard light microscopy, is characterized by the presence of different components of the extracellular matrix (different type of collagens mainly type III, but also types I and IV, proteoglycans, laminin, and fibronectin). Fibrillar collagens such as collagen types I and III are orderly distributed to form a supporting framework, whereas other components such as collagen type IV, proteoglycans, and laminin are distributed in order to form a matrix allowing the exchange of macromolecules between the sinusoidal blood and the hepatocytes. The caliber of the sinusoids is variable, typically 6–30 µm, but can increase up to 180 µm. Periportal sinusoids are narrow and tortuous facilitating solute–capillary wall interaction, whereas perivenous sinusoids are straighter and wider. The changes of the caliber seem to be mostly passive, depending on regional flow and volume changes but depends also on active contraction of HSC, and changes in the diameter of sinusoidal fenestrations as it will be further expanded.

There are two types of sphincter-like structures at the entering sites of hepatic sinusoids. One is located at the junction between the terminal portal venule and the sinusoid, and is characterized by the large endothelial cells surrounded with Ito cells (HSCs). The other is located at the junction between the terminal hepatic arteriole and the sinusoid, and corresponds to the precapillary sphincter because our enzymohistochemical demonstration of arterial capillaries in close association with the sinusoids combined with intravital microscopy has revealed that the terminal hepatic arteriole directly terminates in the sinusoid.

Control of the Intrahepatic Circulation

Under physiological conditions, the liver itself is the main site of resistance to portal flow. It should be emphasized that there is no precise mechanism regulating portal flow into the liver and, in normal conditions, the portal tree is able to accept any amount of blood coming from the splanchnic area. In other words, the liver is not able to control the volume of the portal flow, which is mainly determined by resistance vessels of splanchnic organs that drain into the portal venous system. The principal site of resistance within normal hepatic tissue is still a matter of controversy. There are indeed several structures potentially affecting intrahepatic resistance. These include terminal hepatic venules, small portal venules, and, at the sinusoidal level, the state of tension developed by HSC around sinusoids and the number and diameter of sinusoidal fenestrations. However, an active sinusoidal control of the perfusion still represents a controversial issue, as will be further expanded. Arterial inflow, on the other hand, is a subject of clear and effective control, depending mainly on the actual needs of the liver tissue *(22)*. In addition, compensatory relationships exist between the venous and arterial inflows *(23)*, so arterial flow increases when portal flow decreases. This occurs as a result of communications among main vessels, sinusoids, and peribiliary venules (24) that open in response to nervous and soluble factors (25). In these cases, portal flow blockade has repercussions on the entire territory downstream from the obstruction, following portal dichotomy and producing an arterial reaction strictly confined to that territory and, therefore, with a sectorial, triangular shape. Moreover, in case of bile duct dilatation, a collapse of the peribiliary plexus that surrounds biliary tree like a meshwork and lacks muscular walls is observed. Because this plexus provides an additional flow of portal blood toward the sinusoids, its impairment or failure results in a further decrease in the total amount of portal blood reaching the sinusoids and increase in arterial inflow of these structures.

BIOLOGY OF PORTAL CELLS
INCLUDING SINUSOIDAL ENDOTHELIAL CELLS AND HSCs

Sinusoidal Endothelial Cells (SECs)

Liver sinusoidal endothelial cells (SEC) form a continuous lining of the liver capillaries, or sinusoids, separating parenchymal cells and HSC from sinusoidal blood. SEC differ in fine structure from endothelial cells lining larger blood vessels and from other capillary endothelia in that they lack a distinct basement membrane and also contain open pores, or fenestrae, in the thin cytoplasmic projections that constitute the sinusoidal wall (26). This distinctive morphology supports the protective role played by liver endothelium, the cells forming a general barrier against pathogenic agents and serving as a selective sieve for substances passing from the blood to parenchymal and HSC, and vice versa. Another functional characteristic of SEC is their high endocytotic capacity. This function is reflected by the presence of numerous endocytotic vesicles and by the effective uptake of a wide variety of substances from the blood by receptor-mediated endocytosis (27). This capacity, together with the presence of fenestrae and the absence of a regular basal lamina, makes these cells different and unique from any other type of endothelial cell in the body. Accordingly, SEC can be regarded as a "scavenger system," which clears the blood from many different macromolecular waste products that originate from turnover processes in different tissues.

Beside endocytosis, endothelial transport in the liver sinusoidal endothelium occurs through fenestrae without a diaphragm. During this process, the endosomal and lysosomal compartments are bypassed. The exchange of fluids, solutes, and particles is bidirectional, allowing an intensive interaction between the sinusoidal blood and the microvillus surface of the parenchymal cells. Endothelial fenestrae measure between 150 and 175 nm in transmission electron microscopic preparations, occur at a frequency of 9–13 per μm^2, and occupy about 10% of the wall surface. They are large in zone 1 and smaller but more numerous in zone 3. Endothelial fenestrae do not obstruct most plasmatic macromolecules and enable the exchange of free water and substance within the sinusoids at quite low hydrostatic pressure (2–3 mmHg).

Fenestrae are dynamic structures whose diameter and number vary in response to a variety of hormones, drugs, toxins, diseases, or even to changes in the underlying extracellular matrix. Structural integrity of the fenestrated sinusoidal liver endothelium is essential for the maintenance of a normal exchange of fluids, solutes, particles, and metabolites between the hepatocytes and sinusoidal blood. Changes in the structure and function of fenestrae can have adverse effects on hepatocytes and liver function in general (28).

Sinusoidal fenestrations can change in size in response to various stimuli, including blood pressure, neural impulses, serotonin, endotoxin, alcohol, and nicotine.

Several studies have explored the mechanisms whereby hormones and cytoskeletal-altering drugs change the fenestral diameter and number. From these studies it became clear that drugs which alter the calcium concentration within SEC also change the fenestrae diameter (29). Recent data indicate that both $Ca^{2+}Mg^{2+}$-ATPase and Ca^{2+} pump-ATPase demonstrated on the SEC plasma membrane may be involved in the regulation of intracytoplasmic Ca^{2+} concentration (30). Other studies have shown that drugs which interfere with the SEC-cytoskeleton mainly alter the number of fenestrae (31). Finally, peculiar reports appeared describing fenestral dynamics in various pathological conditions of the liver, such as hypoxia, increasing venous pressure, irradiation, cold storage, and invasion of the liver by metastatic tumor cells or viruses (26).

Some aspects of SEC function may have relevant implications for the regulation of sinusoidal pressure. The filtration of lipoproteins by open pores is the simplest mechanism for steric selection. However, the fenestrae limit the free access to the parenchymal cell by a factor of 10. To overcome the difficulty of bringing solutes and (lipid) particles into the space of Disse and in contact with the parenchymal cells, the mechanisms of "forced sieving" and "endothelial massage" has been postulated (28). The hypothesis of "forced sieving" is based on the consideration that red blood cells unilaterally restrict the space in which lipoproteins move in Brownian motion. Red blood cells therefore increase the chance that lipoprotein droplets will escape through the fenestrae. Taking into account that red blood cells pass by in endless numbers while gently touching the fenestrated lining and, in the meantime, constantly adapting their shape to the dimensions of the sinusoid, it is assumed that red blood cells in their turn exert an important effect on the passage of any molecule larger than water through the liver sieve. According to the hypothesis of endothelial massage, white blood cells plug the sinusoid because they have an average size of 8.5 μm and, therefore, do not fit into a sinusoid, which measures from 5.9 μm in the portal region to 7.1 μm in the centrilobular region. In addition, white blood cells are less plastic than other blood cells and do not easily adapt to obstacles or diameter changes of sinusoids. As a result, white blood cells distend the fenestrated endothelium and the space of Disse. As a consequence, fluid in the space of Disse is pushed downstream and when fenestrae are encountered, fluid will be flushed out of Disse's space. After passage of the white blood cells, the space of Disse resumes its original shape, which causes a suction of fresh fluids into the space. In this way, the homeostasis of sinusoidal pressure is maintained by dispersion of lateral force throughout the sinusoidal sieve. It is implicit that a consistent loss of fenestrations, as it is observed in capillarized sinusoids, represents per se, an initial cause of deregulation of this homeostasis and of increased portal pressure.

HSC

HSC are located in the space of Disse in close contact with hepatocytes and SEC. In human liver, HSC are disposed along the sinusoids with a nucleus-to-nucleus distance of 40 μm, indicating that the sinusoids are equipped with HSC at certain fixed distances (32). These observations suggest that, although the total number of HSC constitutes a small percentage of the total number of liver cells (approx 5–8%), their spatial disposition and spatial extension may be sufficient to cover the entire hepatic sinusoidal microcirculatory network. The most evident ultrastructural feature of HSC in normal adult

Table 1
Action of Vasoactive Agents on Hepatic Stellate Cells

Agent	Contraction	Relaxation	$[Ca^{2+}]i$ increase
Endothelin-1	++++		Coupled
Thrombin	++++		Coupled
Angiotensin-II	+++		Coupled
Substance P	+++		
Adenosine	+++		Coupled
Thromboxane	+++		
Vasopressin	++++		Coupled
Platelet-activating factor	+		Coupled
Cysteinyl leukotrienes	+++		Coupled
Adrenomedullin		++	*
Nitric oxide		++	*
cAMP increasing agents		+++	*
Lipo PGE$_1$		++	
Atrial natriuretic peptide		+++	*
C-type natriuretic peptide		+++	*

*Relaxation associated with an inhibition of vasoconstrictor induced-$[Ca^{2+}]_i$ increase.

liver is the presence of cytoplasmic lipid droplets ranging in diameter from 1 to 2 μm (i.e., "fat-storing cells" or "lipocytes") *(32)*. These lipid droplets are involved in the hepatic storage of retinyl esters because of the key role of HSC in the metabolism and storage of retinoids.

The role of HSC in the progression of liver fibrosis has extensively been characterized. As a consequence of chronic liver tissue damage, HSC, as well as other extracellular matrix-producing cells (e.g., fibroblasts and myofibroblasts constitutively present in the portal tract), undergo a process of activation that leads to a phenotype characterized by increased proliferative, motile, and contractile attitudes.

The recognition that HSC are provided with contractile properties represents a key acquisition in the knowledge of the biology of this cell type *(33)*. Contraction of activated HSC occurs in vitro in response to different vasoconstrictors (Table 1). However, this experimental evidence is likely to be more representative of HSC contractile status in fibrotic liver, where contraction of activated HSC in response to various stimuli may have important implications in the pathogenesis of portal hypertension and in the contraction of mature scar tissue. Following two studies published in 1992 *(34,35)* demonstrating the contraction of HSC in response to different vasoconstrictors, the potential involvement of this cell type in the genesis and progression of portal hypertension has been postulated. Regardless, the potential consequences of the contractile attitude of HSC are still a matter of controversy and some key questions should be addressed before reaching superficial conclusions. These include:

1. Do HSC play a role in the regulation of sinusoidal tone in normal liver?
2. Do HSC influence portal pressure in conditions of developing fibrosis and "capillarization" of sinusoids?
3. Do HSC influence portal pressure in cirrhotic liver?

Because of their anatomical location, ultrastructural features, and similarities with pericytes regulating blood flow in other organs, HSC have been proposed to function as liver-specific pericytes. As already introduced, branches of the autonomic nerve fibers coursing through the space of Disse show a contact surface with HSC *(36)*, and nerve endings containing substance P and vasoactive intestinal peptide have been demonstrated in the vicinity of HSC *(37)*. In both a normal and fibrotic liver, the expression of N-CAM, a typical central nervous system adhesion molecule detected in hepatic nerves, and the expression of glial fibrillary acidic protein (GFAP) are restricted, among liver cell types, to HSC *(38)*. These observations, although reinforcing a potential functional relationship between the autonomic nervous system and HSC, raise a current key issue concerning the origin of this cell type, previously considered to be of myogenic origin because of the expression of desmin and smooth muscle α-actin (α-SMA). Along these lines, activated HSC express nestin, a class VI intermediate filament protein originally identified as a marker for neural stem cells *(39)*. Remarkably, the expression of this cell marker appears to be restricted to HSC and pericytes of brain parenchyma vessels, among all organ-specific pericytes. Another neuroendocrine marker suggesting a combination of mesenchymal and neural/neuroendocrine features in HSC is synaptophysin, a protein involved in neurotransmitter exocytosis. Synaptophysin reactivity is present in perisinusoidal stellate cells in both human and rat normal liver biopsies and the number of synaptophysin-reactive perisinusoidal cells is increased in pathological conditions *(40)*. Recent experimental evidence indicates that rat and human HSC express neurotrophins [including nerve growth factor (NGF), brain-derived neurotrophin, neurotrophin 3, and neurotrophin 4/5] and neurotrophin receptors *(41)*. This information cannot be advocated to support the possible neural/neuroendocrine differentiation of HSC because neurotrophins and the relative receptors have been identified in a variety of mesenchymal cells, such as fibroblasts and myofibroblasts, both in normal tissues and in tissues undergoing acute or chronic wound repair. Expression of neurotrophins in tissues other than the central or peripheral nervous system has classically been considered to be aimed at stimulation of outgrowth and maintenance of the peripheral nervous system. However, an increasing number of experimental reports indicate that the neurotrophin/neurotrophin receptor systems is likely implicated in biological events such as cell differentiation, proliferation, survival, and motility. In addition, a significant positive correlation between NGF synthesis e cell contractility, possibly related to the regulation of intracellular calcium homeostasis, has been reported in vascular smooth muscle cells *(42,43)*. In aggregate, these observations suggest a complex interaction between the pathophysiological role of HSC and the function of the peripheral nervous system.

Although these evidences suggest a role of HSC in the regulation of sinusoidal blood flow in normal liver, this issue is still matter of substantial controversy. From the morphological standpoint, some observations argue against the role of HSC in the regulation of sinusoidal blood flow *(44)*. First, in their in vivo tridimensional disposition, HSC do not have a stellate form (typical of their aspect in bidimensional culture on plastic) but rather a "spider-like" appearance ("arachnocytes") in respect of their small cell body with a series of radiating and parallel slender processes. According to the authors of these observations, cells with this tridimensional disposition are not likely to be "contraction ready." Additional limitations to effective cell contraction are offered by the spatial limitation of the space of Disse, by the intracytoplasmic presence of lipid droplets that prevent microfilaments from assembly in a long span, and by the ultrastructural evidence of a limited development of contractile filaments in quiescent HSC. Regardless, studies evaluating the hepatic microcirculation by intravital microscopy techniques have suggested that HSC could be involved in the regulation of sinusoidal tone in normal liver (45,46). Additional matter of debate is provided by studies aimed at quantitating HSC contraction with techniques able to detect the development of contractile forces in response to vasoconstrictors (47). The results of these studies indicate that the magnitude and kinetics of contraction and relaxation are consistent with the hypothesis that HSC may affect sinusoidal resistance. However, for understandable technical reasons, these data were obtained in rat HSC in primary culture 7 d after isolation, when a certain degree of activation in culture has occurred. In conclusion, although HSC could be proposed as liver-specific pericytes in reason of their location, spatial distribution, relationship with the peripheral nervous system, and ultrastructural features, no conclusive evidence is presently available concerning their role in the regulation of sinusoidal blood flow in physiological conditions.

MAJOR SIGNALING PATHWAYS RELEVANT TO ENDOTHELIAL–SMOOTH MUSCLE CELL INTERACTIONS

Several vasoactive agents have been shown to be effective in modulating activated HSC contractility in culture (see Table 1). The role of two vasoregulatory compounds, namely endothelin 1 (ET-1) and NO, has been particularly highlighted.

Endothelin

Endothelin-1, a potent vasoactive 21-amino-acid peptide secreted by endothelial as well as other cell types, has been shown to exert a multifunctional role in a variety of tissues and cells (48–50), including the liver. Infusion of ET-1 in the isolated perfused rat liver causes a sustained and dose-dependent increase in portal pressure associated with increased glycogenolysis and oxygen consumption (51–53). ET-1 stimulates glycogenolysis, phosphoinositide turnover, and repetitive, sustained intracellular calcium transients in isolated rat hepatocytes (54,55). Other studies indicate that ET-1 may also have important interactions with liver nonparenchymal cells. Cultured sinusoidal endothelial cells isolated from rat liver have been shown to release ET-1 (56), and preferential binding sites for ET-1 have been identified, both in vivo and in vitro (57,58), on HSC. As previously mentioned, ET-1 induces a dose-dependent increase in intracellular free calcium, coupled with cell contraction in this cell type. Importantly, activated rat and human HSC have been shown to express preproET-1 mRNA (59,60) and to release ET-1 in cell supernatants in response to agonists such as angiotensin II, PDGF, TGF-β, and ET-1 itself (61), thus raising the possibility of a paracrine and autocrine action of ET-1 (62). ET-1 synthesis in HSC is regulated through modulation of endothelin converting enzyme-1 (ECE-1), the enzyme that converts precursor ET-1 to the mature peptide, rather than by modulation of the precursor pre-proET-1 (63). Recent evidence suggests that upregulation of 56- and 62-kDa ECE-1 3'-untranslated region (UTR) mRNA binding proteins occurs in HSC after liver injury and during activation in vitro (64). In addition, transforming growth factor-β1, a cytokine integral to the wound healing reaction, stimulates ET-1 production by inducing ECE-1 mRNA stabilization.

Overall, it is increasingly evident that the process of HSC activation and phenotypical modulation is characterized by a close and complex relationship with the ET system. The ability to synthesize and release ET-1 is associated with a progressive shift in the relative predominance of ET_A and ET_B receptors observed during serial subculture: ET_A are predominant in the early phases of activation, whereas ET_B receptors become increasingly more abundant in "myofibroblast-like" cells *(60,65)*. The upregulation of the ET_B receptor is prevented by the incubation of HSC with retinoic acid during the activation process *(66)*, thus confirming that increased expression of this receptor is part of the phenotypical modulation of HSC toward the "myofibroblast-like" phenotype.

The shift in the relative ET receptor densities may be directed at differentiating the possible paracrine and autocrine effects of ET-1 on HSC during the activation process. Indeed, when HSC are provided with a majority of ET_A receptors (early phases of activation), stimulation with ET-1 causes a dose-dependent increase in cell growth, ERK activity, and expression of c-*fos*. These effects, likely related to the activation of the Ras-ERK pathway, are completely blocked by pretreatment with BQ-123, a specific ET_A receptor antagonist *(60)*, and are in agreement with studies performed in other vascular pericytes such as glomerular mesangial cells *(67)*. Conversely, in later stages of activation, when the number of ET_B receptors increases, ET-1 appears to induce a prevalent antiproliferative effect linked to the activation of this receptor subtype *(68)*. In this setting, the activation of the ET_B receptor stimulates the production of prostaglandins, leading to an increase in intracellular cAMP, which in turn reduces the activation of both ERK and JNK *(69)*. In addition, both cAMP and prostaglandins upregulate ET_B binding sites, thus suggesting the possibility of a positive-feedback regulatory loop. In addition, recent studies have further defined the action of cAMP on the ET-1 receptor system. Cyclic AMP rapidly desensitizes ET_A in activated HSC and shifts their ET-1 responsiveness from picomolar to nanomolar concentrations with respect to $Ca^{(2+)}$ signals and HSC contraction. ET_A desensitization also occurs in response to prostaglandin E_2, adenosine, or ET_B stimulation *(70)*.

Concerning the potential involvement of HSC in the development of portal hypertension, it is important to note that, at least in human HSC, ET-1-induced cell contraction occurs at any stage of HSC activation *(60)*. Because HSC contraction is always blocked by ET_A receptor antagonists and never reproduced by selective ET_B agonists, it is conceivable that the signaling pathways regulating HSC contraction require the activation of a small number of ET_A receptors and are somehow divergent from those regulating cell growth.

In aggregate, these observations suggest that ET-1 may act as a potent vasoconstrictor agonist regulating intrahepatic blood flow in cirrhotic liver with a potential role in the pathogenesis of portal hypertension. Along these lines, morphological studies have clearly indicated that ET-1 (both at mRNA and protein levels) is markedly overexpressed in different cellular elements present within cirrhotic liver tissue, and particularly in sinusoidal endothelial and HSC in their activated phenotype located in the sinusoids of the regenerating nodules, at the edges of fibrous septa, and in the ECM embedding neoformed vessels within fibrous bands *(60)*. In addition, clinical studies indicate that a direct relationship exists between ET receptor mRNA abundance and the degree of portal hypertension in cirrhotic patients *(71)*.

NO

NO is a small, relatively stable, free-radical gas that readily diffuses into cells and membranes where it reacts with molecular targets *(72)*. It is important to note that the precise biochemical reactions, which are realized in any biological setting, depend on the concentration of NO achieved and often on subtle variations in the composition of the intra- and extracellular milieu. Accordingly, the biological actions of NO are often defined as a "double-edged sword." NO may act as a key signaling molecule in physiological processes as diverse as host defense, neuronal communication, and regulation of vascular tone. On the other hand, excessive or not adequately regulated NO synthesis has been implicated as causal or contributing to several pathophysiological conditions including vascular shock, diabetes, and chronic inflammation. Although NO is characterized by a very short half-life, its biochemical interactions with oxyradicals lead to the production of longer-lived compounds such as peroxynitrite, with important local effects. NO is produced from L-arginine by one of the three isoforms of nitric oxide synthase (NOS). The "constitutive" forms of NOS, which respond to changes in intracellular calcium concentration and typically produces small amounts of NO, are expressed by endothelial cells and in neurons, whereas a wide variety of other cells express the "inducible" form of this enzyme, that binds calmodulin at virtually all calcium concentrations and produce remarkably higher amounts of NO. The constitutive forms are regulated by hypoxia, shear stretch, or cytokines, whereas the inducible form is regulated by a large variety of stimuli including cytokines and lipopolysaccharide.

Because the intraportal administration of the NOS inhibitor, N^ω-nitro-L-arginine, increases portal pressure *(73)*, NO has been postulated to be a regulator of sinusoidal blood flow in normal liver. Along these lines, in vitro and in vivo evidence indicate that SEC express constitutive nitric oxide synthase (eNOS) and produce NO, and increase their production in response to flow *(74)*. However, an endothelial dysfunction associated with a decreased production of NO in the intrahepatic microcirculation has been documented extensively in cirrhotic liver *(75,76)*, and these defects could directly contribute to the increased intrahepatic resistance typical of portal hypertension. This view is supported by experiments performed in vitro and in animal models by gene transfer of the neuronal NO synthase isoform (nNOS) to sinusoidal endothelial cells or other perisinusoidal cells, such as HSC *(77)*. Expression of nNOS in rat HSC and sinusoidal endothelial cells resulted in increased NO production, and, in HSC, in a reduction of ET-1-induced contractility. Moreover, in two different rat models of cirrhosis and portal hypertension, transduction of livers with recombinant Ad.nNOS significantly reduced intrahepatic resistance and portal pressure.

As in the case of ET-1, circumstantial evidence for a relevance of NO in HSC biology has derived from in vitro studies. Exogenous NO is able not only to prevent ET-1-induced contraction and to relax precontracted cells, but also to reduce the expression of α-SMA *(78)*. In addition, interferon-γ and other cytokines with or without lipopolysaccharide, as well as hyaluronan fragments induce the expression of the inducible form of NOS and the production of NO in HSC *(79,80)*. However, at least in human HSC, this effect is very limited and the possibility of an autocrine action of NO in HSC appears merely speculative. In addition to these effects on HSC contraction and contractile proteins, NO has been shown to reduce the expression of procollagen type I mRNA and the secretion of the encoded protein *(79)*. Therefore, it is possible that NO may influence the progression of portal hypertension by reducing the accumulation of fibrillar matrix in key areas such as the fibrous septa, as suggested by evidence deriving from animal models of liver fibrosis *(81)*. It is also conceivable that the reduced synthesis of NO, typical of cirrhotic liver, may further aggravate the fibrogenic progression of the disease and that administration of orally active NO donors could be proposed as a potential antifibrogenic treatment, as suggested by recent studies performed in human HSC *(82)* and in animal models of liver fibrogenesis *(83)*.

Studies employing patch-clamp techniques have provided additional information on the role of membrane ion channels potential relevant for the action of vasoactive agents in HSC. High-conductance $Ca^{(2+)}$-activated $K^{(+)}$ [BK(Ca)] channels modulate the effects of vasoactive factors in contractile cells. This channels were detected in activated human HSC and may modulate the contractile effect of endothelin-1 and mediate the inhibitory action of NO *(84)*.

Other Vasoactive Agents

Several studies have evaluated the effects of naturally occurring vasodilators on HSC contractility. These include atrial natriuretic peptide (ANP) *(85)* and C-type natriuretic peptide (CNP) *(86)*. Both of these agents have been shown to reduce HSC contraction in response by ET-1 or thrombin. In addition, CNP is able to reduce HSC proliferation induced by PDGF-BB *(86)*.

In addition to ET-1, the potential involvement of other vasoconstrictors synthesized and released within liver tissue has been suggested. Titos et al. *(87)* have reported that in cirrhotic rat liver there is an increased synthesis of cysteinyl leukotrienes (LTs). In this context, hepatocytes exhibit the greatest ability to generate cysteinyl-LTs. It is important to note that these compounds elicit a strong contractile response in activated HSC. These findings further reinforce the concept of an imbalance between vasoconstrictor and vasodilator agents within the intrahepatic circulation of cirrhotic liver. Importantly, the concentration of vasoconstrictors acting on the intrahepatic microvasculature of cirrhotic liver may increase as a consequence of clinical or subclinical events such as infections in the peritoneal cavity, which are clearly associated with a worsening of portal hypertension and with an increased incidence of variceal bleeding *(88)*. This possibility as well other clinical possibilities, including the correct use of the drugs currently indicated in the treatment of portal hypertension *(89)*, should be carefully reconsidered in light of the current knowledge on the cellular and molecular mechanisms of portal hypertension.

REFERENCES

1. Battaglia DM, Wanless IR, Brady AP, Mackenzie RL. Intrahepatic sequestered segment of liver presenting as focal fatty change. Am J Gastroenterol 1995;90:2238–2239.
2. Madding GF, Kennedy PA. Trauma of the liver. In: Calne RY's Liver Surgery with Operative Color Illustrations. WB Saunders, Philadelphia, PA, 1982, p. 5.
3. Douglas BE, Baggenstoss AH, Hollinshead WH. The anatomy of the portal vein and its tributaries. Surg Gynecol Obstet 1979;91:562–576.
4. Bosch J, Navasa M, Garcia-Pagán JC, De Locy AM, Rodes J. Portal hypertension. Med Clin North Am 1989;73:931–953.
5. Popper H, Elias H, Petty DE. Vascular pattern of the cirrhotic liver. Am J Clin Pathol 1952;22:717–722.
6. Vianna A, Hayes PC, Moscoso G, et al. Normal venous circulation of the gastresophageal junction. A route to understanding varices. Gastroenterology 1987;93:876–889.
7. Crissinger KD, Granger DN. Gastrointestinal blood flow. In: Yamada T, et al., eds. Textbook of Gastroenterology. Lippincott-Williams & Wilkins, Philadelphia, PA, 1999, p. 519.
8. Granger DN, Kvietys PR, Korthuis R, Premen AJ. Microcirculation of the intestinal mucosa. In: Wood JD, ed. Handbook of Gastrointestinal Physiology. American Physiological Society, 1989, pp. 1405–1474.
9. Benoit JN, Korthuis RJ, Granger DN, Battarbee HD. Splanchnic hemodynamics in acute and chronic portal hypertension. In: Bonzon A, Blendis LM, eds. Cardiovascular Complications of Liver Disease. CRC, Boca Raton, FL, 1990, p. 179.

10. Jensen JE, Groszmann RJ. Pathophysiology of portal hypertension. In: Kaplowitz N, ed. Liver and Biliary Diseases. Williams & Wilkins, Baltimore, 1992, pp. 494–503.

11. Bioulac-Sage P, Lafon ME, Saric J, Balabaud C. Nerves and persinusoidal cells in human liver. J Hepatol 1990;10:105–112.

12. Wanless IR. Physioanatomic consideration. In: Schiff ER, Sorrel MF, Maddrey WC, ed. Schiff's Diseases of the Liver, 8th ed., Lippincott-Raven, Philadelphia, PA, 1999, pp. 18,19.

13. Wisse E, De Zanger RB, Jacobs R, McCuskey RS. Scanning electron microscope observations on the structure of portal veins, sinusoids and central veins in rat liver. Scan Electron Microsc 1983;3: 1441–1452.

14. Nopanitayo W, Grisham JW, Aghajanian JG, Carso JL. Intrahepatic microcirculation: SEM study of the terminal distribution of the hepatic artery. Scan Electron Microsc 1978;11:837–842.

15. Lautt WW. Relationship between hepatic blood flow and overall metabolism: the hepatic arterial buffer response. Fed Proc 1983;42:1662–1666.

16. Ezzat WR, Lautt WW. Hepatic arterial pressure-flow autoregulation is adenosine mediated. Am J Physiol 1986;252:H836–H845.

17. Shikare SV, Baschir K, Abraham P, Tilve GH. Hepatic perfusion index in portal hypertension of cirrhotic and non cirrhotic aetiologies. Nucl Med Comm 1996;17:520–522.

18. Rappaport AM. The microcirculatory hepatic unit. Microvasc Res 1973;6:212–218.

19. Yamamoto K, Sherman I, Phillips MJ, Fisher MM. Three-dimensional observation of the hepatic arterial terminations in the rat, hamster and human liver by scanning electron microscopy of microvascular casts. Hepatology 1985;5:452–456.

20. Rappaport AM. Physioanatomic consideration. In: Schiff L, Schiff ER, eds. Diseases of the Liver. JB Lippincott, Philadelphia, PA, 1987, pp. 1–46.

21. Sherlock S, Doodley J. The portal venous system and portal hypertension. In: Sherlock S, Doodley J, eds. Disease of the Liver and Biliary System, 7th ed. Blackwell Science, Oxford, UK, 1997.

22. McCuskey RS, Reilly FD. Hepatic microvasculature: dynamic structure and its regulation. Semin Liver Dis 1993;13:1–12.

23. Ternberg JL, Butcher HR Jr. Blood-flow relation between hepatic artery and portal vein. Science 1965; 150:1030,1031.

24. Itai Y, Moss AA, Goldberg HI. Transient hepatic attenuation difference of lobar or segmental distribution detected by dynamic computed tomography. Radiology 1982;144:835–839.

25. Kawasaki T, Carmichael FJ, Saldivia V, Roldan L, Orrego H. Relationship between portal venous and hepatic arterial blood flows. Spectrum of response. Am J Physiol 1990;259:1010–1018.

26. Braet F, Wisse E. Structural and functional aspects of liver sinusoidal endothelial cell fenestrae: a review. Comp Hepatol 2002;1:1–17.

27. De Leeuw AM, Brouwer A, Knook DL. Sinusoidal endothelial cells of the liver: fine structure and function in relation to age. J Electron Microsc Tech 1990;14:218–236.

28. Wisse E, De Zanger RB, Charels K, Van Der Smissen P, McCuskey RS. The liver sieve: considerations concerning the structure and function of endothelial fenestrae, the sinusoidal wall and the space of Disse. Hepatology 1985;5:683–692.

29. Oda M, Kazemoto S, Kaneko H, et al. Involvement of Ca^{++}-calmodulin-actomyosin system in the contractility of hepatic sinusoidal endothelial fenestrae. In: Knook DL, Wisse E, eds. Cells of the Hepatic Sinusoid 4. Kupffer Cell Foundation, Leiden, 1993, pp. 174–178.

30. Yokomori H, Oda M, Ogi M, et al. Hepatic sinusoidal endothelial fenestrae express plasma membrane Ca^{++}pump and $Ca^{++}Mg^{++}$-ATPase. Liver 2000;20:458–464.

31. Steffan AM, Gendrault JL, Kirn A. Increase in the number of fenestrae in mouse endothelial liver cells by altering the cytoskeleton with cytochalasin B. Hepatology 1987;7:1230–1238.

32. Wake K. Liver perivascular cells revealed by gold and silver impregnation methods and electron microscopy. In: Motta P, ed. Biopathology of the Liver, an Ultrastructural Approach. Kluwer, Dordrecht, 1988, pp. 23–26.

33. Pinzani M, Gentilini P. Biology of hepatic stellate cells and their possible relevance in the pathogenesis of portal hypertension in cirrhosis. Semin Liver Dis 1999;397–410.

34. Pinzani M, Failli P, Ruocco C, et al. Fat-storing cells as liver-specific pericytes: spatial dynamics of agonist-stimulated intracellular calcium transients. J Clin Invest 1992;90:642–646.

35. Kawada N, Klein H, Decker K. Eicoesanoid-mediated contractility of hepatic stellate cells. Biochem J 1992;285:367–371.
36. Lafon ME, Bioulac-Sage P, LeBail N. Nerves and perisinusoidal cells in human liver. In: Wisse E, Knook DL, Decker K, eds. Cells of Hepatic Sinusoid. Kupffer Cell Foundation, Riswijk, 1989, pp. 230–234.
37. Ueno T, Inuzuka S, Torimura T, et al. Distribution of substance P and vasoactive intestinal peptide in the human liver. Light and electron immunoperoxidase methods of observation. Am J Gastroenterol 1991;138:1233–1242.
38. Knittel T, Aurisch S, Neubauer K, Eichhorst S, Ramadori G. Cell-type-specific expression of neural cell adhesion molecule (N-CAM) in Ito cells of rat liver. Am J Pathol 1996;149:449–462.
39. Niki T, Pekny M, Hellemans K, et al. Class VI intermediate filament protein nestin is induced during activation of rat hepatic stellate cells. Hepatology 1999;29:520–527.
40. Cassiman D, van Pelt J, De Vos R, et al. Synaptosphysin: a novel marker for human and rat hepatic stellate cells. Am J Pathol 1999;155:1831–1839.
41. Cassiman D, Denef C, Desmet VJ, Roskams T. Human and rat hepatic stellate cells express neurotrophins and neurotrophin receptors. Hepatology 2001;33:148–158.
42. Sherer TB, Neff PS, Hankins GR, Tuttle JB. Mechanisms of increased NGF production in vascular smooth muscle of the spontaneous hypertensive rat. Exp Cell Res 1998;241:186–193.
43. Hasan W, Zhang R, Liu M, Warn D, Smith PG. Coordinate expression of NGF and alpha-smooth muscle actin mRNA and protein in cutaneous wound tissue of developing and adult rats. Cell Tissue Res 2000;300:97–109.
44. Ekataksin W, Kaneda K. Liver microvascular architecture: an insight into the pathophysiology of portal hypertension. Semin Liver Dis 1999;19:359–382.
45. Zhang JX, Pegoli W Jr, Clemens MG. Endothelin-1 induces direct constriction of hepatic sinusoids. Am J Physiol 1994;266:G624–G632.
46. Zhang JX, Bauer M, Clemens MG. Vessel- and target cell-specific actions of endothelin-1 and endothelin-3 in rat liver. Am J Physiol 1995;269:G269–G277.
47. Thimgan MS, Yee HF Jr. Quantitation of rat hepatic stellate cell contraction: stellate cells' contribution to sinusoidal tone. Am J Physiol 1999;277:G137–G143.
48. Yanagisawa M, Masaki T. Endothelin, a novel endothelium-derived peptide. Biochem Pharmacol 1989;38:1877–1883.
49. Simonson MS, Dunn MJ. Endothelins: a family of regulatory peptides. Hypertension 1991;17:856–863.
50. Simonson MS. Endothelins: multifunctional renal peptides. Physiol Rev 1993;73:375–411.
51. Gandhi CR, Stephenson K, Olson MS. Endothelin, a potent peptide agonist in the liver. J Biol Chem 1990;265:17,432–17,435.
52. Roden M, Vierhapper H, Liener K, Waldhausl W. Endothelin-1-stimulated glucose production in vitro in the isolated perfused rat liver. Metabolism 1992;41:290–295.
53. Thran-Thi T-A, Kawada N, Decker K. Regulation of endothelin-1 action on the perfused rat liver. FEBS Lett 1993;318:353–357.
54. Gandhi CR, Behal RH, Harvey SA, Nouchi TA, Olson MS. Hepatic effects of endothelin. Receptor characterization and endothelin-induced signal transduction in hepatocytes. Biochem J 1992;287:897–904.
55. Serradeil-Le Gal C, Jouneaux C, Sanchez-Bueno A, et al. Endothelin action in rat liver. Receptors, free Ca^{2+} oscillations, and activation of glycogenolysis. J Clin Invest 1991;87:133–138.
56. Rieder H, Ramadori G, Meyer zum Buschenfelde KH. Sinusoidal endothelial liver cells in vitro release endothelin: augmentation by transforming growth factor β and Kupffer cell-conditioned media. Klin Wochenschr 1991;69:387–391.
57. Furoya S, Naruse S, Nakayama T, Nokihara K. Binding of ^{125}I-endothelin-1 to fat-storing cells in rat liver revealed by electron microscopic radioautography. Anat Embryol 1992;185:97–100.
58. Gondo K, Ueno T, Masaharu S, Sakisaka S, Sata M, Tanikawa K. The endothelin-1 binding site in rat liver tissue: light- and electron-microscopic autoradiographic studies. Gastroenterology 1993;104:1745–1749.
59. Housset CN, Rockey DC, Bissel DM. Endothelin receptors in rat liver: lipocytes as a contractile target for endothelin 1. Proc Natl Acad Sci USA 1993;90:9266–9270.
60. Pinzani M, Milani S, DeFranco R, et al. Endothelin 1 is overexpressed in human cirrhotic liver and exerts multiple effects on activated hepatic stellate cells. Gastroenterology 1996;110:534–548.

61. Rockey DC, Fouassier L, Chung JJ, et al. Cellular localization of endothelin-1 and increased production in liver injury in the rat: potential for autocrine and paracrine effects on stellate cells. Hepatology 1998;27:472–480.

62. Gabriel A, Kuddus RH, Rao AS, Watkins WD, Ghandi CR. Superoxide-induced changes in endothelin (ET) receptors in hepatic stellate cells. J Hepatol 1998;29:614–627.

63. Shao R, Yan W, Rockey DC. Regulation of endothelin-1 synthesis by endothelin-converting enzyme-1 during wound healing. J Biol Chem 1999;274:3228–3234.

64. Shao R, Shi Z, Gotwals PJ, Koteliansky VE, George J, Rockey DC. Cell and molecular regulation of endothelin-1 production during hepatic wound healing. Mol Biol Cell 2003;14:2327–2341.

65. Reinehr RM, Kubitz R, Peters-Regehr T, Bode JG, Haussinger D. Activation of rat hepatic stellate cells in culture is associated with increased sensitivity to endothelin 1. Hepatology 1998;28:1566–1577.

66. Chi X, Anselmi K, Watkins S, Gandhi CR. Prevention of cultured rat stellate cell transformation and endothelin-B receptor upregulation by retinoic. Br J Pharmacol 2003;139:765–774.

67. Wang YZ, Pouyssegur J, Dunn MJ. Endothelin stimulates mitogen-activated protein kinase activity in mesangial cells through ET(A). J Am Soc Nephrol 1994;5:1074–1080.

68. Mallat A., Fouassier F, Preaux AM, et al. Growth inhibitory properties of endothelin-1 in human hepatic myofibroblastic Ito cells: an endothelin B receptor-mediated pathway. J Clin Invest 1995;96:42–49.

69. Mallat A, Preaux A-M, Serradeil-Le Gal C, et al. Growth inhibitory properties of endothelin-1 in activated human hepatic stellate cells: a cyclic adenosine monophosphate-mediated pathway. J Clin Invest 1996;98:2771–2778.

70. Reinehr R, Fischer R, Haussinger D. Regulation of endothelin-A receptor sensitivity by cyclic adenosine monophosphate in rat hepatic stellate cells. Hepatology 2002;36:861–873.

71. Leivas A, Jimenez W, Bruix J, et al. Gene expression of endothelin-1 and ET(A) and ET(B) receptors in human cirrhosis: relationship with hepatic hemodynamics. J Vasc Res 1998;35:186–193.

72. Gross SS, Wolin MS. Nitric oxide: pathophysiological mechanisms. Annu Rev Physiol 1995;57:737–769.

73. Mittal MK, Gupta TK, Lee FY, Sieber CC, Groszmann RJ. Nitric oxide modulates hepatic vascular tone in normal rat liver. Am J Physiol 1994;267:G416–G422.

74. Shah V, Haddad FG, Garcia-Cardena G, et al. Liver sinusoidal endothelial cells are responsible for nitric oxide modulation of resistance in the hepatic sinusoids. J Clin Invest 1997;100:2923–2930.

75. Rockey DC, Chung JJ. Reduced nitric oxide production by endothelial cells in cirrhotic rat liver: endothelial dysfunction in portal hypertension. Gastroenterology 1998;114:344–351.

76. Gupta TK, Toruner M, Chung MK, Groszmann RJ. Endothelial dysfunction and decreased production of nitric oxide in the intrahepatic microcirculation of cirrhotic rats. Hepatology 1998;28:926–931.

77. Yu Q, Shao R, Qian HS, George SE, Rockey DC. Gene transfer of the neuronal NO synthase isoform to cirrhotic rat liver ameliorates portal hypertension. J Clin Invest 2000;105:741–748.

78. Kawada N, Kuroki T, Uoya M, Inoue M, Kobayashi K. Smooth muscle α-actin expression in rat hepatic stellate cell is regulated by nitric oxide and cAMP. Biochem Biophys Res Comm 1996;229:238–242.

79. Casini A, Ceni E, Salzano R, et al. Neutrophil-derived superoxide anion induces lipid peroxidation and stimulates collagen synthesis in human hepatic stellate cells. Role of nitric oxide. Hepatology 1997;25:361–367.

80. Rockey DC, Chung JJ, McKee CM, Noble PW. Stimulation of inducible nitric oxide synthase in rat liver by hyaluronan fragments. Hepatology 1998;27:86–92.

81. Rockey DC, Chung JJ. Regulation of inducible nitric oxide synthase and nitric oxide during hepatic injury and fibrogenesis. Am J Physiol 1997;273:G124–G130.

82. Failli P, DeFranco RMS, Caligiuri A, et al. Nitric oxide-generating vasodilators inhibit platelet-derived growth factor-induced proliferation and migration of activated human hepatic stellate cells. Gastroenterology 2000;119:479–492.

83. Fiorucci S, Antonelli E, Morelli O, et al. NCX-1000, a NO-releasing derivative of ursodeoxycholic acid, selectively delivers NO to the liver and protects against development of portal hypertension. Proc Natl Acad Sci USA 2001;98:8897–8902.

84. Gasull X, Bataller R, Gines P, et al. Human myofibroblastic hepatic stellate cells express Ca(2+)-activated K(+) channels that modulate the effects of endothelin-1 and nitric oxide. J Hepatol 2001;35:739–748.

85. Gorbig MN, Gines P, Bataller R, et al. Atrial natriuretic peptide antagonizes endothelin-induced calcium increase in cultured human hepatic stellate cells. Hepatology 1999;30:501–509.
86. Tao J, Mallat A, Gallois C, et al. Biological effects of C-type natriuretic peptide in human myofibroblastic hepatic stellate cells. J Biol Chem 1999;274:23,761–23,769.
87. Titos F, Claria J, Bataller R, et al. Hepatocyte-derived cysteinyl leukotrienes modulate vascular tone in experimental cirrhosis. Gastroenterology 2000;119:794–805.
88. Goulis J, Patch D, Burroughs AK. Bacterial infection in the pathogenesis of variceal bleeding. Lancet 1999;353:139–142.
89. Wiest R, Tsai M-H, Groszmann R. Octreotide potentiates PKC-dependent vasoconstrictors in portal-hypertensive rats. Gastroenterology 2001;120:975–983.

3

Cell and Molecular Mechanisms of Increased Intrahepatic Resistance and Hemodynamic Correlates

Don C. Rockey, MD

CONTENTS

THE INTRAHEPATIC MICROCIRCULATION AND PORTAL HYPERTENSION
CELL AND MOLECULAR MECHANISMS AND INCREASED INTRAHEPATIC
    RESISTANCE
ACKNOWLEDGMENTS
REFERENCES

THE INTRAHEPATIC MICROCIRCULATION AND PORTAL HYPERTENSION

The intrahepatic circulatory system consists of three major microvascular components, including: (1) the terminal portal venule (TPV) and hepatic arteriole; (2) the sinusoids (corresponding to the capillary bed); and (3) the terminal hepatic venule (THV). Each of the functional units in theory represents a putative resistance site. The major pre- and postsinusoidal components have been presumed to reflect contraction of vascular smooth muscle cells (TPV and THV). At the sinusoidal level, the major cellular components include endothelial cells and stellate cells, either of which could have a regulatory role. Dynamic changes in endothelial fenestrae have been demonstrated, and raise the possibility that sinusoidal endothelial cells could be involved in blood flow regulation (1). From an ultrastructural standpoint, stellate cells possess long and extensive cytoplasmic processes that essentially encircle many if not all sinusoidal endothelial cells (2,3). This anatomic relationship in the sinusoid suggests that stellate cells function as liver-specific pericytes (pericytes are smooth muscle-like cells that are felt to control capillary blood flow in a wide variety of tissues (4).

Portal pressure is proportional to resistance and flow according to Ohm's law: $\Delta P = Q \times R$, where ΔP is the change in pressure along a vessel, Q is the flow in the vessel, and R is the resistance to that flow. Elevated portal pressure typical of cirrhosis and portal hypertension has been postulated to include components of each increased intrahepatic resistance, as well as increased flow through the splanchnic system (i.e., a hyperdynamic circulation). The level of increased resistance to flow varies with specific forms of liver disease and may occur at presinusoidal or postsinusoidal levels as in schistosomiasis and

From: *Clinical Gastroenterology: Portal Hypertension*
Edited by: A. J. Sanyal and V. H. Shah © Humana Press Inc., Totowa, NJ

Table 1
Agents with Effects on Stellate Cell Contraction

Contract	Relax
Endothelin (1, 2, 3)	Nitric oxide (NO)
Angiotensin II	Carbon monoxide (CO)
Thrombin	PGE_2
Vasopressin	Lipo-PGE_1
Prostaglandin $F_{2\alpha}$	PGI_2 (prostacyclin)
U46619 (Thromboxane A_2)	Adrenomedullin
LPA	
Substance P	
PAF	
Adenosine	
Serum	

venoocclusive disease, respectively. Many forms of liver injury result in "sinusoidal" portal hypertension. Postulated mechanisms for altered blood flow patterns in this process include regenerative nodules, intrahepatic shunts, and hepatocyte swelling *(5–9)*. Furthermore, extinction of typical vascular units after injury and repair *(10)* may lead to increased intrahepatic resistance.

Stellate Cells and Their Contractility

From a conceptual view, the major cellular components capable of causing increases in intrahepatic resistance, and thus sinusoidal portal hypertension, include sinusoidal endothelial cells and stellate cells. Indeed, abundant in vitro data indicate that stellate cells contract *(11–13)*. Additionally, their contractility is enhanced after injury. This enhanced contractility appears to be related to dramatic upregulation of smooth muscle α actin, among other smooth muscle proteins *(9)*. These proteins appear to supply the cellular mach-inery necessary for contraction. Furthermore, studies utilizing in vivo microscopy further indicate that stellate cell contraction plays an important role in modulating sinusoidal dynamics *(14,16)* and, moreover, that *activated* stellate cells, in particular, contribute to the elevated intrahepatic resistance typical of cirrhotic liver *(9,15)*.

A number of compounds have been shown to modulate stellate cell contractility in isolated culture systems (Table 1). Available evidence indicates that the family of endothelins are the most prominent inducers of stellate cell contraction *(17,18)*. Endothelin receptors are detectable on all cell types in rat liver, but are far more numerous on stellate cells than on other hepatic cells (endothelial, Kupffer cells, and hepatocytes) *(19–21)*. After perfusion of the most prominent endothelin species, endothelin-1 (ET-1), into the liver, its localization is consistent with binding to stellate cells *(9.22)*. These data indicate that stellate cells are the major target of endothelin in the liver.

Substances that counter stellate cell contractility include nitric oxide (NO) *(23)* and carbon monoxide (CO) *(24,25)*. NO, in particular, has been shown to be a potent inhibitor of stellate cell contractility *(23)*. Eicosanoids have also been shown to have potent effects on stellate cells, mediating relaxation (as well as contraction) *(26)*.

Vascular Mediators and Their Biology

VASOCONSTRICTORS

Of the multiple known vasoconstrictors, the endothelins appear to have the most prominent effects in the liver. This family of vasoconstrictors is, therefore, reviewed in the most detail.

Endothelins

Introduction: The endothelins comprise a family of potent vasoconstrictors *(27)*, made up of three unique peptides, termed endothelin-1 (ET-1), endothelin-1 (ET-2), and endothelin-1 (ET-3) *(28,29)*. These 21-amino-acid peptides bind to at least two G-protein–coupled receptors termed endothelin A (ET_A) and endothelin B (ET_B) receptors *(30, 31)*. Endothelins are typically produced by endothelial cells and exert paracrine effects on adjacent smooth muscle cells. However, they can also be produced by other cell types.

Endothelin Synthesis and Regulation: The regulation of ET-1 production is complex. ET-1 appears to be regulated, at least in part, at the level of preproendothelin-1 mRNA transcription *(32–35)*. The expression of preproendothelin-1 is stimulated by a variety of extracellular stimuli, including vasopressor hormones such as epinephrine, angiotensin II, and vasopressin, shear stress, ET-1 itself, and cytokines such as interleukin-1. In vascular endothelial cells, once ET-1 is produced, it is secreted in a constitutive manner, without regulation at the level of exocytosis *(36)*. The endothelin peptides arise by proteolytic processing of large precursors (approx 200-amino-acid residues) by furin-like enzymes, a step that appears to be relatively nonspecific. Intermediates termed big ET-1, -2, and -3 (38–41 aa) are excised from prepropeptides by proteases that cleave at sites containing paired basic amino acids. Big endothelins, which have little or no biologic activity, are cleaved at Trp-21-Val/Ile-22 to produce mature 21-residue, biologically active, peptides. The enzyme responsible for the specific cleavage at Trp-21 has been termed endothelin converting enzyme (ECE); it is a neutral membrane-bound metalloprotease with $M_r = 120$ kDa, belonging to the endopeptidase-24.11 family found in brain *(37–39)*.

Two isoforms of ECE have been cloned and termed ECE-1 and ECE-2 *(39,40)*. ECE-1 and ECE-2 are similar in that they convert big ET-1 more efficiently than big ET-2 or big ET-3 *(39,40)*. The ECE isoforms appear to be functionally distinct in that ECE-2 has an acidic pH optimum (pH 5.5 in contrast to the neutral pH optimum of ECE-1) and ECE-2 is much more sensitive to inhibition by phosphoroamidon than is ECE-1. Additionally, several alternatively spliced variants of ECE-1, exist and may exhibit distinct intracellular sorting patterns (although this point is controversial), implying specific functional consequences of each pattern *(41)*. ECE-1b has been reported to exist primarily in endothelia, whereas ECE-1a has been identified in cultured smooth muscle cells *(42)*.

Endothelin Receptors: The two known endothelin receptor subtypes (ET_A and ET_B) mediate a range of biologic effects *(43)*. ET_A receptors are found predominantly on vascular smooth muscle cells and are preferentially activated by ET-1. Rank order affinities are ET-1 > ET-2 >>> ET-3; the affinity of ET-1 for the ET_A receptor is more than 100-fold that of ET-3 *(30,43–45)*. ET_B receptors are widely distributed and have equal affinity for ET-1, ET-2, and ET-3 *(30,43–45)*. ET_B receptor stimulation appears to bring about divergent responses, depending on the cell type expressing the receptor. Stimulation of ET_B receptors on endothelial cells results in NO release and vascular smooth muscle relaxation. It has been proposed that endothelium-dependent relaxation and smooth muscle vasoconstriction mediated by the ET_B receptor are brought about by two different ET_B receptors on smooth muscle cells, termed "ET_{B1}" and "ET_{B2}," respectively *(46)*.

Other ET receptors have been proposed, such as ET_C and ET_{AX} receptors, found in *Xenopus* dermal melanophores and *Xenopus* heart, respectively *(47,48)*. These receptors have approx 50–60% homology to ET_A/ET_B receptors, and appear to be preferentially activated by ET-3 (affinity ET-3 >> ET-1 > ET-2). Finally, a "super-high affinity" receptor related to ET_B has been proposed based on binding studies *(49)*.

Regulation of Endothelin in Wound Healing and Liver Injury: A key feature of injury and wound healing is increased production (and interaction) of multiple different compounds such as cytokines, growth factors, and peptides *(50)*. For example, TGF-b1 production during liver injury is increased in injured tissue *(51)*; this cytokine, in turn, plays an important role in mesenchymal cell-mediated fibrogenesis. Recent data suggest that other compounds, such as biologically active peptides, are also part of the injury and wounding response. Indeed, a large body of work now indicates that the endothelins are involved in the wound-healing response; abundant evidence indicates that endothelin-1 levels are elevated in diverse forms of injury and wound-healing including in patients with cirrhosis *(52–63)*. Available data further indicate that the source of ET-1 is the injured tissue (i.e., as in the liver) itself *(52,64)*.

The mechanism underlying the increased production of endothelin in the injured liver is complex. In the normal liver, endothelin is produced primarily by endothelial cells; after injury, however, endothelin is derived largely from stellate cells (Fig. 1). In the liver, production of precursor ET-1 is increased in stellate cells after injury *(65)*. Furthermore, endothelin production appears to be closely tied to ECE-1 *(66)*. ECE-1 levels in stellate cells is increased at least in part because ECE-1 mRNA is stabilized via 3' UTR binding proteins *(67)*. The regulation of ECE-1 in this system is remarkably complex. For example, transforming growth factor β mediates increased production of ET-1 after liver injury and stellate cell activation, in part by ECE-1 stablization *(67)*.

The Role of Endothelin in Regulation of Intrahepatic Resistance: The importance of endothelins in portal hypertension and regulation of intrahepatic resistance liver disease has been emphasized in a number of recent studies. First, the data emphasizing the potent effect of ET-1 on isolated stellate cells support this role. Additionally, in vivo microscopic data suggest an important role in intrahepatic microvascular dynamics. After perfusion of ET-1 into the liver, it localizes to stellate cells *(9,68)*, suggesting that stellate cells are the major target of endothelin in the liver. Furthermore, data demonstrating that inhibition of ET-1 signaling reduces portal pressure suggests an important role for ET-1 in intrahepatic resistance and the pathogenesis of portal hypertension *(9,69,70)*. Finally, in vivo physiologic data indicate that perfusion of ET-1 into the liver has a potent effect on sinusoidal constriction *(14,71–73)*.

Angiotensin. Angiotensin II, produced by cleavage of angiotensin I to angiotensin II by angiotensin converting enzyme (ACE), has multiple biologic activities *(74)*. Angiotensin II synthesis is a result of the action of renin–angiotensin–aldosterone system (RAAS). In this pathway, renin converts the inactive plasma protein, angiotensinogen, into angiotensin I. The mature active peptide, angiotensin II, has prominent effects on vascular smooth muscle cells, resulting in contraction, proliferation, and extracellular matrix synthesis. Angiotensin II binds to angiotensin receptors on smooth muscle cell receptors, known as AT1 and AT2 receptors *(75)*. The known physiologic effects of angiotensin II appear to be mediated by the AT1 receptor.

The role of angiotensin II in liver is linked to the finding that stellate cells possess AT1 receptors and that its binding induces cellular contraction and proliferation *(76)*. Fur-

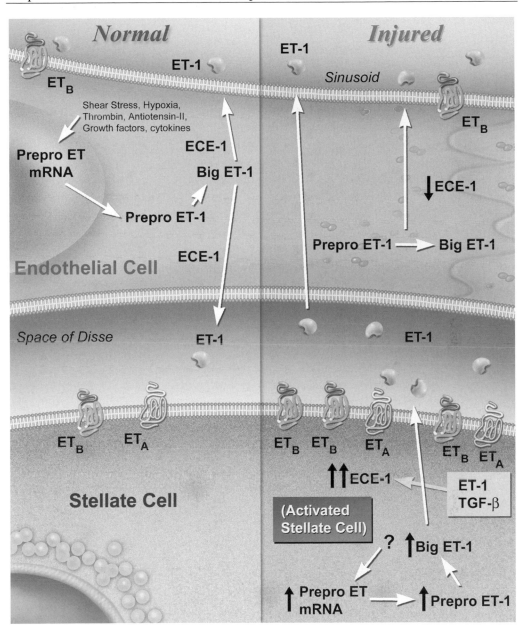

Fig. 1. *Endothelin synthesis in normal and injured liver.* Under normal conditions, control of endothelin synthesis in the sinusoid mirrors that in the systemic vasculature. Hormones, other vascular mediators, and flow conditions appear to modulate precursor endothelin-1 synthesis in endothelial cells. In this state, proteolytic processing of precursor endothelins leads to production of mature endothelin-1. Endothelin-1 then has paracrine physiologic effects on neighboring stellate (or smooth muscle) cells. After liver injury, stellate cell undergo "activation" (see text for details) and synthesis of endothelin-1 shifts dramatically to activated stellate cells. The mechanism underlying enhanced endothelin-1 synthesis appears to largely involve up-regulation of ECE-1, the enzyme responsible for conversion of big endothelin-1 to the mature peptide. In the injured liver, a host of factors, including components in the wounding milieu such as TGF-β, endothelin-1 itself, and other elements are likely to modulate endothelin-1 synthesis. Endothelin-1 in turn has prominent effects on key cellular effectors. Notably, other vasoactive mediators may ultimately be found to have parallel regulatory pathways. From Ref. *18.* (Illustration appears in color following p. 112.)

thermore, recent evidence suggests that the major cellular source of angiotensin II in the liver is the stellate cell (via synthesis of angiotensinogen and expression of ACE) *(77)*. Moreover, its synthesis is upregulated after liver injury, apparently because of pronounced upregulation of ACE *(77)*. Thus, in the injured liver, increased local production of angiotensin II appears to parallel that for endothelin synthesis and the primary effect of angiotensin II in the liver appears to be in extracellular matrix synthesis and wound healing *(78–80)*. The role of angiotensin in intrahepatic vasoregulation is less well defined. Two recent studies, each in small numbers of cirrhotic patients, found that the angiotensin II receptor antagonist, losartan, had divergent effects on portal pressure *(81,82)*.

Eicosanoids. The eicosanoids represent a family of arachidonic acid derivatives that arise from the action of diverse enzymes. The compounds have received great attention in many aspects of general vascular biology, suggesting that they are also likely to be important in hepatic vascular homeostasis. A number of constrictor compounds have been described, including the leukotrienes (products of 5-lipoxygenase), thromboxane $(Tx)A_2$, PGF_{2a}, and epoxyeicosatrienoids (EETs). Unfortunately, the cell biology surrounding their synthesis, regulation of the pathways responsible for their production, and specific cellular effects in the liver are currently poorly understood.

Although the data are limited, it appears that eicosanoids may have in vivo physiologic effects. For example, administration of 8-iso-PGF_{2a} to isolated cirrhotic rat livers resulted in increased portal pressure *(83)*. Such data suggest that eicosanoids, derived from oxidative injury in vivo, could modulate intrahepatic resistance.

Catecholamines. Extensive research indicates that catecholamines have profound effects on vascular smooth muscle (by virtue of binding to a well-defined group of G protein–coupled receptors classified as a or b and in the vasculature. In addition, they have important vascular effects within the liver *(84)*. However, as with prostanoids, the cell biology of this system in the liver is not well understood. Finally, it should be emphasized that catecholamines appear to function largely as circulating hormones, whereas the majority of other vasoactive compounds (i.e., ET-1, NO, CO), act in a paracrine or autocrine fashion.

Others. A number of vasoactive compounds have vasoconstrictive (and relaxing) effects in a variety of circulatory beds and it is likely that they are active in the liver. Such compounds include purinergic agents (adenosine, serotonin, and so on), adrenomedullin, arginine vasopressin, substance P, urotensin-II, atrial natriuretic peptide (ANP), and as yet unidentified factors. However, their function and biology requires further investigation.

VASODILATORS

Multiple vasorelaxing substances have been identified in the vascular bed, several of which appear to be important in the liver. NO has received the greatest attention; it is therefore emphasized.

NO

Introduction: NO is produced from L-arginine by one nitric oxide synthase (NOS) *(85)*. As of this writing, three isoforms, encoded by at least three different genes, have been identified *(86–88)* and fall into two families of enzymes. Endothelial cells (eNOS) and neurons (nNOS) each contain "constitutive" NOS, whereas the inducible form (iNOS) is found in a wide variety of cells *(85)*.

NOS and Regulation: Recent evidence indicates that regulation of NOS expression is complex. Regulation occurs at both transcriptional and posttranslational levels. Multi-

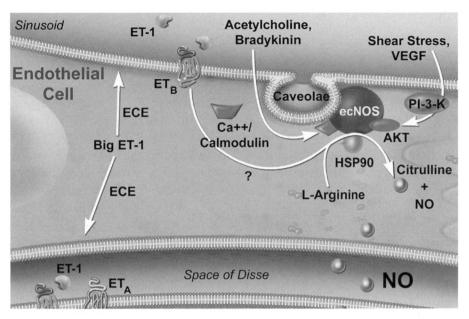

Fig. 2. *Signaling pathways in sinusoidal endothelial cells.* A simplified version of NO signaling pathways is shown. NO is produced after activation of eNOS. Although NO production has been typically thought to be triggered by changes in intracellular Ca^{2+} and activation of Ca^{2+}/calmodulin following stimulation by agonists, eNOS activity is eNOS is extensively post-translationally modified, and its activity can be modulated by many factors. For example, it can be activated and NO synthesis triggered via a signaling pathway involving phosphatidylinositol-3-OH kinase (PI-3-K) and the serine-threonine kinase, AKT. AKT phosphorylation, stimulated by factors such as shear stress and growth factors, leads to eNOS phosphorylation and NO production. Not shown is the effect of NO, in which it binds to guanylate cyclase and leads to production of cGMP which in turn leads to dephosphorylation of myosin and cellular relaxation. From Ref. *18*. (Illustration appears in color following p. 112.)

ple factors stimulate transcription of iNOS *(85)*. Although nNOS and eNOS have often been reported to be "constitutive" isoforms, their levels may be modulated *(89–93)*. For example, eNOS mRNA expression is increased by shear stress, and shear stress response elements have been identified in the eNOS promoter *(94)*. The regulation of eNOS is particularly complex as it is extensively regulated by posttranslational interactions and events *(95–102)*. For example, caveolin-1, the major protein found in caveolae interacts with eNOS and reduces its activity *(95–97)*. Additionally, the protein kinase, Akt (also known as protein kinase B or PKB), phosphorylates eNOS and stimulates its activity *(98)* (Fig. 2).

The Role of NO in Regulation of Intrahepatic Resistance: NO has diverse biologic effects, including its prominent role in the vasculature *(85)*. NO is produced by eNOS in endothelial cells; abnormalities in endothelial production of NO have been described in a number of disorders including in atherosclerosis, diabetes, and hypertension *(85)*. Furthermore, mice lacking eNOS exhibit elevated basal blood pressure, emphasizing the critical role of this enzyme in vascular homeostasis *(103)*.

In the liver, sinusoidal endothelial cells produce NO *(104)*, and production increases in response to flow *(105)*. In vivo physiologic studies, as well as those examining isolated cells, emphasize that NO clearly modulates intrahepatic resistance (25,105–107), and see ref. 108 for review). One of the most important contributions in the field is the finding that endothelial cell synthesis of NO is reduced in the injured liver (104).

A growing body of work has focused on this cellular defect in the injured liver. Interestingly, ecNOS mRNA and protein levels are unaltered after liver injury; thus, the defect in endothelial-derived NO production appears to be related to its extensive posttranslational modifications (104) (Fig. 2), in particular after injury to sinusoidal endothelial cells. For example, increased binding of caveolin to ecNOS in the injured liver is associated with reduced ecNOS activity (109). The finding that caveolin-1 protein levels are markedly increased in the cirrhotic liver (109) supports the possibility that such posttranslational modification of ecNOS is important in portal hypertension.

CO. CO can stimulate guanylate cyclase and cGMP production, leading to smooth muscle relaxation, although the potency that which CO stimulates cGMP production is less than for NO (110,111). Thus, CO may play a role in regulation of vascular resistance, in a fashion analogous to NO. The highly conserved enzyme, heme oxygenase (HO), is responsible for breakdown of heme into equimolar amounts of biliverdin, iron, and CO. Three HO isoforms (HO-1,-2,-3) have been identified. The most prominent isoform, HO-1, can be induced (by heme, other metalloporphyrins, transition metals, and stimuli that induce cellular stress). In contrast, HO-2 is present mainly in the brain and testes and is constitutively expressed. The biologic importance of HO-3 remains unclear.

Endogenously produced CO appears to serve as a vasorelaxant in the hepatic sinusoid (25). Furthermore, CO-dependent dilation in the sinusoid appears to co-localize with hepatic stellate cells (24). Overexpression of CO in the liver reduces intrahepatic vascular resistance (24). Interestingly, within the sinusoid, expression of HO-1 appears to be localized largely to Kupffer cells, particularly in the cirrhotic liver (112) and raises the possibility of paracrine signaling of CO for stellate and endothelial cells.

Prostaglandins. A number of prostaglandins with relaxing capability have been described. These include PGD_2, PGE_2, and PGI_2 (prostacylcin) PGD_2, each of which is produced in the liver, but also which appear to be reduced after liver injury and in cirrhosis, consistent with the tendency toward increased intrahepatic vasoconstriction (26). PGI_2 in particular is produced by endothelial cells, and has effects on stellate cells (11); it appears to lead to vasodilation of the hepatic microcirculation. PGE_2 species are also produced by endothelial cells, and like PGI_2, have effects on stellate cells (11) and also appear to have vasodilatory effects in the liver. However, their cell and molecular biology in the liver is poorly understood.

Cannabanoids. Recent studies have demonstrated that the endogenous cannabinoid anandamide causes vasodilation and systemic hypotension when administered to anesthetized rats. When administered to normal rat liver, anandamide caused an increase in portal flow and portal venous pressure (113). Notably, the rise in portal pressure was less than expected given the increase in portal flow, suggesting that anandamide decreases resistance to flow through the hepatic sinusoids. Additionally, in rats with experimentally induced cirrhosis, their (low) blood pressure was elevated by a specific cannabanoid (CB1) receptor antagonist (114). These data suggest that anandamide and vascular CB1 receptors further play an important role in the vasodilated state in advanced cirrhosis.

Other. A number of other compounds such as bradykinin, vasoactive intestinal peptide, histamines, and acetylcholine, to name a few have been suggested to have effects in the liver. Again however, their cell and molecular biology is not well established.

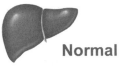
Normal

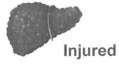
Injured

Vasodilators ≈ Vasoconstrictors   **Vasoconstrictors > Vasodilators**

Normal intrahepatic resistance   **Elevated intrahepatic resistance**

Fig. 3. *An endothelialopathy in liver disease contributes to intrahepatic portal hypertension.* In the normal liver, a balance between vasoconstrictors and vasodilators provides for a low resistance, high flow state. However, after liver injury, concomitant with stellate cell activation, and enhanced stellate cell contractility, increases in vasoconstrictors become pronounced, and moreover, NO production (and perhaps other vasodilators) by sinusoidal endothelial cells is reduced. The net effect is enhanced stellate cell contractility and sinusoidal constriction with an increase in intrahepatic resistance to sinusoidal blood flow.

CELL AND MOLECULAR MECHANISMS AND INCREASED INTRAHEPATIC RESISTANCE

The bulk of the data indicate that with liver injury significant vascular abnormalities exist. Such abnormalities are particularly prominent in the sinusoidal endothelium. In this setting, it appears that an imbalance between vasoconstrictive and vasorelaxing substances occurs (Fig. 3). NO and endothelin-1 are prominent, and serve as a biologically important paradigm. However, other vasoactive compounds play an important role. Not only is ET-1 overproduced in the injured liver *(64,67)*, but NO release by sinusoidal endothelial cells is reduced after cirrhosis *(104,105)*. In the setting of a reduction in other vasodilators (prostanoids and, perhaps, CO) and increases in other vasoconstrictors, an endothelialopathy contributes to portal hypertension. Furthermore, given the prominent increase in stellate cell contractility after liver injury, the data highlight a series of potential molecular mechanisms underlying the well-described increased intrahepatic resistance typical of liver injury. The hemodynamic correlate of these cell and molecular events in portal hypertension.

ACKNOWLEDGMENTS

This work was supported by the NIH (Grants R01 DK50574 and R01 DK54038, both to the author) and the Burroughs Wellcome Fund (DCR).

REFERENCES

1. Oda M, Han JY, Yokomori H. Local regulators of hepatic sinusoidal microcirculation: recent advances. Clin Hemorheol Microcirc 2000;23:85–94.
2. Ekataksin W, Kaneda K. Liver microvascular architecture: an insight into the pathophysiology of portal hypertension. Semin Liver Dis 1999;19:359–382.
3. Wake K. Perisinusoidal stellate cells (fat-storing cells, interstitial cells, lipocytes), their related structure in and around the liver sinusoids, and vitamin A-storing cells in extrahepatic organs. Int Rev Cytol 1980;66:303–353.
4. Shepro D, Morel NM. Pericyte physiology. FASEB J 1993;7:1031–1038.
5. Lautt WW, Greenway CV. Conceptual review of the hepatic vascular bed. Hepatology 1987;7:952–963.

6. Sherman IA, Pappas SC, Fisher MM. Hepatic microvascular changes associated with development of liver fibrosis and cirrhosis. Am J Physiol 1990;258:H460–H465.

7. Blendis LM. Hepatocyte swelling and portal hypertension [comment]. J Hepatol 1992;15:4–5.

8. Lautt WW. The 1995 Ciba-Geigy Award Lecture. Intrinsic regulation of hepatic blood flow. Can J Physiol Pharmacol 1996;74:223–233.

9. Rockey DC, Weisiger RA. Endothelin induced contractility of stellate cells from normal and cirrhotic rat liver: implications for regulation of portal pressure and resistance. Hepatology 1996;24:233–240.

10. Wanless IR, Wong F, Blendis LM, Greig P, Heathcote EJ, Levy G. Hepatic and portal vein thrombosis in cirrhosis: possible role in development of parenchymal extinction and portal hypertension. Hepatology 1995;21:1238–1247.

11. Kawada N, Klein H, Decker K. Eicosanoid-mediated contractility of hepatic stellate cells. Biochem J 1992;285:367–371.

12. Rockey DC, Housset CN, Friedman SL. Activation-dependent contractility of rat hepatic lipocytes in culture and in vivo. J Clin Invest 1993;92:1795–1804.

13. Pinzani M, Failli P, Ruocco C, et al. Fat-storing cells as liver-specific pericytes. Spatial dynamics of agonist-stimulated intracellular calcium transients. J Clin Invest 1992;90:642–646.

14. Zhang JX, Pegoli WJ, Clemens MG. Endothelin-1 induces direct constriction of hepatic sinusoids. Am J Physiol 1994;266:G624–G632.

15. Bauer M, Paquette NC, Zhang JX, et al. Chronic ethanol consumption increases hepatic sinusoidal contractile response to endothelin-1 in the rat. Hepatology 1995;22:1565–1576.

16. Clemens MG, Zhang JX. Regulation of sinusoidal perfusion: in vivo methodology and control by endothelins. Semin Liver Dis 1999;19:383–396.

17. Rockey DC. Characterization of endothelin receptors mediating rat hepatic stellate cell contraction. Biochem Biophys Res Commun 1995;207:725–731.

18. Rockey DC. Vascular mediators in the injured liver. Hepatology 2003;37:4–12.

19. Housset C, Rockey DC, Bissell DM. Endothelin receptors in rat liver: lipocytes as a contractile target for endothelin 1. Proc Natl Acad Sci USA 1993;90:9266–9270.

20. Eakes AT, Howard KM, Miller JE, Olson MS. Endothelin-1 production by hepatic endothelial cells: characterization and augmentation by endotoxin exposure. Am J Physiol 1997;272:G605–G611.

21. Stephenson K, Harvey SA, Mustafa SB, Eakes AT, Olson MS. Endothelin association with the cultured rat Kupffer cell: characterization and regulation. Hepatology 1995;22:896–905.

22. Okumura S, Takei Y, Kawano S, et al. Vasoactive effect of endothelin-1 on rat liver in vivo. Hepatology 1994;19:155–161.

23. Rockey DC, Chung JJ. Inducible nitric oxide synthase in rat hepatic lipocytes and the effect of nitric oxide on lipocyte contractility. J Clin Invest 1995;95:1199–1206.

24. Wakabayashi Y, Takamiya R, Mizuki A, et al. Carbon monoxide overproduced by heme oxygenase-1 causes a reduction of vascular resistance in perfused rat liver. Am J Physiol 1999;277:G1088–G1096.

25. Suematsu M, Goda N, Sano T, et al. Carbon monoxide: an endogenous modulator of sinusoidal tone in the perfused rat liver [see comments]. J Clin Invest 1995;96:2431–247.

26. Birney Y, Redmond EM, Sitzmann JV, Cahill PA. Eicosanoids in cirrhosis and portal hypertension. Prostaglandins Other Lipid Mediat 2003;72:3–18.

27. Yanagisawa M, Kurihara H, Kimura S, et al. A novel potent vasoconstrictor peptide produced by vascular endothelial cells [see comments]. Nature 1988;332:411–415.

28. Inoue A, Yanagisawa M, Kimura S, et al. The human endothelin family: three structurally and pharmacologically distinct isopeptides predicted by three separate genes. Proc Natl Acad Sci USA 1989; 86:2863–2867.

29. Hocher B, Thone-Reineke C, Bauer C, Raschack M, Neumayer HH. The paracrine endothelin system: pathophysiology and implications in clinical medicine [see comments]. Eur J Clin Chem Clin Biochem 1997;35:175–189.

30. Elshourbagy NA, Korman DR, Wu HL, et al. Molecular characterization and regulation of the human endothelin receptors. J Biol Chem 1993;268:3873–3879.

31. Rubanyi GM, Polokoff MA. Endothelins: molecular biology, biochemistry, pharmacology, physiology, and pathophysiology. Pharmacol Rev 1994;46:325–415.

32. Lee ME, Dhadly MS, Temizer DH, Clifford JA, Yoshizumi M, Quertermous T. Regulation of endothelin-1 gene expression by Fos and Jun. J Biol Chem 1991;266:19,034–19,039.

33. Lee ME, Bloch KD, Clifford JA, Quertermous T. Functional analysis of the endothelin-1 gene promoter. Evidence for an endothelial cell-specific cis-acting sequence. J Biol Chem 1990;265:10,446–10,450.

34. Marsen TA, Weber F, Egink G, Suckau G, Baldamus CA. Cyclosporin A induces prepro endothelin-1 gene transcription in human endothelial cells. Eur J Pharmacol 1999;379:97–106.

35. Quehenberger P, Bierhaus A, Fasching P, et al. Endothelin 1 transcription is controlled by nuclear factor-kappaB in AGE-stimulated cultured endothelial cells. Diabetes 2000;49:1561–1570.

36. Yanagisawa M. The endothelin system. A new target for therapeutic intervention [editorial; comment]. Circulation 1994;89:1320–1322.

37. Ohnaka K, Takayanagi R, Nishikawa M, Haji M, Nawata H. Purification and characterization of a phosphoramidon-sensitive endothelin-converting enzyme in porcine aortic endothelium. J Biol Chem 1993; 268:26,759–26,766.

38. Turner AJ, Murphy LJ. Molecular pharmacology of endothelin converting enzymes. Biochem Pharmacol 1996;51:91–102.

39. Xu D, Emoto N, Giaid A, et al. ECE-1: a membrane-bound metalloprotease that catalyzes the proteolytic activation of big endothelin-1. Cell 1994;78:473–485.

40. Emoto N, Yanagisawa M. Endothelin-converting enzyme-2 is a membrane-bound, phosphoramidon-sensitive metalloprotease with acidic pH optimum. J Biol Chem 1995;270:15,262–15,268.

41. Emoto N, Nurhantari Y, Alimsardjono H, et al. Constitutive lysosomal targeting and degradation of bovine endothelin-converting enzyme 1a mediated by novel signals in its alternatively spliced cytoplasmic tail. J Biol Chem 1999;274:1509–1518.

42. Turner AJ, Barnes K, Schweizer A, Valdenaire O. Isoforms of endothelin-converting enzyme: why and where? Trends Pharmacol Sci 1998;19:483–486.

43. Sakurai T, Yanagisawa M, Masaki T. Molecular characterization of endothelin receptors. Trends Pharmacol Sci 1992;13:103–108.

44. Takasuka T, Adachi M, Miyamoto C, Furuichi Y, Watanabe T. Characterization of endothelin receptors ETA and ETB expressed in COS cells. J Biochem (Tokyo) 1992;112:396–400.

45. Masaki T. Historical review: Endothelin. Trends Pharmacol Sci 2004;25:219–224.

46. Clozel M, Gray GA, Breu V, Loffler BM, Osterwalder R. The endothelin ETB receptor mediates both vasodilation and vasoconstriction in vivo. Biochem Biophys Res Commun 1992;186:867–873.

47. Karne S, Jayawickreme CK, Lerner MR. Cloning and characterization of an endothelin-3 specific receptor (ETC receptor) from Xenopus laevis dermal melanophores. J Biol Chem 1993;268:19,126–19,133.

48. Kumar C, Mwangi V, Nuthulaganti P, et al. Cloning and characterization of a novel endothelin receptor from Xenopus heart. J Biol Chem 1994;269:13,414–13,420.

49. Sokolovsky M, Ambar I, Galron R. A novel subtype of endothelin receptors. J Biol Chem 1992;267: 20,551–20,554.

50. Friedman SL, Maher JJ, Bissell DM. Mechanisms and therapy of hepatic fibrosis: report of the AASLD Single Topic Basic Research Conference. Hepatology 2000;32:1403–1408.

51. Czaja MJ, Weiner FR, Flanders KC, et al. In vitro and in vivo association of transforming growth factor-beta 1 with hepatic fibrosis. J Cell Biol 1989;108:2477–2482.

52. Appleton I, Tomlinson A, Chander CL, Willoughby DA. Effect of endothelin-1 on croton oil-induced granulation tissue in the rat. A pharmacologic and immunohistochemical study [see comments]. Lab Invest 1992;67:703–710.

53. Nakamura T, Ebihara I, Fukui M, Tomino Y, Koide H. Effect of a specific endothelin receptor A antagonist on mRNA levels for extracellular matrix components and growth factors in diabetic glomeruli. Diabetes 1995;44:895–899.

54. Tsai YT, Lin HC, Yang MC, et al. Plasma endothelin levels in patients with cirrhosis and their relationships to the severity of cirrhosis and renal function [see comments]. J Hepatol 1995;23:681–688.

55. Park SH, Saleh D, Giaid A, Michel RP. Increased endothelin-1 in bleomycin-induced pulmonary fibrosis and the effect of an endothelin receptor antagonist. Am J Respir Crit Care Med 1997;156: 600–608.

56. Giaid AP, Yanagisawa M, Langleben D, et al. Expression of endothelin-1 in the lungs of patients with pulmonary hypertension. N Engl J Med 1993;328:1732–1739.
57. Saleh D, Furukawa K, Tsao MS, et al. Elevated expression of endothelin-1 and endothelin-converting enzyme-1 in idiopathic pulmonary fibrosis: possible involvement of proinflammatory cytokines. Am J Respir Cell Mol Biol 1997;16:187–193.
58. Kakugawa Y, Giaid A, Yanagisawa M, et al. Expression of endothelin-1 in pancreatic tissue of patients with chronic pancreatitis. J Pathol 1996;178:78–83.
59. Giaid A, Saleh D, Yanagisawa M, Forbes RD. Endothelin-1 immunoreactivity and mRNA in the transplanted human heart. Transplantation 1995;59:1308–1313.
60. Vancheeswaran R, Azam A, Black C, Dashwood MR. Localization of endothelin-1 and its binding sites in scleroderma skin. J Rheumatol 1994;21:1268–1276.
61. Vancheeswaran R, Magoulas T, Efrat G, et al. Circulating endothelin-1 levels in systemic sclerosis subsets—a marker of fibrosis or vascular dysfunction? J Rheumatol 1994;21:1838–1844.
62. Kohan DE. Endothelins in the normal and diseased kidney. Am J Kidney Dis 1997;29:2–26.
63. Forbes RD, Cernacek P, Zheng S, Gomersall M, Guttmann RD. Increased endothelin expression in a rat cardiac allograft model of chronic vascular rejection. Transplantation 1996;61:791–797.
64. Alam I, Bass NM, Bacchetti P, Gee L, Rockey DC. Hepatic tissue endothelin-1 levels in chronic liver disease correlate with disease severity and ascites. Am J Gastroenterol 2000;95:199–203.
65. Rockey DC, Fouassier L, Chung JJ, et al. Cellular localization of endothelin-1 and increased production in liver injury in the rat: potential for autocrine and paracrine effects on stellate cells. Hepatology 1998;27:472–480.
66. Shao R, Yan W, Rockey DC. Regulation of endothelin-1 synthesis by endothelin-converting enzyme-1 during wound healing. J Biol Chem 1999;274:3228–3234.
67. Shao R, Shi Z, Gotwals PJ, Koteliansky VE, George J, Rockey DC. Cell and molecular regulation of endothelin-1 production during hepatic wound healing. Mol Biol Cell 2003;14:2327–2341.
68. Gondo K, Ueno T, Sakamoto M, Sakisaka S, Sata M, Tanikawa K. The endothelin-1 binding site in rat liver tissue: light- and electron-microscopic autoradiographic studies. Gastroenterology 1993; 104:1745–1749.
69. Kojima H, Yamao J, Tsujimoto T, Uemura M, Takaya A, Fukui H. Mixed endothelin receptor antagonist, SB209670, decreases portal pressure in biliary cirrhotic rats in vivo by reducing portal venous system resistance. J Hepatol 2000;32:43–50.
70. Reichen J, Gerbes AL, Steiner MJ, Sagesser H, Clozel M. The effect of endothelin and its antagonist Bosentan on hemodynamics and microvascular exchange in cirrhotic rat liver. J Hepatol 1998;28: 1020–1030.
71. Bauer M, Zhang JX, Bauer I, Clemens MG. ET-1 induced alterations of hepatic microcirculation: sinusoidal and extrasinusoidal sites of action. Am J Physiol 1994;267:G143–G149.
72. Zhang JX, Bauer M, Clemens MG. Vessel- and target cell-specific actions of endothelin-1 and endothelin-3 in rat liver. Am J Physiol 1995;269:G269–G277.
73. Bauer M, Bauer I, Sonin NV, et al. Functional significance of endothelin B receptors in mediating sinusoidal and extrasinusoidal effects of endothelins in the intact rat liver [In Process Citation]. Hepatology 2000;31:937–947.
74. Cody RJ. The integrated effects of angiotensin II. Am J Cardiol 1997;79:9–11.
75. Riordan JF. Angiotensin II: biosynthesis, molecular recognition, and signal transduction. Cell Mol Neurobiol 1995;15:637–651.
76. Bataller R, Gines P, Nicolas JM, et al. Angiotensin II induces contraction and proliferation of human hepatic stellate cells. Gastroenterology 2000;118:1149–1156.
77. Bataller R, Gines P, Lora J, et al. Evidence for a local renin-angiotensin system in human liver: expression in activated hepatic stellate cells. Hepatology 2001;34:399A.
78. Paizis G, Gilbert RE, Cooper ME, et al. Effect of angiotensin II type 1 receptor blockade on experimental hepatic fibrogenesis. J Hepatol 2001;35:376–385.
79. Yoshiji H, Kuriyama S, Yoshii J, et al. Angiotensin-II type 1 receptor interaction is a major regulator for liver fibrosis development in rats. Hepatology 2001;34:745–750.
80. Bataller R, Schwabe RF, Choi YH, et al. NADPH oxidase signal transduces angiotensin II in hepatic stellate cells and is critical in hepatic fibrosis. J Clin Invest 2003;112:1383–1394.

81. De BK, Bandyopadhyay K, Das TK, et al. Portal pressure response to losartan compared with propranolol in patients with cirrhosis. Am J Gastroenterol 2003;98:1371–136.

82. Tripathi D, Therapondos G, Lui HF, Johnston N, Webb DJ, Hayes PC. Chronic administration of losartan, an angiotensin II receptor antagonist, is not effective in reducing portal pressure in patients with preascitic cirrhosis. Am J Gastroenterol 2004;99:390–394.

83. Marley R, Harry D, Anand R, Fernando B, Davies S, Moore K. 8-Isoprostaglandin F2 alpha, a product of lipid peroxidation, increases portal pressure in normal and cirrhotic rats. Gastroenterology 1997; 112:208–213.

84. Bhathal PS, Grossman HJ. Reduction of the increased portal vascular resistance of the isolated perfused cirrhotic rat liver by vasodilators. J Hepatol 1985;1:325–337.

85. Moncada S, Higgs A. The L-arginine-nitric oxide pathway. N Engl J Med 1993;329:2002–2012.

86. Bredt DS, Hwang PM, Glatt CE, Lowenstein C, Reed RR, Snyder SH. Cloned and expressed nitric oxide synthase structurally resembles cytochrome P-450 reductase. Nature 1991;351:714–718.

87. Lowenstein CJ, Glatt CS, Bredt DS, Snyder SH. Cloned and expressed macrophage nitric oxide synthase contrasts with the brain enzyme. Proc Natl Acad Sci USA 1992;89:6711–6715.

88. Lamas S, Marsden PA, Li GK, Tempst P, Michel T. Endothelial nitric oxide synthase: molecular cloning and characterization of a distinct constitutive enzyme isoform. Proc Natl Acad Sci USA 1992;89: 6348–6352.

89. Awolesi MA, Sessa WC, Sumpio BE. Cyclic strain upregulates nitric oxide synthase in cultured bovine aortic endothelial cells. J Clin Invest 1995;96:1449–1454.

90. Weiner CP, Lizasoain I, Baylis SA, Knowles RG, Charles IG, Moncada S. Induction of calcium-dependent nitric oxide synthases by sex hormones. Proc Natl Acad Sci USA 1994;91:5212–5216.

91. Qi WN, Yan ZQ, Whang PG, et al. Gene and protein expressions of nitric oxide synthases in ischemia-reperfused peripheral nerve of the rat. Am J Physiol Cell Physiol 2001;281:C849–C856.

92. Saur D, Seidler B, Paehge H, Schusdziarra V, Allescher HD. Complex regulation of human neuronal nitric-oxide synthase exon 1c gene transcription. Essential role of Sp and ZNF family members of transcription factors. J Biol Chem 2002;277:25,798–25,814.

93. Damy T, Ratajczak P, Shah AM, et al. Increased neuronal nitric oxide synthase-derived NO production in the failing human heart. Lancet 2004;363:1365–1367.

94. Ranjan V, Xiao Z, Diamond SL. Constitutive NOS expression in cultured endothelial cells is elevated by fluid shear stress. Am J Physiol 1995;269:H550–H555.

95. Garcia-Cardena G, Martasek P, Masters BS, et al. Dissecting the interaction between nitric oxide synthase (NOS) and caveolin. Functional significance of the nos caveolin binding domain in vivo. J Biol Chem 1997;272:25,437–25,440.

96. Feron O, Saldana F, Michel JB, Michel T. The endothelial nitric-oxide synthase-caveolin regulatory cycle. J Biol Chem 1998;273:3125–3128.

97. Feron O, Dessy C, Moniotte S, Desager JP, Balligand JL. Hypercholesterolemia decreases nitric oxide production by promoting the interaction of caveolin and endothelial nitric oxide synthase. J Clin Invest 1999;103:897–905.

98. Fulton D, Gratton JP, McCabe TJ, et al. Regulation of endothelium-derived nitric oxide production by the protein kinase Akt. Nature 1999;399:597–601.

99. Garcia-Cardena G, Fan R, Shah V, et al. Dynamic activation of endothelial nitric oxide synthase by Hsp90. Nature 1998;392:821–824.

100. Kou R, Greif D, Michel T. Dephosphorylation of endothelial nitric-oxide synthase by vascular endothelial growth factor. Implications for the vascular responses to cyclosporin A. J Biol Chem 2002; 277:29,669–29,673.

101. Gonzalez E, Kou R, Lin AJ, Golan DE, Michel T. Subcellular targeting and agonist-induced site-specific phosphorylation of endothelial nitric-oxide synthase. J Biol Chem 2002;277:39,554–39,560.

102. Cao S, Yao J, McCabe TJ, et al. Direct interaction between endothelial nitric-oxide synthase and dynamin-2. Implications for nitric-oxide synthase function. J Biol Chem 2001;276:14,249–14,256.

103. Huang PL, Huang Z, Mashimo H, et al. Hypertension in mice lacking the gene for endothelial nitric oxide synthase [see comments]. Nature 1995;377:239–242.

104. Rockey DC, Chung JJ. Reduced nitric oxide production by endothelial cells in cirrhotic rat liver: endothelial dysfunction in portal hypertension. Gastroenterology 1998;114:344–351.

105. Shah V, Haddad FG, Garcia-Cardena G, et al. Liver sinusoidal endothelial cells are responsible for nitric oxide modulation of resistance in the hepatic sinusoids. J Clin Invest 1997;100:2923–2930.
106. Mittal MK, Gupta TK, Lee FY, Sieber CC, Groszmann RJ. Nitric oxide modulates hepatic vascular tone in normal rat liver. Am J Physiol 1994;267:G416–G422.
107. Gupta TK, Toruner M, Chung MK, Groszmann RJ. Endothelial dysfunction and decreased production of nitric oxide in the intrahepatic microcirculation of cirrhotic rats. Hepatology 1998;28:926–931.
108. Wiest R, Groszmann RJ. The paradox of nitric oxide in cirrhosis and portal hypertension: too much, not enough. Hepatology 2002;35:478–491.
109. Shah V, Toruner M, Haddad F, et al. Impaired endothelial nitric oxide synthase activity associated with enhanced caveolin binding in experimental cirrhosis in the rat. Gastroenterology 1999;117: 1222–1228.
110. McMillan K, Bredt DS, Hirsch DJ, Snyder SH, Clark JE, Masters BS. Cloned, expressed rat cerebellar nitric oxide synthase contains stoichiometric amounts of heme, which binds carbon monoxide. Proc Natl Acad Sci USA 1992;89:11,141–11,145.
111. Denninger JW, Marletta MA. Guanylate cyclase and the .NO/cGMP signaling pathway. Biochim Biophys Acta 1999;1411:334–350.
112. Makino N, Suematsu M, Sugiura Y, et al. Altered expression of heme oxygenase-1 in the livers of patients with portal hypertensive diseases. Hepatology 2001;33:32–42.
113. Garcia N Jr, Jarai Z, Mirshahi F, Kunos G, Sanyal AJ. Systemic and portal hemodynamic effects of anandamide. Am J Physiol Gastrointest Liver Physiol 2001;280:G14–G20.
114. Batkai S, Jarai Z, Wagner JA, et al. Endocannabinoids acting at vascular CB1 receptors mediate the vasodilated state in advanced liver cirrhosis. Nat Med 2001;7:827–832.

4

Molecular Mechanisms of Systemic Vasodilation and Hyperdynamic Circulatory State of Cirrhosis

Richard Moreau, MD and Didier Lebrec, MD

CONTENTS

INTRODUCTION
NITRO OXIDE (NO)
ENDOCANNABINOIDS
OTHER MOLECULES
CONCLUSION
REFERENCES

INTRODUCTION

Portal hypertension due to cirrhosis is associated with a chronic hyperkinetic syndrome *(1–3)*. This syndrome is characterized by elevated cardiac output, low arterial pressure, and low systemic vascular resistance *(2,3)*. Splanchnic circulation is also hyperdynamic, i.e., blood flow is elevated and vascular resistance is low in arteries that supply splanchnic organs *(1,4)*. Systemic and splanchnic alterations are interrelated: decreased systemic vascular resistance (systemic vasodilation) is largely due to the decrease in splanchnic arterial resistance (splanchnic vasodilation) *(5)*. Finally, in cirrhosis, there is in vivo and ex vivo arterial hyporeactivity to different receptor-dependent and -independent vasoconstrictors *(6–14)*. A hyperkinetic syndrome also occurs in extrahepatic portal hypertension *(15)*, but it is less marked than that observed in cirrhosis.

The aim of this chapter is to summarize recent progress in understanding molecular mechanisms underlying cirrhosis-associated arterial alterations in systemic and splanchnic territories.

NITRIC OXIDE (NO)

An arterial overproduction of the vasorelaxant NO plays a major role in the pathogenesis of systemic and splanchnic arterial alterations in patients with cirrhosis and in portal hypertensive rats *(16–49)*.

From: *Clinical Gastroenterology: Portal Hypertension*
Edited by: A. J. Sanyal and V. H. Shah © Humana Press Inc., Totowa, NJ

Consequences of NO Overproduction in Arterial Smooth Muscle

Under normal conditions, vasoconstrictors such as angiotensin II, norepinephrine, endothelin-1, and vasopressin are extracellular signals that must bind cognate surface receptors to induce effects in arterial smooth muscle cells (SMCs) *(50)*. Receptors for vasoconstrictors have seven-transmembrane configuration and belong to the superfamily of guanine nucleotide-binding protein (G protein)–coupled receptors (GPCR) *(51)*. Receptors for vasoconstrictors are AT-1 receptors for angiotensin II, α1-adrenoceptors for norepinephrine, ET-A or ET-B receptors for endothelin-1, and V1a-receptor for vasopressin *(50,52)*. GPCR used by vasoconstrictors are coupled to heterotrimeric G proteins, i.e., G proteins that are composed of three polypeptide subunits denoted α, β, and γ *(53)*. The G protein subunit that binds and hydrolyzes GTP is the Gα subunit *(51)*. The Gα subunits used to relay constrictor signals are Gαq or Gα11 subunits of the Gq class *(54)*. Engagement of receptors activate G proteins that stimulate intracellular effectors. One of these effectors is the plasma membrane phospholipase C (PLC)-β, which hydrolyzes phosphatidylinositol 4,5-biphosphate to give the soluble messenger inositol 1,4,5-trisphosphate (IP3), which diffuses in the cytosol, and the endogenous protein kinase C (PKC) activator diacylglycerol (DAG), which remains in the plasma membrane *(50–54)*. In the cytosol, IP3 binds to and activates IP3 receptor, which is located in the membrane of the sarcoplasmic reticulum. IP3 receptor activation causes intracellular Ca^{2+} mobilization, from the sarcoplasmic reticulum to the cytosol *(50,54)*. This causes increased cytosolic free Ca^{2+} concentrations ($[Ca^{2+}]_i$) *(54,55)*. Then, increased $[Ca^{2+}]_i$ induces PKC translocation (which is a first step of PKC activation) from cytosol to the plasma membrane where the enzyme is further activated by DAG *(54–56)*. Activated PKC plays a crucial role in agonist-induced sustained SMC contraction. Indeed, it stimulates the entry of extracellular Ca^{2+} by directly activating plasmalemmal voltage-dependent Ca^{2+} channels (L-type Ca^{2+} channels) *(55)*. PKC is also known to activate L-type Ca^{2+} channels by inducing membrane depolarization *(50)*. Enhanced Ca^{2+} entry contributes to increased $[Ca^{2+}]_i$ *(50–56)*. Then, the complex Ca^{2+}/calmodulin stimulates myosin light-chain kinase to phosphorylate myosin light chain (MLC) *(55)*. Phosphorylated MLC causes SMC contraction. In addition to its effect on the Ca^{2+}-dependent pathway, activated PKC may sensitize the contractile apparatus to Ca^{2+} by inhibiting myosin phosphatase *(55)*. Among PKC isoforms, two are important for SMC contraction: PKC-α (a classic PKC which is dependent on Ca^{2+} and DAG) and PKC-δ (which does not depend on Ca^{2+}) *(57)*.

Portal hypertension-associated hyporeactivity to vasoconstrictors is mainly due to NO *(10,19–21,23,25,26,28,36,37,39,40,43,44)*. The molecular mechanisms of NO-induced portal hypertensive SMC hyporesponsiveness are not well understood *(50,52,58)*. In normal SMC, NO stimulates soluble guanylyl cyclase to produce the second messenger cyclic 3',5'-guanosine monophosphate (cGMP) *(59)*. cGMP then activates a cGMP-dependent serine–threonine protein kinase called PKG *(59)*. PKG has been shown to inhibit the GPCR/Gq/11/PLC-β signaling pathway used by vasoconstrictors. Indeed, PKG may phosphorylate GPCR and thereby uncouple the receptor and G-proteins *(58)*. PKG may also bind to and phosphorylate regulator of G-protein signaling-2 (RGS-2), which increases GTPase activity of Gq/11, terminating vasoconstrictor signaling *(60)*. PLC-β may also be inhibited by PKG in COS cells, although the significance of this pathway in vivo is unknown *(61)*. In portal hypertensive SMC, one of these mechanisms, or more, may be used by NO to inhibit the vasoconstrictor-elicited membrane transduction pathway leading to PKC activation. Indeed, in portal hypertensive arteries, there is a decrease in the ex vivo production of IP3 and DAG in response to vasoconstrictors using GPCR *(62)*. Moreover, in portal hypertensive aortas, PKC-α protein levels are decreased in vivo *(63–65)*. In addition, under ex vivo conditions, in normal aortas, there is a significant decrease in translocation (i.e., activation) of PKC-α and PKC-δ in response to phenylephrine *(64)*. Moreover, ex vivo enzymatic activities of PKC-α and PKC-δ are significantly decreased in cirrhotic SMC *(64)*.

In normal arteries, the NO/cGMP/PKG may relax SMC through several other mechanisms leading to decreased $[Ca^{2+}]_i$. (reviewed in refs. *50* and *58*). First, PKG is known to decrease intracellular Ca^{2+} release by inhibiting the IP3 receptor. Second, PKG may phosphorylate and activate plasmalemmal high-conductance, Ca^{2+}-sensitive K^+ (BKCa) channels. This causes membrane hyperpolarization, which inhibits L-type Ca^{2+} channels and decreases Ca^{2+} entry. PKG may also decrease Ca^{2+} entry by directly inhibiting L-type Ca^{2+} channels. Finally, PKG may favor Ca^{2+} extrusion outside the cytosol, by stimulating Ca^{2+}-ATPases located in the plasma membrane and in the membrane of the sarcoplasmic reticulum. On the other hand, PKG may phosphorylate and activate myosin phosphatase, an effect known to cause desensitization of the contractile apparatus to Ca^{2+} *(58)*. None of these mechanisms have been investigated in portal hypertensive SMC.

In portal hypertension, ex vivo arterial hyporeactivity to vasoconstrictors may differ from one vascular bed to another. For example, in cirrhotic rats, hyporeactivity occurs in the aorta and the superior mesenteric artery whereas reactivity to vasoconstrictors is normal for the carotid artery *(39)*.

The endothelium-denuded human hepatic artery from cirrhotic patients exposed ex vivo to several receptor-dependent vasoconstrictors is hyporeactive to certain vasoconstrictors but not to others *(66–68)*. This suggests that, in addition to endothelium-dependent mechanisms (see below), alterations may occur within SMC.

ROLE OF NITRIC-OXIDE SYNTHASES (NOSs) IN PORTAL HYPERTENSION

NOSs are hemoproteins that produce NO from L-arginine (see reviews in refs. *69* and *70*). There are three isoforms of NOS that are regulated by distinct genes. Neuronal NOS (nNOS), also known as NOS-1, is found in neuronal and some nonneuronal tissues. Inducible NOS (iNOS or NOS-2) was first found in macrophages but has been identified in other cell types (e.g., SMC). Endothelial NOS (eNOS or NOS-3) was first identified as the enzyme-producing endothelium-derived relaxing factor. Both nNOS and eNOS are constitutively expressed. iNOS is not a constitutive enzyme and its expression may be induced by stimuli such as lipopolysaccharide (LPS, endotoxin) or proinflammatory cytokines [i.e., tumor necrosis factor alpha (TNF-α), interleukin-1, and interferon-γ]. A role of the three NOS isoforms has been suggested in portal hypertension.

Increased NOS Activity as an Adpatation to High Arterial Blood Flow. In normal rats, chronic exercise induces a sustained increase in cardiac ouput causing chronic increases in shear stress forces perceived at the surface of arterial endothelial cells *(71)*. In response to chronic shear stress, there is an increase in the expression and catalytic activity of eNOS. Endothelial NO is a gas which diffuses rapidly in underlying SMC to induce their relaxation allowing an increase in vessel diameter and a reduction in the vascular resistance to elevated arterial flow *(69)*. In portal hypertension, NO-induced arterial hyporeactivity occurs in vascular beds with high blood flow (see above) *(39)*. Moreover, in portal hypertensive rats, high cardiac output is associated with increased in vivo aortic levels of eNOS mRNA *(44)* and eNOS protein *(44,72)*. Interestingly, among portal hypertensive rats, aortic eNOS protein is significantly higher in cirrhotic than in portal vein–stenosed rats *(72)*. In both models of portal hypertension, a 7-d administration of the nonselective β-blocker, propranolol (which is known to significantly reduce cardiac output), induces a significant decrease in in vivo aortic eNOS mRNA *(44)*, in eNOS protein *(44, 72)*, and in ex vivo aortic NOS activity *(44,72)*. Finally, in portal vein–stenosed rats treated with propranolol, there is normalization of ex vivo aortic reactivity to vasoconstrictors *(44)*. Together, these findings suggest that portal hypertensive aortas exposed to chronic shear stress overexpress eNOS in vivo, which plays a role in increased NO production. In the mesenteric vasculature of portal hypertensive rats, there is an in vivo increase in eNOS protein levels *(40)*, which is probably related, at least in part, to high mesenteric blood flow. However, this hypothesis has not yet been verified, for example, by evaluating the effects of the nonselective β-blockade-induced reduction in mesenteric hyperdynamic circulation on the local level of eNOS expression.

In normal animals, there is evidence that shear stress controls eNOS mRNA transcription (by modulating eNOS promoter activity) and also regulates posttranscriptional processes that determine eNOS mRNA stability *(73)*. These mechanisms have not yet been studied in portal hypertension.

Under physiological conditions, shear stress is also known to regulate eNOS through posttranslational mechanisms involving interaction of eNOS with other proteins such as caveolin-1, calmodulin, and the chaperone heat shock protein 90 (Hsp90) (reviewed in refs. *74–76*). Caveolin-1 inhibits eNOS whereas calmodulin and Hsp90 stimulate eNOS activity. Endothelial cells express a plasmalemmal small-conductance, Ca^{2+}-sensitive K^+ (SKCa) channel whose opening is induced by shear stress *(77)*. SKCa channel opening induces endothelial membrane hyperpolarization, which favors the entry of extracellular Ca^{2+} through voltage-independent Ca^{2+} channels. The resulting Ca^{2+} entry increases $[Ca^{2+}]_i$. Then, Ca^{2+} binds to calmodulin and the complex Ca^{2+}/calmodulin binds to eNOS and activates the enzyme by displacing the inhibitory protein caveolin-1 *(74–77)*. In cirrhotic rat aortas, endothelial SKCa channels are overexpressed and overactive *(78)*. Indeed, in cirrhotic aortas, selective SKCa channel blockade induces significant decreases in ex vivo eNOS activity and hyporeactivity to vasoconstrictors *(78)*. Thus, in cirrhosis, activation of endothelial SKCa channels may be used by shear stress to stimulate the Ca^{2+}/calmodulin/eNOS pathway. It should be emphasized that the levels of protein expression of caveolin-1 and calmodulin have not yet been studied in portal hypertensive vessels.

Under normal conditions, fluid shear stress may induce Hsp90 *(74,75)*. Moreover, shear stress stimulates the binding of eNOS to Hsp90, and Hsp90 increases eNOS activity in a concentration-dependent manner *(74,75)*. In aortas, in vivo Hsp90 protein levels are significantly higher in portal hypertensive rats than in normal rats *(72)*. Hsp90 levels are significantly higher in cirrhotic aortas than in portal vein-stenosed aortas *(72)*. Hsp90 regulation of endothelial nitric oxide synthase contributes to control of mesenteric vasculature in portal vein–stenosed rats *(43)*. Together, these findings suggest that, in portal hypertensive aortas, under in vivo conditions, enhanced shear stress uses Hsp90 to stimulate eNOS catalytic activity.

Under normal conditions, shear stress–induced posttranslational regulation of eNOS activity may occur not only through protein–protein interactions but also via protein phosphorylation (reviewed in refs. *75* and *76*). For example, shear stress may activate the serine/threonine kinase Akt, which phosphorylates eNOS at serine 1177 (Ser^{1177}). Ser^{1177} phosphorylation is known to stimulate eNOS catalytic activity. Shear stress may also induce eNOS phosphorylation at residues other than Ser^{1177}. However, eNOS phosphorylation and its regulation have not yet been investigated in cirrhotic aortas.

NOS Activity as a Cause of High Arterial Blood Flow. There is evidence that eNOS may initiate hyperdynamic circulation in portal hypertension. In portal vein–stenosed rats, vasoconstriction of the superior mesenteric artery is the earliest hemodynamic event that precedes by 4–5 d the development of hyperkinetic circulation *(49)*. In arteries, vasoconstriction per se may induce shear stress and activate eNOS catalytic activity. In fact, an increase in mesenteric eNOS activity becomes evident as early as 10 h after portal vein stenosis *(49)*. NO overproduction by eNOS precedes hyperdynamic circulation in portal vein–stenosed rats *(41)*. Interestingly, an Akt-dependent eNOS phosphorylation at Ser^{1177} may contribute to the early increase in eNOS activity after portal vein stenosis *(46)*. Together, these findings suggest that mesenteric arterial vasoconstriction plays a triggering role in the upregulation of eNOS catalytic activity in the superior mesenteric artery of portal vein–stenosed rats. This early eNOS overactivity may play a causal role in the subsequent development of splanchnic hyperdynamic circulation. Studies are needed to determine whether early vasoconstriction and subsequent eNOS upregulation occur in the splanchnic circulation of cirrhotic rats.

A key role for eNOS in the development of hyperdynamic circulation is also suggested by the finding that the hyperkinetic syndrome occurs in portal vein–stenosed mice lacking eNOS (eNOS–/–) but not in portal vein–stenosed mice lacking iNOS *(79)*. However, this hypothesis is not supported by the results of another study showing that hyperkinetic syndrome induced by portal vein stenosis occurred in eNOS–/– mice lacking eNOS or in those lacking both eNOS and iNOS (double knock-out mice) *(80)*. In addition, in rats that received an NOS inhibitor, systemic and splanchnic vascular resistance remains significantly lower in portal hypertensive animals than in controls *(27,35)*. Nevertheless, these studies do not rule out a central role of eNOS in the hyperkinetic syndrome because compensatory vasodilators may replace NO to induce this syndrome in portal hypertensive animals (see below).

Endothelial NOS may be activated by stimuli other than shear stress. For example, endothelin-1–induced activation of endothelial ET-B receptors may stimulate eNOS by increasing $[Ca^{2+}]_i$ *(81)*. On the other hand, in endothelial cells, eNOS is known to be inhibited by the interaction with unstimulated ET-B receptors *(75,76)*. Stimulation of ET-B receptors by endothelin-1 may induce the dissociation of eNOS from the ET-B receptor and an increase in NO production *(75,76)*. Because plasma endothelin-1 concentrations are increased in cirrhosis *(82)*, an ET-B-receptor–mediated pathway might contribute to eNOS overactivity.

Because NOS activity is suppressed by interaction with NO-interacting protein (also known as NOSIP) *(75,76)*, there may be a decrease in NOSIP-induced eNOS inhibition in portal hypertension. On the other hand, because dynamin-2 (a GTP-binding protein) *(83)* and porin (an anion channel) *(76)* directly interact with eNOS and activate it, dynamin-2 or porin or both may contribute to eNOS overactivity in portal hypertension. Together, these findings indicate that interactions of NOSIP, dynamin-2, and porin, on one hand, and eNOS, on the other hand, should be studied in portal hypertension.

In conditions other than portal hypertension, vascular endothelial growth factor (VEGF) stimulates eNOS activity through a mechanism that involves Hsp90 activation and eNOS phosphorylation at Ser^{1177} *(75,76)*. However, in cirrhosis, a role for VEGF in eNOS upregulation is unlikely for several reasons. First, VEGF protein expression is significantly lower in aortas from portal hypertensive rats than in aortas from normal rats *(72)*. In addition, among portal hypertensive rats, VEGF protein expression is significantly lower in cirrhotic aortas than in portal hypertensive aortas *(72)*. Moreover, in patient with cirrhosis, plasma VEGF concentrations are decreased *(84)*. Because shear stress and NO are known to downregulate VEGF expression *(85)*, this may explain decreased levels of VEGF in portal hypertensive aortas. Second, following ex vivo exposure to VEGF, aortic NOS activity is more marked in normal aortas than in portal hypertensive aortas *(72)*.

Intestinal translocation of Gram negative bacteria causing endotoxemia without overt sepsis is common in cirrhosis *(40,47)*. This "nonseptic endotoxemia" results in increased plasma concentrations of proinflammatory cytokines such as tumor necrosis factor (TNF)-α *(40)*. The hyperkinetic syndrome is more marked in cirrhotic rats with bacterial translocation than in those without *(40)*. The administration of norfloxacin, an antibiotic that causes selective intestinal decontamination and inhibits bacterial translocation, has been shown to decrease plasma TNF-α levels and systemic hyperdynamic syndrome in patients *(86)* and rats with cirrhosis *(47)*. Moreover, in portal hypertensive rats without overt bacterial sepsis, treatments that decrease TNF-α production *(87)* or action *(38,42, 48,88)* or both *(89)* are known to decrease the hyperkinetic syndrome. Finally, NO overproduction in systemic and splanchnic territories is significantly higher in cirrhotic rats with bacterial translocation than in those without *(40)*. Together, these findings suggest that mechanisms related to bacterial translocation aggravate the hyperkinetic syndrome by increasing NO overproduction. Because endotoxin or TNF-α or both are known to induce iNOS *(90)*, it is not surprising that iNOS protein is found in aortas from cirrhotic rats but not in those from normal rats *(72)*. Interestingly, in cirrhotic rats, chronic norfloxacin therapy is associated with a decrease in aortic iNOS (R Moreau, D Lebrec, unpublished results). Because iNOS produces a large amount of NO *(69)*, iNOS-derived NO, as well as eNOS-derived NO, may play a role in cirrhosis-associated systemic hyperkinetic syndrome. On the other hand, because no iNOS is found in the splanchnic vasculature from cirrhotic rats with bacterial translocation *(40)*, the difference in splanchnic NO production between these rats and those without translocation is probably due to differences in eNOS activity. In cirrhotic mesenteric vasculature, bacterial translocation upregulates GTP-cyclohydrolase I (GTPCH-I) *(91)*, a key enzyme involved in the production of tetrahydrobiopterin (BH4) *(92)*, which is an essential, rate-limiting cofactor in the synthesis of NO by eNOS. Thus, in cirrhotic rats, bacterial translocation may stimulate eNOS activity by increasing the GTPCH-I/BH4 pathway. However, another mechanism may explain that bacterial translocation activates eNOS. Indeed, in rat portal hypertensive gastric mucosa, TNF-α has been shown to activate eNOS by stimulating Akt to phosphorylate eNOS at Ser^{1177} *(48)*.

Aortic nNOS protein expression is higher in cirrhotic rat aortas than in control aortas *(45)*. Treatment of cirrhotic rats for 7 d with a specific nNOS inhibitor normalizes the systemic hyperkinetic syndrome and decreases the aortic levels of nNOS and cGMP *(45)*. Together, these results suggest that nNOS-derived NO may contribute to the development of the systemic hyperkinetic syndrome in cirrhosis. nNOS expression has not yet been studied in the superior mesenteric artery from portal hypertensive rats.

ENDOCANNABINOIDS

In cirrhotic rats, the administration of the cannabinoid CB1 receptor antagonist SR141716A increases arterial pressure *(93,94)* and decreases both portal hypertension and high superior mesenteric artery blood flow *(93)*. Monocytes from cirrhotic, but not control patients or rats, elicit SR141716A-sensitive hypotension in normal recipient rats and have significantly elevated levels of the endocannabinoid anandamide, a CB1 receptor agonist *(93,94)*. The finding that administration of exogenous anandamide decreases arterial pressure in normal rats and has no effect in cirrhotic rats *(93)* suggests a maximal activation of vascular CB1 receptors by an endogenous ligand (possibly anadamide) in the former animals. Together, these results suggest that anandamide and vascular CB1 vascular receptors are involved in cirrhosis-induced vasodilation. Interestingly, in cultured human arterial endothelial cells anandamide increases eNOS catalytic activity by stimulating CB1 receptors *(95)*. Because anandamide-induced hypotension is reduced by 50% in normal rats pretreated with a NOS inhibitor, anandamide-evoked NO production also occurs under in vivo conditions *(93)*. Therefore, in cirrhotic rats, engagement of vascular CB1 receptors by endocannabinoids may play a role in eNOS overactivity *(93)*. However, this hypothesis is not supported by the finding of a decrease in arterial pressure following administration of cirrhotic monocytes to normal recipients rats pretreated with an NOS inhibitor *(94)*.

Moreover, in vitro experiments suggest that CB1 receptors may activate NOS-independent mechanisms (e.g., K^+ channel activation) that may also contribute to the in vivo response to endocannabinoids *(95)*. Studies are needed to elucidate the mechanism of endocannabinoid-induced vasodilation in cirrhosis.

In normal rats, activation of CB1 vascular receptors by endocannabinoid of myeloid origin plays a role in endotoxin-induced hypotension *(96)*. Because endotoxemia is common in cirrhosis (see above), this may be involved in the activation of the endocannabinoid/CB1 receptor pathway in chronic liver disease.

OTHER MOLECULES

Following administration of NOS-inhibitors, systemic and splanchnic vascular resistance remain lower in cirrhotic rats than in normal rats (see above), suggesting the implication of vasorelaxants other than NO. First candidates for this are endothelium-derived prostaglandins.

In normal endothelial cells, cytosolic Ca^{2+}-dependent phospholipase A_2 ($cPLA_2$) hydrolyzes membrane phospholipids to produce arachidonic acid (AA) *(97)*. Then, AA may be metabolized by cyclooxygenase (COX) to produce prostacyclin (PGI_2), a vasodilator prostaglandin (PG) *(98)*. In SMC, PGI_2 engages a GPCR coupled to Gs, which stimulates adenylyl cyclase to produce cyclic 3',5'-adenosine monophosphate (cAMP) *(98)*. cAMP may activate two kinases: cAMP-dependent protein kinase (PKA) *(98)* and PKG *(50)*. PKA- or PKG-induced activation of ATP-sensitive K^+ (K_{ATP}) channels and subsequent membrane hyperpolarization contributes to PGI_2-induced SMC *(99)*. Several studies suggest that the $cPLA_2$/COX/PGI_2 pathway is upregulated in portal hypertension. First, $cPLA_2$ activity is significantly increased in cirrhotic aortas *(100)*. Moreover, in cirrhosis, there are stimuli for $cPLA_2$ overreactivity such as increased fluid shear stress and elevated plasma levels of endogenous vasoconstrictors (e.g., norepinephrine) *(50)*. Second, in portal vein–stenosed rats, COX-1 (the constitutive form of COX) is overexpressed in the aorta (at the early stage of portal hypertension) and in the superior mesenteric artery (at a later stage) *(101)*. COX-2 is not induced in portal hypertensive vessels *(101)*. Third, plasma levels of 6-keto-$PGF_{1\alpha}$, a stable PGI_2 metabolite, are increased in patients and rats with portal hypertension *(102–104)*. Finally, COX inhibition with indomethacin in patients or rats with portal hypertension induces systemic and splanchnic vasoconstriction $(104–106)$. In cirrhotic rats, activation of arterial K_{ATP} channels may contribute to PGI_2-induced vasorelaxation. Indeed, in these rats, the administration of glibenclamide, a selective K_{ATP} channel blocker, induces systemic and splanchnic vasoconstriction, an effect that is suppessed in indomethacin-pretreated rats (107).

In portal vein–stenosed rats, the splanchnic vasoconstrictor effect caused by the combined administration of a NOS inhibitor and indomethacin is equivalent to the addition of their respective effects when administered alone (106). Thus, both NO and PGI_2 may be involved in the baseline splanchnic vasodilation, via nonredundant mechanisms. It should be emphasized that splanchnic arterial resistance after a combination of COX/NOS inhibitors is still significantly lower in portal hypertensive rats than in corresponding controls (106), suggesting that, in addition to NO and PGI_2, other vasorelaxant signals are involved.

Plasma glucagon concentrations are increased in portal hypertension (108). Because glucagon is known to stimulate a GPCR/Gs/adenylyl cyclase/cAMP pathway, it may induce SMC relaxation in portal hypertension (50).

In normal arterial walls exposed to NOS/COX inhibitors, acetylcholine or shear stress induces the release of an endothelium-derived relaxing factor (EDRF) (109). This NOS/COX-inhibitors-insensitive EDRF has been called endothelium-derived hyperpolarizing factor (EDHF) because it elicits arterial SMC relaxation by inducing membrane hyperpolarization in these cells. In the normal superior mesenteric artery exposed to NOS/COX inhibitors, acetylcholine activates apamin- and charybdotoxin-sensitive K^+ channels located in the plasma membrane of endothelial cells (110). The resulting efflux of K^+ outside the cells increases myoendothelial K^+ concentration ($[K^+]$). Increased myoendothelial $[K^+]$, in turn, activates barium-sensitive K^+ channels and the ouabain-sensitive sodium–potassium–adenosine triphosphatase (Na^+/K^+ ATPase) located in the plasma membrane of underlying SMC. Activation of barium-sensitive K^+ channels and Na^+/K^+ ATPase leads to plasma membrane hyperpolarization and SMC relaxation (110). Together, these findings indicate that K^+ released by endothelial apamin- and charybdotoxin-sensitive K^+ channels is an EDHF. In cirrhotic rats, EDHF is released by the superior mesenteric artery but not the aorta (111). In the cirrhotic superior mesenteric artery, EDHF-induced SMC relaxation is abolished by a combination of apamin and charybdotoxin and decreased by exposure to barium or ouabain. Thus, in the superior mesenteric artery from cirrhotic rats, EDHF may be K^+ ion released by endothelial apamin- and charybdotoxin-sensitive K^+ channels; K^+ then activating barium-sensitive K^+ channels and Na^+/K^+ ATPase in SMC. Whether or not EDHF is involved in the alterations in splanchnic circulation associated with portal hypertension remains to be elucidated.

Heme oxygenase (HO) opens the heme ring, resulting in the liberation of equimolar quantities of biliverdin, free iron, and carbon monoxide (CO) (112). CO, like NO, is a gas that may stimulate soluble guanylyl cyclase and activate the cGMP/PKG pathway leading to SMC relaxation (58). There are at least to HO isoforms: HO-1, which is inducible, and HO-2, which is constitutive (112). There is evidence that HO hyperactivity may contribute to portal hypertension–induced NOS-inhibitor-insensitive splanchnic vasodilation. First, $HO-1$ gene expression is increased in splanchnic organs from portal vein–stenosed rats (113). $HO-1$ gene expression also occurs in the liver in patients with cirrhosis (114). Second, HO activity is significantly increased in splanchnic organs from rats with portal vein stenosis (115). Third, in perfused mesenteric vascular beds, in the absence of NOS inhibition, the HO inhibitor zinc mesoporphyrin (ZnMP) has no effect on hypo-reactivity to the vasoconstrictor action induced by elevated extracellular potassium chloride concentrations. Vascular hyporeactivity to potassium chloride is only decreased by a NOS-inhibitor and suppressed by a combination of a NOS-inhibitor and ZnMP *(115)*. Together, these findings suggest that, in portal hypertension, a product of HO-1 activity (probably CO) may explain NO-independent SMC hyporeactivity to potassium chloride. Because HO-1 is inducible by several stimuli, including endotoxin and cytokines, future studies are needed to identify the mechanisms of HO-1 induction in portal hypertension.

Patients with cirrhosis have increased plasma levels of natriuretic peptides [i.e., atrial natriuretic peptide (ANP), brain natriuretic peptide (BNP), and C-type natriuretic peptide (CNP)] *(116–119)*. Natriuretic peptides stimulate specific surface receptors coupled to guanylyl cyclases and thus elicit cGMP/PKG-induced SMC relaxation *(120)*. Together, these findings suggest that antriuretic peptides may be involved in vasodilation associated with cirrhosis.

Because patients with cirrhosis have increased plasma levels of vasorelaxant peptides such as adrenomedullin *(121)*, calcitonin gene–related peptide *(122)*, substance P *(123)*, and vasoactive intestinal peptide *(124)*, these peptides might contribute to vasodilation in cirrhosis. It should be noted that these peptides stimulate specific GPCR to induce relaxing mechanisms that have not yet been clearly identified: certain studies suggest an activation of the NO/cGMP pathway and others a stimulation of cAMP production *(125)*.

Studies are needed to clarify the role of natriuretic peptides and neuropeptides in circulatory alterations associated with portal hypertension.

CONCLUSION

NO is the main vasorelaxant molecule involved in the hyperkinetic syndrome in cirrhosis. Aortic overproduction of eNOS-derived NO is a homeostatic response resulting in a decrease in vascular resistance opposed to chronically increased cardiac output. This mechanism may also occur in the superior mesenteric artery. On the other hand, at least in cirrhotic rats with intestinal bacterial translocation, mechanisms elicited by bacterial products may induce iNOS-derived NO (in the aorta but not the superior mesenteric artery) and further increase production of eNOS-derived NO (in the superior mesenteric artery and perhaps the aorta). These mechanisms related to bacterial translocation may thus aggravate the hyperkinetic syndrome. Increased production of nNOS-derived NO (in the aorta and perhaps the superior mesenteric artery) may also play a role in the systemic hyperkinetic syndrome. Finally, molecules other than NO such as endocannabinoids, COX-derived products, or carbon monoxide may be involved; however, their respective role com-pared to NO should be clarified.

REFERENCES

1. Groszmann R. Hyperdynamic circulation of liver disease forty years later: pathophysiology and clinical consequences. Hepatology 1994;20:1359–1363.
2. Moreau R, Lee SS, Soupison T, Roche-Sicot J, Sicot C. Abnormal tissue oxygenation in patients with cirrhosis and liver failure. J Hepatol 1988;7:98–105.
3. Braillon A, Cales P, Valla D, Gaudy D, Geoffroy P, Lebrec D. Influence of the degree of liver failure on systemic and splanchnic haemodynamics and on response to propranolol in patients with cirrhosis. Gut 1986;27:1204–1209.

4. Lebrec D, Blanchet L. Effects of two models of portal hypertension on splanchnic organ blood flow in the rat. Clin Sci 1985;68:23–28.
5. Fernandez-Seara J, Prieto J, Quiroga J, et al. Systemic and regional hemodynamics in patients with liver cirrhosis and ascites with and without functional renal failure. Gastroenterology 1989;97:1304–1312.
6. Murray BM, Paller MS. Pressor resistance to vasopressin in sodium depletion, potassium depletion, and cirrhosis. Am J Physiol 1986;251:R525–R530.
7. Pinzani M, Marra F, Fusco BM, et al. Evidence for α-adrenoreceptor hyperresponsiveness in hypotensive cirrhotic patients with ascites. Am J Gastroenterol 1991;86:711–714.
8. Braillon A, Cailmail S, Gaudin C, Lebrec D. Reduced splanchnic vasoconstriction to angiotensin II in conscious rats with biliary cirrhosis. J Hepatol 1993;17:86–90.
9. Ryan J, Sudhir K, Jennings G, Esler M, Dudley F. Impaired reactivity of the peripheral vascular to pressor agents in alcoholic cirrhosis. Gastroenterology 1993;105:1167–1172.
10. Hartleb M, Moreau R, Cailmail S, Gaudin C, Lebrec D. Vascular hyporesponsiveness to endothelin-1 in rats with cirrhosis. Gastroenterology 1994;107:1085–1093.
11. Hartleb M, Moreau R, Gaudin C, Lebrec D. Lack of vascular hyporesponsiveness to the L-type calcium channel activator, Bay K 8644, in rats with cirrhosis. J Hepatol 1995;22:202–207.
12. Liao J, Yu PC, Lin HC, Lee FY, Kuo JS, Yang MCM. Study on the vascular reactivity and α-adrenoceptors of portal hypertensive rats. Br J Pharmacol 1994;111:439–444.
13. Huang YT, Wang GF, Yang MCM, Chang SP, Lin HC, Hong CY. Vascular hyporesponsiveness in aorta from portal hypertensive rats: possible sites of involvement. J Pharmacol Exp Ther 1996;278:535–541.
14. Sogni P, Sabry S, Moreau R, Gadano A, Lebrec D, Din-Xuan AT. Hyporeactivity of mesenteric resistance arteries in portal hypertensive rats. J Hepatol 1996;24:487–490.
15. Moreau R, Cailmail S, Lebrec D. Haemodynamic effects of vasopressin in portal hypertensive rats receiving clonidine. Liver 1994;14:45–49.
16. Pizcueta P, Piqué JM, Bosch J, Whittle BJR, Moncada S. Effects of inhibiting nitric oxide biosynthesis on the systemic and splanchnic circulation of rats with portal hypertension. Br J Pharmacol 1992;105:184–190.
17. Claria J, Jiménez W, Ros J, Asbert M, Castro A, Arroyo V, Rivera F, Rodès J. Pathogenesis of arterial hypotension in cirrhotic rats with ascites: role of endogenous nitric oxide. Hepatology 1992;15:343–349.
18. Sogni P, Moreau R, Ohsuga M, et al. Evidence for a normal nitric oxide-mediated vasodilator tone in conscious rats with cirrhosis. Hepatology 1992,16:980–983.
19. Lee FY, Albillos A, Colombato LA, Groszmann RJ. The role of nitric oxide in the vascular hyporesponsiveness to methoxamine in portal hypertensive rats. Hepatology 1992;16:1043–1048.
20. Sieber CC, Groszmann RJ. In vitro hyporeactivity to methoxamine in portal hypertensive rats: reversal by nitric oxide blockade. Am J Physiol 1992;262:G996–G1001.
21. Sieber CC, Groszmann RJ. Nitric oxide mediates hyporeactivity to vasopressors in mesenteric vessels of portal hypertensive rats. Gastroenterology 1992;103:235–239.
22. Pizcueta P, Piqué JM, Fernandez M, et al. Modulation of the hyperdynamic circulation of cirrhotic rats by nitric oxide inhibition. Gastroenterology 1992;103:1909–1915.
23. Castro A, Jiménez W, Claria J, et al. Impaired responsiveness to angiotensin II in experimental cirrhosis: role of nitric oxide. Hepatology 1993;18:367–372.
24. Guarner C, Soriano G, Tomas A, et al. Increased serum nitrite and nitrate levels in patients with cirrhosis: relationship to endotoxemia. Hepatology 1993;18:1139–1143.
25. Sieber CC, Lopez-Talavera JC, Groszmann RJ. Role of nitric oxide in the in vitro splanchnic vascular hyporeactivity in ascitic cirrhotic rats. Gastroenterology 1993;104:1750–1754.
26. Claria J, Jiménez W, Ros J, et al. Increased nitric oxide-dependent vasorelaxation in aortic rings of cirrhotic rats with ascites. Hepatology 1994;20:1615–1621.
27. Garcia-Pagan JC, Fernandez M, Bernadich C, et al. Effects of continued NO inhibition on portal hypertensive syndrome after portal vein stenosis in rat. Am J Physiol 1994;267:G984–G990.
28. Michielsen PP, Boeckxstaens GE, Sys SU, Herman AG, Pelckmans PA. Role of nitric oxide in hyporeactivity to noradrenaline of isolated aortic rings in portal hypertensive rats. Eur J Pharmacol 1995;273:167–174.

29. Niederberger M, Ginès P, Tsai P, et al. Increased aortic cyclic guanosine monophosphate concentration in experimental cirrhosis in rats: evidence for a role of nitric oxide in the pathogenesis of arterial vasodilation in cirrhosis. Hepatology 1995;21:1625–1631.

30. Cahill PA, Foster C, Redmond EM, et al. Enhanced nitric oxide synthase activity in portal hypertensive rabbits. Hepatology 1995;22:598–606.

31. Kanwar S, Kubes P, Tepperman BL, Lee SS. Nitric oxide synthase activity in portal-hypertensive and cirrhotic rats. J Hepatol 1996;25:85–89.

32. Martin PY, Xu DL, Niederberger M, et al. Upregulation of endothelial constitutive NOS: a major role in the increased NO production in cirrhotic rats. Am J Physiol 1996;270:F494–F499.

33. Morales-Ruiz M, Jiménez W, Pérez-Sala D, et al. Increased nitric oxide synthase expression in arterial vessels of cirrhotic rats with ascites. Hepatology 1996;24:1481–1486.

34. Pilette C, Moreau R, Sogni P, et al. Haemodynamic and hormonal responses to long-term inhibition of nitric oxide synthesis in rats with portal hypertension. Eur J Pharmacol 1996;312:63–68.

35. Pilette C, Kirstetter P, Sogni P, Cailmail S, Moreau R, Lebrec D. Dose-dependent effects of a nitric oxide biosynthesis inhibitor on hyperdynamic circulation in two models of portal hypertension in conscious rats. J Gastroenterol Hepatol 1996;11:1–6.

36. Gadano AC, Sogni P, Yang S, et al. Endothelial calcium-calmodium dependent nitric oxide synthase in the in vitro vascular hyporeactivity of portal hypertensive rats. J Hepatol 1997;26:678–686.

37. Atucha NM, Ortiz MC, Fortepiani LA, Ruiz FM, Martinez C, Garcia-Estan J. Role of cyclic guanosine monophosphate and K^+ channels as mediators of the mesenteric vascular hyporesponsiveness in portal hypertensive rats. Hepatology 1998;27:900–905.

38. Ohta M, Tarnawski AS, Itani R, et al. Tumor necrosis factor α regulates nitric oxide synthase expression in portal hypertensive gastric mucosa of rats. Hepatology 1998;27:906–913.

39. Pateron D, Oberti F, Lefilliatre P, et al. Relationship between vascular reactivity in vitro and blood flows in rats with cirrhosis. Clin Sci 1999;97:313–318.

40. Wiest R, Das S, Gadelina G, Garcia-Tsao G, Milstien S, Groszmann RJ. Bacterial translocation in cirrhotic rats stimulates eNOS-derived NO production and impairs mesentenric vascular contractility. J Clin Invest 1999;104:1223–1233.

41. Wiest R, Shah V, Sessa WC, Groszmann RJ. NO overproduction by eNOS precedes hyperdynamic splanchnic circulation in portal hypertensive rats. Am J Physiol 1999;276.G1043–G1051.

42. Munoz J, Albillos A, Perez-Paramo M, Rossi I, Alvarez-Mon M. Factors mediating the hemodynamic effects of tumor necrosis factor-alpha in portal hypertensive rats. Am J Physiol 1999;276.G687–G693.

43. Shah V, Wiest R, Garcia-Cardena G, Cadelina G, Groszmann RJ, Sessa WC. Hsp90 regulation of endothelial nitric oxide synthase contributes to vascular control in portal hypertension. Am J Physiol 1999;277:G463–G468.

44. Pateron D, Tazi KA, Sogni P, et al. Role of aortic nitric oxide synthase 3 (eNOS) in the systemic vasodilation of portal hypertension. Gastroenterology 2000;119:196–200.

45. Xu L, Carter EP, Ohara M, et al. Neuronal nitric oxide synthase and systemic vasodilation in rats with cirrhosis. Am J Physiol 2000;279:F1110–F1115.

46. Iwakiri Y, Tsai MH, McCabe TJ, et al. Phosphorylation of eNOS initiates excessive NO production in early phases of portal hypertension. Am J Physiol 2002;282:H2084–H2090.

47. Rabiller A, Nunes H, Lebrec D, et al. Prevention of Gram-negative translocation reduces the severity of hepatopulmonary syndrome. Am J Respir Crit Care Med 2002;166:514–517.

48. Kawanaka H, Jones MK, Szabo IL, et al. Activation of eNOS in rat portal hypertensive gastric mucosa is mediated by TNF-alpha via the PI 3-kinase-Akt signaling pathway. Hepatology 2002;35:393–402.

49. Tsai MH, Iwakiri Y, Cadelina G, Sessa WC, Groszmann RJ. Mesenteric vasoconstriction triggers nitric oxide overproduction in the superior mesenteric artery of portal hypertensive rats. Gastroenterology 2003;125:1452–1461.

50. Moreau R, Lebrec D. Endogenous factors involved in the control of arterial tone in cirrhosis. J Hepatol 1995;22:370–376.

51. Pierce KL, Premont RT, Lefkowitz RJ. Seven-transmembrane receptors. Nat Rev Mol Cell Biol 2002;3:639–650.

52. Bomzon A, Huang YT. Vascular smooth muscle cell signaling in cirrhosis and portal hypertension. Pharmacol Ther 2001;89:255–272.

53. Clapham DE. The G-protein nanomachine. Nature 1996;379:297–299.
54. Clapham DE. Calcium signaling. Cell 1995;80:259–268.
55. Somlyo AP, Somlyo AV. Signal transduction and regulation in smooth muscle. Nature 1994;372: 231–236.
56. Ron D, Kazanietz G. New insights into the regulation of protein kinase C and novel phorbol ester receptors. FASEB J 1999;13:1658–1676.
57. Ohanian V, Ohanian J, Shaw L, Scarth S, Parker PJ, Heagerty AM. Identification of protein kinase C isoforms in rat mesenteric small arteries and their possible role in agonist-induced contraction. Circ Res 1996;78:806–812.
58. Moreau R. Heme oxygenase: protective enzyme or portal hypertensive molecule? J Hepatol 2001;34: 936–939.
59. Lincoln TM, Cornwell TL. Intracellular cyclic GMP receptor proteins. FASEB J 1993;7:328–338.
60. Tang M, Wang G, Lu P, et al. Regulator of G-protein signaling-2 mediates vascular smooth muscle relaxation and blood pressure. Nat Med 2003;9:1506–1512.
61. Xia C, Bao Z, Yue C, Sanborn BM, Liu M. Phosphorylation and regulation of G-protein-activated phospholipase C-beta 3 by cGMP-dependent protein kinases. J Biol Chem 2001;276:19,770–19,777.
62. Huang YT, Chang S, Lin HC, Yang MCM, Hong CY. Inositol phosphate responses in portal veins from portal hypertensive rats: receptor- and nonreceptor-mediated responses. J Hepatol 1997;26:376–381.
63. Chagneau C, Tazi KA, Heller J, et al. The role of nitric oxide in the reduced contractile response induced by protein kinase C activation in aortae from rats with portal hypertension. J Hepatol 2000; 33:26–32.
64. Tazi KA, Moreau R, Heller J, Poirel O, Lebrec D. Changes in protein kinase C isoforms in association with vascular hyporeactivity in cirrhotic rat aortas. Gastroenterology 2000;119:201–210.
65. Tazi KA, Barrière E, Moreau R, Poirel O, Lebrec D. Relationship between protein kinase C alterations and nitric oxide overproduction in cirrhotic rats aortas. Liver 2002;22:178–183.
66. Heller J, Schepke M, Gehnen N, et al. Altered adrenergic responsiveness of endothelium-denuded hepatic arteries and portal veins in patients with cirrhosis. Gastroenterology 1999;116:387–393.
67. Islam MZ, Williams BC, Madhavan KK, Hayes PC, Hadoke PWF. Selective alteration of agonist-mediated contraction in hepatic arteries isolated from patients with cirrhosis. Gastroenterology 2000; 118:765–771.
68. Schepke M, Heller J, Paschke S, et al. Contractile hyporesponsiveness of hepatic arteries in humans with cirrhosis: evidence for a receptor-specifid mechanism. Hepatology 2001;34:884–888.
69. Moncada S, Palmer RMJ, Higgs EA. Nitric oxide: physiology, pathophysiology, and pharmacology. Pharmacol Rev 1991;43:109–142.
70. Davis KL, Martin E, Turko IV, Murad F. Novel effects of nitric oxide. Annu Rev Pharmacol Toxicol 2001;41:203–236.
71. Nadaud S, Philippe M, Arnal JF, Michel JB, Soubrier F. Sustained increase in aortic endothelial nitric oxide synthase expression in vivo in a model of chronic high blood flow. Circ Res 1996;79:857–863.
72. Tazi KA, Barrière E, Moreau R, et al. Role of shear stress in aortic eNOS up-regulation in rats with biliary cirrhosis. Gastroenterology 2002;122:1869–1877.
73. Förstermann U, Boissel JP, Kleinert H. Expressional control of the 'constitutive' isoforms of nitric oxide synthase (NOS I and NOS III). FASEB J 1998;12:773–790.
74. Shaul PW. Regulation of endothelial nitric oxide synthase: location, location, location. Annu Rev Physiol 2002;64:749–774.
75. Fleming I, Busse R. Molecular mechanisms involved in the regulation of the endothelial nitric oxide synthase. Am J Physiol 2003;284:R1–R12.
76. Boo YC, Jo H. Flow-dependent regulation of endothelial nitric oxide synthase: role of protein kinases. Am J Physiol 2003;285:C499–C508.
77. Nilius B, Viana F, Droogmans G. Ion channels in vascular endothelium. Annu Rev Physiol 1997;59: 145–170.
78. Barrière E, Tazi KA, Pessione F, et al. Role of small-conductance Ca^{2+}-dependent K^+ channels in in vitro NO-mediated aortic hyporeactivity to α-adrenergic vasoconstriction in rats with cirrhosis. J Hepatol 2001;35:350–357.
79. Theodorakis NG, Wang YN, Skill NJ, et al. The role of nitric oxide synthase isoforms in extrahepatic portal hypertension: studies in gene-knockout mice. Gastroenterology 2003;124:1500–1508.

80. Iwakiri Y, Cadelina G, Sessa WC, Groszmann RJ. Mice with targeted deletion of eNOS develop hyperdynamic circulation associated with portal hypertension. Am J Physiol 2002;283:G1074–G1081.

81. Rich S, McLaughlin VV. Endothelin receptor blockers in cardiovascular disease. Circulation 2003; 108:2184–2190.

82. Moore K, Wendon J, Frazer M, Karani J, Williams R, Badr K. Plasma endothelin immunoreactivity in liver disease and the hepatorenal syndrome. N Engl J Med 1992;327:1774–1778.

83. Cao S, Yao J, Shah V. The proline-rich domain of dynamin-2 is responsible for dynamin-dependent in vitro potentiation of endothelial nitric-oxide synthase activity via selective effects on reductase domain function. J Biol Chem 2003;278:5894–5901.

84. Desideri G, Ferri C. Circulating vascular endothelial growth factor levels are decreased in patients with chronic hepatitis and liver cirrhosis depending on the degree of hepatic damage. Clin Sci 2000; 99:159–160.

85. Tsurumi Y, Murohara T, Krasinski K, et al. Reciprocal relation between VEGF and NO in the regulation of endothelial integrity. Nat Med 1997;3:879–886.

86. Albillos A, de la Hera A, Gonzalez M, et al. Increased lipopolysaccharide binding protein in cirrhotic patients with marked immune and hemodynamic derangement. Hepatology 2003;37:208–217.

87. Lopez-Talavera JC, Cadelina G, Olchowski J, Merrill W, Groszmann RJ. Thalidomide inhibits tumor necrosis factor alpha, decreases nitric oxide synthesis, and ameliorates the hyperdynamic circulatory syndrome in portal-hypertensive rats. Hepatology 1996;23:1616–1621.

88. Lopez-Talavera JC, Merrill WW, Groszmann RJ. Tumor necrosis factor alpha: a major contributor to the hyperdynamic circulation in prehepatic portal-hypertensive rats. Gastroenterology 1995;108: 761–767.

89. Lopez-Talavera JC, Levitzki A, Martinez M, Gazit A, Esteban R, Guardia J. Tyrosine kinase inhibition ameliorates the hyperdynamic state and decreases nitric oxide production in cirrhotic rats with portal hypertension and ascites. J Clin Invest 1997;100:664–670.

90. Moreau R, Barriere E, Tazi KA, et al. Terlipressin inhibits in vivo aortic iNOS expression induced by lipopolysaccharide in rats with biliary cirrhosis. Hepatology 2002;36:1070–1078.

91. Wiest R, Cadelina G, Milstien S, McCuskey RS, Garcia-Tsao G, Groszmann RJ. Bacterial translocation up-regulates GTP-cyclohydrolase I in mesenteric vasculature of cirrhotic rats. Hepatology 2003; 38:1508–1515.

92. Govers R, Rabelink TJ. Cellular regulation of endothelial nitric oxide synthase. Am J Physiol 2001; 280:F193–F206.

93. Batkai S, Jarai Z, Wagner JA, et al. Endocannabinoids acting at vascular CB_1 receptors mediate the vasodilated state in advanced liver cirrhosis. Nat Med 2001;7:827–832.

94. Ros J, Claria J, To-Figueras J, et al. Endogenous cannabinoids: a new system involved in the homeostasis of arterial pressure in experimental cirrhosis in the rat. Gastroenterology 2002;122:85–93.

95. Howlett AC, Barth F, Bonner TI, et al. International union of pharmacology. XXVII. Classification of cannabinoid receptors. Pharmacol Rev 2002;54:161–202.

96. Varga K, Wagner JA, Bridgen DT, Kunos G. Platelet- and macrophage-derived endogenous cannabinoids are involved in endotoxin-induced hypotension. FASEB J 1998;12:1035–1044.

97. Balsinde J, Balboa MA, Insel PA, Dennis EA. Regulation and inhibition of phospholipase A_2. Annu Rev Pharmacol Toxicol 1999;39:175–189.

98. Breyer MD, Breyer RM. G protein-coupled prostanoid receptors and the kidney. Annu Rev Physiol 2001;63:579–605.

99. Nelson MT, Quayle JM. Physiological roles and properties of potassium channels in arterial smooth muscle. Am J Physiol 1995;268:C799–C822.

100. Niederberger M, Ginès P, Martin PY, et al. Increased renal and vascular cytosolic phospholipase A_2 activity in rats with cirrhosis and ascites. Hepatology 1998;27:42–47.

101. Hou MC, Cahill PA, Zhang S, et al. Enhanced cyclooxygenase-1 expression within the superior mesenteric artery of portal hypertension rats: role in the hyperdynamic circulation. Hepatology 1998;27: 20–27.

102. Guarner F, Guarner C, Prieto J, et al. Increased synthesis of systemic prostacyclin in cirrhotic patients. Gastroenterology 1986;90:687–694.

103. Guarner C, Soriano G, Such J, et al. Systemic prostacyclin in cirrhotic patients. Relationship with portal hypertension and changes after intestinal decontamination. Gastroenterology 1992;102:203–309.

104. Oberti F, Sogni P, Cailmail S, Moreau R, Pipy B, Lebrec D. Role of prostacyclin in hemodynamic alterations in conscious rats with extrahepatic or intrahepatic portal hypertension. Hepatology 1993; 18:621–627.
105. Wu Y, Burns RC, Sitzmann JV. Effects of nitric oxide and cyclooxygenase inhibition on splanchnic hemodynamics in portal hypertension. Hepatology 1993;18:1416–1421.
106. Fernandez M, Garcia-Pagan JC, Casadevall M, et al. Acute and chronic cyclooxygenase blockage in portal-hypertensive rats: influence on nitric oxide biosynthesis. Gastroenterology 1996;110:1529–1535.
107. Moreau R, Komeichi H, Kirstetter P, Ohsuga M, Cailmail S, Lebrec D. Altered control of vascular tone by adenosine triphosphate-sensitive potassium channels in rats with cirrhosis. Gastroenterology 1994;106:1016–1023.
108. Pizcueta MP, Casamitjana R, Bosch J, Rodes J. Decreased systemic vascular sensitivity to norepinephrine in portal hypertensive rats: role of hyperglucagonism. Am J Physiol 1990;258:G191–G195.
109. Vanhoutte PM. Old-timer makes a comeback. Nature 1998;396:213–215.
110. Edwards G, Dora KA, Gardener MJ, Garland CJ, Weston AH. K^+ is an endothelium-derived hyperpolarizing factor in rat arteries. Nature 1998;396:269–272.
111. Barrière E, Tazi KA, Rona JP, et al. Evidence for an endothelium-derived hyperpolarizing factor in the superior mesenteric artery from rats with cirrhosis. Hepatology 2000;32:935–941.
112. Maines MD. The heme oxygenase system: a regulator of second messenger gases. Annu Rev Pharmacol Toxicol 1997;37:517–554.
113. Fernandez M, Bonkovsky HL. Increased heme oxygenase-1 gene expression in liver cells and splanchnic organs from portal hypertensive rats. Hepatology 1999;29:1672–1679.
114. Makino N, Suematsu M, Sugiura Y, et al. Altered expression of heme oxygenase-1 in the livers of patients with portal hypertensive diseases. Hepatology 2001;33:32–42.
115. Fernandez M, Lambrecht RW, Bonkovsky HL. Increased heme oxygenase activity in splanchnic organs from portal hypertensive rats: role in modulating mesenteric vascular reactivity. J Hepatol 2001; 34:812–817.
116. Ginès P, Jiménez W, Arroyo V, et al. Atrial natriuretic factor in cirrhosis with ascites: plasma levels, cardiac release and splanchnic extraction. Hepatology 1988:8:636–642.
117. Moreau R, Hadengue A, Pussard E, et al. Relationships between plasma atrial natriuretic peptide and hemodynamics and hematocrit in patients with cirrhosis. Hepatology 1991;14:1035–1039.
118. La Villa G, Romanelli RG, Raggi VS, et al. Plasma levels of brain natriuretic peptide in patients with cirrhosis. Hepatology 1992;16:156–161.
119. Gülberg V, Møller S, Henriksen JH, Gerbes AL. Increased renal production of C-type natriuretic peptide (CNP) in patients with cirrhosis and functional renal failure. Gut 2000;47:852–857.
120. Chinkers M, Garbers DL. Signal transduction by guanylyl cyclases. Annu Rev Biochem 1991;60: 553–575.
121. Guevara M, Ginès P, Jiménez W, et al. Increased adrenomedullin levels in cirrhosis: relationship with hemodynamic abnormalities and vasoconstrictor systems. Gastroenterology 1998;114:336–343.
122. Bendtsen F, Schifter S, Henriksen JH. Increased circulating calcitonin gene-related peptide (CGRP) in cirrhosis. J Hepatol 1991;12:118–123.
123. Lee FY, Lin HC, Tsai YT, et al. Plasma substance P levels in patients with liver cirrhosis: relationship to systemic and portal hemodynamics. Am J Gastroenterol 1997;92:2080–2084.
124. Henriksen JH, Staun-Olsen P, Fahrenkrug J, Ring-Larsen H. Vasoactive intestinal polypeptide (VIP) in cirrhosis: arteriovenous extraction in different vascular beds. Scand J Gastroenterol 1980;15:787–792.
125. Bevan JA, Brayden JE. Nonadrenergic neural vasodilator mechanisms. Circulation Research 1987; 60:309–326.

5

Mechanisms of Sodium Retention, Ascites Formation, and Renal Dysfunction in Cirrhosis

*Andrés Cárdenas, MD, MMSc
and Pere Ginès, MD*

CONTENTS

INTRODUCTION
LOCAL FACTORS INVOLVED IN ASCITES FORMATION
HEMODYNAMIC EVENTS LEADING TO RENAL FUNCTION ABNORMALITIES
FUNCTIONAL RENAL ABNORMALITIES
THEORIES OF ASCITES FORMATION
SUMMARY
REFERENCES

INTRODUCTION

The mechanisms responsible for ascites formation in liver disease have aroused interest throughout the history of medicine. The Egyptians and Greeks believed that there was a relationship between liver disease and ascites. In 300 BC, Erasitratus of Cappadoccia described ascites as a consequence of "hardness of the liver" or liver disease. Several centuries later, physicians discovered the relationship between advanced liver disease and the development of ascites. Numerous studies addressing this issue have discovered that alterations in systemic and splanchnic circulation, as well as functional renal abnormalities, are the culprit of this dreaded complication of cirrhosis. Renal abnormalities occur in the setting of a hyperdynamic state characterized by an increased cardiac output, a reduction in total vascular resistance and an activation of neurohormonal vasoactive systems. This circulatory dysfunction, a consequence of intense arterial vasodilation in the splanchnic circulation, is considered a primary feature in the pathogenesis of ascites. The main factor responsible for local vasodilation seems to be the overproduction of extra-hepatic nitric oxide (NO). Splanchnic vasodilation by decreasing effective arterial blood volume causes homeostatic activation of vasoconstrictor and antinatriuretic factors triggered to compensate for a relative arterial underfilling. The net effect is avid retention of sodium and water as well as renal vasoconstriction in advanced stages. The mechanisms of ascites formation and sodium and water retention in patients with cirrhosis are discussed in this chapter.

From: *Clinical Gastroenterology: Portal Hypertension*
Edited by: A. J. Sanyal and V. H. Shah © Humana Press Inc., Totowa, NJ

LOCAL FACTORS INVOLVED IN ASCITES FORMATION

Portal Hypertension

Portal hypertension is necessary for ascites to occur; as a matter of fact, it commonly occurs in diseases causing sinusoidal portal hypertension, such as cirrhosis, Budd–Chiari syndrome, hepatic venoocclusive disease, or acute alcoholic hepatitis *(1)*. Similar to what occurs with the development of esophageal varices, ascites develops only when the hepatic venous pressure gradient (the gradient between wedged and free hepatic venous pressures) is above 12 mmHg *(2)*. On the other hand, ascites is uncommon in liver diseases causing presinusoidal portal hypertension, such as schistosomiasis, idiopathic portal hypertension, congenital hepatic fibrosis, or hepatic sarcoidosis *(1)*. In addition, studies in experimental cirrhosis with rats have demonstrated the relationship between portal hypertension and ascites formation *(3)*. Rats with carbon tetrachloride–induced cirrhosis will accumulate ascites with advanced liver failure *(4)*. Probably the best evidence that portal hypertension is crucial for ascites formation derives from clinical experience with cirrhotic patients with ascites subjected to portosystemic shunting either by surgical portocaval shunts or transjugular portosystemic shunting. In this setting, portal hypertension is reduced and ascites invariably decreases with increase in diuresis and urinary sodium excretion in patients with ascites and cirrhosis *(5,6)*.

Lymph Formation

Ascites in cirrhosis is the result of an increased extravasation of fluid from the splanchnic microcirculation. In the initial phases of the disease, this is compensated by an increase in lymph return. Thoracic duct lymph flow, which in normal conditions is lower than 1 L/d, may increase up to more than 20 L/d in cirrhotic patients with portal hypertension *(7)*. When lymph formation overcomes lymph production, ascites develops.

Experimental studies in animals submitted to an acute obstruction of hepatic veins demonstrate increased leakage of fluid from the hepatic surface into the abdominal cavity *(8)*. Hepatic sinusoids which by nature do not have a basement membrane are widely permeable to proteins. Consequently, small increases in hydrostatic pressure are associated with a marked increase in lymph production. This lymph has a protein concentration similar to that of plasma *(9,10)*. In contrast, splanchnic capillaries are poorly permeable to proteins and have a low concentration when compared to hepatic lymph. Any increase of hydrostatic pressure in these capillaries induces an initial extravasation of lymph with a low protein concentration *(11)*. Although ascites formation has been considered to arise from the hepatic sinusoids with little contribution of the intestinal capillaries *(12)*, there are two arguments against this concept.

One is the process of capillarization of the hepatic sinusoids that occurs in cirrhosis *(13)*. This term refers to collagen deposition in the space of Disse with disappearance of the large hepatic fenestrae leaving the sinusoid with an appearance and function of a normal capillary (Fig. 1). The hepatic sinusoid permeability to proteins (i.e., albumin) and concentration of proteins in the hepatic lymph becomes markedly reduced in cirrhosis *(14)*. As a consequence, the protein concentration in the ascitic fluid of patients with cirrhosis is lower than the protein concentration in the hepatic lymph, suggesting that a great part of the ascitic fluid in cirrhosis derives from the splanchnic capillaries (a vascular bed with lower permeability to plasma proteins) *(1,7)*. The other is that in cirrhosis there is marked vasodilation in the splanchnic arterioles secondary to portal hypertension (see

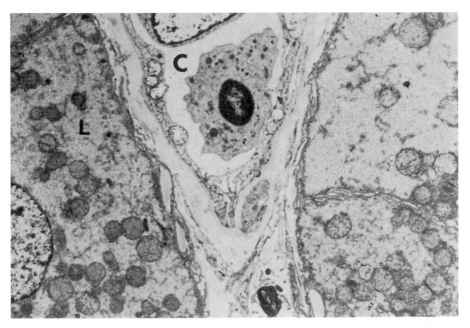

Fig. 1. Electron micrograph showing the capillarization occurring in the sinusoids of a rat with cirrhosis. The sinusoidal lumen (C) is separated from the liver cells (L) by a nonfenestrated endothelial cell membrane, a basement membrane, and a layer of fibrillary collagen. (From Huet et al. J Clin Invest 1982;70:1234–1244 with permission.)

below). This leads to a large inflow of blood at high pressure into the splanchnic capillaries with a rise in hydrostatic pressure due to both a forward increase in flow and a backward transmission of high portal pressure *(15)*. Splanchnic arterial vasodilation also has effects on increasing the permeability of capillaries *(11)*. The net effect of both processes is a marked production of lymph from the splanchnic capillaries. Thus, ascitic fluid in cirrhosis probably derives from both the hepatic sinusoids and the splanchnic capillaries.

HEMODYNAMIC EVENTS LEADING TO RENAL FUNCTION ABNORMALITIES

Systemic Circulatory Derangements

Cirrhotic patients with ascites show a severe disturbance in their systemic hemodynamics, characterized by a low arterial blood pressure, high cardiac output, and a decreased total systemic vascular resistance consequence of an intense splanchnic arterial vasodilation *(16)*. By contrast, other vascular beds such as the cerebral, upper and lower limbs, and renal circulation are constricted in cirrhotic patients *(17–19)*. These circulatory abnormalities increase with the progression of liver disease, and become very pronounced in patients with functional renal failure in the late stages of the disease. Experimental models of cirrhosis and ascites have clearly shown that the circulatory changes precede sodium and water retention and ascites accumulation, supporting the so-called arterial vasodilation theory of ascites formation and renal dysfunction (see later) (Fig. 2) *(20)*.

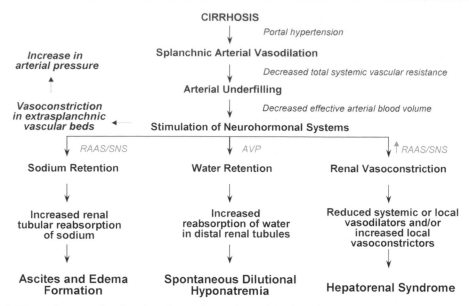

Fig. 2. The pathogenesis of ascites formation and renal dysfunction according to the arterial vaso-dilation theory. The neurohumoral effects of the renin-angiotensin-aldosterone system (RAAS), sympathetic nervous system (SNS), and arginine vasopressin (AVP) on systemic circulation and renal function in cirrhosis with ascites are responsible for sodium and water retention as well as hepatorenal syndrome. The levels of these vasoconstrictors are highest in patients with hepatorenal syndrome.

Local Circulatory Derangements

A key element in the pathophysiology of portal hypertension is an increase in vascular resistance to portal blood flow occurring in the hepatic microcirculation. Recent studies indicate that increased hepatic vascular resistance in cirrhosis is not merely a mechanical consequence of a distorted architecture but there is also an active and dynamic process secondary to contraction of myofibroblasts and activated stellate cells in the intrahepatic circulation *(21)*. Intrahepatic vascular tone is regulated by high levels of endogenous vaso-constrictors (endothelin, leukotrienes, thromboxane A_2, angiotensin II, and others) *(21–25)* and low levels of intrahepatic NO *(26,27)*. In cirrhosis an increased hepatic vascular resistance is probably caused by an imbalance between vasodilator and vasoconstrictor factors, the latter being predominant *(26)*. Another important factor is that of increased blood flow from the portal venous system; this is a constant feature with chronic increase in portal pressure and plays a major role in the increased pressure in the portal venous sys-tem *(28)*. This is mainly caused by splanchnic arterial vasodilation which contributes to an increase in portal pressure that remains elevated despite the development of porto-systemic collateral formation *(29)*. This vasodilation is caused by a disproportional release of endogenous vasodilators (mainly NO) that perpetuate elevated portal pressure *(30–32)*. For a detailed discussion of the events leading to the development of splanchnic vasodila-tion in cirrhosis, refer to Chapter 5.

Neurohormonal Activation

Several neurohumoral systems with vasoactive properties, namely the renin–angioten-sin–aldosterone system (RAAS), sympathetic nervous system (SNS), and arginine vaso-

Table 1
Neurohormonal Factors Potentially
Implicated in Ascites Formation in Cirrhosis

- Renin-angiotensin-aldosterone system (RAAS)
- Sympathetic nervous system (SRS)
- Arginine vasopressin (AVP)
- Endothelin
- Atrial natriuretic peptide
- Arachidonic acid metabolites
- Adenosine

pressin (AVP), are directly implicated in ascites formation and renal dysfunction in cirrhosis (Table 1). The activity of these vasoconstrictor systems is increased in a large proportion of cirrhotic patients with ascites, particularly in those with end-stage liver disease and hepatorenal syndrome (HRS) as a homeostatic response to maintain arterial blood pressure within normal limits. However, this may contribute to the progression of liver disease by worsening hepatic hemodynamics and mediate a progressive renal vasoconstriction (Fig. 2).

A large body of evidence indicates that the RAAS is activated in cirrhosis and is involved in circulatory homeostasis and ascites formation *(33,34)*. Plasma renin activity (PRA), a marker of RAAS activation, is markedly increased in most patients with cirrhosis and ascites; in addition, the plasma levels of angiotensin II and aldosterone, the two main effectors of the RAAS that mediate vasoconstriction and sodium retention, respectively, are also increased in cirrhosis *(34)*. RAAS inhibition, either by the administration of angiotensin-converting enzyme (ACE) inhibitors, angiotensin II antagonists, or angiotensin II receptor blockers, is accompanied by a fall in arterial pressure or in some cases a deterioration of renal function *(35–37)*. Activation of the SNS is also present in patients with advanced liver disease as evidenced by increased levels of norepinephrine (NE) and epinephrine *(38)*. Measurements of NE release and spillover in specific vascular beds have shown that the activity of the SNS is increased in many vascular territories, including kidneys, splanchnic organs, heart, and muscle and skin, supporting the concept of a generalized activation of the SNS *(39–43)*. As occurs with RAAS, inhibition of the SNS in human and experimental cirrhosis results in marked arterial hypotension, suggesting that the SNS is also activated as a homeostatic response to maintain blood pressure in cirrhosis *(44)*. Additionally, the SNS also contributes to sodium retention (see below). Aside from water retention in cirrhosis, AVP is also a vasoconstrictor that probably contributes to the maintenance of arterial pressure in cirrhosis.

Other substances that play a role in the hemodynamic derangement of advanced cirrhosis are endothelin (ET) and the natriuretic hormones. The plasma levels of endothelin, an endothelial-derived powerful vasoconstrictor peptide, are increased in patients with cirrhosis, particularly in those with HRS *(45)*. Because of its powerful vasoactive effects, ET has been implicated in the pathogenesis of arterial hypertension and other conditions associated with increased vascular resistance and reduced organ perfusion. Despite the great efforts aimed at elucidating the role of ET in cirrhosis its relevance in circulatory homeostasis in cirrhosis is unclear, because the antagonization of endothelin receptors in cirrhotic rats with ascites is not associated with significant changes in arterial pressure

(46–48). Nonetheless, when the endothelin ET_A receptor blocker BQ123 was used to treat a small number of patients with HRS, there was an improvement in renal function *(49)*. Further studies are needed to understand and characterize the role of endothelin in advanced cirrhosis.

The natriuretic hormones, represented by the atrial natriuretic peptide (ANP) and brain natriuretic peptide (BNP) are increased in patients with cirrhosis and ascites *(50,51)*. High plasma levels of ANP in cirrhosis with ascites are caused by increased cardiac secretion of the peptide and not reduced hepatic or systemic catabolism, as cardiac production of ANP is increased in cirrhotic patients with ascites and splanchnic and peripheral extraction are normal *(50,52)*. Consistent with these observations is the finding of increased mRNA expression for ANP in ventricles from cirrhotic rats with ascites *(53)*. The cardiac production and release of ANP in cirrhosis with ascites can be increased further by maneuvers that increase the central blood volume, such as insertion of a peritoneovenous shunt *(54)* or TIPS *(55)*. The presence of increased plasma levels of ANP in cirrhosis with ascites sufficient to have a natriuretic effect in healthy subjects, together with the presence of renal sodium retention, indicates a renal resistance to the effects of ANP. This renal resistance has been confirmed in studies in human and experimental cirrhosis in which pharmacological doses of natriuretic peptides (ANP or BNP) were administered *(56–60)*. In these investigations, patients with activation of antinatriuretic systems (RAAS and SNS) had a blunted or no natriuretic response after ANP infusion. This blunted response can be reversed by procedures that increase distal sodium delivery in human cirrhosis or by bilateral renal denervation in experimental cirrhosis, suggesting that the renal resistance to ANP in cirrhosis is related to the increased activity of antinatriuretic systems *(61,62)*.

The role of natriuretic peptides in cirrhosis is not entirely clear. Although most of these peptides have vasodilator properties, a role in the pathogenesis of arterial vasodilation in cirrhosis has been proposed but not proved. By contrast, data from experimental studies suggest that they play an important role in the maintenance of renal perfusion and modulation of RAAS activity, as the selective blockade of the natriuretic peptide A and B receptors causes renal vasoconstriction and increased PRA and aldosterone levels in experimental cirrhosis *(63)*. It could be speculated, therefore, that the cardiac synthesis of ANP and BNP is increased in an attempt to maintain renal perfusion within normal levels and limit the activation of the RAAS. The mechanism(s) leading to this increased synthesis of natriuretic peptides remains unknown.

Renal Factors

A significant number of local renal factors participate in the pathogenesis of ascites formation. The presence of arachidonic acid metabolites, adenosine, and NO, exert powerful effects on the renal circulation and tubular reabsorption of sodium and water. In cirrhosis, one of the arachidonic acid metabolites, the prostaglandins (PGs), normally produced in the kidney via the cycloxygenase pathway, seem to protect the kidney from the vasoconstrictor effects of the SNS, RAAS, and AVP. The renal PGs namely, PGI2 and PGE2, have vasodilator properties in the kidney and are increased in cirrhosis with ascites *(64,65)*. This increased production of PG contributes to the maintenance of renal hemodynamics.

Adenosine, an endogenous nucleoside produced locally in most cells by the intracellular degradation of adenosine triphosphate, is a potent vasodilator in most vascular beds, except the kidneys, where it causes vasoconstriction. Adenosine-1 receptors are present on the afferent arteriole in the kidney and cells of the proximal tubules, whereas adenosine-2 receptors are found in the systemic vasculature. Stimulation of adenosine-1 receptors leads to renal vasoconstriction and sodium and water retention, whereas that of adenosine-2 receptors cause vasodilation *(66)*. The possible role of adenosine in the pathogenesis of renal functional abnormalities in human cirrhosis was evaluated by giving aminophylline (a methylxanthine), that acts as nonspecific adenosine antagonist, to patients with cirrhosis and ascites . This agent caused an increase in renal blood flow (RBF), glomerular filtration rate (GFR), and sodium and water excretion in patients with ascites *(67)*, although the acute administration of an adenosine-1 receptor antagonist to patients with cirrhosis and ascites induces a marked increase in sodium excretion and urine flow, without changes in renal hemodynamics *(68)*. Conversely, the acute administration of dipyridamole, a drug that acts, at least in part, by increasing the levels of adenosine in the extracellular fluid caused by inhibition of the cellular uptake of this substance, is associated with renal vasoconstriction and increased sodium and water retention, particularly in patients with ascites and increased activity of the RAAS *(66)*. A role for intrahepatic adenosine causing changes in portal venous blood flow and triggerring an hepatorenal reflex to regulate sodium and water excretion has been recently proposed (see Chapter 7).

The renal production of NO also participates in the regulation of renal function *(69)*. Under normal circumstances, NO plays a role in the regulation of glomerular microcirculation by modulating the arteriolar tone and the contractility of mesangial cells. Moreover, NO facilitates natriuresis in response to changes in renal perfusion pressure, and regulates renin release *(69)*. The inhibition of NO synthesis in rats with cirrhosis and ascites does not result in renal vasoconstriction but induces a marked rise in urinary prostaglandin excretion *(70)*. However, the simultaneous inhibition of NO and PGs synthesis results in a marked renal vasoconstriction suggesting that NO interacts with PGs to maintain renal hemodynamics in cirrhosis *(71)*.

FUNCTIONAL RENAL ABNORMALITIES

The most common functional renal abnormalities in cirrhotic patients are an impaired ability to excrete sodium and water and a reduction of RBF and GFR, the latter two being secondary to renal vasoconstriction. Sodium retention is a key factor in ascites and edema formation, whereas an impairment in solute-free water excretion (water retention) is responsible for the development of dilutional hyponatremia. Renal vasoconstriction, when severe, leads to HRS. Chronologically, sodium retention is the earliest alteration of kidney function observed in patients with cirrhosis, whereas dilutional hyponatremia and HRS are late findings *(1,7,72,73)* (Fig. 3). In most patients, functional renal abnormalities worsen as liver disease progresses. However, in some patients a spontaneous improvement or even normalization of sodium and, less frequently, water excretion may occur during the course of their disease *(74)*. Improvement of water excretion is associated with an increase or normalization of serum sodium concentration. Normalization of renal function abnormalities is seen after alcohol abstinence in some patients with alcoholic cirrhosis or alcoholic hepatitis, but it may occur spontaneously in patients with nonalcoholic cirrhosis as well, although this is unusual.

Sodium Retention

Cirrhosis with ascites is one of the clinical conditions associated with more avid sodium retention. It is the most common abnormality of kidney function in patients with cirrhosis and ascites and plays a fundamental role in the formation of ascites and edema *(1,7)*. As

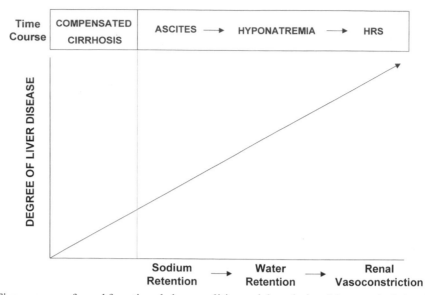

Fig. 3. Time-course of renal functional abnormalities and the relationship to underlying degree of liver disease in patients with cirrhosis. HRS: hepatorenal syndrome.

in other sodium-retaining states, the total amount of sodium retained by cirrhotic patients, and the subsequent gain of extracellular fluid, depends on the balance between sodium intake and sodium excretion. If the amount of sodium excreted in the urine is lower than that ingested, patients accumulate extracellular fluid as ascites and/or edema. By contrast, if the amount of sodium excreted in the urine is greater than that ingested, patients lose extracellular fluid and ascites and/or edema decrease. The important role of sodium retention in the pathogenesis of ascites formation is further supported by the fact that ascites can disappear by reducing sodium intake in some patients or by increasing urinary sodium excretion with the administration of diuretics in others. Although no studies assessing the chronological relationship between sodium retention and the formation of ascites have been performed in patients with cirrhosis, studies in experimental animals have provided conclusive evidence indicating that sodium retention precedes ascites formation, further emphasizing the important role of this abnormality of renal function in the pathogenesis of ascites in cirrhosis *(72,73)*. This observation suggests that sodium retention is a cause and not a consequence of ascites formation in cirrhosis

Sodium is retained along with water iso-osmotically in the kidney (i.e., 1 L of water for each 135 mEq of sodium). As a consequence, sodium retention is associated with fluid retention, leading to the expansion of extracellular volume and an increased amount of fluid in the interstitial tissue. The severity of sodium retention varies among cirrhotic patients; some have a near-normal urine sodium excretion and some others have severe sodium retention *(75,76)* (Fig. 4). Most patients who require hospitalization because of large ascites have marked sodium retention (<10 mEq/d) on a low-sodium diet and without diuretic therapy *(76)*. In those with mild or moderate ascites, the majority excrete > 10 mEq/d spontaneously (without diuretic therapy). The response to diuretics is usually better in patients with moderate sodium retention than in those with marked sodium retention *(77)*. The role of sodium retention in the pathogenesis of ascites is at least demonstrated by two clinical observations; one is that sodium restriction in some cirrhotic patients

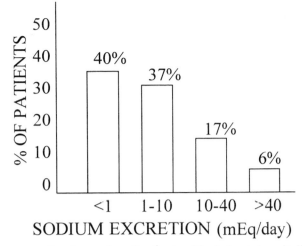

SODIUM EXCRETION (mEq/day)

Fig. 4. Urinary sodium excretion in a series of patients with cirrhosis hospitalised for treatment of ascites. (From Ginés P, Fernández Esparrach G, Arroyo V, et al. Pathophysiology of ascites. Semin Liver Dis 1997;17:175, with permission.)

with ascites may be sufficient to eliminate ascites and edema and the other is that diuretics, by increasing sodium excretion, relieve ascites, and edema *(76)*.

In cirrhotic patients without ascites or in the preascitic stage there is also evidence of subtle sodium retention *(78–81)*. The main findings in these patients relate to increased blood volume *(78,82)*, inability to handle a sodium load *(83)*, and lack of escape to the sodium-retaining effect of mineralocorticoids *(79)*. In preascites, most patients have an increased intravascular fluid volume, which suggests they have experienced transient episodes of sodium retention *(78,80,82,84)*. Additionally, a high-sodium diet or intravenous saline may lead to the accumulation of ascites in preascitic cirrhotic patients *(83)*. Healthy subjects treated with mineralocorticoids for several days show an early phase characterized by sodium retention that results in increased extracellular fluid volume and plasma expansion, followed by increased sodium excretion with return of extracellular fluid volume and plasma volume to normal values despite the persistent administration of mineralocorticoids. This escape phenomenon is aimed at preventing a persistent sodium retention and subsequent development of edema and is caused by the suppression of sodium retaining mechanisms together with activation of natriuretic mechanisms. When mineralocorticoids are given to patients with compensated cirrhosis, approx 20% of patients do not show this escape phenomenon and develop marked sodium retention with formation of ascites and edema *(79)*. Another important feature of preascitic cirrhosis is the abnormal natriuretic responses to changes in posture. Cirrhotic patients retain sodium while upright, and show marked natriuresis when lying down as compared to normal subjects *(85)*. A role for antinatriuretic systems such as the RAAS has been implicated in the pathogenesis of sodium retention in preascitic cirrhosis *(81,86)*.

Sites of Sodium Retention

Sodium retention in cirrhosis is mainly caused by an increased renal tubular reabsorption of sodium because it occurs in the presence of normal or slightly reduced GFR *(75,76)*.

The exact contribution of each segment of the nephron is unknown but both experimental and clinical studies suggest that both proximal and distal tubules are involved *(87)*. Sodium retention is usually more intense in patients with ascites and renal failure than in those without renal failure. This is because of a reduction in the amount of sodium filtered and possibly a greater increase in tubular sodium reabsorption. The potential mediators for this increase in tubular reabsorption include changes in hydrostatic and colloid pressure in the peritubular capillaries and increased activity of the two main sodium-retaining systems that account for the increased sodium retention in cirrhosis: the RAAS and SNS. The baroreceptor-mediated activation of these systems arising from a decrease in effective arterial blood volume constitutes a homeostatic response in an attempt to maintain arterial pressure within normal limits. Several studies indicate that the activation of RAAS contributes to sodium retention in cirrhosis *(86,88–90)*. In addition, there is also an intrarenal activation of RAAS *(81)*. The two final effectors of this system, angiotensin II and aldosterone, induce marked sodium reabsorption by acting in the proximal tubule and the collecting duct, respectively *(88)*. Patients with cirrhosis and ascites have increased urine excretion or plasma levels of aldosterone, which correlate with renal sodium excretion *(91)*. Nonetheless, the strongest evidence for the role of RAAS in sodium derives from the use of medications that antagonize these systems. The administration of aldosterone antagonists successfully promotes diuresis and natriuresis and decreases ascites in cirrhotics *(92)*. In addition, administration of angiotensin II blockers like losartan also induce natriuresis when given at low doses *(86,93)*. The SNS is also commonly activated in advanced cirrhosis and stimulates sodium reabsorption in the proximal tubule, loop of Henle, and distal and collecting tubules *(38,94)*. There are elevated levels of norepinephrine in plasma and increased rates of norepinephrine spillover from different organs in advanced liver disease *(38)*. Additionally, there is an increase in the α-adrenergic receptor tone, which results in an enhanced proximal tubular reabsorption of sodium and an elevation in the β-adrenergic receptor tone, which causes an increase in renin secretion *(95)*.

An unanswered question is why a significant proportion of patients with cirrhosis and ascites present sodium retention despite normal plasma levels of renin, aldosterone, and norepinephrine, and increased circulating levels of natriuretic peptides *(96)*. Most of these patients have normal renal plasma flow and GFR. Therefore, sodium retention cannot be explained on the basis of an impaired renal perfusion or a decreased filtered sodium load. It has been suggested that an unknown mechanism (renal or extrarenal), extremely sensitive to changes in effective arterial blood volume would induce sodium retention at the early stages of decompensated cirrhosis *(81)*. This mechanism(s) would be more sensitive than the traditional sodium-retaining systems and, consequently, would be activated earlier in the course of the liver disease (see Chapter 7).

Water Retention

A derangement in the renal capacity to regulate water balance commonly occurs in advanced cirrhosis *(97)*. The major clinical consequence of this impairment is the appearance of dilutional hyponatremia (sodium serum sodium <130 mEq/L), which occurs despite avid sodium retention because water is retained in excess of sodium. The estimated prevalence of spontaneous hyponatremia in hospitalized patients with cirrhosis and ascites is near 30–35% *(98,99)*. However, this figure increases to nearly 70% when water retention is measured as an inability to excrete water after a water load *(76,100)* (Fig. 5).

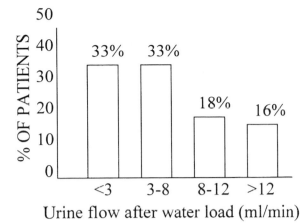

Fig. 5. Urine flow after a water load (20 mL/kg body weight of 5% dextrose IV) in a series of patients with cirrhosis and ascites. Normal values for healthy subjects are between 8–18 mL/min. (From Ginés P, Fernández Esparrach G, Arroyo V, et al. Pathophysiology of ascites. Semin Liver Dis 1997;17:175, with permission.)

In preascitic cirrhosis, patients display similar water handling mechanisms when compared to healthy subjects. Impaired water handling is common in cirrhotics with ascites; as a matter of fact more than two thirds of hospitalized cirrhotics have an abnormal renal water handling mechanism as indicated by an impaired ability to generate solute-free water after a water load (Fig. 5) *(100)*. Water retention in cirrhosis usually occurs late in the disease, follows sodium retention, and is a poor prognostic indicator *(100)*. The pathogenesis of increased water retention in cirrhosis is complex and involves several factors, including high levels of AVP and reduced delivery of filtrate to the ascending limb of the loop of Henle.

Among these factors, AVP is probably the most important factor in the pathogenesis of water retention in cirrhosis with ascites. The high-plasma AVP levels seen in cirrhosis are likely to be secondary to a reduced effective intravascular volume. The hemodynamic changes occurring in cirrhosis (low arterial blood pressure, high cardiac output, and low total systemic vascular resistance) cause arterial hypotension which unloads the high-pressure baroreceptors and stimulate a nonosmotic release of AVP with the subsequent increase in water reabsorption (Fig. 2) *(97)*.

The biological effects of AVP are mediated through three types of receptors present in target cells *(101)*. These receptors belong to the superfamily of GPCR and are known as V1a, V1b, and V2. V1a and V1b are associated to the phosphoinositol signaling pathway with intracellular calcium as second messenger. V1a is responsible for vascular smooth muscle cell contraction, platelet aggregation, and hepatic glycogenolysis and V1b is expressed in the anterior pituitary where it mediates adrenocorticotropin release *(102)*. The V2 receptors are located on the basolateral (capillary) membrane of the principal cells of the collecting ducts and are responsible for the AVP-induced water reabsorption *(102)*. The effect of AVP on these receptors is mediated by selective water channels, called aquaporins (AQP). The most important one is AQP2. This water channel has been characterized in human and rat kidneys and is expressed almost exclusively in the principal cells of the collecting ducts *(103,104)*. The binding of AVP to the V2 receptor stimulates adenyl cyclase via the stimulatory G protein and promotes the formation of cyclic AMP (cAMP). This cAMP binds to a regulatory subunit of protein kinase A, which in turn phosphorylates AQP2, which is then translocated from vesicular bodies present in the cytosol to the luminal (apical) plasma membrane of the collecting duct cells, and acts as a water channel thereby increasing water permeability. The water entering the cell by the luminal plasma membrane leaves the cell through the basolateral membrane and enters the capillaries that are in close contact with tubular cells. AQP 3 and AQP 4 mediate the exiting of water from the cells. In contrast with AQP2, which is translocated from the cytosol to the luminal membrane by the action of AVP, AQP3 and AQP4 are constitutively expressed in the basolateral membrane and their action is not regulated by AVP *(103,104)*. The administration of newly designed V2 receptor antagonists increases free water excretion and improves dilutional hyponatremia in patients with cirrhosis *(105)*.

Another important mechanism for impaired water excretion in cirrhosis is a reduced delivery of filtrate to the ascending limb of the loop of Henle, the distal diluting segment of the nephron *(105)*. To produce solute-free water, tubular fluid has to be delivered to the distal nephron where sodium is reabsorbed without water. Lithium clearance, which estimates distal delivery of filtrate, is reduced in patients with cirrhosis and ascites *(106)*. Also in cirrhotics with ascites, water clearance correlates closely with the GFR, this along with sodium reabsorption is the main determinant of distal delivery of filtrate. Therefore, decreased glomerular filtrate and excessive proximal sodium reabsorption may play a significant role in the impaired free water excretion seen in cirrhosis and ascites.

In most patients, dilutional hyponatremia is asymptomatic, but in some it may be associated with symptoms such as anorexia, headache, poor concentration, lethargy, nausea, vomiting, and, occasionally, seizures. Presently, there is no pharmacological therapy for dilutional hyponatremia and the only therapeutic measure that improves or stops the progressive decrease in serum sodium concentration is water restriction to approx 1 L/d. The administration of hypertonic saline solutions is not recommended because it invariably leads to further expansion of extracellular fluid volume and accumulation of ascites and edema. Preliminary studies show that two types of aquaretics drugs selectively increase water excretion in hyponatremic patients with cirrhosis. The first are antagonists of the V2 receptor of AVP and the second are selective kappa opioid agonists. The former group of drugs antagonize selectively the water-retaining effect of AVP in the cortical collecting duct whereas the latter inhibit AVP release from the neurohypophysis. The beneficial effects of a V2 receptor antagonist (VPA-985) were recently reported in two phase II multicenter, randomized, placebo-controlled trials in patients with cirrhosis and dilutional hyponatremia *(107,108)*. These compounds when available for use in clinical practice will offer a novel therapeutic approach for the treatment of water retention and dilutional hyponatremia in patients with ascites.

Renal Vasoconstriction

Renal vasoconstriction as manifested by the development of HRS is the latest renal functional abnormality in patients with cirrhosis and ascites and its pathogenesis involves several mechanisms, including increased activity of vasoconstrictor factors and probably a reduced activity of renal vasodilator factors. The degree of renal vasoconstriction may range from a modest renal impairment which can be detected only by measuring GFR and renal plasma flow by clearance techniques to a severe renal failure with elevation of blood urea nitrogen and serum creatinine concentration *(109,110)*. The pathogenesis of

Table 2
Vasoactive Factors
Potentially Involved in Regulation Renal
Perfusion and Renal Vasoconstriction in Cirrhosis

Vasodilators
    Prostaglandin E2
    Nitric oxide
    Prostacyclin
    Atrial natriuretic peptide
    Kallikrein-kinin system
Vasoconstrictors
    Angiotensin II
    Norepinephrine
    Neuropeptide Y
    Endothelin-1
    Adenosine
    Thromboxane A2
    Cysteinyl leukotrienes
    F2-isoprostanes

renal vasoconstriction in cirrhosis is related to changes in systemic hemodynamics. The most accepted theory considers that renal vasoconstriction is the consequence of the extreme underfilling of the arterial circulation present in the latter stages of cirrhosis *(20)*. The pathophysiologic hallmark of HRS is a vasoconstriction of the renal circulation *(111–113)*. Studies of renal perfusion with renal arteriography, ^{133}Xe washout technique, para-aminohippuric acid excretion, or, more recently, duplex Doppler ultrasonography, have demonstrated the existence of marked vasoconstriction in the kidneys of patients with HRS, with a characteristic reduction in renal cortical perfusion *(114,115)*. The functional nature of HRS has been conclusively demonstrated by the lack of significant morphological abnormalities in the kidney histology and normalization of renal function after liver transplantation *(112,113)*.

The mechanism of this vasoconstriction is incompletely understood and possibly multifactorial involving changes in systemic hemodynamics, increased pressure in the portal venous system, activation of vasoconstrictor factors, and suppression of vasodilator factors acting on the renal circulation. Other vascular beds, besides the renal circulation, are also vasoconstricted in patients with HRS, including the brachial and femoral circulation and the cerebral circulation *(16–19,116)*. This indicates the existence of a generalized arterial vasoconstriction in nonsplanchnic vascular beds of patients with HRS and suggests that the main vascular bed responsible for arterial vasodilation and reduced total systemic vascular resistance in cirrhosis with HRS is the splanchnic circulation.

The major factors mediated in vasoconstriction and vasodilation of the kidney vasculature in cirrhosis are listed in Table 2. Among these the effectors of the RAAS (angiotensin) and SNS (norepinephrine) play a role causing significant renal vasoconstriction, although direct inhibition of these systems carries the risk of inducing hypotension. Other vasoconstrictors such as adenosine, cysteinyl leukotrienes seem to play a role in renal vasoconstriction. On the other hand, renal vasodilators such as PGs, NO, and natriuretic peptides struggle to maintain renal perfusion. As disease ensues, the maximal stimulation of vasoconstrictor factors cannot be counterbalanced by either systemic or renal vasodilators and, as a consequence, severe vasoconstriction of renal vessels occurs and HRS ensues (see Chapter 23).

THEORIES OF ASCITES FORMATION

The arterial vasodilation theory was described in an attempt to explain the pathogenesis of ascites and renal dysfunction in cirrhosis *(20)*. It is a rational explanation as to why the hemodynamic changes that occur in cirrhosis are directly related to the development of ascites and renal failure. This theory (Fig. 2) considers that the primary event of renal sodium and water retention in cirrhosis is splanchnic arterial vasodilation secondary to portal hypertension. In the preascitic stage, circulatory homeostasis is maintained by the development of hyperdynamic circulation (high plasma volume, cardiac index, and heart rate). However, as the disease progresses and splanchnic arterial vasodilation increases, this compensatory mechanism is insufficient to maintain circulatory homeostasis. Arterial pressure decreases causing stimulation of baroreceptors with a homeostatic increase in the sympathetic nervous activity, renin–angiotensin system activity, and circulating levels of AVP. This leads to renal sodium and water retention. Sinusoidal portal hypertension by virtue of causing splanchnic vasodilation produces systemic arterial vascular underfilling and a "forward" increase in the splanchnic capillary pressure and filtration coefficient. In patients with compensated cirrhosis, the degree of portal hypertension and splanchnic arterial vasodilation is moderate. Arterial underfilling is compensated for by an increase in plasma volume and cardiac output. In these patients, the lymphatic system is able to return the moderate increase in lymph produced to the systemic circulation, thus preventing leakage of fluid into the abdominal cavity. As cirrhosis progresses, portal hypertension and decreased splanchnic vascular resistance turn progressively worse and a critical point is reached in which the consequences of this intense splanchnic arterial vasodilation cannot be compensated for by increasing lymph return, plasma volume, and cardiac output. The maintenance of arterial pressure then requires persistent activation of RAAS, SNS, and AVP, which produce continuous sodium and water retention. The retained fluid is, however, ineffective in refilling the dilated arterial vascular bed because it escapes from the intravascular compartment, owing to an imbalance between the excessive lymph production and the ability of the lymphatic system to return it to the systemic circulation. The final consequence of both disorders is persistent renal sodium and water retention with ongoing leakage of fluid into the abdominal cavity and the formation of ascites (Fig. 6).

SUMMARY

Ascites is the most common complication of cirrhosis and its existence is associated with profound changes in the splanchnic and systemic circulation, as well as renal abnormalities. The development of ascites is related to the existence of severe sinusoidal portal hypertension that causes marked splanchnic arterial vasodilation and a forward increase in the splanchnic production of lymph. Additionally, splanchnic arterial vasodilation decreases effective arterial blood volume and leads to fluid accumulation and renal function abnormalities which are a consequence of the homeostatic activation of vasoconstrictor and antinatriuretic factors triggered to compensate for a relative arterial underfilling.

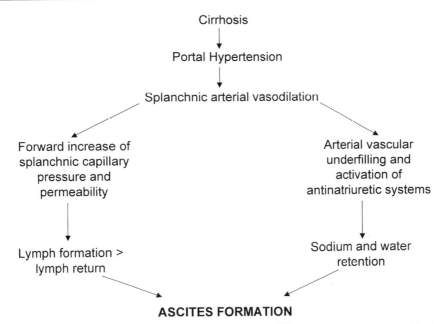

Fig. 6. Events leading to a forward increase in splanchnic capillary pressure and arterial underfilling that ultimately lead to ascites formation in cirrhosis.

Table 3
Areas of Future Research in the Area of Ascites Formation

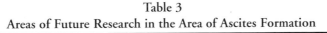

1. Identification of other mechanisms and neurohormonal factors that may play an additional role in the pathogenesis of sodium and water retention will help to better treat patients with ascites
2. New therapies targeted at treating portal hypertension before the development of functional renal abnormalities are needed.
3. In patients with ascites and portal hypertension, new pharmacological therapies aimed at blocking NO production may help elucidate the role of this factor in cirrhosis.
4. Use of V2 receptor antagonists in dilutional hyponatremia with large-scale efficacy and safety trials are needed in order validate their use in dilutional hyponatremia.

In addition to changes in splanchnic hemodynamics, cirrhotics with ascites develop a hyperdynamic circulatory state characterized by reduced systemic vascular resistance with low arterial pressure, and increased cardiac output. As a consequence of splanchnic vasodilatation, central baroreceptors sense decreased plasma volume triggering RAAS, SNS, and AVP. The net effect is avid retention of sodium and water. The major clinical consequence of impaired solute-free water excretion is dilutional hyponatremia. Renal vasoconstriction develops late in the disease and manifests as HRS with elevated creatinine, oliguria, and azotemia. Future areas of investigation that are still needed to help elucidate the role of various substances that contribute to ascites formation and target therapies for ascites and renal functional abnormalities in cirrhosis are outlined in Table 3.

REFERENCES

1. Arroyo V, Ginès P, Planas R, Rodés J. Pathogenesis, diagnosis and treatment of ascites in cirrhosis. In: Bircher J, Benhamou JP, McIntyre N, Rizzetto M, Rodés J, eds. Oxford Textbook of Clinical Hepatology, 2nd ed. Oxford University Press, Oxford, 1999, pp. 697–732.
2. Bosch J, Arroyo V, Betriu A. Hepatic hemodynamics and the renin-angiotensin-aldosterone system in cirrhosis. Gastroenterology 1980;78:92–99.
3. Jiménez W, Clària J, Arroyo V. Experimental cirrhosis and pathogenesis of ascites formation in chronic liver disease. In: Holstege A, Hahn EG, Scholmerich J, eds. Portal Hypertension. Kluwer Academic, Dordrecht, 1995, pp. 15–25.
4. Clària J, Jiménez W. Renal dysfunction and ascites in carbon tetrachloride induced cirrhosis in rats. In: Arroyo V, Ginès P, Rodés J, Schrier RW, eds. Ascites and Renal Dysfunction in Liver Disease. Blackwell Science, Malden, 1999, pp. 378–396.
5. Castells A, Saló J, Planas R, et al. Impact of shunt surgery for variceal bleeding in the natural history of ascites in cirrhosis: a retrospective study. Hepatology 1994;20:584–591.
6. Arroyo V, Cárdenas A. TIPS in the treatment of refractory ascites. In: Arroyo V, Bosch J, Brugera M, Rodés J, Sánchez-Tapias JM, eds. Treatment of Liver Diseases. Masson, Barcelona, 1999, pp. 43–51.
7. Cárdenas A, Bataller R, Arroyo V. Mechanisms of ascites formation. Clin Liver Dis 2000;4:447–465.
8. Laine GA, Hall JT, Laine SH, et al. Transinusoidal fluid dynamics in canine liver during venous hypertension. Circ Res 1979;45:317–323.
9. Witte CL, Witte MH, Dumont AE, et al. Lymph protein and experimental hepatic and portal venous hypertension. Ann Surg 1968;168:567–577.
10. Witte CL, Witte MH, Dumont AE. Lymph imbalance in the genesis and perpetuation of the ascites syndrome in hepatic cirrhosis. Gastroenterology 1980;78:1059–1068.
11. Harris NR, Granger DN. Alterations of hepatic and splanchnic microvascular exchange in cirrhosis: local factors in the formation of ascites. In: Arroyo V, Ginès P, Rodés J, Schrier RW, eds. Ascites and Renal Dysfunction in Liver Disease. Blackwell Science, Malden, 1999, pp. 351–362.
12. Levy M. Pathophysiology of ascites formation. In: Epstein M, ed. The Kidney in Liver Disease, 4th ed. Hanley and Belfus, Philadelphia, 1996, pp. 179–220.
13. Huet PM, Goresky CA, Villenueve JP, et al. Assessment of liver microcirculation in human cirrhosis. J Clin Invest 1982;70:1234–1244.
14. Witte CL, Witte MH, Dumont AE. Estimated net transcapillary water and protein flux in the liver and intestine of patients with portal hypertension from hepatic cirrhosis. Gastroenterology 1981;80:265–272.
15. Korthuis RJ, Kinden DA, Brimer GE, et al. Intestinal capillary filtration in acute and chronic portal hypertension. Am J Physiol 1988;254:G339–G345.
16. Arroyo V. Comment: Hecker R, Sherlock S. Electrolyte and circulatory changes in terminal liver failure [Lancet 1956;2:1221–1225]. J Hepatol 2002;36:315–320.
17. Menon K, Kamath P. Regional and systemic hemodynamic disturbances in cirrhosis. Clin Liver Dis 2001;5:617–627.
18. Guevara M, Bru C, Ginès P, et al. Increased cerebral vascular resistance in cirrhotic patients with ascites. Hepatology 1998;28:39–44.
19. Maroto A, Ginès P, Arroyo V, et al. Brachial and femoral artery blood flow in cirrhosis: relationship to kidney dysfunction. Hepatology 1993;17:788–793.
20. Schrier RW, Arroyo V, Bernardi M, et al. Peripheral arterial vasodilation hypothesis: a proposal for the initiation of renal sodium and water retention in cirrhosis. Hepatology 1988;8:1151–1157.
21. Reynaert H, Thompson MG, Thomas T, Geerts A. Hepatic stellate cells: role in microcirculation and pathophysiology of portal hypertension. Gut 2002;50:571–581.
22. Rockey D, Weisiger R. Endothelin induced contractility of stellate cells from normal and cirrhotic rat liver: implications for regulation of portal pressure and resistance. Hepatology 1996;24:233–240.
23. Titós E, Clària J, Bataller R, et al. Hepatocyte-derived cysteinyl leukotrienes modulate vascular tone in experimental cirrhosis. Gastroenterology 2000;119:794–805.
24. Graupera M, Garcia-Pagan JC, Abraldes JG, et al. Cyclooxygenase-derived products modulate the increased intrahepatic resistance of cirrhotic rat livers. Hepatology 2003;37:172–181.
25. Bataller R, Sancho-Bru P, Ginès P, et al. Activated human hepatic stellate cells express the renin-angiotensin system and synthesize angiotensin II. Gastroenterology 2003;125:117–125.

26. Wiest R, Groszmann R. The paradox of nitric oxide in cirrhosis and portal hypertension: too much, not enough. Hepatology 2002;35:478–491.

27. Rockey DC, Chung JJ. Reduced nitric oxide production by endothelial cells in cirrhotic rat liver: endothelial dysfunction in portal hypertension. Gastroenterology 1998;114:344–351.

28. Vorobioff J, Bredfeldt JE, Groszmann RJ. Hyperdynamic circulation in portal-hypertensive rat model: a primary factor for maintenance of chronic portal hypertension. Am J Physiol 1983;244:G52–G57.

29. Benoit JN, Granger DN. Intestinal microvascular adaptation in chronic portal hypertension in the rat. Gastroenterology 1988;94:471–476.

30. Martin PY, Ginès P, Schrier RW. Nitric oxide as a mediator of hemodynamic abnormalities and sodium and water retention in cirrhosis. N Engl J Med 1998;339:533–541.

31. Wiest R, Groszmann R. Nitric oxide and portal hypertension: its role in the regulation of intrahepatic and splanchnic vascular resistance. Semin Liver Dis 1999;19:411–426.

32. Moller S, Bendtsen F, Henriksen JH. Vasoactive substances in the circulatory dysfunction of cirrhosis. Scand J Clin Lab Invest 2001;61:421–429.

33. Bernardi M, Trevisani F, Gasbarrini A, Gasbarrini G. Hepatorenal disorders: the role of the renin-angiotensin-aldosterone system. Semin Liver Dis 1994;14:23–34.

34. Asbert M, Jiménez W, Gaya J, et al. Assessment of the renin-angiotensin system in cirrhotic patients. Comparison between plasma renin activity and direct measurement of immunoreactive renin. J Hepatol 1992;15:179–183.

35. Schroeder ET, Anderson GH, Goldman SH, Streeten DHP. Effect of blockade of angiotensin II on blood pressure, renin and aldosterone in cirrhosis. Kidney Int 1976;9:511–519.

36. Arroyo V, Bosch J, Mauri M, et al. Effect of angiotensin-II blockade on systemic and hepatic haemodynamics and on the renin-angiotensin-aldosterone system in cirrhosis with ascites. Eur J Clin Invest 1981;11:221–229.

37. Schneider AW, Kalk JF, Klein CP. Effect of losartan, an angiotensin II receptor antagonist, on portal pressure in cirrhosis. Hepatology 1999;29:334–339.

38. Henriksen JH, Moller S, Ring Larsen H, et al. The sympathetic nervous system in liver disease. J Hepatol 1998;29:328–341.

39. Willett I, Esler M, Burke F, et al. Total and renal sympathetic nervous system activity in alcoholic cirrhosis. J Hepatol 1985;1:639–648.

40. Henriksen JH, Ring-Larsen H, Christensen NJ. Hepatic intestinal uptake and release of catecholamines in alcoholic cirrhosis. Evidence of enhanced hepatic intestinal sympathetic nervous activity. Gut 1987; 28:1637–1642.

41. MacGilchrist AJ, Howes LG, Hawksby C, et al. Plasma noradrenaline in cirrhosis: a study of kinetics and temporal relationship to ascites formation. Eur J Clin Invest 1991;21:238–243.

42. Esler M, Dudley F, Jennings G, et al. Increased sympathetic nervous activity and the effects of its inhibition with clonidine in alcoholic cirrhosis. Ann Intern Med 1992;116:446–455.

43. Henriksen JH, Ring-Larsen H, Kanstrup IL, et al. Splanchnic and renal elimination and release of catecholamines in cirrhosis. Evidence of enhanced sympathetic nervous activity in patients with decompensated cirrhosis. Gut 1984;25:1034–1043.

44. Esler M, Dudley F, Jennings G, et al. Increased sympathetic nervous activity and the effects of its inhibition with clonidine in alcoholic cirrhosis. Ann Inten Med 1992;116:446–455.

45. Moore K, Wendon J, Frazer M, et al. Plasma endothelin immunoreactivity in liver disease and the hepatorenal syndrome. N Engl J Med 1992;327:1774–1778.

46. Leivas A, Jiménez W, Lamas S, et al. Endothelin-1 does not play a major role in the homeostasis of arterial pressure in cirrhotic rats with ascites. Gastroenterology 1995;108:1842–1848.

47. Sogni P, Moreau R, Gomola A, et al. Beneficial hemodynamic effects of bosentan, a mixed ET(A) and ET(B) receptor antagonist, in portal hypertensive rats. Hepatology 1998;28:655–659.

48. Kogima H, Yamao J, Tsujimoto T, Uemura M, Takaya A, Fukui H. Mixed endothelin receptor antagonist, SB209670, decreases portal pressure in biliary cirrhotic rats in vivo by reducing portal venous system resistance. J Hepatol 2000;32:43–50.

49. Soper CP, Latif AB, Bending MR. Amelioration of hepatorenal syndrome with selective endothelin-A antagonist. Lancet 1996;347:1842–1843.

50. Ginès P, Jiménez W, Arroyo V, et al. Atrial natriuretic factor in cirrhosis with ascites: plasma levels, cardiac release and splanchnic extraction. Hepatology 1988;8:636–642.

51. La Villa G, Romanelli RG, Casini Raggi V, et al. Plasma levels of brain natriuretic peptide in patients with cirrhosis. Hepatology 1992;16:156–161.

52. Henriksen JH, Bendtsen F, Schutten HJ, et al. Hepatic-intestinal disposal of endogenous human alpha atrial natriuretic factor 99-126 in patients with cirrhosis. Am J Gastroenterol 1990;85:1155–1159.

53. Poulos JE, Gower WR, Fontanet HL, et al. Cirrhosis with ascites: increased atrial natriuretic peptide messenger RNA expression in rat ventricle. Gastroenterology 1995;108:1496–1502.

54. Epstein M, Loutzeinhiser R, Norsk P, et al. Relationship between plasma ANF responsiveness and renal sodium handling in cirrhotic humans. Am J Nephrol 1989;9:133–143.

55. Ginès P, Uriz J, Calahorra B, et al. Transjugular intrahepatic portosystemic shunting versus paracentesis plus albumin for refractory ascites in cirrhosis. Gastroenterology 2002;123:1839–1847.

56. Salerno F, Badalamenti S, Incerti P, et al. Renal response to atrial natriuretic peptide in patients with advanced liver cirrhosis. Hepatology 1988;8:21–26.

57. López C, Jiménez W, Arroyo V, et al. Role of altered systemic hemodynamics in the blunted renal response to atrial natriuretic peptide in rats with cirrhosis and ascites. J Hepatol 1989;9:217–226.

58. Beutler JJ, Koomans HA, Rabelink TJ, et al. Blunted natriuretic response and low blood pressure after atrial natriuretic factor in early cirrhosis. Hepatology 1989;10:148–153.

59. Laffi G, Pinzani M, Meacci E, et al. Renal hemodynamic and natriuretic effects of human atrial natriuretic factor infusion in cirrhosis with ascites. Gastroenterology 1989;96:167–177.

60. La Villa G, Riccardi D, Lazzeri C, et al. Blunted natriuretic response to low-dose brain natriuretic peptide infusion in nonazotemic cirrhotic patients with ascites and avid sodium retention. Hepatology 1995;22:1745–1750.

61. Abraham WT, Lauwaars M, Kim J, et al. Reversal of atrial natriuretic peptide resistance by increasing distal tubular sodium delivery in patients with decompensated cirrhosis. Hepatology 1995;22:737–743.

62. Koepke J, Jones S, DiBona G. Renal nerves mediate blunted natriuresis to atrial natriuretic peptide in cirrhotic rats. Am J Physiol 1987;252:R1019–R1023.

63. Angeli P, Jiménez W, Arroyo V, et al. Renal effects of natriuretic peptide receptor blockade in cirrhotic rats with ascites. Hepatology 1994;20:948–954.

64. Pérez-Ayuso RM, Arroyo V, Camps J, et al. Evidence that renal prostaglandins are involved in renal water metabolism in cirrhosis. Kidney Int 1984;26:72–80.

65. Laffi G, La Villa G, Pinzani M, et al. Arachidonic acid derivatives and renal function in liver cirrhosis. Semin Nephrol 1997;17:530–548.

66. Llach J, Ginès P, Arroyo V, et al. Effect of dipyridamole on kidney function in cirrhosis. Hepatology 1993;17:59–64.

67. Milani L, Merkel C, Gatta A. Renal effect of aminophylline in hepatic cirrhosis. Eur J Clin Pharmacol 1983;24:757–760.

68. Stanley AJ, Forrest EH, Dabos K, Bouchier IAD, Hayes PC. Natriuretic effect of an adenosine-1 receptor antagonist in cirrhotic patients with ascites. Gastroenterology 1998;115:406–411.

69. Blantz RC, Deng A, Lortie M, et al. The complex role of nitric oxide in the regulation of glomerular ultrafiltration. Kidney Int 2002;61:782–785.

70. Clària J, Jiménez W, Ros J, et al. Pathogenesis of arterial hypotension in cirrhotic rats with ascites: role of endogenous nitric oxide. Hepatology 1992;15:343–349.

71. Ros J, Clària J, Jiménez W, et al. Role of nitric acid and prostaglandin in the control of renal perfusion in experimental cirrhosis. Hepatology 1995;22:915–920.

72. Jiménez W, Martínez-Pardo A, Arroyo V, et al. Temporal relationship between hyperaldosteronism, sodium retention and ascites formation in rats with experimental cirrhosis. Hepatology 1985;5:245–250.

73. Levy M, Allotey JB. Temporal relationships between urinary salt retention and altered systemic hemodynamics in dogs with experimental cirrhosis. J Lab Clin Med 1978;92:560–569.

74. Pecikyan R, Kanzaki G, Berger EY. Electrolyte excretion during the spontaneous recovery from the ascitic phase of cirrhosis of the liver. Am J Med 1967;42:359–367.

75. Arroyo V, Rodés J. A rational approach to the treatment of ascites. Postgrad Med J 1975;51:558–562.

76. Ginès P, Fernández-Esparrach G, Arroyo V, et al. Pathogenesis of ascites in cirrhosis. Semin Liver Dis 1997;17:175–189.

77. Bernardi M, Laffi G, Salvagnini M, et al. Efficacy and safety of the stepped care medical treatment of ascites in liver cirrhosis: a randomized controlled clinical trial comparing two diets with different sodium content. Liver 1993;13:156–162.
78. Papper S, Rosenbaum JD. Abnormalities in the excretion of water and sodium in "compensated cirrhosis of the liver. J Lab Clin Med 1952;40:523–530.
79. La Villa G, Salmerón JM, Arroyo V, et al. Mineralocorticoid escape in patients with compensated cirrhosis and portal hypertension. Gastroenterology 1992;102:2114–2119.
80. Wong F, Liu P, Allidina Y, et al. Pattern of sodium handling and its consequences in patients with preascitic cirrhosis. Gastroenterology 1995;108:1820–1827.
81. Bernardi M. Renal sodium retention in preascitic cirrhosis: expanding knowledge, enduring uncertainties. Hepatology 2002;35:1544–1547.
82. Bernardi M, Trevisani F, Santini C, et al. Aldosterone related blood volume expansion in cirrhosis before and after the early phase of ascites formation. Gut 1983;24:761–766.
83. Caregaro L, Lauro S, Angeli P, et al. Renal water and sodium handling in compensated liver cirrhosis: mechanism of the impaired natriuresis after saline loading. Eur J Clin Invest 1985;15:360–365.
84. Reynolds TB, Lieberman FI., Redeker AG. Functional renal failure with cirrhosis. The effect of plasma expansion therapy. Medicine (Baltimore) 1967;46:191–196.
85. Bernardi M, Di Marco C, Trevisani F, et al. Renal sodium retention during upright posture in preascitic cirrhosis. Gastroenterology 1993;105:188–193.
86. Wong F, Liu P, Blendis L. The mechanism of improved sodium homeostasis of low-dose losartan in preascitic cirrhosis. Hepatology 2002;35:1449–1458.
87. Angeli P, Gatta A, Caregaro L, et al. Tubular site of renal sodium retention in ascitic liver cirrhosis evaluated by lithium clearance. Eur J Clin Invest 1990;20:111–117.
88. Bernardi M, Trevisani F, Caraceni P. The renin-angiotensin-aldosterone system in cirrhosis. In: Arroyo V, Ginès P, Rodés J, Schrier RW, eds. Ascites and Renal Dysfunction in Liver Disease. Blackwell Science, Malden, 1999, pp. 175–197.
89. Girgrah N, Liu P, Collier J, et al. Haemodynamic, renal sodium handling, and neurohormonal effects of acute administration of low dose losartan, an angiotensin II receptor antagonist, in preascitic cirrhosis. Gut 2000;46:114–120.
90. Helmy A, Jalan R, Newby DE, et al. Role of angiotensin II in regulation of basal and sympathetically stimulated vascular tone in early and advanced cirrhosis. Gastroenterology 2000;118:565–572.
91. Trevisani F, Bernardi M, DePalma R, et al. Circadian variation in renal sodium and potassium handling in cirrhosis. The role of aldosterone, cortisol, sympathoadrenergic tone, and intratubular factors. Gastroenterology 1989;96:1187–1198.
92. Pérez-Ayuso RM, Arroyo V, Planas R, et al. Randomized comparative study of furosemide versus spironolactone in patients with liver cirrhosis and ascites. Relationship between the diuretic response and the activity of the renin-aldosterone system. Gastroenterology 1983;84:961–968.
93. Yang YY, Lin HC, Lee WC, et al. One-week losartan administration increases sodium excretion in cirrhotic patients with and without ascites. J Gastroenterol 2002;37:194–199.
94. Dudley FJ, Esler MD. The sympathetic nervous system in cirrhosis. In: Arroyo V, Ginès P, Rodés J, Schrier RW, eds. Ascites and Renal Dysfunction in Liver Disease. Blackwell Science, Malden, 1999, pp. 198–219.
95. Esler M, Kaye D. Increased sympathetic nervous system activity and its therapeutic reduction in arterial hypertension, portal hypertension and heart failure. J Auton Nerv Syst 1998;72:210–219.
96. Salò J, Ginés A, Anibarro L, et al. Effect of upright posture and physical exercise on endogenous neurohormonal systems in cirrhotic patients with sodium retention and normal supine plasma renin, aldosterone and norepinephrine levels. Hepatology 1995;22:479–487.
97. Arroyo V, Clària J, Saló J, Jiménez W. Antidiuretic hormone and the pathogenesis of water retention in cirrhosis with ascites. Semin Liver Dis 1994;14:44–58.
98. Arroyo V, Rodés J, Gutiérrez-Lizarraga MA, Revert L. Prognostic value of spontaneous hyponatremia in cirrhosis with ascites. Am J Dig Dis 1976;21:249–256.
99. Porcel A, Diaz F, Rendon P, et al. Dilutional hyponatremia in patients with cirrhosis and ascites. Arch Intern Med 2002;162:323–328.

100. Fernández-Esparrach G, Sánchez-Fueyo A, Ginès P, et al. A prognostic model for predicting survival in cirrhosis with ascites. J Hepatol 2001;34:46–52.
101. Thibonnier M, Conarty DM, Preston JA, Wilkins PL, Berti-Mattera LN, Mattera R. Molecular pharmacology of human vasopressin receptors. Adv Exp Med Biol 1998;449:251–276.
102. Verbalis J. Vasopressin V2 receptor antagonists. J Mol Endocrinol 2002;29:1–9.
103. Kwon TH, Hager H, Nejsum LN, Andersen ML, Frokiaer J, Nielsen S. Physiology and pathophysiology of renal aquaporins. Semin Nephrol 2001;21:231–238.
104. Nielsen S, Frokiaer J, Marples D, Kwon TH, Agre P, Knepper MA. Aquaporins in the kidney: from molecules to medicine. Physiol Rev 2002;82:205–244.
105. Cárdenas A, Ginès P. Pathogenesis and treatment of dilutional hyponatremia in cirrhosis. In: Arroyo V, Forns X, Garcia-Pagan JC, Rodés J, eds. Progress in the Treatment of Liver Diseases. Ars Medica, Barcelona, 2003, pp. 31–42.
106. Angeli P, De Bei E, Dalla Pria M, et al. Effects of amiloride on renal lithium handling in nonazotemic ascitic cirrhotic patients with avid sodium retention. Hepatology 1992;15:651–654.
107. Wong F, Blei AT, Blendis LM, Thuluvath PJ. A vasopressin receptor antagonist (VPA-985) improves serum sodium concentration in patients with hyponatremia: a multicenter, randomized, placebo-controlled trial. Hepatology 2003;37:182–191.
108. Gerbes AL, Gulberg V, Ginès P, et al. VPA Study Group. Therapy of hyponatremia in cirrhosis with a vasopressin receptor antagonist: a randomized double-blind multicenter trial. Gastroenterology 2003; 124:933–939.
109. Caregaro L, Menon F, Angeli P, et al. Limitations of serum creatinine level and creatinine clearance as filtration markers in cirrhosis. Arch Intern Med 1994;154:201–205.
110. Sherman DS, Fish DN, Teitelbaum I. Assessing renal function in cirrhotic patients: problems and pitfalls. Am J Kidney Dis 2003;41:269–278.
111. Epstein M, Berck DP, Hollemberg NK, et al. Renal failure in the patient with cirrhosis. The role of active vasoconstriction. Am J Med 1970;49:175–185.
112. Cárdenas A, Uriz J, Ginès P, Arroyo V. Hepatorenal syndrome. Liver Transpl 2000;6(4 Suppl 1): S63–S71.
113. Dagher L, Moore K. The hepatorenal syndrome. Gut 2001;49:729–737.
114. Platt JF, Marn CS, Baliga PK, et al. Renal dysfunction in hepatic disease: early identification with renal Duplex Doppler US in patients who undergo liver transplantation. Radiology 1992;183:801–806.
115. Maroto A, Ginès A, Saló J, et al. Diagnosis of functional renal failure of cirrhosis by Doppler sonography. Prognostic value of resistive index. Hepatology 1994;20:839–844.
116. Newby D, Hayes PC. Hyperdynamic circulation in liver cirrhosis: not peripheral vasodilatation but 'splanchnic steal'. QJM 2002;95:827–830.

6 Hepatic Hemodynamics in Portal Hypertension

Compliance, Hepatic Arterial Buffer Response, Hepatorenal Syndrome, and Liver Regeneration

W. Wayne Lautt and Zhi Ming

CONTENTS

INTRODUCTION
HEPATIC COMPLIANCE
HABR
THE HEPATORENAL REFLEX
BLOOD FLOW REGULATION OF HEPATIC CELL MASS
CONCLUSION
ACKNOWLEDGMENTS
REFERENCES

INTRODUCTION

This chapter will discuss some consequences of the hepatic hemodynamic disturbances that accompany portal hypertension. Fibrosis or other mechanisms that lead to a restriction of blood flow through the liver have enormous consequences to the entire cardiovascular system, endocrine processing system, and metabolic homeostasis in general. Many systems have evolved to compensate for the disturbances that result from portal hypertension but some regulatory systems result in a worsening of homeostasis as a result of confusion at the afferent end of the signaling process. For example, does the liver respond to a decrease in portal blood flow the same if the decrease is caused by vasoconstriction of the superior mesenteric artery and subsequent reduction in intestinal blood flow as it does if blood flow to the hepatic parenchymal cells is reduced because of portacaval shunt formation? This chapter represents a conceptual focus on our own areas of expertise with no attempt to provide a detailed literature review. Although the references are few, more detailed references are available in the cited reviews and original articles. The approach taken is to evaluate the effects of increases and decreases in intrahepatic portal flow on four vital hepatic areas: the hepatic blood reservoir, hepatic arterial blood flow, the hepatorenal reflex, and liver cell mass.

From: *Clinical Gastroenterology: Portal Hypertension*
Edited by: A. J. Sanyal and V. H. Shah © Humana Press Inc., Totowa, NJ

Normally, the liver serves a significant stabilizing cardiovascular volume buffer function. A decrease in portal blood flow will result in a reduction in intrahepatic pressure proximal to the hepatic veins. The decreased pressure within this extremely compliant vascular bed results in a passive recoil and a decrease in stressed hepatic blood volume that results in a transfusion of hepatic blood volume into the central venous compartment thereby tending to increase venous return and cardiac output. The increased cardiac output will elevate splanchnic blood flow and portal venous flow will be partially corrected as a consequence. This mechanism may be completely absent in the presence of hepatic fibrosis and portacaval shunting.

The hepatic arterial buffer response (HABR) theory supplanted the previous view that metabolic activity of the liver controlled hepatic arterial blood flow in a similar manner to that regulating the blood flow in other organs. Hepatic arterial blood flow, although affected by hepatic sympathetic nerves and numerous circulating substances, is primarily regulated on a moment-to-moment basis by the HABR. The HABR is the inverse arterial response to changes in portal blood flow and is independent of hepatic oxygen supply and demand. The HABR is regulated as a result of washout of adenosine from a restricted vascular space, the space of Mall, by the portal venous flow. If portal flow decreases, adenosine accumulates and results in arterial vasodilation, which tends to counteract the impact of portal flow changes on total hepatic blood flow. This response tends to maintain total hepatic blood flow relatively constant on a moment-to-moment basis, which is suggested to have important consequences for endocrine homeostasis by virtue of blood flow–dependent clearance of numerous hormones. Hormonal homeostasis is maintained by a balance between hormone production and destruction, with destruction generally being regulated through the liver and often in a blood flow–dependent manner.

The third area of discussion deals with an autonomic reflex that has hepatic portal flow as the afferent signal and renal salt and water absorption as the efferent limb. Through this proposed mechanism, decreases in intrahepatic portal blood flow result in accumulation of adenosine (in a manner consistent with the role of adenosine in the HABR) with adenosine accumulation resulting in activation of hepatic sensory nerves and a reflex activation of salt and water retention in the kidneys. Although this mechanism is useful to maintain cardiac output and portal flow in healthy conditions, activation subsequent to portacaval shunting is proposed to account for salt and water retention in liver cirrhosis and the hepatorenal syndrome in the final stages of the disease process.

The reduced hepatic portal inflow that occurs by virtue of the induction of portacaval shunts leads to hepatic parenchymal cell atrophy. Normally, there is a relationship between total portal inflow and hepatic cell mass that is regulated by the effect of portal flow on vascular shear stress and the resultant release of nitric oxide. For example, if portal blood flow through a mass of liver tissue is increased as a result of surgical removal of part of the liver (portal flow is not controlled by the liver so the entire portal flow must pass through the remaining liver mass) the increased blood flow-to-liver mass results in a shear stress–induced release of nitric oxide and initiation of the liver regeneration cascade. When the liver volume returns to normal levels, thus restoring shear stress, the proliferative mechanism is turned off and liver mass remains at a stable level.

Portacaval shunting provides a false signal of reduced portal flow thus resulting in intrahepatic accumulation of adenosine and activation of hepatic arterial dilation, activation of the hepatorenal reflex and salt and water retention, and hepatic atrophy and hepatocyte cell mass appropriate for the reduced flow.

HEPATIC COMPLIANCE

The liver is highly vascularized with hepatic parenchymal cells arranged as a syncytium of hepatocyte plates generally consisting of a single layer of hepatocytes bordered by sinusoidal cells and blood flow on two sides of the hepatocyte. Approximately 25% of liver volume is accounted for by blood volume. The large blood volume of the liver serves an active and dynamic reservoir function with both active and passive changes in hepatic volume being able to result in expulsion of up to 50% of the total hepatic blood volume thus leading to a potential transfusion to the central venous compartment of approx 7% of the total body blood volume. This response is dramatically activated during hemorrhage and is regulated through both active means including hepatic sympathetic nerves and circulating catecholamines acting to decrease unstressed venous capacitance, and through the passive effect of reduced intrahepatic flow leading to reduced pressure and subsequently reduced stressed volume.

The concept of stressed and unstressed capacitance with specific reference to the role of the splanchnic circulation has previously been reviewed (1). Unstressed volume is a hypothetical volume of blood that would remain within the organ at a vascular pressure of zero. This measurement is obtainable only through extrapolation of pressure volume curves through the zero pressure axis. The subtle interaction between stressed and unstressed volume is beyond the purview of this chapter. Suffice it to summarize that all known active constrictors of hepatic blood volume do so through changes in the unstressed volume. Changes in hepatic blood volume that are caused by altered hepatic blood inflow or passive venous congestion result in changes in intrahepatic pressure with subsequent changes in stressed hepatic volume determined entirely by the effect of intrahepatic pressure and hepatic compliance.

In diseased states, hepatic autonomic nerve dysfunction is common and can result in reduced hepatic sympathetic neural expulsion of hepatic blood volume (2). Interestingly, when the active compensation for hemorrhage is reduced, the decrease in cardiac output and blood pressure caused by hemorrhage is magnified which results in a more severe decrease in portal blood flow and an increased passive capacitance effect. The proportion of hepatic blood volume response caused by active or passive effects is extremely difficult to quantify but it has been demonstrated that the reduction in hepatic blood volume that occurs during hemorrhage is associated with a dramatic decrease in portal blood flow. If the portal blood flow is passively reduced through the use of mechanical occluders on the superior mesenteric artery, the hepatic blood volume changes can essentially be duplicated (3). Partial occlusion of the superior mesenteric artery in dogs led to a reduction of 2.8 mmHg in portal pressure and a rise of 19% in cardiac output (4). That is, if portal blood flow is decreased either by hemorrhage or by mechanical means, the decrease in hepatic blood volume is similar.

The passive response to decreased portal blood flow is dependent upon two parameters, intrahepatic distending pressure and hepatic compliance. Compliance is defined as the change in volume per unit change in pressure. The liver is an extremely compliant organ whose blood volume can more than double as a result of an increase in intrahepatic pressure of approx 8 mmHg (5). The distending blood pressure of relevance is determined by the relationship between intrahepatic vascular resistance and hepatic blood inflow. Although somewhat controversial, we have argued extensively that the primary resistance to hepatic portal blood flow is at hepatic venous sites (6). Blood pressure upstream from the hepatic venous resistance sites is therefore determined by the resistance and by the amount of flow presented to the resistance sites so that an increase in portal flow will result in an increase in intrahepatic distending pressure and an expansion in hepatic blood volume. The observation that equal decreases in portal inflow and arterial inflow will cause equal decreases in hepatic volume provides strong support for the argument that the resistance site of relevance is postsinusoidal *(7)*. Additional complexities in this equation arise as a result of the extreme distensibility of the intrahepatic venous resistance sites. The passive high venous resistance distensibility is a mechanism that leads to passive autoregulation of portal venous pressure *(6)*. For example, if portal blood flow is doubled, portal venous pressure only increases by approx 2 mmHg as a result of the increases in distending pressure at the resistance site causing a large passive decrease in resistance. The relationship between the distending pressure and the resistance has been previously described mathematically in a way that allows a differentiation between active and passive venous resistance. Resistance is inversely related to the cube of distending pressure, which is calculated as the mean of the pressure above and below the resistance site *(8)*.

In the presence of portal hypertension but absence of significant portacaval shunts, changes in portal blood flow will result in substantially greater changes in portal pressure if the diseased state results in reduced vascular distensibility. Compliance (volume) and resistance site distensibility responses to both volume expansion *(9)* and to blood loss would be expected to be reduced in fibrosed livers. The area of research relating the diseased hepatic vasculature to altered venous distensibility and altered responses to stressed and unstressed capacitance regulation has not been carried out; however, in the presence of extensive portacaval shunting, it is clear that the passive blood volume buffering role of the liver in response to changes in intrahepatic portal flow will be completely lost thereby removing a powerful and versatile stabilizer of overall cardiovascular status.

HABR

Lautt *(10)* reviewed the historical perspective of the development of the modern hepatic arterial buffer concept. Prior to 1977 *(11)* it was the consensus strongly and commonly stated in textbooks and reviews that hepatic metabolic supply and demand regulated hepatic arterial blood flow in the same manner as arterial blood flow was regulated in other organs. A survey of the literature indicates that there does not appear to ever have existed experimental evidence to support this contention. Although many extrinsic factors such as hepatic sympathetic nerves, circulating hormones and nutrients may dramatically affect hepatic arterial blood flow, the primary intrinsic regulator of the arterial flow appears to be the inverse reaction to changes in portal blood flow. The earliest studies reporting an effect of changes in portal perfusion on hepatic arterial flow were credited by Child *(12)* to Betz in 1863 *(13)* and Gad in 1873 *(14)*. The discovery of the mechanism of the HABR is an example of pure serendipity where it was observed that hemodilution resulting in a dramatic decrease in hepatic oxygen delivery did not result in the anticipated dilation of the hepatic artery to compensate. Subsequent studies showed that both increases and decreases in hepatic metabolic activity were without the anticipated effects on hepatic arterial blood flow and that the only parameter that appeared to correlate with changes in hepatic arterial blood flow were the opposite changes in portal flow *(11)*. A number of alternate hypotheses were tested and rejected prior to demonstration of the adenosine washout theory *(15)*.

The intrahepatic vasculature transports arterial and portal blood to the liver through progressive parallel divisions of these vessels that eventually travel as their terminal branches through a small space referred to as the space of Mall, which is surrounded by a limiting plate of hepatocytes. In the space of Mall, the hepatic artery is intimately intertwined with the portal venule. The two vessels eventually drain into the hepatic sinusoids. Adenosine appears to be produced at a constant rate, independent of oxygen supply or demand, and is secreted into the space of Mall where it serves as a powerful dilator of the hepatic artery. The concentration of adenosine is regulated by the rate of washout into the blood vessels that pass through the space of Mall. According to this theory, a decrease in portal blood flow results in a reduced washout of adenosine and the accumulated adenosine concentration results in dilation of the hepatic artery thus partially compensating for the decrease in portal blood flow and often compensating fully for the decrease in oxygen delivery *(10)* even in cirrhotic livers *(16)*.

The role of adenosine as the regulator of the HABR initially appears inconsistent with the statement that the hepatic artery is generally not controlled by the oxygen supply or demand to the liver, especially considering the known primary regulators of adenosine as being the breakdown from ATP to ADP, AMP, and, finally, adenosine or the breakdown of cyclic AMP to adenosine. However, a less-recognized oxygen-independent pathway leading to adenosine production by demethylation of S-adenosylhomocysteine *(17)* that accounts for basal adenosine production in the heart could also account for the production in the liver. Evidence consistent with the adenosine hypothesis includes the observation that adenosine is an extremely potent dilator of the hepatic artery. The hypothesis also requires that portal blood must have access to the arterial resistance vessels so that portal flow can wash away adenosine from the area of the resistance vessels. This is shown by the observation that adenosine administered into the portal blood has ready access to the arterial resistance vessel sites and therefore should also be able to remove adenosine from the relevant site. Potentiators of the effects of exogenous adenosine also potentiate the buffer response and blockers of the effects of exogenous adenosine also inhibit the buffer response. Dose-response studies indicate the classically recognized ability to block exogenously administered substances using selective receptor antagonists is substantially more effective than the ability to block endogenously released substances. Nevertheless, full dose-response studies indicate that a complete and selective blockade of the dilator effect of adenosine can be achieved using 8-phenyltheophylline (8-PT), which leaves the response to other dilators, including isoproterenol, intact *(18,19)*.

One area of confusion related to the adenosine hypothesis is based upon the unusual anatomy of the hepatic microcirculation. The terminal branches of the hepatic portal venules and arterioles drain into the center of the microvascular unit of the liver, the hepatic acinus, which represents a sphere of hepatic tissue of approx 2 mm in diameter. Blood flows concurrently in adjacent sinusoids and passes approx 16 hepatocytes prior to draining into the terminal hepatic venules. The microvascular anatomy is such that this unique separation of inlet and outlet vessels precludes diffusion of products produced by the hepatocytes from moving upstream to act on the arterial resistance vessels. Thus, although the liver is capable of producing huge amounts of adenosine in response to hypoxia or hemorrhage, this adenosine is produced by hepatocytes that export the adenosine into the sinusoidal blood that flows downstream and away from the resistance vessels such that the resistance vessels are not affected by hepatic parenchymal cell adenosine production or by other dilator substances released from these sites. It should be noted that the putative

urine production. These studies provided direct evidence, for the first time, that the change in intrahepatic portal flow is involved in the regulation of renal function through a hepatorenal reflex.

To propose hepatic flow as the afferent signal, it is necessary to also propose a mechanism by which portal flow can serve as an activator of an afferent reflex limb. Our prior studies related to the hepatic arterial buffer response indicated that adenosine in the space of Mall was directly controlled by intrahepatic blood flow. The observation that the hepatic perivascular region is also rich in sensory nerve endings *(38)* supported the feasibility of an adenosine-mediated afferent limb. Adenosine has previously been shown to activate sensory nerves in the carotid body *(39)* and in the heart *(40)*. Stimulation of myocardial adenosine A1 receptors increased the discharge of cardiac afferent fibers and resulted in an increase in neural discharge of the renal sympathetic efferent fibers in anesthetized dogs *(40,41)*. It seemed possible, therefore, that a decrease in intrahepatic portal blood flow through the reduced washout of adenosine and resultant accumulation of adenosine in the space of Mall could activate hepatic sensory nerves to trigger the hepatorenal reflex. Intrahepatic adenosine infusion significantly decreased urine flow and urinary sodium excretion in the absence of changes in glomerular filtration rate. In contrast, intravenous adenosine at the same dose was without any effect on renal function thereby indicating that the effect of the infused adenosine was through the liver and not direct action on the kidney. Intrahepatic application of the adenosine receptor antagonist, 8-PT, abolished the renal response to intraportal adenosine. Further, both hepatic and renal denervation abolished the renal response to adenosine thereby proving the reflex connection *(42)*.

Thus, these data, taken together, are consistent with the hypothesis that reductions in intraportal blood flow lead to an adenosine-mediated activation of hepatic afferent nerves that result in a sympathetic reflex to the kidneys causing fluid retention. This response would serve a useful function in normal physiological conditions where the reduced portal flow would cause fluid retention thereby increasing the circulating blood volume and cardiac output. The elevated cardiac output would result in elevated portal flow thus correcting the flow imbalance to the liver. In the diseased state with portacaval shunts existing, the signal would be anticipated to occur as a result of the decreased intrahepatic portal flow; however, the salt and water retention would not lead to a correction of the intrahepatic flow, but, rather, would lead to elevated cardiac output and elevated portal inflow which would simply bypass the liver through the shunts leading to a progressive, inappropriate reflex accumulation of fluid.

Although our first studies *(37,42)* demonstrated clearly that the hepatorenal reflex was mediated by adenosine as the afferent activator responding to reduced hepatic blood flow, the relationship to the diseased liver state could not be assumed. In a recent study (unpublished observations), we used the liver disease model produced by chronic administration of the hepatotoxic thioacetamide. Severe fibrosis was demonstrated consistent with advanced liver disease. Reduced basal urine flow and a reduced ability to excrete a saline load were demonstrated. The renal dysfunction was partially corrected by intrahepatic administration of the adenosine receptor antagonist, 8-PT. Thus the hypothesis tested in the healthy state was consistent with the data from the diseased state. However, at this point, it must be cautioned that it is not clear whether the adenosine-mediated hepatorenal reflex seen in the cirrhotic liver was actually secondary to shunt-induced decreases in intrahepatic blood flow or whether adenosine may have been increased as a result of a metabolic imbalance induced by the disease. Further studies are required to clarify the mechanism of adenosine production but the data strongly support a therapeutic approach treating the early renal dysfunction and, perhaps, even the late stage hepatorenal syndrome through the blockade of intrahepatic adenosine receptors.

BLOOD FLOW REGULATION OF HEPATIC CELL MASS

Similar to the previous section, the relationship between hepatic blood flow and liver cell mass represents a recent breakthrough that has not previously been reviewed and, therefore, requires provision of additional technical information. The liver is well recognized to have a unique ability to rapidly regenerate. Perhaps even the ancient Greeks knew of this remarkable ability because the legend of Prometheus describes the wrathful punishment by Zeus for the sin of revealing the secret of fire to mankind by the unique torture of the chained Prometheus having his liver plucked out by an eagle by day to be regenerated by night, thus perpetuating his torment indefinitely. Although the extent of hepatic liver regeneration is exaggerated by this legend, it remains a striking observation that following a two-thirds partial hepatectomy to rats, full restoration of liver volume can be attained within approx 1 wk and 50% of the recovery occurs within 48 h. In a review of hepatic regeneration, Michalopoulos and DeFrancis (43) indicated that, despite over 100 years of research, the trigger of liver regeneration remained unknown and that the discovery of this trigger would be akin to the big bang theory of evolution of the universe.

Prior to 1954, there were a number of studies that were compatible with the hypothesis that hepatic blood flow regulated liver cell mass but a few poorly conducted and improperly interpreted studies led to a rapid consensus that hepatic blood flow was not a significant regulator of liver mass. However, in the process of preparing an extensive review on hepatic circulation, Greenway and Lautt (44) suggested that the coincidence of enzyme induction and elevated portal blood flow that had been interpreted to suggest that an increase in hepatic metabolism and liver volume led to an increase in portal flow were inconsistent with several clearly defined studies demonstrating that the liver cannot directly control portal blood flow thereby suggesting that the blood flow may have controlled liver cell mass. A reasonable mechanism explaining how hepatic blood flow could regulate liver mass was suggested by the demonstration that portal blood flow caused shear-induced release of nitric oxide thereby suggesting the possibility that either adenosine (see the Hepatic Arterial Buffer Response section) or nitric oxide could serve as a blood flow–dependent regulator. Early studies quickly demonstrated that adenosine was not a viable regulator but nitric oxide was.

The hypothesis suggesting vascular shear stress regulation of hepatic cell mass is based upon the observation that increases in vascular shear stress in the liver release nitric oxide which can be shown to have significant impact on vascular responses and metabolic responses to the sympathetic nerves (45) and on the fact that the liver does not control portal blood flow. With a two-thirds partial hepatectomy, all of the portal blood flow is forced to pass through the remaining liver mass thereby increasing the flow-to-mass ratio by 300%. The suggestion was, therefore, that the hemodynamic consequences of partial hepatectomy led to shear stress–induced release of nitric oxide, which served as the initial trigger for the hepatic regeneration cascade.

For a finite event to be proposed as a trigger for the regeneration cascade, the even must occur immediately after the partial hepatectomy and serve as a trigger for an entire cascade.

The first studies were based on the previous observation that a wide range of hepatic proliferating factors appeared in the plasma of animals that had been subjected to a partial hepatectomy at varying time points after the removal of liver mass. A bioassay was used to detect the presence of proliferating factors by the ability of plasma from a rat with a partial hepatectomy to stimulate hepatocyte proliferation in vitro. Partial hepatectomy was demonstrated to result in elevation of proliferating factors that peaked at approx 4 h after the partial hepatectomy and which could be completely blocked by inhibition of hepatic nitric oxide synthase. The response could be restored by provision of a nitric oxide donor to the liver *(46,47)*.

Subsequent studies evaluated the earliest and latest stages of the regeneration cascade. At the early stage, we utilized the expression of an immediate early gene that had previously been shown to reach a peak activation 15 min after partial hepatectomy and was dependent on the degree of partial hepatectomy performed *(48)*. C-*fos* activation was shown to occur in the remnant liver following partial hepatectomy and not in sham-operated animals *(49)*. c-*fos* mRNA expression was prevented by blocking hepatic nitric oxide synthase activation and by blocking prostaglandin production, both of which are regulated by shear stress (Smith-Schoen and Lautt, unpublished observations). Furthermore, a nitric oxide donor, a phosphodiesterase antagonist, and prostaglandin I_2 potentiated c-*fos* mRNA expression following partial hepatectomy. Similar pharmacological manipulation resulted in potentiation of liver weight restoration 48 h after partial hepatectomy. The relation between blood flow and this trigger was supported by the demonstration that prevention of shear stress following partial hepatectomy blocked the trigger. Occlusion of the superior mesenteric artery decreases hepatic blood flow by approximately two-thirds and a two-thirds partial hepatectomy increases hepatic blood flow per remaining liver mass by three times. Therefore, occlusion of the superior mesenteric artery following a two-thirds partial hepatectomy should prevent the development of shear stress in the liver. This was shown by a lack of activation of c-*fos* in this model *(49)*.

Selective ligation of portal venous lobar veins leads to decreased portal flow in the ligated lobes with compensatory arterial dilation and "elevated" flow to the unligated lobes. Liver volume adjusts so that flow per unit liver weight is restored by 1 wk and the hepatic arterial buffer response is maintained *(50)*.

The selective ligation of the left branch of the portal vein resulted in increased portal flow to the unligated two-thirds of the liver and led to similar elevation in portal pressure as was achieved by two-thirds partial hepatectomy of the same lobes thus indicating similar elevations of shear stress. The resultant elevations in c-*fos* in the unligated lobes and the appearance of proliferating factors in plasma were similar and could be blocked by nitric oxide synthase antagonists *(49)*.

These hemodynamic relationships to shear stress and liver volume have not been studied in liver disease but the presence of portacaval shunts and altered intrahepatic hemodynamics could be a major cause of reduced hepatic regenerative capacity in disease states.

CONCLUSION

Intrahepatic circulation is disrupted at the earliest stage of liver disease and becomes dramatically dysfunctional with progression of the disease state culminating in the formation of portacaval shunts and potential complete absence of portal blood flow to the liver. Considering the important hemodynamic and metabolic position of the liver, it is not unanticipated that there should be a number of quite predictable severe consequences to this circulatory disruption. In this brief overview, we have described dysfunction of a number of systems that are normally regulated to maintain hepatic blood flow constant relative to liver mass. The decrease in the hepatic blood volume reservoir function primarily affects cardiovascular stability by removing a powerful blood volume buffer. The hepatic arterial buffer response is important for cardiovascular homeostatic and endocrine homeostasis and, although still functioning in severely diseased livers, may be anticipated to be fully activated in conditions of maximal portacaval shunting thereby removing the buffering capacity of this mechanism. The establishment of portacaval shunts results in reduced intrahepatic blood flow, which activates the normal physiological compensatory hepatorenal reflex. However, in the presence of the portacaval shunts, the fluid retention triggered by this reflex does not correct the signaled deficit and, rather, leads to a progressive and, eventually, devastating cardiovascular disturbance. Finally, the delicate balance between hepatic blood flow and liver hepatocyte mass would be anticipated to be dramatically altered in situations where portacaval shunts occur. The impact of this latter mechanism in the severely diseased liver is unknown as there may be other more powerful mechanisms accounting for lack of liver regeneration capacity in the diseased liver.

ACKNOWLEDGMENTS

Funding of this work by the authors was from the Canadian Institutes of Health Research, the Heart and Stroke Foundation of Manitoba and Saskatchewan, and the Manitoba Kidney Foundation. The contribution of numerous technicians and trainees is acknowledged in the original publications. Manuscript preparation by Karen Sanders is greatly appreciated.

REFERENCES

1. Greenway CV, Lautt WW. Blood volume, the venous system, preload, and cardiac output. Can J Physiol Pharmacol 1986;64:383–387.
2. Schafer J, d'Almeida MS, Weisman H, Lautt WW. Hepatic blood volume responses and compliance in cats with long-term bile duct ligation. Hepatology 1993;18:969–977.
3. Lautt WW, Brown LC, Durham JS. Active and passive control of hepatic blood volume responses to hemorrhage at normal and raised hepatic venous pressure in cats. Can J Physiol Pharmacol 1980;58:1049–1057.
4. Groszmann RJ, Blei AT, Kniaz JL, Storer EH, Conn HO. Portal pressure reduction induced by partial mechanical obstruction of the superior mesenteric artery in the anesthetized dog. Gastroenterology 1978;75:187–192.
5. Lautt WW, Greenway CV. Hepatic venous compliance and role of liver as a blood reservoir. Am J Physiol 1976;231:292–295.
6. Lautt WW, Legare DJ. Passive autoregulation of portal venous pressure: distensible hepatic resistance. Am J Physiol 1992;263:G702–G708.
7. Bennett TD, Rothe CF. Hepatic capacitance responses to changes in flow and hepatic venous pressure in dogs. Am J Physiol 1981;240:H18–H28.
8. Lautt WW, Greenway CV, Legare DJ. Index of contractility: quantitative analysis of hepatic venous distensibility. Am J Physiol 1991;260:G325–G332.
9. Hadengue A, Moreau R, Gaudin C, Bacq B, Champigneulle B, Lebrec D. Lack of response to volume expansion in patients with decompensated cirrhosis is related to abnormal venous compliance (abstract). Hepatology 1990;12:851.
10. Lautt WW. The 1995 Ciba-Geigy Award Lecture. Intrinsic regulation of hepatic blood flow. Can J Physiol Pharmacol 1996;74:223–233.

11. Lautt WW. The hepatic artery: subservient to hepatic metabolism or guardian of normal hepatic clearance rates of humoral substances. Gen Pharmacol 1977;8:73–78.
12. Child CG. The Hepatic Circulation and Portal Hypertension. W.B. Saunders, Philadelphia, 1954.
13. Betz W. The circulation within the liver, especially that of the hepatic artery. Zeitschrift fuer rat Med 1863;18:44–60.
14. Gad J. Studies on the relations of the blood stream of the portal vein to the blood stream in the hepatic artery. Dissertation, G. Schade, Berlin, 1873.
15. Lautt WW. Role and control of the hepatic artery. In: Lautt WW, ed. Hepatic Circulation in Health and Disease. Raven, New York, 1981, pp. 203–226.
16. Mucke I, Richter S, Menger MD, Vollmar B. Significance of hepatic arterial responsiveness for adequate tissue oxygenation upon portal vein occlusion in cirrhotic livers. Int J Colorectal Dis 2000;15: 335–341.
17. Lloyd HE, Schrader J. The importance of the transmethylation pathway for adenosine metabolism in the heart. In: Gerlach E, Becker BF, eds. Topics and Perspectives in Adenosine Research. Springer-Verlag, Berlin, 1987.
18. Lautt WW, Legare DJ. The use of 8-phenyltheophylline as a competitive antagonist of adenosine and an inhibitor of the intrinsic regulatory mechanism of the hepatic artery. Can J Physiol Pharmacol 1985; 63:717–722.
19. Richter S, Vollmar B, Mucke I, Post S, Menger MD. Hepatic arteriolo-portal venular shunting guarantees maintenance of nutritional microvascular supply in hepatic arterial buffer response of rat livers. J Physiol 2001;531:193–201.
20. Henderson JM, Gilmore GT, Mackay GJ, Galloway JR, Dodson TF, Kutner MH. Hemodynamics during liver transplantation: the interactions between cardiac output and portal venous and hepatic arterial flows. Hepatology 1992;16:715–718.
21. Bolognesi M, Sacerdoti D, Bombonato G, et al. Change in portal flow after liver transplantation: effect on hepatic arterial resistance indices and role of spleen size. Hepatology 2002;35:601–608.
22. Iwao T, Toyonaga A, Shigemori H, et al. Hepatic artery hemodynamic responsiveness to altered portal blood flow in normal and cirrhotic livers. Radiology 1996;200:793–798.
23. Richter S, Mucke I, Menger MD, Vollmar B. Impact of intrinsic blood flow regulation in cirrhosis: maintenance of hepatic arterial buffer response. Am J Physiol Gastrointest Liver Physiol 2000;279:G454–G462.
24. Gulberg V, Haag K, Rossle M, Gerbes AL. Hepatic arterial buffer response in patients with advanced cirrhosis. Hepatology 2002;35:630–634.
25. Messerli FH, Nowaczynski W, Honda M, et al. Effect of angiotensin II on steroid metabolism and hepatic blood flow in man. Circ Res 1977;40:204–207.
26. Zimmon DS, Kessler RE. Effect of portal venous blood flow diversion on portal pressure. J Clin Invest 1980;65:1388–1397.
27. Burchell AR, Moreno AH, Panke WF, Nealon TJ Jr. Hepatic artery flow improvement after portacaval shunt: a single hemodynamic clinical correlate. Ann Surg 1976;184:289–302.
28. Dauzat M, Lafortune M, Patriquin H, Pomier-Layrargues G. Meal induced changes in hepatic and splanchnic circulation: a noninvasive Doppler study in normal humans. Eur J Appl Physiol 1994;68: 373–380.
29. Lafortune M, Dauzat M, Pomier-Layrargues G, et al. Hepatic artery: effect of a meal in healthy persons and transplant recipients. Radiology 1993;187:391–394.
30. Sato N, Hayashi N, Kawano S, Kamada T, Abe H. Hepatic hemodynamic in patients with chronic hepatitis or cirrhosis as assessed by organ-reflectance spectrophotometry. Gastroenterology 1983;84: 611–616.
31. Gines P, Arroyo V. Hepatorenal syndrome. J Am Soc Nephrol 1999;10:1833–1839.
32. Bosch B, Garcia-Pagan CG. Complication of cirrhosis. I. Portal hypertension. J Hepatol 2000;32(Suppl 1):141–156.
33. Kawasaki T, Moriyasu F, Kimura T, et al. Hepatic function and portal hemodynamics in patients with liver cirrhosis. Am J Gastroenterol 1990;85:1160–1164.
34. Koyama S, Kanai K, Aibiki M, Fujita T. Reflex increase in renal nerve activity during acutely altered portal venous pressure. J Auton Nerv Syst 1988;23:55–62.

35. Levy M, Wexler MJ. Renal sodium retention and ascites formation in dogs with experimental cirrhosis but without portal hypertension or increased splanchnic vascular capacity. Lab Clin Med 1978;91: 520–536.
36. Liang CC. The influence of hepatic portal circulation on urine flow. J Physiol 1977;214:571–581.
37. Ming Z, Smyth DD, Lautt WW. Decreases in portal flow trigger a hepatorenal reflex to inhibit renal sodium and water excretion in rats: role of adenosine. Hepatology 2002;35:167–175.
38. Niijima A. An electrophysiological study on hepatovisceral reflex: the role played by vagal hepatic afferents from chemosensors in the hepatoportal region. In: Haussinger D, Jungermann K, eds. Liver and Nervous System. Kluwer Academic, U.K., 1998, pp. 159–172.
39. Vandier C, Conway AF, Landauer RC, Kumar P. Presynaptic action of adenosine on a 4-aminopyridine-sensitive current in the rat carotid body. J Physiol 1999;515:419–429.
40. Thames MC, Kinugawa T, Dibner-Dunlap ME. Reflex sympathoexcitation by cardiac sympathetic afferents during myocardial ischemia: role of adenosine. Circulation 1993;87:1698–1704.
41. Montano N, Lombardi F, Ruscone TG, Contini M, Guazzi M, Malliani A. The excitatory effect of adenosine on the discharge activity of the afferent cardiac sympathetic fibers. Cardiologia 1991;36: 953–959.
42. Ming Z, Smyth DD, Lautt WW. Intrahepatic adenosine triggers a hepatorenal reflex to regulate sodium and water excretion. Auton Neurosci 2001;93:1–7.
43. Michalopolous GK, DeFrances MC. Liver regeneration. Science 1997;276:60–66.
44. Greenway CV, Lautt WW. Hepatic Circulation. In: Schultz SG, Wood JD, Rauner BB, eds. Handbook of Physiology. The Gastrointestinal System I. Vol. 1, Part 2, chap 41. American Physiological Society. Oxford University Press, New York, 1989, pp. 1519–1564.
45. Macedo MP, Lautt WW. Shear-induced modulation of vasoconstriction in the hepatic artery and portal vein by nitric oxide. Am J Physiol 1998;274:G253–G260.
46. Wang H, Lautt WW. Does nitric oxide (NO) trigger liver regeneration? Proc West Pharmacol Soc 1997; 40:17,18.
47. Wang H, Lautt WW. Evidence of nitric oxide, a flow-dependent factor, being a trigger of liver regeneration in rats. Can J Physiol Pharmacol 1998;76:1072–1079.
48. Moser MJ, Gong Y, Zhang MN, et al. Immediate-early oncogene expression and liver function following varying extents of partial hepatectomy in the rat. Dig Dis Sci 2001;46:907–914.
49. Schoen JM, Wang HH, Minuk GY, Lautt WW. Shear stress-induced nitric oxide release triggers the liver regeneration cascade. Nitric Oxide: Biol Chem 2001;5:453–464.
50. Rocheleau B, Ethier C, Houle R, Huet PM, Bilodeau M. Hepatic artery buffer response following left portal vein ligation: its role in liver tissue homeostasis. Am J Physiol 1999;277:G1000–G1007.

7

Neovascularization, Angiogenesis, and Vascular Remodeling in Portal Hypertension

Manuel Morales-Ruiz
and Wladimiro Jiménez, PhD

CONTENTS

BASIC MECHANISMS OF NEW BLOOD VESSEL FORMATION
BASIC MECHANISMS OF VASCULAR REMODELING
PATHOPHYSIOLOGICAL INDUCTION OF LONG-TERM STRUCTURAL
    VASCULAR CHANGES IN PORTAL HYPERTENSION
ACKNOWLEDGMENTS
REFERENCES

BASIC MECHANISMS OF NEW BLOOD VESSEL FORMATION

The cardiovascular system mainly develops during embryogenesis and only to a limited extent in postnatal life. This is a complex process that involves proliferation, migration, and differentiation of endothelial cells and, in a final step, recruitment of smooth muscle cells to form mature vessels. These are key events in the formation of new vessels that are spatially and temporally orchestrated through two very-well-differentiated mechanisms of new blood vessel formation: vasculogenesis and angiogenesis.

Vasculogenesis

The term vasculogenesis refers to the *de novo* differentiation of endothelial cells from mesodermal precursors and the subsequent formation of an early capillary plexus. In the developing embryo, vasculogenesis begins when cells derived from the mesoderm form cellular aggregates termed blood islands that fuse to form the yolk sac capillary network. In these aggregates, the inner cell population differentiates into hematopoietic stem cells and the peripheral cell population develops endothelial cell precursors known as angioblasts *(3,4)*. Although vasculogenesis mainly takes place during embryonic development, it has recently been demonstrated that circulating bone-marrow endothelial progenitor cells (EPCs) may also contribute to vasculogenesis through their incorporation into sites of active neovascularization such as ischemic myocardium, tumor vasculature, wound healing, or injured corneas in adult species. Moreover, postnatal vasculogenesis has been

From: *Clinical Gastroenterology: Portal Hypertension*
Edited by: A. J. Sanyal and V. H. Shah © Humana Press Inc., Totowa, NJ

demonstrated to be involved in the physiological replacement of endothelium in mature vessels *(5,6)*. However, whether differentiation of EPCs plays an important role in adult neovascularization still needs to be defined.

Angiogenesis

Angiogenesis is the main process of new vessel formation in postnatal stages and is defined as the mechanisms by which new capillaries are formed from a preexisting capillary network without the participation of endothelial cell precursors. In adults, this process is fundamental in reproduction and wound healing and is highly regulated in physiological conditions. However, when the balance between angiogenic and antiangiogenic factors is abnormal, angiogenesis becomes an important pathophysiological agent in a large number of diseases. For instance, some disorders are characterized by excessive angiogenesis such as rheumatoid arthritis, tumor growth, psoriasis, or retinopathies, which are often associated with diabetes. Furthermore, insufficient angiogenesis may lead to a worsening of ulcerations, pulmonary fibrosis, or Crohn's disease, among others *(7–11)*. Owing to the wide-spectrum applicability of a therapeutic control in disregulated angiogenesis, a great effort and resources have been dedicated to understand the fundamental aspects of angiogenesis. In this regard, two different mechanisms of angiogenesis have been described so far. The first describes the process by which angiogenesis is generated through the sprouting of a preexisting vessel and the second refers to the splitting or intussusception of a vessel into two new capillaries. Initially, the construction of a vascular network by sprouting angiogenesis requires the activity of proteolytic enzymes (metalloproteinases, plasmin, collagenase, plasminogen activator) that catalyze the degradation of extracellular matrix and basement membranes located between the preexisting vessel and the adjacent tissue. After that, endothelial cells undergo morphogenesis, migration, adhesion, and proliferation to form a vascular sprout, which, in a later phase, is stabilized by the recruitment of mural cells and by the production of a highly specific basement membrane. All these processes are required in the final sprout to form a functional, mature vasculature *(3)*. By contrast, intussusceptive angiogenesis is formed by internal division of preexisting vessels through the formation of transcapillary tissue pillars resulting in two new vascular entities. Stabilization of pillars, and as a result the newly formed blood vessels, occurs by invagination of surrounding pericytes and extracellular matrix. The successive repetition of this process contributes to the expansion of the capillary network *(12)*.

Vascular Endothelial Growth Factor

Vasculogenesis and angiogenesis are complex processes that require coordination between a number of growth factors and receptor systems that govern proliferation, chemotaxis, and morphogenesis (Table 1). A considerable amount of information has emerged in the last decade exploring the mechanism of action of these systems in vascular development. Thus, it is impossible to thoroughly explore every aspect of the subject in this chapter. Accordingly, a basic overview of the VEGF family has been given preference over other growth factors due to the fact that VEGF plays an irreplaceable role in the development of the vascular system. Thus, it should be considered that its biological function must always be placed in a provasculogenic or proangiogenic context of a plethora of endothelial and mural cell stimuli.

The VEGF system is absolutely required for differentiative, proliferative, and chemotactic responses in vasculogenic and angiogenic processes. This statement is highlighted

Table 1
Example of Molecules Governing Angiogenesis

	Putative roles		
Molecules	Proliferation	Chemotaxis	Morphogenesis
VEGF	Yes	Yes	Yes
PlGF	Weak	Yes	?
bFGF	Yes	Yes	Yes
PDGF	Yes	Yes	?
Angiopoietin-1	No	Yes	Yes
Nitric oxide	Yes	Yes	?
Integrin $\alpha v \beta 3$	Yes	Yes	Yes
MMP's	No	Yes	Yes
Akt	No	Yes	Yes
GM-CSF	Yes	Yes	?
HIF-1	Yes	Yes	Yes
TGF-β	Inhibition	No	Yes
VCAM-1	No	Yes	?
TNF-α	?	No	
Adrenomedullin	Yes	Yes	?

VEGF, vascular endothelial growth factor; PlGF, placenta growth factor; bFGF, basic fibroblast growth factor; PDGF, platelet-derived growth factor; MMPs, matrix metalloproteinases; GM-CSF, granulocyte-macrophage-colony stimulating factor; HIF- 1, hypoxia-inducible factor; TGF-β, transforming growth factor β; VCAM-1, vascular cell adhesion molecule-1; TNF-α, tumor necrosis factor-α *(3,8,15,26,47,66)*.

by the fact that embryos lacking a single VEGF allele presented abnormal blood vessel development *(13,14)*. The VEGF family comprises six known members of structurally related dimeric glycoproteins: VEGF-A, VEGF-B, VEGF-C, VEGF-D, VEGF-E (from orf parapox virus), and placental growth factor (PlGF). In addition, alternative exon splicing of the VEGF-A gene generates at least five VEGF isoforms, with 121, 145, 165, 189, or 206 amino acid residues with different bioavailability and with VEGF-A_{121} and VEGF-A_{165} being the most frequently expressed form. $VEGF_{121}$ does not bind heparin and is highly diffusible. In contrast, the higher-molecular-weight species (189 and 206 amino acid isoforms) contain increasingly basic and heparin-binding residues that mediate their sequestration in cellular membrane or in ECM from where they can be released by protease activation and cleavage *(15–18)*.

This family of growth factors binds and activates three VEGF transmembrane tyrosine kinase receptors: VEGFR-1 (Flt-1), VEGFR-2 (KDR/Flk-1), and VEGFR-3 (Flt- 4), which differ in their ligand specificities (Fig. 1). For example, VEGFR-1 is activated with VEGF-A, VEGF-B, and PlGF homodimers, whereas VEGFR-2 binds VEGF-A, VEGF-C, VEGF-D, and VEGF-E. These two receptors are predominantly expressed on vascular endothelium. By contrast VEGFR-3, which is localized mainly in lymphatic endothelial cells, binds VEGF-C and VEGF-D with high affinity. In addition, there are two more receptors that lack tyrosine kinase activity. The first is a soluble form of the VEGFR-1 (sVEGFR-1) and the second is a cell surface glycoprotein that has also been identified

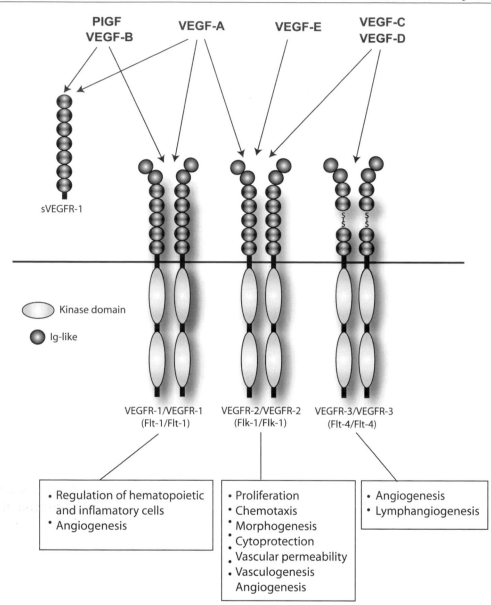

Fig. 1. Schematic overview of the VEGF family and their interaction with VEGF receptors. The VEGF family comprises six known members: VEGF-A, VEGF-B, VEGF-C, VEGF-D, VEGF-E, and placental growth factor (PlGF). This family of growth factors binds and activates three VEGF tyrosine kinase receptors: VEGFR-1 (Flt-1), VEGFR-2 (KDR/Flk-1), and VEGFR-3 (Flt-4), which differ in their ligand specificities and biological functions.

as the VEGF165 receptor, neuropilin-1. However, in contrast with the other VEGFRs, neuropilin is expressed abundantly by both endothelial and nonendothelial cells *(15,18)*.

Gene knockout studies for VEGFR-1 or VEGFR-2 have demonstrated that one of the most prominent defects in these mutant embryos is the incomplete development of the vasculature. Close analysis of the mutants revealed that embryos homozygous for the

VEGFR-2 gene were defective in vasculogenesis and failed to develop blood islands. By contrast, VEGFR-1 deficient embryos have endothelial cells, but showed a defective re-organization of endothelium into normal vascular channels, suggesting a differential mechanism of signal transduction between the two receptors (19–21). Effectively, numerous studies have shown that kinase activity of VEGFR-1 is low compared to VEGFR-2 (22). These findings have led to the hypothesis that VEGFR-1 plays a negative role by acting as a suppressing signaling receptor for the VEGF system. However, recent studies imply a positive regulatory role of VEGFR-1 in the regulation of hematopoietic and inflammatory cells (23). VEGF-C and VEGF-D regulate lymphangiogenesis, through their specific receptor activation (VEGFR-3), which has been linked to human hereditary lymphoedema (24). However, as occurs with VEGFR-1 and -2, VEGFR-3 appears to have an essential role in the development of functional vascular network during embryonary stages, when it is still expressed on endothelial cells. Gene-targeting studies have shown that VEGFR-3 knockout mice display early embryonic lethality due to cardiovascular failure and defects in maturation of large vessels (25).

Apart from a wide range of growth factors and cytokines, hypoxia is one of the major stimulators of VEGF-A production through both gene transcription and mRNA stabilization, thus providing a compensatory mechanism by which tissues can bypass an inadequate oxygen supply through the induction of vasculogenesis or angiogenesis (26).

BASIC MECHANISMS OF VASCULAR REMODELING

Many diseases affecting the mature cardiocirculatory system are associated with structural modifications of the vessel wall. Systemic and pulmonary hypertension, ischemia, atherosclerosis, arteriovenous fistula, and aneurysm are among the pathological conditions in which vascular remodeling phenomena have been well documented (27–30). This active process occurs in response to long-term modifications in hemodynamic conditions (28). The cellular signals involved in this process are not fully elucidated. However, it is widely recognized that, as the primary sensor of the hemodynamic changes, endothelial cells play a prominent role (27,30). Recent advances in the understanding of the mechanisms that govern structural modifications of blood vessels during collateral vessel growth and chronic changes in blood flow will be discussed.

Collateral Circulation

Native collateral circulation is an effective resource system constituted by preexisting arterioles that increase in size after stenosis or increased tissular resistance to blood flow. The aim of this rescue system is to protect tissues from the harmful effects of hypoxia and ischemia acting as new conductance blood vessels. It is worth noting that in the last few decades, the concept that describes collaterals as a passive network of preexisting blood vessels has been modified by a more dynamic definition. Nowadays, a vast majority of publications have demonstrated that collateral vessels have an adaptive and active growth depending on blood perfusion deficits (7,31,32). However, the dynamic phenomenon of collateral growth is not necessarily included within the definition of angiogenesis because distinct patterns of mechanisms coordinate each process separately. This affirmation is based on the facts that first, the morphology of collateral vessels (preexisting mature arterioles or venules which differentiate into functional arteries or venules) contrast with the definition of angiogenesis (which is the formation of new capillaries from a preexisting capillary network). Second, collateral growth is not dependent on hypoxic conditions, and third, collateral vessel growth is absolutely dependent on inflammatory stimuli whereas angiogenesis may also occur with noninflammatory conditions *(7,32)*.

Endothelial cells not only have an essential role in vasculogenesis and angiogenesis, but their activation is also a necessary step in collateral vessel growth. Further insight into these complex mechanisms has come from studies showing that increased flow velocity in collaterals after decompression of the vascular system is associated with augmented shear stress (defined as the frictional wall pressure promoted by a laminal flow pattern), which is the trigger factor for endothelial cell activation *(33–35)*. Although the precise mechanism as to how endothelium is able to sense shear stress is still unclear, it is known that this process mediates regulation of gene transcription through shear stress–responsive elements, such as endothelial NOS and some cytokines *(36,37)*, located in the promoter regions of various genes. As a result of endothelium activation, monocyte chemotactic protein-1 (MCP-1), granulocyte-macrophage colony-stimulating factor (GM-CSF), and endothelial surface receptors are expressed in endothelial cells promoting the recruitment of circulating monocytes to the vascular wall, which is an obligatory step in collateral growth. After activated monocytes adhere and invade the blood vessel, an inflammatory environment is locally created [composed of bFGF, tumor necrosis factor-α (TNF-α), PDGF-B, TGF-β1, fibronectin, metalloproteinases and plasmin, among other factors], thereby inducing the remodeling of the extracellular matrix and allowing vessel enlargement through endothelial and smooth muscle cell growth *(3,13,31,32)*.

NO and Vascular Remodeling

Endothelial cells provide a large surface area that functions as a transductor of mechanical stimuli into biochemical events that regulate vascular tone and structure *(28,33, 38,39)*. The identification of the biological factor that acts as a link between sensing and transduction of signals has been widely studied and although this/these factor/s have not been fully characterized, it is obvious that NO produced by the endothelium has many of the requirements that fulfill the condition of being a mediator of vessel remodeling. This concept is supported by studies in eNOS knockout mice that were performed to analyze the role of eNOS in vivo. This gene disruption resulted in fertile, viable eNOS–/– with a hypertensive phenotype an increase in smooth muscle cell growth in response to vascular injury, predisposition to form neointimal proliferation, and a poor response to growth factor–stimulated angiogenesis *(40–42)*. In addition, several studies in endothelial cells have demonstrated that frictional wall pressure promoted by a laminal flow of blood causes the activation of eNOS and induces its gene expression *(43,44)*. Recently, several reports have convincingly indicated that eNOS activity controls vascular remodeling in vivo *(30,45)*. Following a chronic increase in arterial pressure, the vascular wall undergoes important changes, including augmentation of the muscle mass, rearrangement of cells, augmentation of the wall thickness, and diminution of the vessel lumen. Conversely, a maintained reduction in blood flow usually results in a diminution of the muscular mass of the vessel *(28)*. Consequently, Rudic et al. *(30)* demonstrated that ligation of the left external carotid artery in wild-type mice was associated with a reduction in lumen diameter and smooth muscle cell number of the ipsilateral common carotid artery. By contrast, the ligation of the left external carotid artery in eNOS knockout mice did not correlate with a reduction in lumen diameter in the vessel sensing the remodeling stimulus. In addition, vessel wall thickness in abnormally remodeled vessels from eNOS knockout mice were thicker because of an increase in smooth muscle cell proliferation. Similar results were reported by Moroi et al., assessing the response to injury in a model of cuff placement around the femoral artery of mice that mimics features of human atherosclerosis. In wild-type animals, cuff placement causes a pronounced and reproducible intimal proliferation that was calculated based on the ratio between the thickness of the intima and media. Interestingly, this pathophysiological response was greatly exaggerated in eNOS knockout mice that had a much greater degree of intimal growth (45). These studies confirm that eNOS is required as a sensor for physiological vascular adaptation to blood flow and, thus, impaired NO production in blood vessels can promote abnormal vascular remodeling that may be responsible for pathological changes in vessel wall morphology.

PATHOPHYSIOLOGICAL INDUCTION OF LONG-TERM STRUCTURAL VASCULAR CHANGES IN PORTAL HYPERTENSION

Angiogenesis

Angiogenesis and structural alterations in the blood vessels are of major importance under circumstances of adult tissue repair and remodeling such as wound healing, bone repair, ischemic heart and peripheral vascular disease, tumor growth, and metastasis (7, 9). Therefore, no doubts have been raised as to the existence of important angiogenic processes in the human cirrhotic liver with a superimposed hypervascular tumor such as hepatocellular carcinoma. However, whether these changes also occur in advanced liver disease in the absence of hepatic tumorogenic activity has been the subject of discussion for the last decades. This possibility is supported by several observations showing that portal hypertensive rats do experience angiogenic processes. Prominent persistent abnormalities in the microangioarchitecture of gastric mucosa of portal vein ligated rats have been described, which could explain the hypertrophic gastropathy observed in cirrhotic patients (46). Moreover, in vivo mesenteric angiogenesis assays have shown that portal hypertension is accompanied by a significant increased in NO-dependent angiogenesis (47,48), in agreement with the fact that NO is recognized as an important in vivo and in vitro angiogenic substance. Intravital microscopy studies have also found that following partial portal vein ligation, an extensive neovascularization occurs in the rat hepatic arterial system (49). On the other hand, increased angiogenesis and permeability has very recently been reported in the peritoneal circulation of rats with portal hypertension and cirrhosis (50).

ACTIVATION OF ANGIOGENIC FACTORS

Ascites is the most common complication of patients with advanced liver disease and consists in the accumulation of fluid in the peritoneal cavity (51). Ascites has the characteristic of a transudate, with a protein concentration ranging from 0.5 to more than 6 g/dL, and contains mesothelial cells, leukocytes, and red blood cells (52). Because of this relatively simple composition, ascites has generally been considered to have little influence on the hemodynamic, renal, and host defense abnormalities occurring in cirrhotic patients. This concept, however, has recently been challenged by several investigations describing significant amounts of proinflammatory cytokines, growth factors, vasoactive agents, or extracellular matrix-forming proteins in ascites of human cirrhotics (53–58). In addition, several studies have demonstrated that the cellular component of ascites might, to a great extent, influence the concentration of these substances. Under proper stimulus, resident cells in the peritoneal cavity could regulate nonspecific immune response and vascular permeability and angiogenesis in this area, or in adjacent territories such as the splanchnic vascular bed. For example, peritoneal macrophages of cirrhotic patients are able to markedly increase VEGF-A protein secretion into ascites in response to cytokines and lipopolysaccharide treatment (Fig. 2) or hypoxic stimulation (59,60). Interestingly enough, this seems to be a specific characteristic of resident macrophages of cirrhotic patients because this response was not reproduced by peripheral blood monocytes isolated from healthy subjects. All these conditions may be present during the natural history of decompensated cirrhosis and, accordingly, overproduction of NO, VEGF-A, and adrenomedulin (ADM) has been described in peritoneal macrophages from cirrhotic patients (59–61).

Spontaneous bacterial peritonitis (SBP) is a relatively common, severe complication of patients with cirrhosis and ascites (62). Ascites of SBP patients contains larger amounts of cytokines than that of cirrhotics without peritonitis (63). These patients commonly develop an accentuation of the circulatory dysfunction already present before infection. The mechanisms underlying this life-threatening complication are poorly known although the implication of some local factor/s mainly acting on the splanchnic vasculature could be suspected, because arteriolar vasodilation and increased vessel permeability mainly occurs in this territory (64). This hypothesis has been fueled by investigations showing that peritoneal macrophages of SBP patients also express and produce significant amounts of NO and VEGF (61,65). In fact, when peritoneal macrophages of cirrhotic patients with SBP are cultured in vitro; they release detectable amounts of NO and produce huge quantities of VEGF, although cells from noninfected patients with ascites do not produce NO and release significantly lower quantities of VEGF. Furthermore, peritoneal macrophages from cirrhotic patients with SBP, express the iNOS mRNA and protein whereas those obtained from ascites of patients without peritonitis do not (61). VEGF mRNA and protein expression are higher in peritoneal macrophages of patients with SBP that in noninfected cirrhotics, as well. Moreover, enhanced endothelial cell proliferation induced by conditioned medium of macrophages isolated from the ascites of SBP patients is abolished by anti-VEGF antibody and peritoneal tissue of cirrhotic patients expresses both VEGF receptors, Flt-1 and KDR (65). These results are consistent with the concept that locally released VEGF may result in increased vascular proliferation and linkage in peritoneal vessels of cirrhotics with SBP.

Hypoxia has also been demonstrated to be an inducer of vasodilator agents with angiogenic properties in human peritoneal macrophages. In vitro studies recently showed that an O_2 tension within the range of that found in the ascites fluid is able to promote the synthesis of VEGF and ADM in macrophages of cirrhotic patients, likely through HIF-1 enhanced transcriptional activity (59). Thus, this study lends support to the notion that hypoxia-induced release of ADM and VEGF in peritoneal macrophages may serve as an endogenous mediator of vascular neoformation and angiogenesis in human cirrhosis.

Collectively, these data indicate that ascites is, under different pathological circumstances, a liquid containing remarkable concentrations of substances with proangiogenic properties, suggesting, therefore, that ascites accumulation in the peritoneal cavity may markedly influence the structure and development of the circulatory tree in this territory. In this regard, recent in vivo and in vitro experiments have demonstrated that ascites of cirrhotic patients behaves as a powerful inducer of angiogenesis, a phenomenon in which activation of the phosphoinositide 3-kinase/AKT signaling pathway seems to be of major relevance (66).

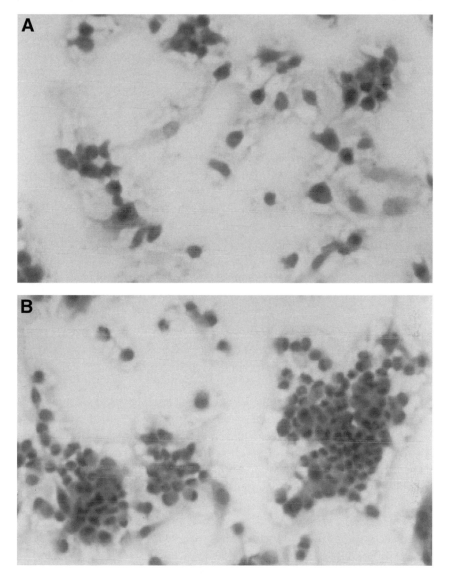

Fig. 2. Immunocytochemical localization of VEGF-A protein in human peritoneal macrophages. Cells were obtained by paracentesis, centrifuged, and seeded on slides. After fixation, cells were stained for VEGF-A. (**A**) Peritoneal macrophages of a cirrhotic patient cultured for 48 h. (**B**) Peritoneal macrophages of the same patient cultured for 48 h in the presence of tumor necrosis factor-α, interleukin-1β, and lipopolysaccharide (original magnification ×400). Reprinted with permission from ref. *65*.

Vascular Collateralization

The development of portal–systemic collateral vessels between the portal vasculature and the systemic venous system is one of the major causes of complications of portal hypertension. However, it has been a matter of discussion whether the development of the portal collateral venous system is exclusively dependent on portal pressure or portal venous inflow. In this regard, early work by Halvorsen et al. *(67)* proposed that collateral vessels arise from the passive dilatation of preexisting venous channels in portal vein–

ligated rats. More recently, increased flow and pressure through preexisting collateral vessels have been shown in mice with schistosomiasis, a natural disease model of portal hypertension (68). It should be noted, however, that this is not a passive phenomenon merely explained by the increased pressure in the intrahepatic vascular tree. As in other territories, the endothelial cell monolayer accurately regulates vessel tonicity in this area. In situ portal–systemic collateral perfusion models have demonstrated that the NO synthase activity inhibitor, L-NNA, prevents the acethylcholine-induced dilatation of the collaterals in portal hypertensive rats (69). Further indications for a role of NO in the regulation of collateral circulation development and function have arisen from studies performed by two independent laboratories showing that NO inhibition reduces portal–systemic shunting and enhances the constrictive response of collateral vessels to vasopressin, without affecting portal pressure (70,71). Finally, antiangiogenic treatments have proven to be efficacious in reducing the formation of portal systemic collateral vessels and splanchnic vasodilation in portal hypertensive rats (72). Therefore, there is a substantial amount of information strongly indicating that, in addition to the opening of preexisting vessels, development of collateral channels or shunts in portal hypertension is also associated with active mechanisms promoting vascular neoformation and angiogenesis.

Vascular Remodeling in Conductance Vessels

Reduced arterial pressure, high cardiac output, low peripheral resistance, endothelial dysfunction, altered vascular reactivity, and increased circulating levels of endogenous vasoactive substances are characteristic features in advanced liver disease (1,73). In most cases, this marked cardiovascular dysfunction develops over a long period of time, thus making the existence of vascular remodeling processes in the circulatory tree of patients with decompensated cirrhosis extremely likely. Because endothelium-derived NO plays a central role in regulating the structure of the vessel wall, this contention is further supported by numerous investigations showing increased NO-dependent vasorelaxation (74), higher production of endothelium-derived NO (75), and increased vascular expression of eNOS mRNA and protein (73) in humans and rats with cirrhosis.

Studies performed in rats with CCl_4-induced cirrhosis and ascites recently demonstrated that these animals undergo an intense process of vascular remodeling (76). The most remarkable features of this phenomenon are a decrease in the thickness and the total area of the vascular wall (Fig. 3). In addition, a reduction in the vascular production of NO resulted in a significant improvement in the architectural distortions observed in the arterial vessels of these animals indicating that endothelium-derived NO also has an important role in the control of vascular morphology in experimental cirrhosis. These results also raise the hypothesis that the hyperdynamic circulation in cirrhosis, results in a chronic increase in endothelium-derived NO in large conductive vessels which promotes an important architectural modification in structure of these vessels further contributing to the aggravation of the circulatory dysfunction already existing in this disease.

ACKNOWLEDGMENTS

This work was supported by Grants from the Ministerio de Ciencia y Tecnología (SAF 99-0016, SAF 2001-2585, SAF 2003-02597), the Fondo de Investigación Sanitaria (01/ 1514), and Fundació la Marató de TV3 (000610). M. Morales-Ruiz is an investigator of the Programa Ramón y Cajal (Ministerio de Ciencia y Tecnología).

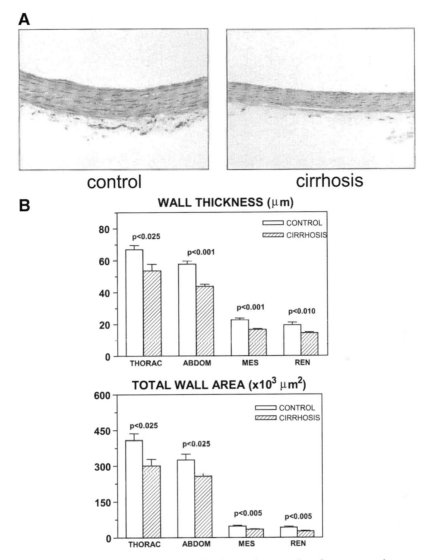

Fig. 3. Vascular remodeling in cirrhotic rats. (**A**) Photomicrographs of representative cross sections of aorta from a control rat and a cirrhotic rat with ascites. Note the marked reduction in wall thickness and the diminution in the number of nuclei in the cirrhotic vessel (H&E staining; original magnifications, ×200). (**B**) Wall thickness, and total wall area in control rats and in cirrhotic rats with ascites. THORAC, thoracic aorta; ABDOM, abdominal aorta; MES, mesenteric artery; REN, renal artery. Data are mean ± SE. Reprinted with permission from ref. *76*.

REFERENCES

1. Arroyo V, Jimenez W. Complications of cirrhosis. II. Renal and circulatory dysfunction. Lights and shadows in an important clinical problem. J Hepatol 2000;32(1 Suppl):157–170.
2. Bosch J, Garcia-Pagan JC. Pathophysiology of portal hypertension and its complications. In: Bircher J, Benhamou JP, McIntyre N, Rizzetto M, Rodes J, eds. Oxford Textbook of Clinical Hepatology. Oxford University Press, New York, 1999, pp. 653–660.
3. Carmeliet P. Mechanisms of angiogenesis and arteriogenesis. Nat Med 2000;6(4):389–395.
4. Risau W, Flamme I. Vasculogenesis. Annu Rev Cell Dev Biol 1995;11:73–91.

5. Asahara T, Murohara T, Sullivan A, Silver M, van der ZR, Li T, et al. Isolation of putative progenitor endothelial cells for angiogenesis. Science 1997;275(5302):964–967.
6. Rafii S, Lyden D. Therapeutic stem and progenitor cell transplantation for organ vascularization and regeneration. Nat Med 2003;9(6):702–712.
7. Carmeliet P. Angiogenesis in health and disease. Nat Med 2003;9(6):653–660.
8. Ferrara N, Alitalo K. Clinical applications of angiogenic growth factors and their inhibitors. Nat Med 1999;5(12):1359–1364.
9. Folkman J. Angiogenesis in cancer, vascular, rheumatoid and other disease. Nat Med 1995;1(1):27–31.
10. Hyder SM, Stancel GM. Regulation of angiogenic growth factors in the female reproductive tract by estrogens and progestins. Mol Endocrinol 1999;13(6):806–811.
11. Risau W. Mechanisms of angiogenesis. Nature 1997;386(6626):671–674.
12. Djonov V, Baum O, Burri PH. Vascular remodeling by intussusceptive angiogenesis. Cell Tissue Res 2003;314(1):107–117.
13. Carmeliet P, Ferreira V, Breier G, et al. Abnormal blood vessel development and lethality in embryos lacking a single VEGF allele. Nature 1996;380(6573):435–439.
14. Ferrara N, Carver-Moore K, Chen H, et al. Heterozygous embryonic lethality induced by targeted inactivation of the VEGF gene. Nature 1996;380(6573):439–442.
15. Ferrara N. Vascular endothelial growth factor: molecular and biological aspects. Curr Top Microbiol Immunol 1999;237:1–30.
16. Meyer M, Clauss M, Lepple-Wienhues A, et al. A novel vascular endothelial growth factor encoded by Orf virus, VEGFE, mediates angiogenesis via signalling through VEGFR-2 (KDR) but not VEGFR-1 (Flt-1) receptor tyrosine kinases. EMBO J 1999;18(2):363–374.
17. Ogawa S, Oku A, Sawano A, Yamaguchi S, Yazaki Y, Shibuya M. A novel type of vascular endothelial growth factor, VEGF-E (NZ-7 VEGF), preferentially utilizes KDR/Flk-1 receptor and carries a potent mitotic activity without heparinbinding domain. J Biol Chem 1998;273(47):31,273–31,282.
18. Veikkola T, Alitalo K. VEGFs, receptors and angiogenesis. Semin Cancer Biol 1999;9(3):211–220.
19. Fong GH, Rossant J, Gertsenstein M, Breitman ML. Role of the Flt-1 receptor tyrosine kinase in regulating the assembly of vascular endothelium. Nature 1995;376(6535):66–70.
20. Fong GH, Zhang L, Bryce DM, Peng J. Increased hemangioblast commitment, not vascular disorganization, is the primary defect in flt-1 knock-out mice. Development 1999;126(13):3015–3025.
21. Shalaby F, Rossant J, Yamaguchi TP, et al. Failure of blood-island formation and vasculogenesis in Flk-1-deficient mice. Nature 1995;376(6535):62–66.
22. Shibuya M, Ito N, Claesson-Welsh L. Structure and function of vascular endothelial growth factor receptor-1 and -2. Curr Top Microbiol Immunol 1999;237:59–83.
23. Luttun A, Tjwa M, Moons L, et al. Revascularization of ischemic tissues by PlGF treatment, and inhibition of tumor angiogenesis, arthritis and atherosclerosis by anti-Flt1. Nat Med 2002;8(8):831–840.
24. Jeltsch M, Tammela T, Alitalo K, Wilting J. Genesis and pathogenesis of lymphatic vessels. Cell Tissue Res 2003;314(1):69–84.
25. Dumont DJ, Jussila L, Taipale J, et al. Cardiovascular failure in mouse embryos deficient in VEGF receptor-3. Science 1998;282(5390):946–949.
26. Pugh CW, Ratcliffe PJ. Regulation of angiogenesis by hypoxia: role of the HIF system. Nat Med 2003; 9(6):677–684.
27. Dzau VJ, Horiuchi M. Vascular remodeling—the emerging paradigm of programmed cell death (apoptosis): the Francis B. Parker lectureship. Chest 1998;114(1 Suppl):91S–99S.
28. Gibbons GH, Dzau VJ. The emerging concept of vascular remodeling. N Engl J Med 1994;330(20): 1431–1438.
29. Mulvany MJ. Vascular remodelling of resistance vessels: can we define this? Cardiovasc Res 1999; 41(1):9–13.
30. Rudic RD, Shesely EG, Maeda N, Smithies O, Segal SS, Sessa WC. Direct evidence for the importance of endothelium-derived nitric oxide in vascular remodeling. J Clin Invest 1998;101(4):731–736.
31. Schaper W, Pasyk S. Influence of collateral flow on the ischemic tolerance of the heart following acute and subacute coronary occlusion. Circulation 1976;53(3 Suppl):I57–I62.
32. Schaper W, Ito WD. Molecular mechanisms of coronary collateral vessel growth. Circ Res 1996;79(5): 911–919.

33. Kamiya A, Togawa T. Adaptive regulation of wall shear stress to flow change in the canine carotid artery. Am J Physiol 1980;239(1):H14–H21.

34. Unthank JL, Fath SW, Burkhart HM, Miller SC, Dalsing MC. Wall remodeling during luminal expansion of mesenteric arterial collaterals in the rat. Circ Res 1996;79(5):1015–1023.

35. Zarins CK, Zatina MA, Giddens DP, Ku DN, Glagov S. Shear stress regulation of artery lumen diameter in experimental atherogenesis. J Vasc Surg 1987;5(3):413–420.

36. Lehoux S, Tedgui A. Cellular mechanics and gene expression in blood vessels. J Biomech 2003;36(5): 631–643.

37. Shyy JY, Chien S. Role of integrins in endothelial mechanosensing of shear stress. Circ Res 2002;91(9): 769–775.

38. Davies PF. Flow-mediated endothelial mechanotransduction. Physiol Rev 1995;75(3):519–560.

39. Kohler TR, Kirkman TR, Kraiss LW, Zierler BK, Clowes AW. Increased blood flow inhibits neointimal hyperplasia in endothelialized vascular grafts. Circ Res 1991;69(6):1557–1565.

40. Lee PC, Salyapongse AN, Bragdon GA, et al. Impaired wound healing and angiogenesis in eNOS-deficient mice. Am J Physiol 1999;277(4 Pt 2):H1600–H1608.

41. Murohara T, Asahara T, Silver M, et al. Nitric oxide synthase modulates angiogenesis in response to tissue ischemia. J Clin Invest 1998;101(11):2567–2578.

42. Shesely EG, Maeda N, Kim HS, et al. Elevated blood pressures in mice lacking endothelial nitric oxide synthase. Proc Natl Acad Sci USA 1996;93(23):13,176–13,181.

43. Awolesi MA, Sessa WC, Sumpio BE. Cyclic strain upregulates nitric oxide synthase in cultured bovine aortic endothelial cells. J Clin Invest 1995;96(3):1449–1454.

44. Uematsu M, Ohara Y, Navas JP, et al. Regulation of endothelial cell nitric oxide synthase mRNA expression by shear stress. Am J Physiol 1995;269(6 Pt 1):C1371–C1378.

45. Moroi M, Zhang L, Yasuda T, et al. Interaction of genetic deficiency of endothelial nitric oxide, gender, and pregnancy in vascular response to injury in mice. J Clin Invest 1998;101(6):1225–1232.

46. Albillos A, Colombato LA, Enriquez R, Ng OC, Sikuler E, Groszmann RJ. Sequence of morphological and hemodynamic changes of gastric microvessels in portal hypertension. Gastroenterology 1992; 102(6):2066–2070.

47. Sieber CC, Sumanovski LT, Stumm M, Van der KM, Battegay E. In vivo angiogenesis in normal and portal hypertensive rats: role of basic fibroblast growth factor and nitric oxide. J Hepatol 2001;34(5): 644–650.

48. Sumanovski LT, Battegay E, Stumm M, Van der KM, Sieber CC. Increased angiogenesis in portal hypertensive rats: role of nitric oxide. Hepatology 1999;29(4):1044–1049.

49. Yokoyama Y, Baveja R, Sonin N, Clemens MG, Zhang JX. Hepatic neovascularization after partial portal vein ligation: novel mechanism of chronic regulation of blood flow. Am J Physiol Gastrointest Liver Physiol 2001;280(1):G21–G31.

50. Geerts A, Colle I, De Vriese A, et al. Increased angiogenesis and permeability in the peritoneal microcirculation of rats with portal hypertension and cirrhosis. J Hepatol 2004 (Abstract).

51. Arroyo V, Gines P, Jimenez W, Rodes J. Ascites, renal failure, and electrolyte disorders in cirrhosis. Pathogenesis, diagnosis and treatment. In: McIntyre N, Benhamou JP, Bircher J, Rizzetto M, Rodes J, eds. Textbook of Clinical Hepatology. Oxford University Press, Oxford, 1991, pp. 427–470.

52. Hoefs JC. Characteristics of ascites. In: Arroyo V, Gines P, Rodes J, Schrier RW, eds. Ascites and Renal Dysfunction in Liver Disease: Pathogenesis, Diagnosis and Treatment. Blackwell Science, Malden, MA, 1999, pp. 14–35.

53. Gerbes AL, Jungst D, Xie YN, Permanetter W, Paumgartner G. Ascitic fluid analysis for the differentiation of malignancy-related and nonmalignant ascites. Proposal of a diagnostic sequence. Cancer 1991; 68(8):1808–1814.

54. Jin-no K, Tanimizu M, Hyodo I, Kurimoto F, Yamashita T. Plasma level of basic fibroblast growth factor increases with progression of chronic liver disease. J Gastroenterol 1997;32(1):119–121.

55. Martinez-Bru C, Gomez C, Cortes M, et al. Ascitic fluid interleukin-8 to distinguish spontaneous bacterial peritonitis and sterile ascites in cirrhotic patients. Clin Chem 1999;45(11):2027–2028.

56. Mesquita RC, Leite-Mor MM, Parise ER. Fibronectin in the ascitic fluid of cirrhotic patients: correlation with biochemical risk factors for the development of spontaneous bacterial peritonitis. Braz J Med Biol Res 1997;30(7):843–847.

57. Navasa M, Follo A, Filella X, et al. Tumor necrosis factor and interleukin-6 in spontaneous bacterial peritonitis in cirrhosis: relationship with the development of renal impairment and mortality. Hepatology 1998;27(5):1227–1232.
58. Shimizu I, Ichihara A, Nakamura T. Hepatocyte growth factor in ascites from patients with cirrhosis. J Biochem (Tokyo) 1991;109(1):14–18.
59. Cejudo-Martin P, Morales-Ruiz M, Ros J, et al. Hypoxia is an inducer of vasodilator agents in peritoneal macrophages of cirrhotic patients. Hepatology 2002;36(5):1172–1179.
60. Perez-Ruiz M, Ros J, Morales-Ruiz M, et al. Vascular endothelial growth factor production in peritoneal macrophages of cirrhotic patients: regulation by cytokines and bacterial lipopolysaccharide. Hepatology 1999;29(4):1057–1063.
61. Jimenez W, Ros J, Morales-Ruiz M, et al. Nitric oxide production and inducible nitric oxide synthase expression in peritoneal macrophages of cirrhotic patients. Hepatology 1999;30(3):670–676.
62. Hall JC, Heel KA, Papadimitriou JM, Platell C. The pathobiology of peritonitis. Gastroenterology 1998; 114(1):185–196.
63. Rimola A, Navasa M. Infections in liver disease. In: Bircher J, Benhamou JP, McIntyre N, Rizzetto M, Rodes J, eds. Oxford Textbook of Clinical Hepatology. Oxford University Press, Oxford, 1999, pp. 1862–1874.
64. Guarner C, Soriano G. Spontaneous bacterial peritonitis. Semin Liver Dis 1997;17(3):203–217.
65. Cejudo-Martin P, Ros J, Navasa M, et al. Increased production of vascular endothelial growth factor in peritoneal macrophages of cirrhotic patients with spontaneous bacterial peritonitis. Hepatology 2001; 34(3):487–493.
66. Morales-Ruiz M, Cejudo-Martin P, Ros J, et al. Ascites from cirrhotic patients is an in vitro and in vivo inducer of angiogenesis through the activation of the phosphoinositide 3-kinase (PI3-k)/Akt signalling pathway. Hepatology 2002;36:139A (Abstract).
67. Halvorsen JF, Myking AO. The porto-systemic collateral pattern in the rat. An angiographic and anatomical study after partial occlusion of the portal vein. Eur Surg Res 1974;6(3):183–195.
68. Sarin SK, Groszmann RJ, Mosca PG, et al. Propranolol ameliorates the development of portal-systemic shunting in a chronic murine schistosomiasis model of portal hypertension. J Clin Invest 1991; 87(3):1032–1036.
69. Mosca P, Lee FY, Kaumann AJ, Groszmann RJ. Pharmacology of portalsystemic collaterals in portal hypertensive rats: role of endothelium. Am J Physiol 1992;263(4 Pt 1):G544–G550.
70. Chan CC, Lee FY, Wang SS, et al. Effects of vasopressin on portal-systemic collaterals in portal hypertensive rats: role of nitric oxide and prostaglandin. Hepatology 1999;30(3):630–635.
71. Lee FY, Colombato LA, Albillos A, Groszmann RJ. Administration of N omeganitro-L-arginine ameliorates portal-systemic shunting in portal-hypertensive rats. Gastroenterology 1993;105(5):1464–1470.
72. Fernandez M, Vizzutti F, Garcia-Pagan JL, Rodes J, Bosch J. Anti-VEGF receptor-2 monoclonal antibody prevents portal-systemic collateral vessel formation in portal hypertensive mice. Gastroenterology 2004;126(3):886–894.
73. Morales-Ruiz M, Jimenez W, Perez-Sala D, et al. Increased nitric oxide synthase expression in arterial vessels of cirrhotic rats with ascites. Hepatology 1996;24(6):1481–1486.
74. Claria J, Jimenez W, Ros J, et al. Increased nitric oxide-dependent vasorelaxation in aortic rings of cirrhotic rats with ascites. Hepatology 1994;20(6):1615–1621.
75. Ros J, Jimenez W, Lamas S, et al. Nitric oxide production in arterial vessels of cirrhotic rats. Hepatology 1995;21(2):554–560.
76. Fernandez-Varo G, Ros J, Morales-Ruiz M, et al. Nitric oxide synthase 3-dependent vascular remodeling and circulatory dysfunction in cirrhosis. Am J Pathol 2003;162(6):1985–1993.

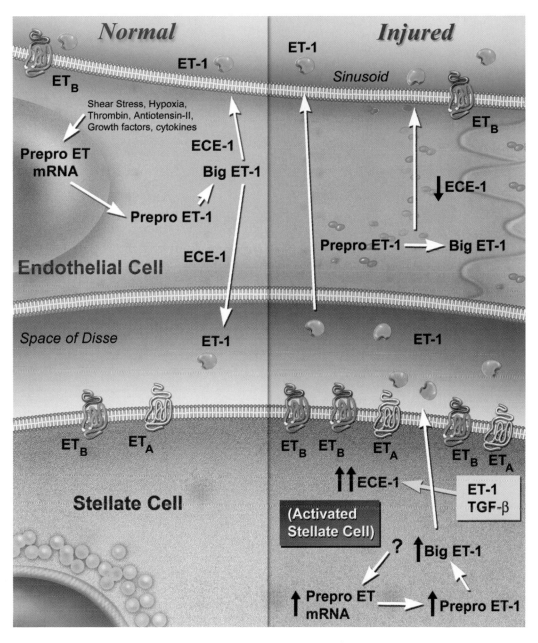

Color Plate 1, Fig. 1. (*See* full caption and discussion in Ch. 3, p. 41). Endothelin synthesis in normal and injured liver.

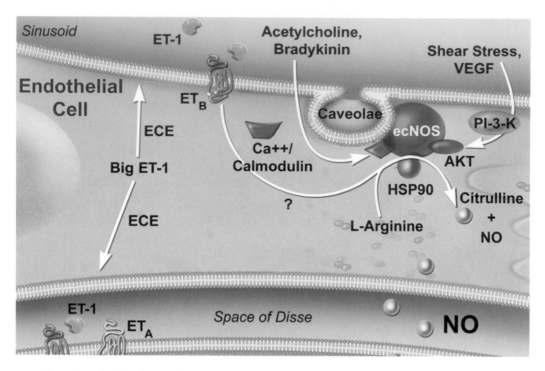

Color Plate 2, Fig. 2. (*See* full caption and discussion in Ch. 3, p. 43). Signaling pathways in sinusoidal endothelial cells.

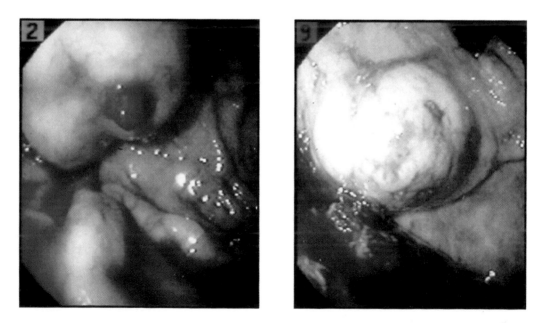

Color Plate 3, Fig. 2. (*See* caption and discussion in Ch. 18, p. 273). Gastric varices. Actively bleeding gastric varix (left panel); the same gastric varix after injection of cyanoacrylate (right panel).

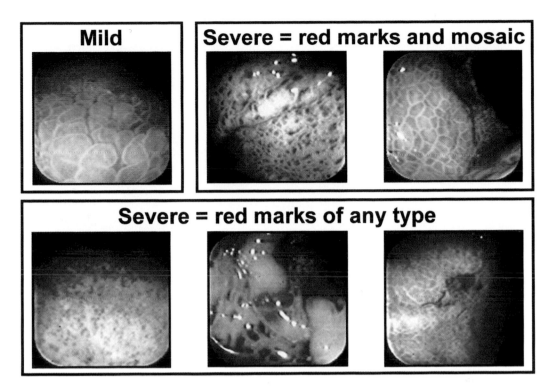

Color Plate 4, Fig. 3. (*See* full caption and discussion in Ch. 18, p. 273). Severity of portal hypertensive garstopathy.

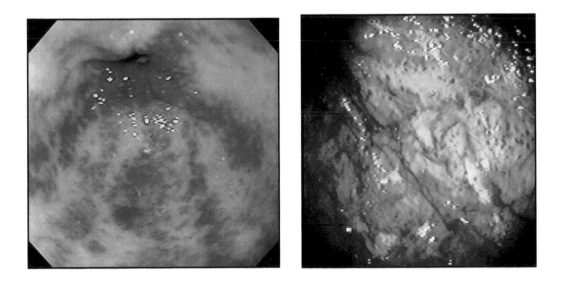

Color Plate 5, Fig. 4 (Left) *(see* full caption and discussion in Ch. 18, p. 274). Endothelin synthesis in normal and injured liver. **Fig. 5 (Right)** (see full caption and discussion in Ch. 18. p. 275). Diffuse gastric vascular ectasia.

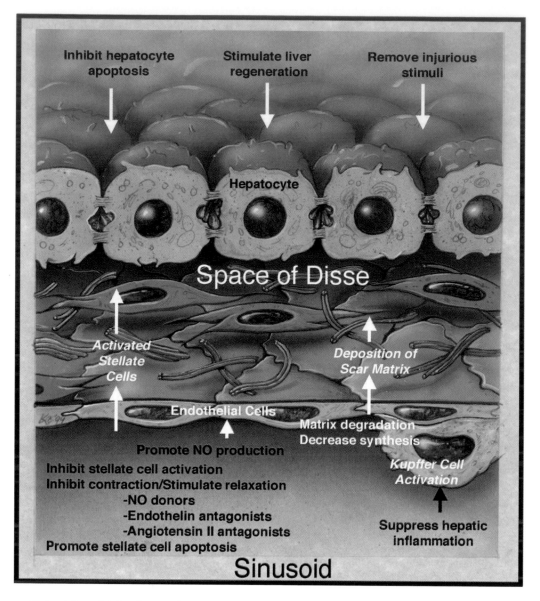

Color Plate 6, Fig. 2. (*See* full caption and discussion in Ch. 29, p. 488). Potential targets for antifibrotics and agents that modulate intrahepatic vascular resistance.

8

Mechanisms of Cardiopulmonary Hemodynamics and Dysfunction in Portal Hypertension

Michael B. Fallon, MD

CONTENTS

INTRODUCTION
CIRRHOTIC CARDIOMYOPATHY
HEPATOPULMONARY SYNDROME
PORTOPULMONARY HYPERTENSION
CONCLUSION
REFERENCES

INTRODUCTION

The concept that chronic liver disease and portal hypertension are accompanied by widespread alterations in vascular tone that have important clinical consequences has developed over the last 50 yr and relevant mechanisms for systemic vascular changes are outlined in Chapter 5. However, it has been only over the last 15 yr that specific cardiopulmonary abnormalities associated with the presence of liver disease and portal hypertension have been widely appreciated and submitted to investigation. These abnormalities include cirrhotic cardiomyopathy and two distinct alterations in the pulmonary vasculature: the hepatopulmonary syndrome (HPS) characterized by microvascular dilatation and portopulmonary hypertension (POPH) characterized by vasoconstriction and remodeling. These entities may share pathogenetic mechanisms with systemic vascular alterations and with each other, although each has unique features. Here, we will address our current understanding of the pathogenesis of these cardiopulmonary complications of portal hypertension.

CIRRHOTIC CARDIOMYOPATHY

Clinical Studies

Following the recognition of the hyperdynamic circulatory state in liver disease, studies performed in alcoholic cirrhosis *(1,2)* revealed a subnormal cardiac contractile response

From: *Clinical Gastroenterology: Portal Hypertension*
Edited by: A. J. Sanyal and V. H. Shah © Humana Press Inc., Totowa, NJ

in situations of increased demand. The initial assumption was that alcohol was the cause of the observed cardiac dysfunction. Over the last 20 yr, it has been established that the cardiac response to physiologic and pharmacologic stresses may be impaired in many different etiologies of human cirrhosis and also in experimental models (for review, see refs. *3* and *4)*. These observations have resulted in the recognition that a unique form of high output cardiac dysfunction occurs in liver disease. Cardiac dysfunction is often mild or latent in cirrhosis, a finding some have attributed to the afterload-reducing effects of systemic vasodilatation that decrease cardiac work *(5)*. Impairment in both systolic function under stress and diastolic filling have been reported in humans *(6–9)*. Cardiac abnormalities have been found commonly in both compensated and decompensated liver disease and in noncirrhotic portal fibrosis *(6–10)*, but no studies have evaluated prehepatic portal hypertensive patients.

Experimental Studies

The pathogenesis of abnormalities in cardiac function in liver disease has largely been investigated in experimental models and a number of alterations have been described. In carbon tetrachloride–induced cirrhosis, cardiac output fails to rise after volume loading *(11)* and in common bile duct ligation (CBDL) cirrhosis and partial portal vein ligation (PVL), blunted chronotropic responses to β-adrenergic agonists are observed *(12,13)*. These findings are similar to the impaired systolic function under stress seen in human studies. The finding that both prehepatic portal hypertension and cirrhosis models have altered cardiac responses to stress suggests that portal hypertension may be an important underlying event. However, the cardiac abnormalities described in PVL animals differ from those seen in cirrhosis models. Specific alterations described in cardiac myocytes in these experimental models are summarized below (Fig. 1).

β-ADRENERGIC RECEPTOR SIGNALING

Alterations in cardiac myocyte β-adrenergic signaling have been found in human and CBDL cirrhosis *(12,14,15)* and correlate with the blunted cardiac responsiveness to agonists. Specifically in CBDL, a decrease in β-adrenergic receptor and stimulatory G_S-protein membrane levels and function *(16)*, uncoupling of the receptor–ligand complex from G-protein *(15)* and decreased activity of adenylate cyclase have been found *(16, 17)*. Some of the functional changes have been attributed to altered myocyte membrane fluidity *(17)*. These results were not accompanied by compensatory increases in cardiac muscarinic receptors *(18)*. In contrast, in PVL animals, the decrease in responsiveness to β-adrenergic agonists was not associated with the above alterations but was associated with downstream effects on cellular calcium signaling (see below, *19–21*).

CELLULAR CALCIUM AND POTASSIUM KINETICS

Cardiac myocyte calcium signaling has been found to be inhibited in both the CBDL and PVL models *(21,22)*. After CBDL, a decrease in membrane L-type calcium channel content and function were shown whereas intracellular calcium signaling was unaffected *(22)*. In PVL animals, similar effects on L-type calcium channels were observed, but in contrast, the caffeine-sensitive sarcoplasmic reticulum calcium pool was found to be decreased *(21)*. Ventricular myocyte K^+ currents are also diminished in CBDL animals and are proposed as a mechanism for the prolonged Q-T interval seen on electrocardiograms in cirrhotic patients *(23)*.

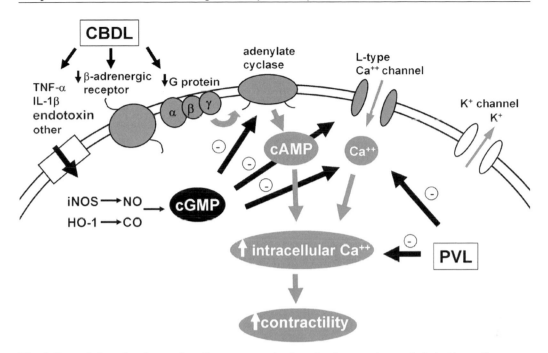

Fig. 1. Potential mechanisms of cardiac myocyte dysfunction in experimental cirrhotic cardiomyopathy. See text for details. PVL, partial portal vein ligation; CBDL, common bile duct ligation; TNF-α, tumor necrosis factor alpha; IL-1β, interleukin-1 beta; cAMP, cyclic adenosine monophosphate; cGMP, cyclic guanosine monophosphate; iNOS, inducible nitric oxide synthase; HO-1, heme oxygenase 1; NO, nitric oxide; CO, carbon monoxide.

Nitric Oxide (NO)

Nitric oxide (NO) has been established to play a multifaceted role in physiologic and pathophysiologic regulation of cardiac contractility and this area is evolving and has been extensively reviewed *(24,25)*. In noncirrhotic models of heart failure both endothelial nitric oxide synthase (eNOS) and inducible nitric oxide synthase (iNOS) overexpression have been implicated in depressed contractility, largely through effects on β-adrenergic stimulation *(25)*. Specifically, enhanced cGMP mediated degradation of cAMP and inhibition of L-type calcium channels and intracellular calcium release have been observed *(24,25)*. The administration of a NOS inhibitor to isolated cardiac preparations from CBDL animals resulted in improved contractility supporting a role for NO in cirrhotic cardiac dysfunction *(26)*. Subsequent studies documented iNOS, but not eNOS, overexpression in CBDL hearts with increased cardiac cGMP levels (27). Circulating levels of tumor necrosis factor alpha (TNF-α) and interleukin-1 β (IL-1β) were increased in these animals and were presumed to be the stimulus for increased myocyte iNOS expression. In papillary muscle preparations, NOS inhibition improved basal and IL-1β–mediated decreased contractility while exogenous NO depressed contractility *(27)*. In contrast, in PVL animals, cardiac iNOS alterations were not observed and NO did not appear to play a role in the observed cardiac dysfunction *(28)*. Together, these results demonstrate a role for NO in depressed cardiac contractility in CBDL animals and suggest that cytokine-mediated iNOS expression may be involved. The observation that PVL animals do not have iNOS overexpression is in line with the findings by some that bacterial translocation does not occur at later time points after PVL *(29)*. This difference from cirrhotic animals could also provide one hypothesis to explain the recent finding that echocardiographic findings are less apparent in patients with noncirrhtoic portal fibrosis than in those with cirrhosis *(10)*. However, the mechanisms through which PVL influences cellular calcium signaling remain undefined. Finally, whether oxidative stress and NO-derived reactive oxygen species contribute to myocyte dysfunction in human or experimental cirrhotic cardiomyopathy as has been postulated in noncirrhotic cardiomyopathy has not been explored *(25)*.

HEME OXYGENASE AND CARBON MONOXIDE

Much less is known about the role of heme oxygenase (HO) in cardiac function. To date, experimental studies support that expression of the inducible form of the enzyme, HO-1, is protective in cardiac ischemia–reperfusion injury *(30,31)*. However, HO can also increase cGMP levels through production of carbon monoxide (CO) and activation of soluble guanylate cyclase resulting in effects similar to those described for NOS. In CBDL animals, left ventricular HO-1 expression and HO activity have been found to be significantly increased *(32)*. The cellular source of HO-1 has not been identified, but is assumed to be the myocyte. Treatment with zinc protoporphyrin, an inhibitor of HO activity, in vivo decreased ventricular cGMP content and in isolated papillary muscle preparations improved contractility. Furthermore, administration of CO depressed papillary muscle contractility. These findings suggest that HO-1 overexpression may contribute to impaired contractility in experimental cirrhotic cardiomyopathy.

Summary

Recognition of cirrhotic cardiomyopathy has increased. Human studies demonstrate both systolic and diastolic cardiac abnormalities. Experimental studies have identified multiple abnormalities within myocytes including abnormalities in β-adrenergic signaling and plasma membrane and intracellular calcium kinetics possibly mediated through increased iNOS and HO-1 expression and cGMP generation in cirrhotic models. These studies also suggest that the pathogenesis of changes in cardiac myocyte contractility may be different in noncirrhotic and cirrhotic portal hypertension. However, whether similar changes occur in human disease and how the observed experimental findings contribute to diastolic abnormalities seen in humans remain unknown.

HEPATOPULMONARY SYNDROME

Clinical Studies

The association between liver disease and vascular abnormalities in the lung has been recognized for more than 100 yr *(33)*. However, the term "hepatopulmonary syndrome" was not used until 1977 *(34)* to describe what is now recognized as pulmonary microvascular dilatation resulting in impaired oxygenation *(35)*. HPS develops in 15–20% of patients with cirrhosis *(35,36)* and is generally progressive. Mortality is increased in cirrhotic patients with HPS relative to cirrhotic patients without HPS *(37)*. There have been few studies evaluating the pathogenesis of human HPS and to date, NO is the only mediator that has been assessed. Early work demonstrated that exhaled NO levels, used as a measure of pulmonary production, are increased in patients with HPS and normalize after transplantation as HPS resolves *(38–40)*. However, exhaled NO levels may also be increased in cirrhosis in the absence of HPS *(38)*. In more recent work, the acute administration of methylene blue, an inhibitor of the action of NO through soluble guanylate cycl-ase and inhaled N^G-nitro-L-arginine methyl ester, a NOS inhibitor, transiently improved oxygenation in HPS *(41,42)*. Finally, in one cohort, elevated circulating progesterone levels, which can modulate eNOS-mediated NO production in vitro, were found to cor-relate with the presence of intrapulmonary vasodilatation and gas exchnage abnormalities in patients with HPS *(43,44)*. These studies support that NO contributes to pulmonary vasodilatation in human HPS, although the stimulus for and source of increased NO pro-duction remain incompletely characterized. In addition, whether other mediators influence pulmonary vascular tone has not been evaluated.

One hypothesis for the pathogenesis of HPS is that the mechanisms that trigger HPS are the same as those that trigger systemic vascular alterations in cirrhosis and portal hypertension. However, it has recently been appreciated that HPS can occur across a spectrum of liver disorders in the absence of established cirrhosis or portal hypertension. Specifically, HPS has been reported in hepatic venous outflow obstruction without cirrhosis *(45)*, in extrahepatic portal venous obstruction *(46)*, and in acute *(47)* and chronic (48) hepatitis. Together, these studies suggest that the pathogenesis of HPS may involve distinct mechanisms from those associated with systemic vasodilatation in cirrhosis.

Experimental Studies

The recognition by Chang et al. that CBDL cirrhosis also results in a decrease in pulmonary vascular resistance and gas exchange abnormalities analogous to human disease provided a model system to study HPS *(49)*. These early studies found an influx of pulmonary intravascular macrophages in CBDL cirrhosis, and suggested that vasoconstrictive eicosanoid production might contribute to lung abnormalities but did not directly measure intrapulmonary vasodilatation *(50)*. Extension of these findings using an in vivo awake microsphere technique to size the pulmonary microcirculation documented the development of progressive pulmonary microvascular dilatation and gas exchange abnormalities without lung injury *(51)*. The onset of HPS after CBDL occurs prior to the development of cirrhosis and in advance of the full expression of portal hypertension or systemic vasodilatation *(51)*. In contrast, PVL resulting in portal hypertension in the absence of cirrhosis and thioacetamide (TAA)–induced hepatocellular cirrhosis do not result in the development of HPS *(52)*. These studies suggest that experimental biliary cirrhosis results in a unique sequence of abnormalities leading to HPS. Studies over the last 6 yr, described below, have begun to identify and characterize this sequence of events (Fig. 2).

NO

Based on findings in humans, the role of NO in experimental HPS has been investigated. Increased pulmonary vascular endothelial eNOS levels and enhanced NO activity in lung and pulmonary artery segments are found after CBDL and correlate with the development of HPS *(53)*. Increased pulmonary iNOS expression, localized to intravascular macrophages, has also been found in some but not all studies *(53–55)*. A recent detailed analysis of changes in NOS expression over time after CBDL has documented a transient significant increase in iNOS expression in intravascular macrophages in 3 wk CBDL animals that is not sustained while eNOS levels remain elevated and correlate with vasodilatation and gas-exchange abnormalities *(55)*. In addition, two studies have shown that

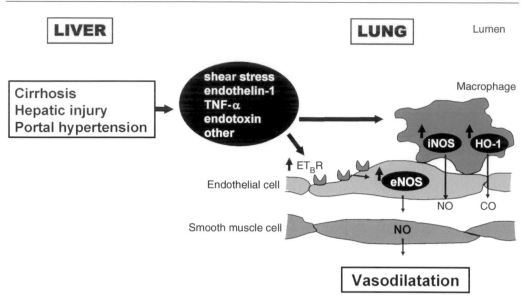

Fig. 2. Potential mechanisms of intrapulmonary vasodilatation in experimental hepatopulmonary syndrome. See text for details. TNF-α, tumor necrosis factor alpha; $ET_B R$, endothelin B receptor; iNOS, inducible nitric oxide synthase; eNOS, endothelial nitric oxide synthase; HO-1, heme oxygenase 1; NO, nitric oxide; CO, carbon monoxide.

the administration of NOS inhibitors can prevent or improve experimental HPS, confirming a role for enhanced NO production in pathogenesis *(54,56)*. Finally, no increase in pulmonary eNOS or iNOS expression is seen in PVL animals and only a small increase in pulmonary intravascular macrophage iNOS expression is seen in TAA animals, two models where HPS does not develop *(52)*. Together, these studies support an important role for NOS derived NO in experimental HPS although the precise contribution of endothelial eNOS and macrophage iNOS in producing NO remains controversial.

HO-1 AND CO

HO-1 has important protective effects on oxidant injury in the lung and can influence vascular tone through its enzymatic products, most notably CO *(57)*. Expression of HO-1 can be modulated by a wide range of agents increased in liver disease, including inflammatory cytokines and NO *(57)*. Based on these observations, HO-1 expression in the lung has been evaluated in experimental HPS. Lung HO-1 expression is markedly increased after CBDL and appears to contribute to the blunted hypoxic pulmonary vasoconstrictive response based on the fact that the response is partially restored by HO inhibition *(58)*. Furthermore, chronic NOS inhibition in vivo blocked the increase in HO-1 expression suggesting that NO may drive HO-1 expression. Subsequent studies documented that the increase in HO-1 occurs predominately in pulmonary intravascular macrophages as HPS progresses and is associated with increased lung HO activity and increased circulating carboxyhemoglobin levels *(59)*. In vivo HO inhibition for 1 wk with tin protoporphyrin decreased intrapulmonary vasodilatation, improved gas exchange, and normalized lung HO activity and carboxyhemoglobin levels in CBDL animals. Treatment did not result in appreciable lung injury over the timeframe studied. In addition, HO inhibition resulted in an increase in macrophage iNOS levels supporting that CO may also inhibit macrophage iNOS expression. Increased HO-1 expression was not seen in PVL- or TAA-induced cirrhosis *(52)*. These findings support a role for HO-1 overexpression in pulmonary intravascular macrophages in the progression of experimental HPS, presumably through CO mediated cGMP production. In addition, they support that NO and CO may influence HO-1 and iNOS expression, respectively.

ENDOTHELIN-1 (ET-1) AND HPS

Endothelin-1 (ET-1) is classically recognized as a locally produced vasoconstrictor acting through the vascular smooth muscle endothelin A receptor (ET_A) *(60)*. It was initially evaluated in CBDL animals to define if a defect in lung vascular production contributed to pulmonary vasodilatation. However, lung levels were not altered after CBDL, whereas hepatic production and plasma levels of ET-1 significantly increased within 1 wk, prior to the development of cirrhosis or a hyperdynamic state *(52,61)*. The magnitude of the increase in plasma ET-1 levels after CBDL correlated with the rise in pulmonary eNOS levels, the degree of intrapulmonary vasodilatation, and the severity of gas-exchange abnormalities *(62,63)* suggesting that circulating ET-1 might contribute to vasodilatation rather than vasoconstriction in the lung. Although hepatic production *(62–64)* and circulating levels of ET-1 *(63,65,66)* are increased in other forms of experimental and human cirrhosis, levels are lower in these situations and are found only in advanced disease in the presence of marked hyperdynamic changes and ascites. Hepatic production and plasma ET-1 levels were not increased in PVL animals or in TAA cirrhosis where HPS does not develop *(52)*. Furthermore, proliferating biliary epithelium and reflux of biliary cyst fluid into the circulation were postulated to be important and unique sources of circulating ET-1 after CBDL *(63,67)*.

Subsequent studies revealed that chronic ET-1 infusion increased pulmonary eNOS levels and triggered HPS in PVL, but not in normal, animals, supporting that portal hypertensive animals are uniquely susceptible to ET-1–mediated pulmonary vasodilatation. Similarly, exogenous ET-1 increased eNOS levels and NO production in isolated pulmonary artery segments from PVL and CBDL animals but not normals and in cultured pulmonary microvascular endothelial cells *(61,63,68)*. The effects of exogenous ET-1 were prevented by inhibition of the endothelin B (ET_B) receptor, which is recognized to activate eNOS in the endothelium. Recently, a selective increase in pulmonary microvascular endothelial ET_B receptor expression has been found in experimental cirrhosis and portal hypertension (CBDL, PVL, and TAA) compared to normals *(52,61)*. These findings support that increased pulmonary endothelial ET_B receptor expression in the setting of cirrhosis or portal hypertension may be the event that predisposes animals to ET-1 mediated eNOS activation and intrapulmonary vasodilatation. However, the mechanisms underlying ET_B receptor alterations in liver disease remain undefined.

BACTERIAL TRANSLOCATION, TNF-α, INTRAVASCULAR MACROPHAGES, AND HPS

The observation that bacterial translocation from the gut to mesenteric lymph nodes increases in cirrhosis and contributes to the production of proinflammatory cytokines, including TNF-α, that induce splanchnic endothelial eNOS overexpression *(69)* and can modulate iNOS expression prompted evaluation in experimental HPS. CBDL has been found to cause increased translocation of Gram-Positive and Gram-Negative organisms to mesenteric lymph nodes *(70)*. Oral treatment with norfloxacin, beginning at the time of

CBDL surgery, decreased Gram-Negative translocation, reduced the number of pulmonary intravascular macrophages and iNOS levels, and improved HPS. HO-1 and CO were not evaluated. Of note, treatment was not associated with amelioration of the hyperdynamic state or a reduction in pulmonary eNOS levels. This finding supports that bacterial translocation modulates the accumulation of intravascular macrophages and iNOS levels and contributes to HPS after CBDL. Subsequent studies demonstrated that macrophage accumulation begins within 1 wk after CBDL, but is not associated with iNOS or HO-1 expression until 3 wk after ligation *(59)*. This observation suggests that the initial adhesion of macrophages may occur through different mechanisms than the subsequent activation. Finally, evaluation of circulating TNF-α levels in relation to the development of HPS has been undertaken in the CBDL and TAA models and after chronic ET-1 infusion in PVL animals. In TAA cirrhosis, circulating TNF-α levels are significantly greater than those seen after CBDL and are associated with a modest increase in macrophage accumulation but not with the development of HPS *(52)*. In addition, ET-1 infusion in PVL animals is associated with an increase in TNF-α levels and an increase in lung intravascular macrophage accumulation suggesting that interplay between ET-1 and TNF-α may be important in the full expression of experimental HPS. However, whether bacterial translocation and TNF-α modulate hepatic or circulating ET-1 or influence ET_B receptor expression is not known.

Summary

Excess NO production appears to play a central role in both human and experimental HPS. In experimental HPS, pulmonary endothelial expression and activation of eNOS and intravascular macrophage accumulation and production of iNOS have been identified as sources of NO production. In addition, recent studies support that macrophage HO-1 and CO production may be important in the progression of vasodilatation. The mechanisms underlying the sequence of molecular alterations in experimental HPS are under investigation. Early hepatic production and release of ET-1 and increased pulmonary endothelial ET_B receptor expression appear to trigger eNOS after CBDL and correlate with the onset of vasodilatation. Bacterial translocation and TNF-α production appear to enhance intravascular macrophage accumulation and iNOS and HO-1 expression and contribute to progression of vasodilatation. Recent work suggests that ET-1 and TNF-α may interact to contribute to the full expression of experimental HPS. Defining the precise interactions between ET-1 and TNF-α in the pathogenesis of experimental HPS and determining if similar mechanisms and alterations are in play in human HPS are important ongoing areas of investigation.

PORTOPULMONARY HYPERTENSION

Clinical Studies

The initial observation that pulmonary arterial hypertension can occur in the setting of cirrhosis and portal hypertension was made more than 50 yr ago *(71)*. Since that time, POPH has evolved from a rare complication of liver disease to an increasingly important and relatively common disorder *(72)*. POPH is now established to occur in both cirrhotic and noncirrhotic portal hypertension and portal hypertension has been assumed to be a key underlying event. However, POPH has also been recognized in the absence of portal hypertension *(73)*. The prevalence of POPH does not appear to correlate with the sever-

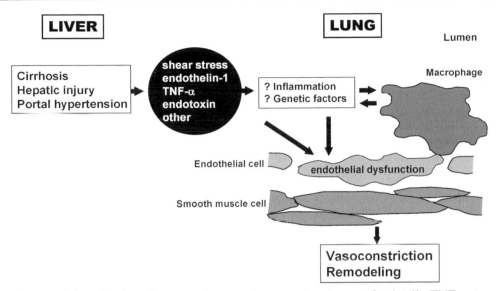

Fig. 3. Potential mechanisms in portopulmonary hypertension. See text for details. TNF-α; tumor necrosis factor alpha.

ity of underlying liver disease, although there is controversy over whether it correlates with the degree of portal hypertension (72). In addition, recent studies suggest that POPH is more commonly recognized in patients undergoing evaluation for liver transplantation or in those with refractory ascites (74). There are no specific human studies on pathogenesis of POPH, though a recent study has found that circulating ET-1 levels are higher in cirrhotic patients with refractory ascites and POPH than in those without POPH (74). Because POPH and HPS both may develop in the setting of underlying cirrhosis and portal hypertension, it is reasonable to postulate that they may share some common mediators and mechanisms.

Experimental Studies

There are no identified models of portopulmonary hypertension, although an array of potential contributors have been considered and reviewed based in large part on data from primary pulmonary hypertension (72,75). A general framework places pulmonary endothelial dysfunction or injury at the center of the vasoproliferative response leading to pulmonary arterial hypertension (Fig. 3). In addition to genetic factors and specific vasoactive mediators implicated in primary pulmonary hypertension, increased shear stress, inflammatory cytokines, and an imbalance of vasoactive mediators in liver disease and portal hypertension have been proposed to contribute to endothelial dysfunction. Of note, both the PVL and CBDL models have been evaluated and have not been found to develop POPH (54,76,77). These results suggest that factors in addition to alterations in flow, vasoactive mediators and cytokines are needed for experimental POPH to develop. Although speculative, the concept that the pulmonary endothelial response in the setting of cirrhosis or portal hypertension may define whether HPS or POPH develops has emerged and could explain the development of divergent vascular responses in similar situations. For instance, if the endothelium is intact and functional, then circulating ET-1 and intravascular macrophages could trigger NO and CO overproduction leading to microvascu-

31. Yet S-F, Tian R, Layne MD, et al. Cardiac-specific expression of heme oxygenase-1 protects against ischemia and reperfusion injury in transgenic mice. Circ Res 2001;89(2):168–173.

32. Liu H, Song D, Lee SS. Role of heme oxygenase-carbon monoxide pathway in pathogenesis of cirrhotic cardiomyopathy in the rat. Am J Physiol Gastrointest Liver Physiol 2001;280(1):G68–G74.

33. Fluckiger M. Vorkommen von trommelschagel formigen fingerendphalangen ohne chronische veranderungen an der lungen oder am herzen. Wien Med Wochenschr 1884;34:1457.

34. Kennedy TC, Knudson RJ. Exercise aggregated hypoxemia and orthodeoxia in cirrhosis. Chest 1977; 72:305.

35. Lange PA, Stoller JK. The hepatopulmonary syndrome. Ann Intern Med 1995;122:521–529.

36. Fallon M, Abrams G. The hepatopulmonary syndrome. Progr Liver Dis 1997;15,247–15,264.

37. Schenk P, Schoniger-Hekele M, Fuhrmann V, Madl C, Silberhumer G, Muller C. Prognostic significance of the hepatopulmonary syndrome in patients with cirrhosis. Gastroenterology 2003;125:1042–1052.

38. Rolla G, Brussino L, Colagrande P. Exhaled nitric oxide and impaired oxygenation in cirrhotic patients before and after liver transplantation. Ann Intern Med 1998;129:375–378.

39. Rolla G, Brussino L, Colagrande P, et al. Exhaled nitric oxide and oxygenation abnormalities in hepatic cirrhosis. Hepatology 1997;26:842–847.

40. Cremona G, Higenbottam TW, Mayoral V, et al. Elevated exhaled nitric oxide in patients with hepatopulmonary syndrome. Eur Respir J 1995;8:1883–1885.

41. Rolla G, Bucca C, Brussino L. Methylene blue in the hepatopulmonary syndrome. N Engl J Med 1994; 331:1098.

42. Schenk P, Madl C, Rezale-Majd S, Lehr S, Muller C. Methylene blue improves the hepatopulmonary syndrome. Ann Int Med 2000;133:701–706.

43. Aller R, de Luis DA, Moreira V, et al. The effect of liver transplantation on circulating levels of estradiol and progesterone in male patients: parallelism with hepatopulmonary syndrome and systemic hyper-dynamic circulation improvement. J Endocrinol Invest 2001;24(7):503–509.

44. Aller R, Moya JL, Avila S, et al. Implications of estradiol and progesterone in pulmonary vasodilatation in cirrhotic patients. J Endocrinol Invest 2002;25(1):4–10.

45. Binay K, Sen S, Biswas PK, Sanyal R, Jumdar DM, Biswas J. Hepatopulmonary syndrome in inferior vena cava obstruction responding to cavoplasty. Gastroenterology 2000;118(1):192–196.

46. Gupta D, Vijaya DR, Gupta R, et al. Prevalence of hepatopulmonary syndrome in cirrhosis and extrahepatic portal venous obstruction. Am J Gastroenterol 2001;96(12):3395–3399.

47. Regev A, Yeshurun M, Rodriguez M, et al. Transient hepatopulmonary syndrome in a patient with acute hepatitis A. J Viral Hep 2001;8:83–86.

48. Teuber G, Teupe C, Dietrich C, Caspary W, Buhl R, Zeuzem S. Pulmonary dysfunction in non-cirrhotic patients with chronic viral hepatitis. Eur J Intern Med 2002;13:311–318.

49. Chang S-W, O'Hara N. Pulmonary circulatory dysfunction in rats with biliary cirrhosis. Am Rev Respir Dis 1992;148:798–805.

50. Chang SW, Ohara N. Chronic biliary obstruction induces pulmonary intravascular phagocytosis and endotoxin sensitivity in rats. J Clin Invest 1994;94(5):2009–2019.

51. Fallon MB, Abrams GA, McGrath JW, Hou Z, Luo B. Common bile duct ligation in the rat: a model of intrapulmonary vasodilatation and hepatopulmonary syndrome. Am J Physiol 1997;272 (Gastrointest Liver Physiol 35):G779–G784.

52. Luo B, Liu L, Tang L, Zhang J, Ling Y, Fallon MB. ET-1 and TNF-α in hepatopulmonary syndrome: analysis in prehepatic portal hypertension, biliary and nonbiliary cirrhosis in rats. Am J Physiol 2004; 286 (Gastrointest Liver Physiol):G294–G303.

53. Fallon MB, Abrams GA, Luo B, Hou Z, Dai J, Ku DD. The role of endothelial nitric oxide synthase in the pathogenesis of a rat model of hepatopulmonary syndrome. Gastroenterology 1997;113:606–614.

54. Nunes H, Lebrec D, Mazmanian M, et al. Role of nitric oxide in hepatopulmonary syndrome in cirrhotic rats. Am J Resp Crit Care Med 2001;164(5):879–885.

55. Zhang F, Kaide JI, Yang L, et al. Carbon monoxide modulates the pulmonary vascular response to acute hypoxia: relation to endothelin. Am J Physiol Heart Circ Physiol 2003;00678.2002.

56. Zhang X-J, Katsuta Y, Akimoto T, Ohsuga M, Aramaki T, Takano T. Intrapulmonary vascular dilatation and nitric oxide in hypoxemic rats with chronic bile duct ligation. J Hepatol 2003;39(5):724–730.

57. Morse D, Choi AM. Heme oxygenase-1: the "emerging molecule" has arrived. Am J Resp Cell Molec Biol 2002;27(1):8–16.
58. Carter EP, Hartsfield CL, Miyazono M, Jakkula M, Morris KG Jr, McMurtry IF. Regulation of heme oxygenase-1 by nitric oxide during hepatopulmonary syndrome. Am J Physiol-Lung Cell Molec Physiol 2002;283(2):L346–L53.
59. Zhang J, Ling Y, Luo B, et al. Analysis of pulmonary heme oxygenase-1 and nitric oxide synthase alterations in experimental hepatopulmonary syndrome. Gastroenterology 2003;125:1441–1451.
60. Filep JG. Endothelin peptides: biological actions and pathophysiological significance in the lung. Life Sciences 1992;52:119–133.
61. Luo B, Liu L, Tang L, et al. Increased pulmonary vascular endothelin B receptor expression and responsiveness to endothelin-1 in cirrhotic and portal hypertensive rats: a potential mechanism in experimental hepatopulmonary syndrome. J Hepatol 2003;38:556–563.
62. Rockey D, Fouassier L, Chung J, et al. Cellular localization of endothelin-1 and increased production in liver injury in the rat: potential for autocrine and paracrine effects on stellate cells. Hepatology 1998; 27:472–480.
63. Luo B, Abrams GA, Fallon MB. Endothelin-1 in the rat bile duct ligation model of hepatopulmonary syndrome: correlation with pulmonary dysfunction. J Hepatol 1998;29:571–578.
64. Pinzani M, Milani S, DeFranco R, et al. Endothelin 1 is overexpressed in human cirrhotic liver and exerts multiple effects on activated hepatic stellate cells. Gastroenterology 1996;110(2):534–548.
65. Moore K, Wendon J, Frazer M, Krani J, Williams R, Badr K. Plasma endothelin immunoreactivity in liver disease and the hepatorenal syndrome. N Engl J Med 1992;327:1774–1777.
66. Asbert M, Gines A, Gines P, et al. Circulating levels of endothelin in cirrhosis. Gastroenterology 1993; 104:1485–1491.
67. Liu L, Zhang M, Luo B, Abrams GA, Fallon MB. Biliary cyst fluid from common bile duct ligated rats stimulates eNOS in pulmonary artery endothelial cells: a potential role in hepatopulmonary syndrome. Hepatology 2001;33:722–727.
68. Zhang M, Luo B, Chen SJ, Abrams GA, Fallon MB. Endothelin-1 stimulation of endothelial nitric oxide synthase in the pathogenesis of hepatopulmonary syndrome. Am J Physiol 1999;277:G944–G952.
69. Wiest R, Das S, Cadelina G, Garcia-Tsao G, Milstien S, Groszmann R. Bacterial translocation in cirrhotic rats stimulates eNOS-derived NO production and impairs mesenteric vascular contractility. J Clin Invest 1999;104:1223–1233.
70. Rabiller A, Nunes H, Lebrec D, et al. Prevention of gram-negative translocation reduces the severity of hepatopulmonary syndrome. Am J Resp Crit Care Med 2002;166(4):514–517.
71. Mantz FA, Craig E. Portal axis thrombosis with spontaneous portacaval shunt and resultant cor pulmonale. Arch Pathol Lab Med 1951;52:91–97.
72. Budhiraja R, Hassoun PM. Portopulmonary hypertension: a tale of two circulations. Chest 2003;123(2): 562–576.
73. Yoshida EM, Erb SR, Ostrow DN, Ricci DR, Scudamore CH, Fradet G. Pulmonary hypertension associated with primary biliary cirrhosis in the absence of portal hypertension: a case report. Gut 1994; 35(2):280–282.
74. Benjaminov FS, Prentice M, Sniderman KW, Siu S, Liu P, Wong F. Portopulmonary hypertension in decompensated cirrhosis with refractory ascites. Gut 2003;52(9):1355–1362.
75. Herve P, Lebrec D, Brenot F, et al. Pulmonary vascular disorders in portal hypertension. Eur Respir J 1998;11:1153–1166.
76. Kibria G, Smith P, Heath D, Sagar S. Observations on the rare association between portal and pulmonary hypertension. Thorax 1980;35(12):945–949.
77. Carter EP, Sato K, Morio Y, McMurtry IF. Inhibition of K(Ca) channels restores blunted hypoxic pulmonary vasoconstriction in rats with cirrhosis. Am J Physiol-Lung Cell Molec Physiol 2000;279(5): L903–L910.

III METHODOLOGY TO ASSESS PORTAL HYPERTENSION IN HUMANS

9

Measurement of Hepatic Venous Pressure Gradient:

Methods, Interpretation, and Pitfalls

G. Pomier-Layrargues, MD
and P.-Michel Huet, MD, PhD

CONTENTS

INFORMATION AND COMPARISON OF AVAILABLE METHODS TO ASSESS PORTAL HYPERTENSION IN HUMANS

Definition

Portal hypertension is defined as an increased pressure in the portal vein, but is better evaluated by the pressure gradient between the portal vein and the inferior vena cava, with a normal value lower than 5 mmHg. This gradient represents the real perfusion pressure within the portal and hepatic circulation, which is, under normal conditions, a high-flow/low-resistance system, considering the high portal blood flow (between 700 and 1000 mL/min). The various causes of an increased portal venous resistance, which are discussed in specific chapters in this book, are characterized by changes in the anatomic architecture (fibrous scars delineating nodules, distal venous thrombosis, collagenization of the space of Disse, and loss of the normal elasticity of the sinusoidal endothelium), changes in splanchnic hemodynamics (increased splanchnic blood flow), and changes in the intra-hepatic vascular resistance (vasoconstriction of the sinusoids related to the transformation of stellate cells into myofibroblasts).

From: *Clinical Gastroenterology: Portal Hypertension*
Edited by: A. J. Sanyal and V. H. Shah © Humana Press Inc., Totowa, NJ

Pathophysiologic and Anatomical Considerations

Once pressure is increased in the portal vein, the splanchnic blood flow circulation will face resistance within the liver and will have to reach another venous territory with a low resistance, before going back to the central circulation. In most instances, blood will be directed toward venous circulation originating from the stomach and the esophagus via collaterals derived from preexisting venous connections between coronary and/or short gastric veins (with a reversal of the blood normally flowing toward the portal vein) and the azygos vein (blood returning to the superior vena cava). This collateral circulation will divert part of the splanchnic blood away from the liver and will lead to the development of gastric and esophageal varices, which may rupture and bleed when located under the mucosal layer of the gastroesophageal epithelium. Other collaterals may develop in different venous territories but have less clinical implications because they are usually located under the serous layer of the intestinal epithelium with a much lower risk of bleeding. All of these portosystemic collaterals may contribute to the onset of portosystemic encephalopathy, because they allow neurotoxic gut-derivated substances to bypass the liver. Ascites is also a clinical manifestation of portal hypertension and is directly related to increased pressure in the splanchnic venous bed.

At first glance, the hemodynamic evaluation of portal hypertension may appear redundant in patients who have already developed complications such as ascites, portosystemic encephalopathy, and variceal bleeding. In this situation, measurement of the portohepatic gradient will seem only to confirm portal hypertension but may in fact help determine the prognosis of patients with chronic liver diseases. In the absence of clinical symptoms, however, pressure measurements provide useful information that may lead to the detection of esophageal varices and eventually to a prophylaxis of bleeding. Upper gastrointestinal endoscopy, echo Doppler ultrasonography, helicoidal computed tomography, and magnetic resonance imaging can all be used in conjunction with manometric studies to detect the presence and evaluate the severity of portal hypertension. Portal systemic collaterals, subclinical ascites, and splenomegaly can be demonstrated by these techniques.

In a given patient, there are two majors reasons for a more thorough investigation of portal hypertension: the first is to demonstrate the patency of the portal vein or to determine the site of partial or total obstruction of the portal venous system before any surgery either for portacaval shunts, for liver transplantation, or, nowadays, before radiological transvenous intrahepatic portacaval shunts (TIPS). The second reason is to evaluate the indication, and eventually, to monitor a pharmacological treatment of gastroesophageal varices before the first bleeding episode or to prevent recurrent bleeding.

Anatomical evaluation of the portal vein is not so simple: because of its particular localization in the abdomen, the portal vein is not directly accessible from a peripheral vein as is the case for other venous territories in the body. Indeed, the portal vein drains toward the liver all blood coming from the splanchnic area, including upper and lower abdominal portions of the digestive track, the pancreas, and the spleen. This situation creates a "portal" system, i.e., a venous territory between two capillary systems, as observed in the venous system of the pituitary gland. Most techniques used to visualize the portal vein were more or less invasive, which justified the development of noninvasive imaging techniques as discussed further in the following chapters. Unfortunately, although they generally give a good indication of the portal vein patency with a valid evaluation of the presence, direction, and velocity of blood flow in the portal vein and its tributaries, these

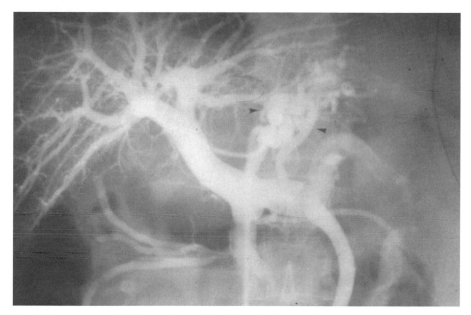

Fig. 1. Umbilicoportography in a patient with cirrhosis showing the portal venous system and large oeso-gastric varices fed by two left gastric veins (arrows).

noninvasive techniques are not always able to demonstrate unequivocally the anatomical integrity of the portal venous system. In addition, they cannot give a good evaluation of the severity of the portal hypertension. The same comments are true for the venous phase of celiac and/or splenic arteriography which was commonly performed before the availability of noninvasive imaging techniques and provided in most cases a good visualisation of the portal vein and its tributaries.

Visualisation of the Portal Vein with Measurement of Portal Vein Pressures

UMBILICAL PORTOGRAPHY

During fetal life, the portal vein is connected to the placenta through the umbilical vein, which originates from the left branch of the portal vein and runs through the *ligamentum teres*. At birth, with interruption of the placental circulation, the umbilical (and paraumbilical) veins flatten, remaining with a virtual lumen. These veins can enlarge with portal hypertension and can give rise to the Cruveilhier–Baumgarten syndrome. These veins, even when not dilated, can be found in a cordlike structure under the skin near the umbilicus and can be catheterized by surgical dissection *(1,2)*. Umbilical vein catheterization allowed for the first time a direct access to the portal system and provided excellent venograms of the portal venous system and a direct measurement of the portal vein pressure (Fig. 1) *(3)*, but required a skilled surgeon and could only be done under general anaesthesia; it was therefore abandoned.

SPLENOPORTOGRAPHY

Splenoportography was another historical technique to visualize the portal system and provide an indirect evaluation of portal pressure after transcutaneous puncture of the spleen and measurement of the intrasplenic pulp pressure, which is almost identical to the portal vein pressure. However, the risk of splenic hemorrhage is significant and this technique is no longer used in humans; it is still helpful in experimental animals (with the use of biological glue) to assess portal pressure changes under pharmacological treatments.

PERCUTANEOUS TRANSHEPATIC CATHETERIZATION OF THE PORTAL VEIN

This technique, pioneered by Lunderquist et al. *(4)*, consisted in direct cannulation of the portal vein with a catheter, under fluoroscopic guidance, and allowed not only the measurement of portal pressure but also the embolization of bleeding gastrophageal varices with autologous clots or inert material. It was almost abandoned after the introduction of endoscopic variceal sclerotherapy and later, band ligation, which are much safer and can be repeated, particularly in patients with coagulation defects. In addition, variceal embolization had only a short-term protective effect on the risk of rebleeding from varices because recanalization of previously obliterated veins occurred frequently *(5)*.

A modification of this technique was introduced by Boyer et al. *(6)* who used a thin needle (the Chiba needle used for transhepatic cholangiography) to puncture a portal vein branch within the liver, under fluoroscopy, and measure the portal venous pressure. This method is much safer because of the size of the needle (outer diameter: 0.7 mm); it not only allows measurement of portal venous pressure, but also good evaluation of the presence and direction of portal blood flow; in addition, during the same procedure, a branch of an hepatic vein can be punctured, allowing measurement of the pressure in the outflow of the liver and, therefore, evaluation of the pressure gradient across the liver (Fig. 2). This was not possible with the other techniques (umbilical portography, splenoportography, and percutaneous transhepatic catheterization of the portal vein) where only portal venous pressure could be measured. The other advantage of the thin needle technique is that it can be performed in patients already undergoing a percutaneous liver biopsy using the same approach. We have used this method routinely for more than 10 yr, in the prospective evaluation of portal hypertension in a cohort of patients with primary biliary cirrhosis *(7)*, without any complications.

INTRAHEPATIC PRESSURE

The thin needle technique has to be performed under fluoroscopic guidance in order to ascertain that the tip of the needle enters a branch of the portal vein. Intrahepatic pressure measurement using the same thin needle has been advocated as an another indirect but less cumbersome technique for measurement of portal vein pressure that can be performed without fluoroscopic equipment at the patient's bedside *(8)*. Unfortunately, a careful study comparing intrahepatic pressure measurement with portal vein pressure obtained by the direct puncture of a portal vein branch using the thin needle, demonstrated the absence of a consistent relationship between both techniques *(9)*, indicating that the intrahepatic pressure was not a reliable index of portal vein pressure.

HEPATIC VEIN CATHETERIZATION

The hepatic venous system can be catheterized and opacified by introducing an end-hole catheter through an antecubital vein *(10,11)* and, more recently, through a jugular or femoral vein. This technique was developed more than 50 yr ago by Myers and Taylor *(12)* for the measurement of pressures in an hepatic vein (usually the right hepatic vein). The catheter, placed under fluoroscopy in an hepatic vein, allows measurement of free

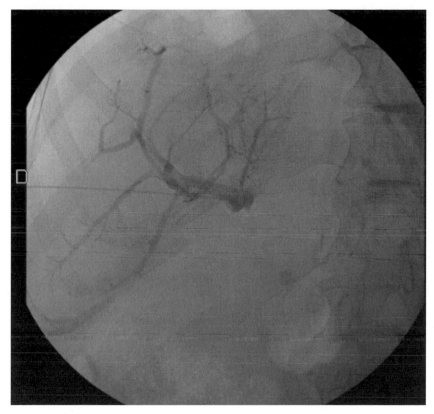

Fig. 2. Transhepatic opacification of a portal vein branch using the thin Chiba needle.

hepatic venous pressure (FHVP). The catheter is then pushed down in the hepatic vein until it cannot be advanced further, which results in a complete obstruction of flow; the pressure recorded in the occluded position is the wedged hepatic venous pressure (WHVP). It was assumed that WHVP gave an accurate estimate of portal pressure and that the difference between both pressures (wedged and free), the hepatic venous pressure gradient (HVPG), could be an accurate index of portal hypertension. Initially, comparison between the wedged hepatic venous pressure and portal venous pressure was obtained during abdominal surgery *(12–15)* and a rather good correlation between both pressures was demonstrated. It was only in 1970 that Viallet et al. *(3)* showed for the first time a close relationship between portal vein pressure (measured through umbilicoportal catheterization) and WHVP (measured simultaneously through hepatic vein catheterization), in a large group of conscious cirrhotic patients, mostly alcoholic cirrhotics. Since then, several studies have confirmed that WHVP was very similar to portal venous pressure (mainly using the thin needle) in most chronic liver diseases, particularly in alcoholic and viral (B and C) cirrhosis *(6,16–18)*. In some patients with nonalcoholic nonviral cirrhosis and primary biliary cirrhosis, the portal venous pressure can be higher than the WHVP, which may then not provide a reliable estimate of the severity of the portal hypertension *(16)* as discussed later. In patients with clinical evidence of portal hypertension, but a normal or slightly elevated WHVP, direct measurement of portal pressure is, therefore, needed to confirm the diagnosis.

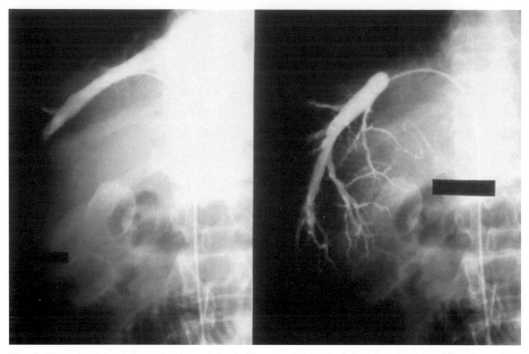

Fig. 3. Hepatic vein catheterization with a balloon catheter. Left-hand panel: opacification of the hepatic vein with a deflated balloon catheter (measurement of the free hepatic venous pressure). Right-hand panel: opacification of the same hepatic vein with a distended balloon catheter (measurement of the wedged hepatic venous pressure). There is no reflux of contrast material around the balloon.

A modification of the technique for measuring WHVP was proposed and validated by Groszmann et al. *(19)* with the use of a balloon catheter allowing inflation and deflation of the balloon within an hepatic vein (and, therefore, measurement of wedged and free pressures), usually in a large right lobar hepatic vein without the need to advance and withdraw the catheter for each WHVP and FHVP determination. This is particularly useful when repeated measurements have to be performed to get an accurate estimation of pressure with or without pharmacological therapy *(20)*. In addition, a wedged position can be obtained in almost every case by using the balloon catheter which is not always possible when using the end-hole catheter, particularly if it is introduced through the femoral vein and cannot be pushed down in a wedged position (Figs. 3 and 4).

Wedged hepatic venography can in some cases allow visualization of the portal vein in a retrograde fashion, particularly in patients with reverse and/or stagnant flow in the portal venous system, which can be difficult to demonstrate even with the new noninvasive imaging techniques. The use of carbon dioxide as a contrast agent might be useful to avoid dye nephrotoxicity (Fig. 5). Although previously used in the evaluation of patients with suspected Budd–Chiari syndrome, hepatic vein catheterization is no longer performed in such cases not only because of the possible migration of clots from the hepatic vein but mainly because the diagnosis can be done readily and safely confirmed by noninvasive imaging techniques such as echo Doppler or magnetic resonance imaging. In addition,

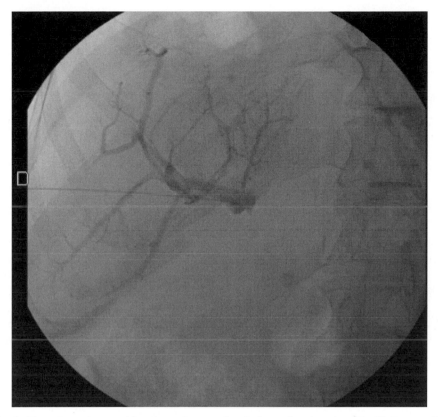

Fig. 2. Transhepatic opacification of a portal vein branch using the thin Chiba needle.

hepatic venous pressure (FHVP). The catheter is then pushed down in the hepatic vein until it cannot be advanced further, which results in a complete obstruction of flow; the pressure recorded in the occluded position is the wedged hepatic venous pressure (WHVP). It was assumed that WHVP gave an accurate estimate of portal pressure and that the difference between both pressures (wedged and free), the hepatic venous pressure gradient (HVPG), could be an accurate index of portal hypertension. Initially, comparison between the wedged hepatic venous pressure and portal venous pressure was obtained during abdominal surgery *(12–15)* and a rather good correlation between both pressures was demonstrated. It was only in 1970 that Viallet et al. *(3)* showed for the first time a close relationship between portal vein pressure (measured through umbilicoportal catheterization) and WHVP (measured simultaneously through hepatic vein catheterization), in a large group of conscious cirrhotic patients, mostly alcoholic cirrhotics. Since then, several studies have confirmed that WHVP was very similar to portal venous pressure (mainly using the thin needle) in most chronic liver diseases, particularly in alcoholic and viral (B and C) cirrhosis *(6,16–18)*. In some patients with nonalcoholic nonviral cirrhosis and primary biliary cirrhosis, the portal venous pressure can be higher than the WHVP, which may then not provide a reliable estimate of the severity of the portal hypertension *(16)* as discussed later. In patients with clinical evidence of portal hypertension, but a normal or slightly elevated WHVP, direct measurement of portal pressure is, therefore, needed to confirm the diagnosis.

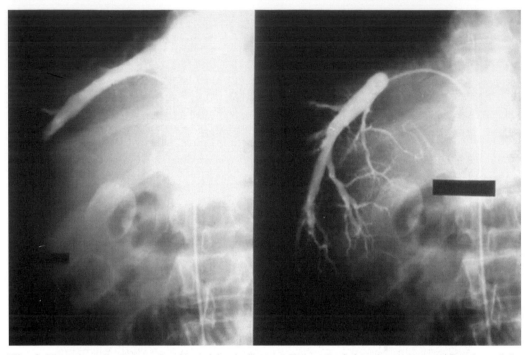

Fig. 3. Hepatic vein catheterization with a balloon catheter. Left-hand panel: opacification of the hepatic vein with a deflated balloon catheter (measurement of the free hepatic venous pressure). Right-hand panel: opacification of the same hepatic vein with a distended balloon catheter (measurement of the wedged hepatic venous pressure). There is no reflux of contrast material around the balloon.

A modification of the technique for measuring WHVP was proposed and validated by Groszmann et al. *(19)* with the use of a balloon catheter allowing inflation and deflation of the balloon within an hepatic vein (and, therefore, measurement of wedged and free pressures), usually in a large right lobar hepatic vein without the need to advance and withdraw the catheter for each WHVP and FHVP determination. This is particularly useful when repeated measurements have to be performed to get an accurate estimation of pressure with or without pharmacological therapy *(20)*. In addition, a wedged position can be obtained in almost every case by using the balloon catheter which is not always possible when using the end-hole catheter, particularly if it is introduced through the femoral vein and cannot be pushed down in a wedged position (Figs. 3 and 4).

Wedged hepatic venography can in some cases allow visualization of the portal vein in a retrograde fashion, particularly in patients with reverse and/or stagnant flow in the portal venous system, which can be difficult to demonstrate even with the new noninvasive imaging techniques. The use of carbon dioxide as a contrast agent might be useful to avoid dye nephrotoxicity (Fig. 5). Although previously used in the evaluation of patients with suspected Budd–Chiari syndrome, hepatic vein catheterization is no longer performed in such cases not only because of the possible migration of clots from the hepatic vein but mainly because the diagnosis can be done readily and safely confirmed by noninvasive imaging techniques such as echo Doppler or magnetic resonance imaging. In addition,

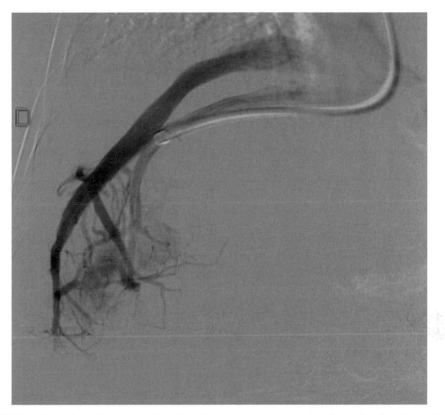

Fig. 4. Wedged hepatic venography showing a large venous to venous shunt distal to the wedged tip of the catheter. In such a case, the wedged hepatic venous pressure underestimates the true sinusoidal pressure.

hepatic vein catheterization allows liver biopsy to be performed in patients with a poor coagulation or ascites.

Finally, as further described in the following chapter, hepatic vein catheterization was the first step in the development of transjugular intrahepatic portosystemic shunts (TIPS) as a nonsurgical treatment of severe portal hypertension *(21)*.

MEASUREMENT OF VARICEAL PRESSURE

During endoscopy, direct measurement of variceal pressure can be obtained by puncture of esophageal varices *(22)* or by using pressure-sensitive gauges applied on the surface of esophageal varices *(23)*. These techniques, although promising, can only be performed in a few highly specialized centers and should still be considered as research tools.

PHYSIOPATHOLOGIC BASIS OF HVPG MEASUREMENT

Classification of Portal Hypertension

As stated earlier, the accuracy and safety of the different methods for the assessment of portal hypertension have been evaluated prospectively. The most popular technique remains the measurement of HVPG (difference between WHVP and FHVP) as proposed by Myers and Taylor *(12)*. It was assumed that the wedged catheter creates stasis within

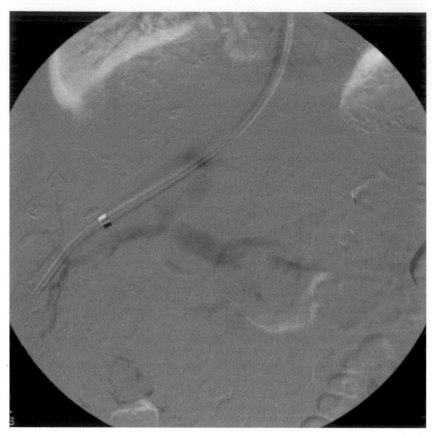

Fig. 5. Retrograde portography obtained after injection of carbon dioxide in a catheter wedged in an hepatic vein.

the occluded hepatic venule that is in equilibrium with the sinusoidal pressure, which itself is a good estimate of the pressure of portal blood entering the sinusoidal bed *(15)*. This assumption was the basis for the first classification of portal hypertension: (a) presinusoidal, when WHVP was normal despite overt signs of portal hypertension; and (b) postsinusoidal, when WHVP was elevated. Portal hypertension can be better classified now according to the major site of increased resistance to portal blood flow: (a) prehepatic, owing to obstruction of the portal vein or of one of its tributaries, particularly the splenic vein; (b) posthepatic, owing to a increased pressure secondary to cardiac insufficiency (mainly right heart failure) or to obstruction of large hepatic veins (Budd–Chiari syndrome); and finally, (c) intrahepatic portal hypertension, which can be subclassified into presinusoidal, sinusoidal, and postsinusoidal *(24)*.

Intrahepatic Portal Hypertension

Depending on the anatomical changes induced by the liver disease, the static column of blood created by the occluding catheter will be in equilibrium with the pressure existing upstream of the obstacle, until the first connection with an area of lower resistance allowing blood flow derivation toward another nonoccluded hepatic vein. Therefore, in intrahepatic portal hypertension, the WHVP is normal in the presinusoidal subtype and elevated in the sinusoidal and postsinusoidal subtypes.

PRESINUSOIDAL INTRAHEPATIC PORTAL HYPERTENSION

In presinusoidal intrahepatic portal hypertension [as found in idiopathic portal hypertension *(25)* or shistosomiasis], the increased resistance to portal blood flow is upstream of normal sinusoids and very far from the occluded vessel; therefore, blood will flow through unimpeded adjacent sinusoids toward the veins. In such cases, the static column will be in equilibrium with sinusoidal pressure, and the WHVP will be in a normal range.

POSTSINUSOIDAL INTRAHEPATIC PORTAL HYPERTENSION

In postsinusoidal intrahepatic portal hypertension (as found in venooclusive disease), the increased resistance to portal flow is downstream of normal sinusoids and very close to the occluded vessel. The static column will be in equilibrium with pressure in a vascular compartment extending up to the portal vein, and WHVP will be similar to FPVP.

SINUSOIDAL INTRAHEPATIC HYPERTENSION

In micronodular cirrhosis, sinusoids are uniformly transformed into rigid tubes by collagen deposition in the space of Disse, with loss of the normal fenestrated endothelial lining (capillarization and collagenization of the sinusoidal bed) *(26)*; in addition, large fibrous scars delineate regenerative nodules, further compressing the sinusoids. In such cases, there is no connection with an hepatic vein having a lower resistance, and the static column of blood will also be in equilibrium with the pressure existing in the vascular compartment extending up to the portal vein. WHVP will be equal to portal vein pressure as found in most alcoholic cirrhosis *(6,16)* and cirrhosis due to virus B, C chronic infection *(17,18)*.

It must be emphasized that WHVP values may differ when measured in different hepatic veins (usually within a range of 1 to 3 mmHg), which is probably a result of the heterogeneity of the cirrhotic process through the liver. This finding is more frequent when the end-hole catheter is wedged in a small hepatic vein and may be minimized by using the balloon catheter, occluding a much larger area of the liver *(19)*.

In addition, in macronodular cirrhosis, the anatomical alterations can be located mainly at a presinusoidal level, whereas some parenchymal lesions are not uniformly distributed throughout the liver, with some areas showing preserved or near normal parenchyma and sinusoids. In such cases, connections may develop through normal sinusoids with hepatic veins having a lower resistance; therefore, the static column of blood will be partly in equilibrium with the pressure existing in the normal sinusoids. Normal or only slightly elevated WHVP can be found in some patients with macronodular cirrhosis despite clinical signs of portal hypertension, particularly at the beginning of the cirrhotic process (e.g., early primary biliary cirrhosis, sarcoidosis, and schistosomiasis) *(16,27)*. With progression of the liver disease, the alterations of sinusoids become more pronounced and WHVP will progressively increase from a normal value to levels similar to that of the portal venous pressure. In such cases, during the early course of the diseases, the HVPG can be less increased than PVPG (gradient between the portal vein and vena cava pressures).

Another anatomical change occurring in long-standing cirrhosis is the development of anastomoses between both afferent (portal veins and hepatic arteries) and efferent (hepatic veins) vessels, particularly within the large fibrous septa surrounding regenerative nodules. These intrahepatic anastomoses can be large (up to 200 μm in diameter) *(28)* and may have a clinical significance in cirrhotic patients, shunting portal blood away from sinusoids *(29)*; there is, however, no evidence that their presence influences the value of WHVP. Occasionally, very high WHVP can be found in a vein draining an hepatocarcinoma, most likely caused by large arteriohepatic fistulas that may be found in these tumors.

Calculation of Hepatic Venous Pressure Gradient (HVPG)

DEFINITION

The HVPG is the difference between the portal vein and the inferior vena cava pressures (IVCP) and represents the real perfusion pressure within the portal and hepatic circulations. Both pressures have to be recorded during the hemodynamic investigation *(30)*. Because pressure in any single vein below the diaphragm is subject to changes in intraabdominal pressure, particularly as caused by ascites, this may lead to falsely elevated results. Because this effect influences both portal vein and vena cava pressures equally, the gradient remains unaffected.

As discussed earlier, the WHVP is a good estimate of portal vein pressure in a majority of patients. However, there is no agreement for using either the FHVP or IVCP above the liver when calculating the HVPG. We personally prefer to use the IVCP as a reference value, because partial obstruction by the catheter of a narrow, flattened vessel may result in falsely elevated free hepatic vein pressure. FHVP is generally higher than IVCP (1–3 mmHg) *(20)*, which leads to underestimation of the HVPG values. This is not a trivial issue because, as we will see below, the expected changes in HVPG during drug therapy are most often in the 2–6 mmHg range in patients considered as responders.

MEASUREMENT OF PRESSURES

Under fluoroscopic guidance and using either the hole-end or the balloon catheter, the HVPG measurement is a safe technique. No serious complications have been reported in the medical literature, and such is our experience after more than 4000 procedures. For accurate interpretation of the HPVG *(20,30)* several criteria most be followed: (a) pressures should be recorded and tracings should be printed; (b) adequate calibration of the strain-gauge transducers should be performed and recorded for each procedure; (c) before measurement, stabilization of pressures should be observed during at least 15 s and tracings obtained during at least 15 s; (d) after measurement, complete occlusion of the hepatic vein must be demonstrated for each determination of WHVP, using either the end-hole or the balloon catheter, by injection of a small amount of contrast material (less than 5 mL) which allows the visualization of sinusoids proximal to the catheter thus ensuring no leakage of contrast material around the catheter/balloon toward the hepatic vein and inferior vena cava. No communication with another hepatic vein should be visualized because the WHVP will underestimate the real pressure existing in the intrahepatic circulation; in such cases, the catheter should be placed in another hepatic vein in order to avoid this source of error; and (e) at least three measurements should be performed and the mean value should be used in the calculations.

INDICATION AND INTERPRETATION OF HVPG IN HUMANS FOR MANAGEMENT OF PHARMACOTHERAPY

As we just emphasized, HVPG measurement is a safe, easy, and reproducible method to assess portal hypertension in humans. This technique has provided useful insights for the pathophysiology of portal hypertension. Initially it was used as a diagnostic tool.

Recently, it has been suggested that it may be useful for prognostic evaluation *(31)* as well as to monitor the effect of drug therapy on portal hypertension *(32,33)* or on the evolution of the liver disease itself *(34)*. However, it has never been incorporated in various prognostic indices (Child–Turcotte, Child–Pugh, or MELD scores) that are used to determine the optimal timing of liver transplantation.

Use of HVPG as a Diagnostic Tool

As stated earlier, portal hypertension may result from increased resistance at a presinusoidal or sinusoidal level. HVPG measurement allows a reliable assessment of portal pressure in a majority of chronic liver diseases particularly in alcoholic and viral cirrhosis *(6,16–18)*; however, HVPG underestimates portal pressure in presinusoidal hypertension either intrahepatic or extrahepatic. Clinical evidence of portal hypertension (presence of esogastric varices or ascites) together with a normal of slightly elevated HVPG should lead to the evaluation of the patency of the portal venous system by echo Doppler examination. If thrombosis is ruled out, portal pressure must be measured directly either by the transhepatic approach using a Chiba needle or by the transjugular route. A liver biopsy performed after pressure measurements allows a definitive diagnosis of pure or mixed intrahepatic presinusoidal portal hypertension caused by various diseases: primary biliary cirrhosis, sarcoidosis, shistosomiasis, or idiopathic portal hypertension.

Use of HVPG as a Prognostic Marker

It has been shown repeatedly that complications of portal hypertension, and particularly bleeding from gastroesophageal varices, almost never occur below a threshold value of 12 mmHg *(35–37)*. Above this value, there is no relationship between HVPG and the risk of bleeding. Some authors, however, have suggested that the measurement of portal pressure early after a variceal bleeding episode may be useful to predict the likelihood of rebleeding *(38 40)*. It has been reported that the risk of rebleeding is higher in patients with HVPG greater than 16 mmHg *(39)* or 20 mmHg *(40)*.

The prognostic value of the HVPG for survival is another controversial matter. Recently, it has been suggested that HVPG might be a prognostic indicator when used in conjunction with other parameters such as the Child–Pugh and MELD scores. Some authors have shown that HVPG measured after bleeding *(39,41)* or sequential HVPG recordings *(42)* may help predict survival whereas others have not found any prognostic value of the HVPG for survival *(43,44)*. In addition, a recent study *(45)* suggested that the value of HVPG may predict the recurrence of varices after eradication by band ligation.

Taken together, all these data strongly suggest that HVPG measurement may provide useful prognostic information in addition to the other more conventional parameters such as the well-validated Pugh score.

Use of HVPG to Monitor Treatment in Chronic Liver Diseases

Treatment of Portal Hypertension

In 1980, pioneer investigations by Lebrec et al. demonstrated for the first time that propranolol can decrease HVPG *(46)*; subsequently, the same group reported a decreased rebleeding rate in cirrhotic patients treated with this drug after a variceal bleeding episode *(47)*. These findings led to the concept of pharmacotherapy of portal hypertension *(48)* and a large number of clinical trials have evaluated the efficacy of vasoactive drugs (mainly β-blockers and nitrates) in primary or secondary prevention of variceal bleeding (49).

Therefore, it was proposed by several groups to use HVPG as a "splanchnic sphygmomanometer" to monitor the effects of vasoactive drugs on portal pressure. However, hepatic vein catheterization is invasive and cannot be done on a routine basis except in highly specialized liver units.

The clinical usefulness of such repeated measurements has been evaluated during the recent years (49). Feu et al. suggested for the first time that a hemodynamic response could be defined as a 20% decrease in HVPG or by a HVPG lower than 12 mmHg on pharmacological treatment (50); they reported that the rate of rebleeding was 8% in responders as compared to 52% in nonresponders. This study evaluated patients treated for prevention of rebleeding and the second HVPG measurement was performed after 3 mo of treatment.

The analysis of the literature is not simple given the heterogeneity of the studied population, the difference in the timing of HVPG measurements, and the fact that drug-induced HVPG changes were evaluated either in primary or secondary variceal bleeding prophylaxis, or both. It is also well known that portal hypertension may improve spontaneously either in alcoholics who become abstinent or within days after a bleeding episode (51,52).

In patients treated for primary prophylaxis, the timing of HVPG measurement is less crucial because patients are usually in stable hemodynamic conditions; a second measurement performed 1–3 mo after the initiation of the treatment appears appropriate.

However, in patients treated for the prevention of rebleeding, the second hemodynamic evaluation must take place early after bleeding as the high incidence of early rebleeding may preclude the measurement of HVPG under pharmacological treatment. Thus, the evaluation of drug-induced changes must be performed within 7–10 d of the index bleed. Interpretation of published data is quite confusing given the high variability of time interval for the second measurement (1–3 mo), which is reflected by the high proportion of patients excluded from this assessment (30–40%) due to premature death or rebleeding. Some authors recently proposed to evaluate the acute hemodynamic effects of a single dose of vasoactive drug and to correlate it with the incidence of rebleeding (53,54). However, the value of this approach is still a matter of controversy.

It is now generally accepted that, when the HVPG decreases below 12 mmHg, the risk of first or recurrent variceal bleeding is virtually nil. Unfortunately, this threshold value is not frequently obtained, except in patients with baseline mildly to moderately elevated baseline HPVG and possibly less at risk of bleeding. A majority of studies reported that a 20% HVPG decrease should be considered as a significant response to therapy, the risk of the first bleeding or of rebleeding being significantly reduced in responders (50,55–59). This target can be obtained in 40–60% of patients treated with β-blockers alone and the rate of response can be increased by the addition of nitrates. Therefore, it has been suggested to evaluate the hemodynamic response by measuring HVPG changes induced by β-blockers and to add nitrates in non responders (59).

Although this approach appears to be quite logical, its usefulness has not been established unequivocally in clinical practice. Some studies failed to reproduce the correlation between the hemodynamic and clinical response as defined earlier (60). In addition, a recent study suggested that measuring HVPG twice or three times (in patients treated with the combination of β-blockers and nitrates) might not be cost effective (61).

The concept of drug therapy of portal hypertension appears promising because it is hoped that reducing the incidence of the first variceal bleed or the rate of rebleeding will translate with improved survival. Surprisingly, only a few clinical trials were able to demonstrate a positive correlation between hemodynamic response and a better survival rate *(55,62)*, whereas others did not *(50,58)*, probably because patients died more often from liver failure than from bleeding itself.

TREATMENT OF CHRONIC LIVER DISEASE

Sequential HVPG measurements might be useful not only to assess the efficacy of vasoactive drugs, but also to evaluate the effects of treatment of various liver diseases used in conjunction with liver biopsy and Child–Pugh score. It is well accepted now that cirrhosis secondary to both hepatitis B virus and hepatitis C virus can improve dramatically with lamivudine or interferon/ribavirin treatment. Indeed, Burroughs et al. *(34)* suggested recently that HVPG measurement could serve as a marker for disease progression or to monitor treatment efficacy in patients with chronic hepatitis C. This parameter can add useful information to liver biopsies, the interpretation of which might be biased by interobserver variation and by sample error.

PITFALLS OF USE

Measurement Error

HVPG calculation results from the difference of two pressures each of which has its own potential measurement error (nearly 1 mmHg). In addition, the technique of HVPG measurement must fulfill several technique requirements as recently pointed out by Groszmann and Wongcharatrawee *(20)* and reemphasized above. Good equipment is needed to obtain reliable pressures and, most importantly, to document them on tracings. This equipment must be calibrated for each measurement. Measurement of wedged hepatic vein pressure must be done preferably by using a balloon catheter which reflects pressure in a wide vascular territory of the liver; interpretation of data recorded must be done on the tracings.

Interpretation of Spontaneous or Drug-Induced Changes

As correctly pointed out by Talheimer et al. *(33)*, interpretation of data on HVPG changes induced by pharmacotherapy are difficult owing to many potential sources of bias. Certain studies have evaluated patients for primary prophylaxis, and others for secondary prophylaxis, with some including both populations. The proportion of active alcoholism is heterogeneous in different investigations and the timing of the second HVPG measurement is highly variable (1–3 mo). In this respect, evaluation of the acute hemodynamic effect of vasoactive drugs appears to be a promising approach as long as this strategy can predict the likelihood of first bleeding or rebleeding *(53,54)*. In addition, it could avoid the need for a second HVPG measurement. Finally, the concept of a target HVPG might be questionable; bleeding is caused by increased variceal tension, which is related to variceal pressure and variceal size, both of which are not evaluated by HPVG measurement.

Clearly, there is a need for further clinical trials to prospectively evaluate the prognostic value of HVPG changes for the risk of bleeding. For secondary prophylaxis, the second measurement must be performed as early as possible to avoid the premature exclusion of patients because of rebleeding. In the meantime, it appears reasonable to evaluate the effects of treatment on the HVPG only in patients enrolled in controlled clinical trials.

However, in such trials, the HVPG should be measured according to a rigid protocol such as the one proposed by Groszmann and Wongcharatrawee *(20)*, preferably by experienced hepatologists and/or well-trained radiologists with a specific interest in hepatology, or both.

REFERENCES

1. Bayly JH, Carbalhaes OG. The umbilical vein in the adult: diagnosis, treatment and research. Ann Surg 1964;30:56–60.
2. Lavoie P, Légaré A, Viallet A. Portal catheterization via the round ligament of the liver. Am J Surg 1967; 114:822–830.
3. Viallet A, Joly JG, Marleau D, Lavoie P. Comparison of the free portal venous pressure and wedged hepatic venous pressure in patients with cirrhosis of the liver. Gastroenterology 1970;59:372–375.
4. Lunderquist A, Wang J. Transhepatic catheterization and obliteration of the coronary vein in patients with portal hypertension and esophageal varices. N Engl J Med 1974;291:646–649.
5. Lunderquist A, Simert G, Tylen U, Wang J. Follow-up of patients with portal hypertension and esophageal varices treated with percutaneous obliteration of gastric coronary vein. Radiology 1977;122:59–63.
6. Boyer TD, Triger DR, Horisawa M, Redeker AG, Reynolds TB. Direct transhepatic measurement of portal vein pressure using a thin needle. Comparison with wedged hepatic vein pressure. Gastroenterology 1977;72:584–589.
7. Huet PM, Huet J, Deslauriers J. Portal hypertension in patients with primary biliary cirrhosis. In: Lindor KD, Heathcote EJ, Poupon R, eds. Primary Biliary Cirrhosis: From Pathogenesis to Clinical Treatment. Kluwer Academic, The Netherlands, 1998, pp. 87–91.
8. Orrego H, Blendis LM, Crossley IR, et al. Correlation of intrahepatic pressure with collagen in the Disse space and hepatomegaly in humans and in the rat. Gastroenterology 1981;80:546–556.
9. Fenyves D, Pomier-Layrargues G, Willems B, Coté J. Intrahepatic pressure measurement: not an accurate reflection of portal vein pressure. Hepatology 1988;8:211–216.
10. Warren JV, Brannon ES. A method of obtaining blood samples directly from the hepatic vein in man. Proc Soc Exper Biol Med 1948;55:144.
11. Bradley SE, Ingelfinger FJ, Bradley GP, Curry JJ. The estimation of hepatic blood flow in man. J Clin Invest 1945;24:890–897.
12. Myers JD, Taylor WJ. An estimation of portal venous pressure by occlusive catheterization of a hepatic venule. J Clin Invest 1951;30:662–663.
13. Welch GE, Emmett R, Craighead CC, Hoeffler G, Browne DC, Rosen I. Simultaneous pressure measurements in the hepatic venule and portal venous system in man. Am J Med Sci 1954;228:643–645.
14. Cohn R, Ordway G, Ellis E. Relation of portal venous pressure to occluded hepatic venous pressure. Arch Surg 1954;69:853–857.
15. Reynolds TB, Balfour DC Jr, Levinson DC, Mikkelsen W, Pattison A. Comparison of wedged hepatic vein pressure with portal vein pressure in human subjects with cirrhosis. J Clin Invest 1955;34:213–218.
16. Pomier-Layrargues G, Kusielewicz D, Willems B, et al. Presinusoidal portal hypertension in nonalcoholic cirrhosis. Hepatology 1985;5:415–418.
17. Lin HC, Tsai YT, Lee FY, et al. Comparison between portal vein pressure and wedged hepatic vein pressure in hepatitis B-related cirrhosis. J Hepatol 1989;9:326–330.
18. Perello A, Escorsell A, Bru C, et al. Wedged hepatic venous pressure adequately reflects portal pressure in hepatitis C virus-related cirrhosis. Hepatology 1999;30:1393–1397.
19. Groszmann R, Glickman M, Blei A, Storer E, Conn HO. Wedged and free hepatic venous pressure measured with a balloon catheter. Gastroenterology 1979;76:253–258.
20. Groszmann RJ, Wongcharatrawee S. The hepatic venous pressure gradient: anything worth doing should be done right. Hepatology 2004;39:280–283.
21. Boyer TD. Transjugular intrahepatic portosystemic shunt: current status. Gastroenterology 2003;124: 1700–1710.
22. Staritz M, Poralla T, Meyer Zum Buschenfelde KH. Intravascular oesophageal variceal pressure (IOVP) assessed by endoscopic fine needle puncture under basal conditions, Valsalva's manœuvre and after glyceryltrinitrate application. Gut 1985;26:525–530.

23. Bosch J, Bordas JM, Rigau J, et al. Non-invasive measurement of the pressure of esophageal varices using an endoscopic gauge: comparison with measurement by variceal puncture in patients undergoing endoscopic sclerotherapy. Hepatology 1986;6:667–672.

24. Genecin P, Groszmann RJ. The biology of portal hypertension. In: Arias IM, Boyer JL, Fausto N, Jakoby WB, Schachter DA, Shafritz DA, eds. The Liver Biology and Pathobiology, 3rd ed. Raven, New York, 1994, pp. 1327–1341.

25. Villeneuve JP, Huet PM, Joly JG, et al. Idiopathic portal hypertension. Am J Med 1976;61:459–464.

26. Schaffner F, Poppper H. Capillarization of the sinusoids. Gastroenterology 1963;44:239–242.

27. Coutinho A. Hemodynamic studies of portal hypertension in schistosomiasis. Am J Med 1968;44: 547–556.

28. Popper H, Elias H, Petty D. Vascular pattern of the cirrhotic liver. Am J Clin Pathol 1952;22:717–729.

29. Huet PM, Villeneuve JP, Pomier-Layrargues G, Marleau D. Hepatic circulation in cirrhosis. In: Benhamou JP, Lebrec D, eds. Clinics in Gastroenterology. Elsevier, Amsterdam, 1985, pp. 155–168.

30. Bosch J, D'Amico G, Garcia-Pagan JC. Portal hypertension. In Schiff's diseases of the liver. Schiff E, Sorrell MF, Maddrey W, eds. 9th ed. Lippincott JB, Philadelphia, 2003, pp. 429–485.

31. Armonis A, Patch D, Burroughs A. Hepatic venous pressure measurement: an old test as a new prognostic marker in cirrhosis. Hepatology 1997;25:245–248.

32. Boyer TD. Changing clinical practice with measurement of portal pressure. Hepatology 2004;39: 283–285.

33. Thalheimer U, Mela M, Patch D, Burroughs AK. Targeting portal pressure measurements, a critical appraisal. Hepatology 2004;39:286–290.

34. Burroughs AK, Groszmann R, Bosch J, et al. Assessment of therapeutic benefit of antiviral therapy in chronic hepatitis C: is hepatic venous pressure gradient a better end-point? Gut 2002;50:425–427.

35. Viallet A, Marleau D, Huet PM, et al. Hemodynamic evaluation of patients with intrahepatic portal hypertension. Relationship between bleeding varices and the portohepatic gradient. Gastroenterology 1975;69:1297–1300.

36. Lebrec D, De Fleury P, Rueff B, Nahum H, Benhamou JP. Portal hypertension, size of esophageal varices, and risk of gastrointestinal bleeding in alchololic cirrhosis. Gastroenterology 1980;79: 1139–1144.

37. Garcia-Tsao G, Groszmann RJ, Fisher RL, Conn HO, Atterbury CE, Glickman M. Portal pressure, presence of gastroesophageal varices and variceal bleeding. Hepatology 1985;5:419–424.

38. Vinel JP, Cassigneul J, Levade M, Voigt JJ, Pascal JP. Assessment of short-term prognosis after variceal bleeding in patients with alcoholic cirrhosis by early measurement of hepatic gradient. Hepatology 1986;6:116–117.

39. Stanley AJ, Robinson I, Forrest EH, Jones AL, Hayes PC. Haemodynamic parameters predicting variceal haemorrhage and survival in alcoholic cirrhosis. QJM 1998;91:19–25.

40. Moithinho E, Escorsell A, Bandi JC, et al. Prognostic value of early measurements of portal pressure in acute variceal bleeding. Gastroenterology 1999;117:626–631.

41. Patch D, Armonis A, Sabin C, et al. Single portal pressure measurement predicts survival in cirrhotic patients with recent bleeding. Gut 1999;44:264–169.

42. Vorobioff J, Groszmann RJ, Picabea E, et al. Prognostic value of hepatic venous pressure gradient measurements in alcoholic cirrhosis: a 10-year prospective study. Gastroenterology 1996;111:701–709.

43. Patch D, Sabin CA, Goulis J, et al. A randomized controlled trial of medical therapy versus endoscopic ligation for the prevention of variceal rebleeding in patients with cirrhosis. Gastroenterology 2002;123: 1013–1019.

44. Delrente P, Rufat P, Hillaire S, et al. Lack of prognostic usefulness of hepatic venous pressures and hemodynamic values in a select group of patients with severe alcoholic cirrhosis. Am J Gastroenterol 2002;97:1187–1190.

45. Alonso S, Banares R, Albillos A, et al. Hepatic venous pressure gradient (HVPG) predicts early recurrence of varices and rebleeding after endoscopic band ligation (EBL) (Abstract). Hepatology 2003;38 (Suppl 1):295A.

46. Lebrec D, Hillon P, Munoz C, Goldfarb G, Nouel O, Benhamou JP. The effect of propranolol on portal hypertension in patients with cirrhosis: a hemodynamic study. Hepatology 1982;2:523–527.

47. Lebrec D, Poynard T, Bernuau J, et al. A randomized controlled study of propranolol for prevention of recurrent gastrointestinal bleeding in patients with cirrhosis: a final report. Hepatology 1984;4:355–358.

48. Bosch J, Mastai R, Kravetz D, et al. Effects of propranolol on azygos venous blood flow and hepatic and systemic hemodynamics in cirrhosis. Hepatology 1984;4:1200–1205.
49. Boyer T. Pharmacologic treatment of portal hypertension: past, present and future. Hepatology 2001; 34:834–839.
50. Feu F, Garcia-Pagan JC, Bosch J, et al. Relation between portal pressure response to pharmacotherapy and risk of recurrent variceal haemorrhage in patients with cirrhosis. Lancet 1995;346:1056–1059.
51. Leevy C, Zinke M, Baber J, Chey WY. Observations on influence of medical therapy on portal hypertension. Ann Int Med 1958;49:837–851.
52. Reynolds TB, Geller HM, Kuzma OT, Redeker AG. Spontaneous decrease in portal pressure with clinical improvement in cirrhosis. N Engl J Med 1960;263:734–739.
53. Aracil C, Lopez-Balaguer JM, Monfort D, et al. Hemodynamic response to beta-blockers and prediction of clinical efficacy in the primary prophylaxis of variceal bleeding in patients with cirhrosis (Abstract). Hepatology 2003;38(Suppl 1):296A.
54. De BK, Sen S, Biswas PK, et al. Propranolol in primary and secondary prophylaxis of variceal bleeding amount cirrhotics in India: a hemodynamic evaluation. Am J Gastroenterol 2000;95:2023–2028.
55. Groszmann RJ, Bosch J, Grace ND, et al. Hemodynamic events in a prospective randomized trial of propranolol versus placebo in the prevention of a first variceal hemorrhage. Gastroenterology 1990;99: 1401–1407.
56. Merkel C, Bolognesi M, Sarcedoti D, et al. The hemodynamic response to medical treatment of portal hypertension as a predictor of clinical effectiveness in the primary prophylaxis of variceal bleeding in cirrhosis. Hepatology 2000;32:930–934.
57. Escorsell A, Bordas JM, Castaneda B, et al. Predictive value of the variceal pressure response to continued pharmacological therapy in patients with cirrhosis and portal hypertension. Hepatology 2000; 31:1061–1067.
58. Villanueva C, Minana J, Ortiz J, et al. Endoscopic ligation compared with combined treatment with nadolol and isosorbide mononitrate to prevent recurrent variceal bleeding. N Engl J Med 2001;30:647–655.
59. Bureau C, Peron JM, Alric L, et al. "À la carte" treatment of portal hypertension: adapting medical therapy to hemodynamic response for the prevention of bleeding. Hepatology 2002;36:1361–1366.
60. McCormick PA, Patch D, Greensdale L, Chin J, McIntyre N, Burroughs AK. Clinical vs haemodynamic response to drugs in portal hypertension. J Hepatol 1998;28:1015–1019.
61. Hicken BL, Sharara AI, Abrams GA, Eloubeidi M, Fallon MB, Argueda MR. Hepatic venous pressure gradient measurements to assess response to primary prophylaxis in patients with cirrhosis: a decision analytical study. Aliment Pharmacol Ther 2003;17:145–153.
62. Abraldes JG, Tarantino I, Turnes J, Garcia-Pagan JC, Rodes J, Bosch J. Hemodynamic response to pharmacological treatment of portal hypertension and long-term prognosis of cirrhosis. Hepatology 2003; 37:902–908.

10

Evaluation of Portal Hemodynamics Using Indicator Dilution and Noninvasive Techniques

Juerg Reichen, MD

CONTENTS

INTRODUCTION
THE MULTIPLE INDICATOR DILUTION TECHNIQUE
INTRAVITAL MICROSCOPY
OTHER TECHNIQUES TO ASSESS IMPAIRED MICROVASCULAR
    EXCHANGE
ESTIMATION OF HEPATIC PERFUSION BY THE CLEARANCE TECHNIQUE
RADIOLOGICAL TECHNIQUES TO ASSESS HEPATIC PERFUSION
ACKNOWLEDGMENT
REFERENCES

INTRODUCTION

Microvascular exchange in the liver is quite peculiar owing to the porosity of the sinusoidal endothelial cells; the pores in the sinusoidal endothelium allow free passage of macromolecules, which allows the hepatocyte to take up tightly protein bound drugs *(1)*. One of the major changes occurring in cirrhosis is sinusoidal capillarization *(2)*, which leads to a profound impediment of passage of substances into the space of Disse. Sinusoidal capillarization was first described by Hans Popper on a morphological level *(2)*; he—rightfully—predicted that this phenomenon would have important bearings on hepatic function. It lasted almost 20 yr until sinusoidal capillarization was demonstrated functionally using the multiple indicator dilution technique *(3)*—this study was quite a feat because it applied this demanding technique to humans before studying the phenomenon in animal models. Another important aspect of altered microvascular exchange is loss of the sinusoidal fenestrations that, at least in alcoholic liver disease, occurs before significant fibrosis is seen *(4)*.

Another important aspect is the regulation of sinusoidal flow, which is profoundly disturbed in cirrhosis. Here tribute has to be paid to the earliest advocates of intravital microscopy, Aaron Rappaport and Robert S. McCuskey. Dr. Rappaport published little, but influenced many. His movies around redistribution of sinusoidal blood flow inspired

From: *Clinical Gastroenterology: Portal Hypertension*
Edited by: A. J. Sanyal and V. H. Shah © Humana Press Inc., Totowa, NJ

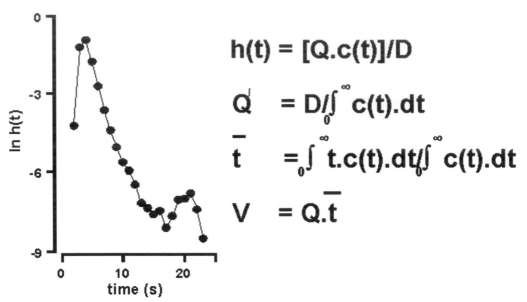

$$h(t) = [Q.c(t)]/D$$

$$Q = D/\int_0^\infty c(t).dt$$

$$\bar{t} = \int_0^\infty t.c(t).dt/\int_0^\infty c(t).dt$$

$$V = Q.\bar{t}$$

Fig. 1. The Stewart-Hamilton principle of calculating flow and volume from the dispersion of an injected indicator, which can be a dye, fluorescent compound, radioactive material, or thermal challenge. The frequency function $h(t)$ is the product of the flow going through the area of interest Q and the concentrations in its outflow divided by the amount injected D. This equation can be solved to derive the flow from the observed concentrations in the outflow, the mean transit time as the ratio of the area under the curve and its first moment. Finally, the volume traversed is the product of flow and mean transit time.

many to study the topic. At the end of his career, he wrote a landmark paper correlating the histological changes of cirrhosis with alterations in flow *(5)*. Robert McCuskey, to my knowledge, is the first to formally describe the technique of modern intravital microscopy with on-line analysis *(6)*.

In this chapter we will consider the main techniques, to probe microvascular exchange, namely, the indicator dilution technique and intravital microscopy. Also, the old clearance techniques, as well as newer radiological noninvasive methods to probe different aspects of portal hypertension, in particular, estimated hepatic blood flow and microvascular exchange, will be reviewed.

THE MULTIPLE INDICATOR DILUTION TECHNIQUE

The indicator dilution technique to determine flow and volume of distribution—also known as the Stewart–Hamilton principle—is quite simple a concept as shown in Fig. 1. Renkin took this a step further by using indicators with different volumes of distribution to calculate surface/permeability coefficients *(7)*. The multiple indicator technique had been pioneered in hepatology by the late Carl Goresky who was the first to describe the formalism of the technique in the liver, to use it to calculate hepatic spaces *(8)*, and to evaluate transport phenomena *(9)*. The principle is simple: a mix of radioactively marked substances with different volumes of distribution is injected into the inflow vessel— either the portal vein or the hepatic artery in case of the liver—and the outflow is collected. The technique is particularly useful in the perfused organ because there the outflow can

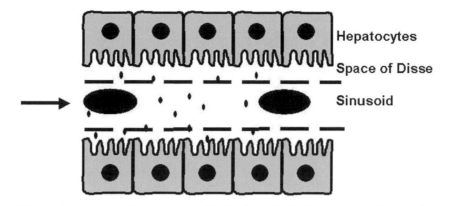

Fig. 2. Schematic representation of a sinusoid. The flow-limited pattern of multiple indicator dilution curves is due to the fact that erythrocytes (large ellipses) are confined to the sinusoid while diffusible molecules such as albumin (small circles) diffuse into the space of Disse and back into the sinusoid.

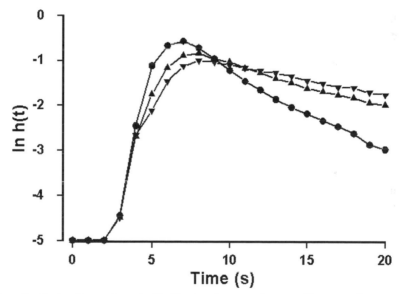

Fig. 3. Flow-limited pattern of a set of indicators in normal mouse liver: erythrocytes (●) peak higher and appear earlier than diffusible labels such as albumin (▲) or sucrose (▼).

be collected quantitatively thereby avoiding recirculation of the indicators. Furthermore, catheter distortion can be minimized and adequately evaluated.

In the liver, erythrocytes are used as the intravascular reference substance because they are confined to the intrasinusoidal space. Albumin or some other large molecule is used to estimate the space of Disse; in cirrhotic liver, a low-molecular-weight substance such as ^{22}Na or sucrose is used to probe the diffusional barrier. What happens then is quite predictable (see Fig. 2): in the sinusoid, erythrocytes are confined to the intravascular space and therefore peak higher and emerge earlier than a diffusible substance such as albumin (Fig. 3) and cross into the space of Disse and are therefore delayed. A typical set of multiple indicator dilution curves in a normal mouse liver is shown in Fig. 3.

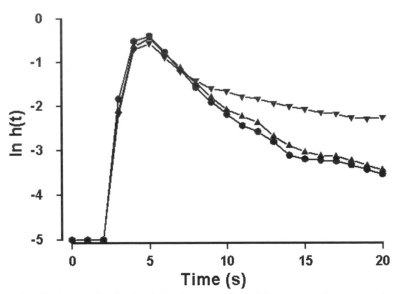

Fig. 4. Multiple indicator dilution in cirrhotic mouse liver: The pattern changes to a barrier-limited pattern as seen in most other vascular beds: The albumin (▲) is virtually superimposed upon the erythrocyte (●) curve since due to sinusoidal capillarization and loss of fenestrae it cannot leave the intravascular space. Sucrose (▼) in contrast shows a biexponential decay due to diffusion across the sinusoidal barrier.

Interestingly, the technique has been applied to patients with cirrhosis before animal cirrhosis models were studied. In a landmark study, Huet et al. described a continuous decrease in the extravascular space accessible to albumin in 23/25 patients; the other two exhibited bimodal outflow curves compatible with pronounced intrahepatic shunting *(3)*.

In cirrhotic rat liver, sinusoidal capillarization has been first described as the emergence of barrier, rather than flow-limited distribution of indicators (Fig. 4) again by P.M. Huet's groups in Montreal *(10)*. The extravascular albumin space is the most important predictor of hepatic function—more important than shunting or functional liver cell mass —in rats with CCl_4-induced cirrhosis *(11)*. Sinusoidal capillarization correlates with the degree of fibrosis *(12)*, volume fraction of hepatic stellate cells *(12)*, and loss of fenestrations *(13)*. The decreased clearance function of the cirrhotic liver is mainly caused by decreased uptake since metabolism is maintained as evidenced by a multiple indicator study in different models of chronic and acute liver injury *(14)*.

Capillarization and loss of fenestrations are not the whole story, however, because there is a reversible component to the decreased extravascular albumin space. Thus, calcium antagonists in high doses are able to increase the space accessible to albumin; this is associated with improved clearance function in the isolated organ *(15)*. The exact nature of this reversible part of impaired microvascular exchange remains to be determined. Chances are good that it is related to endogenous vasoactive compounds, in particular endothelin: endothelins play a major role in fibrogenesis and are markedly elevated in portal hypertension (reviewed elsewhere in this volume). Particularly germane is the finding that endothelin antagonists also are able to partially reverse the altered microvascular exchange *(16)*. In normal animals, endothelin induces a change from flow-limited to barrier-limited microvascular exchange such as that seen in cirrhosis *(16)*. Interestingly, mechanically increasing portal inflow also improves microvascular exchange and clearance function *(17)*.

The multiple indicator dilution technique can also be applied to the hepatic arterial bed; this visualizes the peribiliary plexus and increased cellular volume, presumably the cholangiocyte compartment *(18)*. Hepatic intraarterial injection of indicators into cirrhotic liver demonstrates increased vascular space compared to intraportal injection; this most likely reflects the extended peribiliary plexus but could also be caused by sinusoids accessible only to arterial inflow *(19)*.

INTRAVITAL MICROSCOPY

This powerful tool has become the workhorse of physiologists and pathophysiologists interested in the study of microvascular exchange. It was introduced into liver physiology Robert McCuskey in 1966 *(6)*. The methodology is well described in some review articles by the leaders in the field *(20,21)*. Parameters easily obtained include red cell flow velocity and vascular diameters. In contrast with the multiple indicator dilution technique, it allows single sinusoids to be viewed, to identify the cell type taking part in certain reactions such as vasoconstriction, and to localize the sites where such changes occur. Its only drawbacks are the fact that, in contrast with the multiple indicator dilution technique, only superficial sinusoids can be viewed and that it does not give a distribution of transit times through the whole organ.

A very powerful aspect of intravital microscopy is the possibility to view the interaction of inflammatory cells with resident cells in the liver. Although this has so far been mostly studied in ischemia–reperfusion injury and acute toxicity, a few data in animal models of cirrhosis are available. Thus, Ito et al. have demonstrated that chronic bile duct ligation exacerbates the inflammatory response to endotoxin by hypoperfusion of sinusoids exacerbated by increased adherence of leukocytes *(22)*.

The use of fluorescent dyes and online analysis have added considerably to the possibilities of intravital microscopy (reviewed in ref. *21*). Recently, Paxian et al. have published a technique whereby oxygenation can be measured using a fluorescent dye *(23)*; application of this technique to cirrhotic liver should be quite interesting.

Sherman et al. were among the first to use this technique in portal hypertension; in their landmark paper they identified "fast sinusoids" as a major feature of early and late fibrosis, such sinusoids accounting for 7% and 33% of all sinusoids, respectively, *(24)*; furthermore, a dilatation of terminal hepatic venules was found early on in the process of fibrogenesis. Furthermore, the expansion of hepatic stellate cells could be visualized by their autofluorescence *(24)*. Using similar techniques, these findings were later confirmed by Vollmar et al. *(25)*. The latter authors also demonstrated that blockade of Kupffer cells with $GdCl_3$ attenuated and delayed but did not prevent fibrogenesis *(26)*.

Assessment of microvascular exchange has traditionally been performed using the multiple indicator dilution technique. Use of fluorescent dextrans in the perfused liver has made it possible to calculate diffusion coefficients and permeability for single sinusoids *(27)*. Similarly, such compounds have been used to visualize lymph vessels during cirrhogenesis *(28)*.

Using intravital microscopy, important compensatory mechanisms in different models of portal hypertension, hitherto unknown or only poorly characterized, could be identified.

Thus, after portal vein ligation the sinusoidal blood flow is maintained because of angiogenesis providing the liver with arterial blood *(29)*. In a similar vein, the hepatic arterial buffer response is increased in CCl_4-induced cirrhosis *(30)*.

OTHER TECHNIQUES TO ASSESS IMPAIRED MICROVASCULAR EXCHANGE

Some magnetic resonance techniques with much promise to probe different aspects of microcirculation are emerging. Thus, functional magnetic resonance imaging has been successfully used to monitor oxygenation in vivo *(31)*. An ingenious approach has been described recently using contrast agents of different molecular weight *(32)*. Thereby, van Beers et al. were able to demonstrate diminished access of a large-molecular-weight (52 kDa) compound whereas that of a small-molecular-weight one (6.5 kDa) was increased in livers of fibrotic rabbits. A similar technique for use with computed tomography has been described earlier by the same group *(33)*. Application of this technique in humans appears very promising and such results are eagerly awaited. Interestingly, serum hyaluronate—normally used as a noninvasive marker of fibrosis *(34)*—indicates sinusoidal capillarization when its level exceeds 200 ng/mL *(35)*.

ESTIMATION OF HEPATIC PERFUSION BY THE CLEARANCE TECHNIQUE

Hepatic perfusion can be estimated by the Fick principle; this was introduced 1945 by Stan Bradley and Franz Ingelfinger *(36)* and applied to cirrhotic patients by the same group *(37)*. A bolus or steady-state infusion of a high extraction compound is given; perfusion Q can then be calculated as

$$Q = \text{clearance/extraction.}$$

If an infusion is given, under steady-state conditions, clearance can be set equal to the infusion rate. The method is not truly noninvasive because measurement of extraction has to be performed *(38)*. The compounds most frequently used for this technique are indocyanine green, galactose, and sorbitol. For this method to yield accurate values of hepatic perfusion, the indicator used should have no extra hepatic clearance and have an extraction ratio close to 1.

Indocyanine green is the most widely used compound to estimate hepatic blood flow; it was introduced into clinical research in the early 1960s *(39,40)*. There is virtually no extra-hepatic metabolism of ICG but the second condition, namely, an extraction close to 1 is not achieved. This deteriorates further in the presence of shunting and loss of liver function. Provided extraction is determined *(38,41)*, estimation of hepatic blood flow using indocyanine green remains a valuable tool in particular when evaluating the effects of short-term pharmacological or surgical interventions. Determination of ICG retention has value as a quantitative liver function test *(42)* but does not reflect hepatic perfusion.

Different compounds with higher extraction efficiency have been proposed but none has been able to replace indocyanine green in the leading research centers so far. The one which comes closest to the ideal substance is sorbitol *(43)*, which in healthy volunteers has an extraction ratio of 0.96 *(44)*. In fulminant hepatic failure—where indocyanine green extraction is too low to estimate hepatic blood flow—sorbitol clearance has successfully been employed *(45)*. However, in cirrhotic liver sorbitol clearance underestimates hepatic perfusion to a similar degree as does indocyanine green *(46)*. In the direct comparison to duplex assessment of portal flow, sorbitol clearance shows a decrease while by duplex it is maintained *(47)*. It has been proposed to use the difference between "nutritional" flow—estimated with indocyanine green—and total flow as a measure of shunting *(48)*. However, alternative interpretations which are quite as plausible have been proposed *(49)*.

Where does that leave the value of flow determination by the clearance technique? We have to accept that neither flow nor shunting can be determined accurately by the clearance technique. However, the technique is still valuable to assess pharmacologically or surgically induced changes in hepatic perfusion, provided extraction is measured *(38)*.

RADIOLOGICAL TECHNIQUES TO ASSESS HEPATIC PERFUSION

Sonographic examinations including duplex are standard in the evaluation of patients with portal hypertension. Combining measurement of the cross-sectional area (CSA) of the portal vein with flow velocity (*v*), physical portal flow (*Q*) can be calculated as

$$Q = v \cdot CSA.$$

This assumes that CSA is constant—which it is not because it depends very much on respiration—in a model system up to 53% variation *(50)*. The main problem with this method is that it is very operator dependent with variable intra- and poor interobserver correlation *(51)*. This is mostly because of the uncertainty of the angle at which the signal is transmitted; by just reporting flow velocity, reliability greatly increases *(52)*. This weakness—as well as the dependence on the type of equipment used—can be partially overcome by adherence to a rigorous protocol for sonographic examination and training of the operator *(53)*. Flow velocity measurements are highly sensitive and correlate well with the Child–Pugh classification *(54)*.

Thus, the value of Duplex determination of portal flow or flow velocity is mainly for short-term assessment of physiological changes such as postprandial hyperemia *(55–57)* or of pharmacological interventions *(56)*. If absolute values are required, MR angiography is superior to duplex *(57)*.

MR angiography is a promising technique to evaluate hepatic perfusion in patients with cirrhosis in particular since it allows also determination of transit times *(58)* and absolute volumes of flow can be obtained *(59)*.

Nuclear medicine techniques are complicated because of the dual blood supply of the liver; derivation of flow parameters requires deconvolution analysis or other demanding mathematical techniques. Therefore, they have remained a research tool and never made into daily clinical practice in the research centers interested in portal hypertension; a good overview of nuclear medicine techniques was recently published by Chow et al. *(60)*.

ACKNOWLEDGMENT

The author was supported by a Grant from the Swiss National Foundation for Scientific Research (No. 63476.00).

REFERENCES

1. Reichen J. The role of sinusoidal endothelium in liver function. News Physiol Sci 1999;14:117–120.
2. Schaffner F, Popper H. Capillarization of hepatic sinusoids in man. Gastroenterology 1963;44:239–242.

3. Huet PM, Goresky CA, Villeneuve JP, Marleau D, Lough JO. Assessment of liver microcirculation in human cirrhosis. J Clin Invest 1982;70:1234–1244.
4. Horn T, Christoffersen P, Henriksen JH. Alcoholic liver injury: defenestration in noncirrhotic livers—A scanning electron microscopic study. Hepatology 1987;7:77–82.
5. Rappaport AM, MacPhee PJ, Fisher MM, Phillips MJ. The scarring of the liver acini (cirrhosis). Tridimensional and microcirculatory considerations. Virchow's Arch A Pathol Anat 1983;402:107–137.
6. McCuskey RS. A dynamic and static study of hepatic arterioles and hepatic sphincters. Am J Anat 1966; 119:455–478.
7. Renkin EM. Multiple pathways of capillary permeability. Circ Res 1977;41:735–743.
8. Goresky CA. A linear method for determining liver sinusoidal and extravascular volume. Am J Physiol 1963;204:626–640.
9. Goresky CA, Bach GG, Nadeau BE. On the uptake of material by the intact liver: the transport and net removal of galactose. J Clin Invest 1973;52:991–1009.
10. Varin F, Huet PM. Hepatic microcirculation in the perfused cirrhotic rat liver. J Clin Invest 1985;76:1904–1912.
11. Reichen J, Egger B, Ohara N, Zeltner TB, Zysset T, Zimmermann A. Determinants of hepatic functions in liver cirrhosis in the rat: a multivariate analysis. J Clin Invest 1988;82:2069–2076.
12. Zimmermann A, Zhao DL, Reichen J. Myofibroblasts in the cirrhotic rat liver reflect hepatic remodeling and correlate with fibrosis and sinusoidal capillarization. J Hepatol 1999;30:646–652.
13. Hung DY, Chang P, Cheung K, Winterford C, Roberts MS. Quantitative evaluation of altered hepatic spaces and membrane transport in fibrotic rat liver. Hepatology 2002;36:1180–1189.
14. Gariépy L, Fenyves D, Kassissia I, Villeneuve JP. Clearance by the liver in cirrhosis. 2. characterization of propranolol uptake with the multiple-indicator dilution technique. Hepatology 1993;18:823–831.
15. Reichen J, Le M. Verapamil favourably influences hepatic microvascular exchange and function in rats with cirrhosis of the liver. J Clin Invest 1986;78:448–455.
16. Reichen J, Gerbes AL, Stainer MJ, Sägesser H, Clozel M. The effect of endothelin and its antagonist Bosentan on hemodynamics and microvascular exchange in cirrhotic rat liver. J Hepatol 1998;28:1020–1030.
17. Cardoso JE, Giroux L, Kassissia I, Houssin D, Habib N, Huet PM. Liver function improvement following increased portal blood flow in cirrhotic rats. Gastroenterology 1994;107:460–467.
18. Reichen J. Role of the hepatic artery in canalicular bile formation by the perfused rat liver. A multiple indicator dilution study. J Clin Invest 1988;81:1462–149.
19. Kassissia I, Brault A, Huet PM. Hepatic artery and portal vein vascularization of normal and cirrhotic rat liver. Hepatology 1994;19:1189–1197.
20. McCuskey RS, Reilly FD. Hepatic microvasculature: dynamic structure and its regulation. Semin Liver Dis 1993;13:1–12.
21. Clemens MG, Zhang JX. Regulation of sinusoidal perfusion: in vivo methodology and control by endothelins. Semin Liver Dis 1999;19:383–396.
22. Ito Y, Machen NW, Urbaschek R, McCuskey RS. Biliary obstruction exacerbates the hepatic microvascular inflammatory response to endotoxin. Shock 2000;14:599–604.
23. Paxian M, Keller SA, Cross B, Huynh TT, Clemens MG. High-resolution visualization of oxygen distribution in the liver in vivo. Am J Physiol Gastrointest Liver Physiol 2004;286:G37–G44.
24. Sherman IA, Pappas SC, Fisher MM. Hepatic microvascular changes associated with development of liver fibrosis and cirrhosis. Am J Physiol 1990;258:H460–H465.
25. Vollmar B, Siegmund S, Menger MD. An intravital fluorescence microscopic study of hepatic microvascular and cellular derangements in developing cirrhosis in rats. Hepatology 1998;27:1544–1553.
26. Vollmar B, Siegmund S, Richter S, Menger MD. Microvascular consequences of Kupffer cell modulation in rat liver fibrogenesis. J Pathol 1999;189:85–91.
27. Stock RJ, Cilento EV, McCuskey RS. A quantitative study of fluorescein isothiocyanate-dextran transport in the microcirculation of the isolated perfused rat liver. Hepatology 1989;9:75–82.
28. Vollmar B, Wolf B, Siegmund S, Katsen AD, Menger MD. Lymph vessel expansion and function in the development of hepatic fibrosis and cirrhosis. Am J Pathol 1997;151:169–175.
29. Yokoyama Y, Baveja R, Sonin N, Clemens MG, Zhang JX. Hepatic neovascularization after partial portal vein ligation: novel mechanism of chronic regulation of blood flow. Am J Physiol Gastrointest Liver Physiol 2001;280:G21–G31.

30. Richter S, Vollmar B, Mücke I, Post S, Menger MD. Hepatic arteriolo-portal venular shunting guarantees maintenance of nutritional microvascular supply in hepatic arterial buffer response of rat livers. J Physiol (Lond) 2001;531:193–201.
31. Foley LM, Picot P, Thompson RT, Yau MJ, Brauer M. In vivo monitoring of hepatic oxygenation changes in chronically ethanol-treated rats by functional magnetic resonance imaging. Magn Reson Med 2003;50:976–983.
32. Van Beers BE, Materne R, Annet L, et al. Capillarization of the sinusoids in liver fibrosis: noninvasive assessment with contrast-enhanced MRI in the rabbit. Magn Reson Med 2003;49:692–699.
33. Materne R, Annet L, Dechambre S, et al. Dynamic computed tomography with low- and high-molecular-mass contrast agents to assess microvascular permeability modifications in a model of liver fibrosis. Clin Sci (Lond) 2002;103:213–216.
34. Oberti F, Valsesia E, Pilette C, et al. Noninvasive diagnosis of hepatic fibrosis or cirrhosis. Gastroenterology 1997;113:1609–1616.
35. Ueno T, Inuzuka S, Torimura T, et al. Serum hyaluronate reflects hepatic sinusoidal capillarization. Gastroenterology 1993;105:475–481.
36. Bradley SE, Ingelfinger FJ, Bradley GP, Currey J. The estimation of hepatic blood flow in man. J Clin Invest 1945;24:890–897.
37. Bradley SE, Ingelfinger FJ, Bradley GP. Hepatic circulation in cirrhosis of the liver. Circulation 1952; 5:419–429.
38. Groszman RJ. The measurement of liver blood flow using clearance techniques. Hepatology 1983;3: 1039–1040.
39. Caesar J, Shaldon S, Chiandussi L, Guevara L, Sherlock S. The use of indocyanine green in the measurement of hepatic blood flow and as a test of hepatic function. Clin Sci 1961;21:43–57.
40. Leevy CM, Mendenhall CL, Lesko W, Howard MM. Estimation of hepatic blood flow with indocyanine green. J Clin Invest 1962;41:1169–1179.
41. Clements D, West R, Elias E. Comparison of bolus and infusion methods for estimating hepatic blood flow in patients with liver disease using indocyanine green. J Hepatol 1987;5:282–287.
42. Reichen J. Assessment of hepatic function with xenobiotics. Semin Liver Dis 1995;15:189–201.
43. Molino G, Avagnina P, Cavanna A, et al. Sorbitol clearance: a parameter reflecting liver plasma flow in the rat. Res Comm Chem Pathol Pharmacol 1986;52:119–132.
44. Zeeh J, Lange H, Bosch J, et al. Steady-state extrarenal sorbitol clearance as a measure of hepatic plasma flow. Gastroenterology 1988;95:749–759.
45. Clemmesen JO, Tygstrup N, Ott P. Hepatic plasma flow estimated according to Fick's principle in patients with hepatic encephalopathy: evaluation of indocyanine green and D-sorbitol as test substances. Hepatology 1998;27:666–673.
46. Keiding S, Engsted E, Ott P. Sorbitol as a test substance for measurement of liver plasma flow in humans. Hepatology 1998;28:50–56.
47. Zoli M, Magalotti D, Bianchi G, et al. Functional hepatic flow and Doppler-assessed total hepatic flow in control subjects and in patients with cirrhosis. J Hepatol 1995;23:129–134.
48. Molino G, Avagnina P, Ballare M, et al. Combined evaluation of total and functional liver plasma flows and intrahepatic shunting. Dig Dis Sci 1991;36:1189–1196.
49. Ott P, Clemmesen O, Keiding S. Interpretation of simultaneous measurements of hepatic extraction fractions of indocyanine green and sorbitol—Evidence of hepatic shunts and capillarization? Dig Dis Sci 2000;45:359–365.
50. Chow PK, Yu WK, Ng TH, et al. Influence of respiration and portal pressure on transabdominal duplex Doppler ultrasound measurement of portal blood flow: a porcine model for experimental studies. J Surg Res 2000;89:66–73.
51. Sabba C, Weltin GG, Cicchetti DV, et al. Observer variability in echo-Doppler measurements of portal flow in cirrhotic patients and normal volunteers. Gastroenterology 1990;98:1603–1611.
52. Sabba C, Ferraioli G, Buonamico P, et al. Echo-Doppler evaluation of acute flow changes in portal hypertensive patients: flow velocity as a reliable parameter. J Hepatol 1992;15:356–360.
53. Sabbà C, Merkel C, Zoli M, et al. Interobserver and interequipment variability of echo-Doppler examination of the portal vein: effect of a cooperative training program. Hepatology 1995;21:428–433.
54. Zironi G, Gaiani S, Fenyves D, Rigamonti A, Bolondi L, Barbara L. Value of measurement of mean portal flow velocity by Doppler flowmetry in the diagnosis of portal hypertension. J Hepatol 1992;16:298–303.

55. de Vries PJ, de Hooge P, Hoekstra JBL, Van Hattum J. Blunted postprandial reaction of portal venous flow in chronic liver disease, assessed with duplex Doppler: significance for prognosis. J Hepatol 1994; 21:966–973.

56. Buonamico P, Sabbá C, Garcia-Tsao G, et al. Octreotide blunts postprandial splanchnic hyperemia in cirrhotic patients: a double-blind randomized echo-Doppler study. Hepatology 1995;21:134–139.

57. Nijeholt GJLA, Burggraaf K, Wásser MNJM, et al. Variability of splanchnic blood flow measurements using MR velocity mapping under fasting and post-prandial conditions—Comparison with echo-Doppler. J Hepatol 1997;26:298–304.

58. Annet L, Materne R, Danse E, Jamart J, Horsmans Y, Van Beers BE. Hepatic flow parameters measured with MR imaging and Doppler US: correlations with degree of cirrhosis and portal hypertension. Radiology 2003;229:409–414.

59. Burkart DJ, Johnson CD, Ehman RL, Weaver AL, Ilstrup DM. Evaluation of portal venous hypertension with cine phase—contrast MR flow measurements—high association of hyperdynamic portal flow with variceal hemorrhage. Radiology 1993;188:643–648.

60. Chow PKH, Yu WK, Soo KC, Chan STF. The measurement of liver blood flow: a review of experimental and clinical methods. J Surg Res 2003;112:1–11.

11

Endoscopic Assessment of Portal Hypertension Including Variceal Pressure Measurements

Methods, Interpretation, and Pitfalls

Àngels Escorsell, MD and Jaime Bosch, MD

INTRODUCTION

Portal hypertension is a common complication in liver diseases that should be searched for in all cirrhotic patients, as well as in other chronic liver diseases (1). Its main clinical consequence is bleeding from ruptured esophageal or gastric varices, which constitutes the major cause of death and of liver transplantation in patients with cirrhosis, the leading etiology for portal hypertension.

In the present chapter we review the endoscopic tools to assess portal hypertension (endoscopy, measurement of variceal pressure, and endosonography). These techniques are useful in the diagnosis of portal hypertension and gastroesophageal varices, as well as in the evaluation of the risk of bleeding and the effects of therapy on that risk.

ENDOSCOPY

Upper endoscopy is the best method for evaluating the presence of complications of portal hypertension including gastroesophageal varices and portal hypertensive gastropathy; and is routinely used as a first-level approach to assess this syndrome (1,2).

Esophageal varices are present in about 40% of compensated patients and in 60% of those presenting with ascites at the initial diagnosis of cirrhosis (3,4). Moreover, the incidence of esophageal varices in cirrhotic patients has been estimated in about 5% per year (5). Thus, the estimated 5-yr risk of varices is about 65%. For this reason, in a large consensus conference it was agreed that all patients with cirrhosis should be endoscopically screened

From: *Clinical Gastroenterology: Portal Hypertension*
Edited by: A. J. Sanyal and V. H. Shah © Humana Press Inc., Totowa, NJ

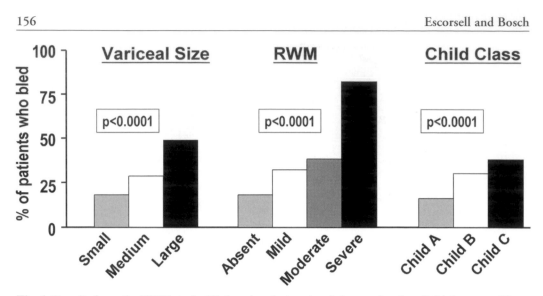

Fig. 1. Results from the NIEC study *(9)* showing that variceal size, variceal wall thickness and liver function (according to the Child–Pugh classification) are factors strongly related to the risk of bleeding.

for the presence of varices at the time of the initial diagnosis *(5,6)*. In patients without varices on initial endoscopy, a second (follow-up) evaluation should be performed to detect the development of varices before these bleed. As we mentioned, and because the expected incidence of newly developed varices is about 5% per year, the general consensus *(5,6)* is that endoscopy should be repeated after 2–3 yr in those patients. In patients with small varices on initial endoscopy, the aim of subsequent evaluations is to detect the progression of small to large varices because of its important prognostic and therapeutic implications. Based on an expected 10–15% per year rate of progression of variceal size, endoscopy should be repeated every 1–2 yr in patients with small varices *(5,7)*.

To correctly interpret the results of clinical studies, it can be useful to standardize the endoscopic assessment of varices (i.e., evaluating its presence and size at full inflation, before removal of the endoscope) and to obtain digital images allowing review and comparison with follow-up studies. Owing to the frequent requirement of the latter, it is also very important to improve the acceptability of the procedure by providing conscious sedation [with drugs proven not to significantly modify portal pressure *(8)*].

Endoscopy also discloses the characteristics of the varices. These are extremely important because they have prognostic value for variceal bleeding. Several studies have shown that the risk of variceal bleeding is directly related to the size of the varices (graded on a scale of I to IV) and to the presence of "red signs" in variceal wall (telangiectasias, red whale marking, or cherry red spots) (Fig. 1) *(7,9,10)*. Both factors, along with the degree of liver impairment as assessed by the Child–Pugh class, constitute one of the most widely used prognostic indexes for variceal bleeding, the North Italian Endoscopic Club (NIEC) index *(9)*. These three parameters, variceal size, red signs, and severity of liver impairment, significantly correlate with variceal pressure *(11,12)*; which in turn is significantly associated with the risk of bleeding and death *(13)*. From a practical point of view, it should be remembered that patients with esophageal varices > 5 mm in diameter and presence of red signs are those with the highest risk of variceal bleeding; especially if they have a Child–Pugh class B or C and ascites (Fig. 1).

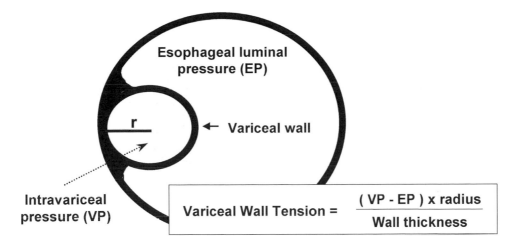

Fig. 2. Calculation of variceal wall tension according to Frank's modification of Laplace's law.

Furthermore, endoscopy informs on the presence of gastric varices and of portal hypertensive gastropathy, conditions responsible for many of the nonesophageal variceal bleeding episodes in cirrhotic patients. The identification of gastric varices at endoscopy may offer some difficulties that have now been overcome by the introduction of endosonography, allowing the identification of gastric varices as roundish, echo-free structures, located mostly in the gastric submucosal layer *(14)*.

Recently, another endoscopic index combining variceal size, the presence of portal hypertensive gastropathy and the presence of gastric varices has been proposed *(15)*. Its value, alone or incorporating additional parameters related with portal hypertension (i.e., spleen size, platelet count), remains to be determined.

MEASUREMENT OF VARICEAL PRESSURE

Longitudinal studies have identified variceal pressure as a prognostic indicator of the bleeding risk and of the response to pharmacological therapy in patients with both cirrhosis *(11,16)* and noncirrhotic portal hypertension *(17)*. Interestingly, higher variceal pressures have been documented in patients with previous variceal bleeding, large varices, and in those with red color signs, which are those more prone to bleed *(11)*.

Variceal pressure, size, and wall thickness are the determinants of the tension in the wall of the varix, which has been identified as the key factor leading to variceal rupture *(11,12,18)*. According to Frank's modification of Laplace's law, variceal wall tension is directly proportional to the transmural variceal pressure (the gradient between variceal and intraesophageal pressures) and the radius of the varix, and is inversely proportional to the thickness of the variceal wall (Fig. 2) *(12)*.

This equation indicates that a large variceal size multiplies the deleterious effects of a high intravariceal pressure increasing the tension exerted on the wall of the varices; a big varix with thin walls will reach a high wall tension (and risk of bleeding) at much lower variceal pressures than a small varix with thick walls. This may explain why large gastric fundal varices may bleed at relatively low portal pressure. Similarly, this equation explains

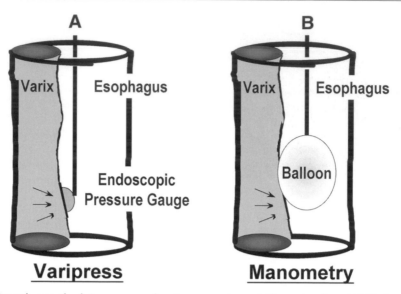

Fig. 3. Noninvasive methods to assess variceal pressure in portal hypertension. (**A**) Varipress (endoscopic pressure gauge). (**B**) Manometry.

the prognostic value of the red color signs (which reflect areas where the wall of the varices is especially thin) *(9,10)*. Furthermore, esophageal varices are more prone to bleed than varices of other locations [ectopic varices, responsible for 1–5% of variceal bleeds *(19)*] because of the negative esophageal luminal pressure during inspiration, and the lack of external tissue support, which decreases the elastic limit of the vessel *(12)*.

The sequence of events leading to variceal hemorrhage is, therefore, initiated by a high portal pressure, which promotes the opening of collaterals and the formation of varices. The maintenance of an increased intravascular pressure, together with a high collateral blood flow causes the dilatation of the varices, and as the varices dilate, their walls become thinner. Once wall tension exceeds the elastic limit of the varices, the patient will experience the first bleeding episode. After this, the patient remains at a high risk of rebleeding unless wall tension is decreased *(20)*.

The assessment of variceal size and wall thickness is better achieved by endoscopy or endosonography (see below). Variceal pressure can be measured by different methods.

Methods of Variceal Pressure Measurement

The "gold standard" is the measurement of intravariceal pressure by direct puncture of the varix with a thin needle. This invasive method carries a high risk of bleeding, which limits its use to patients undergoing endoscopic injection sclerotherapy after the procedure *(21)*. For this reason, noninvasive methods (mainly endoscopic pressure sensitive gauges and manometry) have also been developed (Fig. 3). Noninvasive techniques assume that varices behave as an elastic structure because of their thin walls and lack of external tissue support *(12)*; thus, the pressure needed to compress a varix (which can be sensed by pressure gauges or under direct vision using clear balloons or endosonography) equals the pressure inside the varix. Several studies have shown a good correlation between these techniques and the more aggressive variceal puncture technique *(11,22)*.

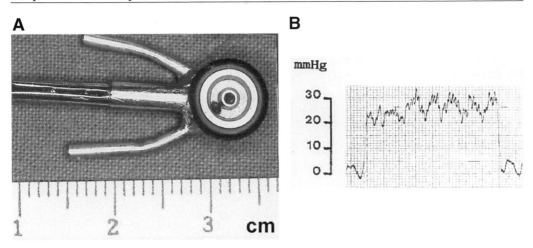

Fig. 4. (**A**) Endoscopic pressure gauge with a measuring surface (central hole) of 2 mm of diameter. (**B**) Correct variceal pressure tracing (note the fluctuations following cardiac and respiratory cycles as well as the stability of the tracing).

ENDOSCOPIC PRESSURE GAUGE (FIGS. 3A AND 4)

The use of the endoscopic pressure gauge was introduced by Mosimann et al. in 1982 *(23)*. Polio et al. *(24,25)* and Bosch et al. *(22,26)* introduced different modifications leading to the present and most commonly used device, the *Varipress* system (Solid Components, Barcelona, Spain) (Fig. 4A). The device consists of a small chamber covered by a thin elastic (latex) membrane, and which is continuously perfused with nitrogen. Owing to the elasticity of the varices, it is assumed that when the gauge is applied over the varix, the pressure needed to perfuse the gauge equals the pressure inside the varix *(23)*. The difference between the pressure needed to perfuse the gauge (equivalent to the pressure inside the varix) and the zero pressure (the pressure recorded when the gauge is free in the esophageal lumen) equals the transmural variceal pressure *(11)*. The *Varipress* gauge, with a measuring surface of 2 mm in diameter (Fig. 4A), showed a close correlation both in vitro (with an artificial varix system) and in vivo (measuring intravariceal pressure by direct puncture) *(22,26)*. In double-blind studies, placebo caused little variation following either acute administration (range: 0–4%) *(22,26–29)* or chronic administration (1–6%) *(30,31)*. Moreover, the small measuring surface makes the gauge suitable for measuring variceal pressure in varices of small size.

Variceal pressure measurements are considered satisfactory only when fulfilling the following predetermined criteria: (a) stable intraesophageal pressure; (b) absence of artifacts caused by esophageal peristalsis; and (c) correct placement of the capsule over the varix, as shown by the fine fluctuations of the pressure tracing according to heart cycle and respiration, for at least 10 s or three respiratory cycles (Fig. 4B) *(26–29)*. These conditions are easily met when the procedure is performed by a skilled endoscopist in a cooperative patient. In addition, 20 mg butyl scopolamine may be administered intravenously at the beginning of endoscopy to diminish artifacts caused by esophageal peristalsis without affecting variceal pressure measurements *(11,26)*.

These strict requirements are the main drawback in using the endoscopic gauge to measure variceal pressure. Actually, about 25% of patients initially scheduled to have variceal pressure measurements must be excluded because of technical difficulties that preclude obtaining correct measurements *(32)*. Of these, two-thirds correspond to patients with small varices.

Most of the studies assessing the utility of variceal pressure measurements (see below) were done using that technique.

ENDOSCOPIC MANOMETRY (FIG. 3B)

Manometry uses an endoscopic balloon to measure variceal pressure *(33–35)*. Up until now, this method relied on the visual appearance of the varices and, therefore, was subjected to observer bias. Recently, a new device combining endosonography and manometry has been introduced by different investigators. This method uses an endosonography probe with *(36)* or without *(37)* power Doppler capability to assess the appearance and disappearance of flow inside the varix. Variceal pressure is considered as the pressure needed by the balloon to cause the disappearance of flow inside the varix during its compression. The method has demonstrated its reliability and accuracy in two in vitro studies *(36,37)*. Clinical studies are waited.

Utility of Variceal Pressure Measurements

Previous studies have shown that variceal pressure correlates significantly with portal pressure and azygos blood flow, an index of blood flow through portocollateral vessels *(11,22)*. Despite these correlations, however, variceal pressure is significantly lower than portal pressure, probably because a significant resistance along the collaterals feeding the varices causes a pressure drop from the portal vein to the varix *(11)*. These findings suggest that collateral circulation (and resistance to blood flow in collaterals) is important in modulating variceal pressure.

ASSESSMENT OF THE RISK AND PROGNOSIS OF VARICEAL BLEEDING

The first evidence of the value of variceal pressure in assessing the risk of variceal bleeding came from the observation that patients who have bled from varices have significantly greater variceal pressure than those who have never bled, despite having similar portal pressures *(11,29,31)*. Moreover, variceal pressure is greater in patients with large varices than in those with small varices, who are known to have a lower risk of bleeding *(22,29, 38)*. This finding further suggests that high variceal pressure is a mechanism that contributes in increasing the size of the varices.

Nevertheless, the most important finding is the identification of variceal pressure as an independent prognostic factor determining the evolution of an acute variceal bleeding episode, the development of the first variceal hemorrhage, and of variceal rebleeding in patients receiving pharmacological therapy (see below).

In fact, Ruiz del Arbol et al. showed that variceal pressures greater than 18 mmHg during the acute bleeding episode were frequently associated with failure to control bleeding and early rebleeding *(39)*. Nevens et al. published the results of a prospective investigation in cirrhotics showing that a variceal pressure above 15.2 mmHg is a strong risk factor predicting the first variceal hemorrhage *(16)*. The same authors demonstrated that variceal pressure is also a strong predictor of variceal bleeding in patients with noncirrhotic portal hypertension, in whom HVPG is not adequate to assess portal pressure *(17)*. In this population, the risk of bleeding is lower than in cirrhotics despite having similar variceal pressure and is related to the progression of the disease.

ASSESSMENT OF THE EFFECTS OF PHARMACOLOGICAL THERAPY

The authors have recently shown that patients receiving pharmacological therapy with propranolol ± isosorbide-5-mononitrate showing a decrease in variceal pressure from baseline of 20% or more have a very low actuarial probability of variceal bleeding on follow-up (7% at 3 yr). Patients considered nonresponders by this measurement have a 46% rate of variceal bleeding during the same time period *(32)*. Furthermore, the results show that the prognostic value of the variceal pressure response is as powerful as that of the HVPG response, although the two methods identify different patients with a favorable outcome and should be considered complementary rather than mutually exclusive *(32)*.

Despite the limited applicability of variceal pressure measurements, mainly because of difficulties achieving correct tracings in small varices and of the presence of artifacts caused by esophageal peristalsis; its use may increase because its noninvasiveness and the potential advantage of being applicable in patients with esophageal varices of any etiology.

ENDOSONOGRAPHY

Endosonography (or endoscopic ultrasonography) allows the visualization of esophageal and gastric varices, the periesophageal and perigastric collateral veins, the portal venous system, and the azygos vein. Nowadays, the clinical use of endosonography is restricted to two main applications: the diagnosis of gastric fundal varices when endoscopy offers doubtful results *(14)* and assessing the risk of variceal recurrence after varices have been eradicated by endoscopic sclerotherapy or banding ligation *(40,41)*. Thus, the finding of grossly dilated periesophageal veins *(14)* or of patent perforating veins below the gastroesophageal junction *(42)* after these eradicative procedures seems to carry a high risk of variceal recurrence.

Recently, Miller et al. *(43)* investigated the value of the cross-sectional area (CSA) of esophageal varices measured by using a 20-MHz endosonographic probe in predicting the risk of variceal bleeding. The authors studied 28 patients with no prior history of variceal bleeding, in whom they calculated the sum of the CSA of all the varices identified at the point where the varices appeared the largest. A cutoff value of CSA of 0.45 cm^2 was identified as that having the highest sensitivity (83%) and specificity (75%) for determining future bleeding. This observation is not surprising considering that the size of the varices, measured by either endoscopy (subjected to observer bias) or endosonography (allowing objective and reproducible measurements) is a key factor determining variceal wall tension according to Laplace's law.

Endosonography has proven useful in pathophysiological and pharmacological research in patients with portal hypertension. The authors combined endosonography, allowing the objective measurement of variceal diameter, and the endoscopic measurement of transmural variceal pressure, to quantitatively estimate variceal wall tension, which is the more relevant parameter with regards to the risk of variceal bleeding. In that regard, we have shown that increasing intra-abdominal pressure, as it occurs in the presence of ascites or during many daily activities, causes a significant increase in variceal pressure, volume (the sum of the CSA of all the varices in the last 5 cm of the esophagus) and wall tension and, by these mechanisms, may contribute to the progressive dilatation that precedes the rupture of the varices *(44)*. In addition, pharmacological therapy with β-blockers resulted in a significant decrease of all these parameters, which correlated with its clinical efficacy *(27)*.

Further studies are required to explore a potential unique contribution of endosonography, such is the objective measurement of variceal wall thickness (with an established prognostic value). If a reliable measurement of variceal wall tension becomes possible, this will probably contribute to further improvement in the assessment of the risk of variceal bleeding.

REFERENCES

1. Bolondi L, Gatta A, Groszmann RJ, et al. Baveno II consensus statements: imaging techniques and hemodynamic measurements in portal hypertension. In: De Franchis R, ed. Portal Hypertension II: Proceedings of the Second Baveno International Consensus Workshop on Definitions, Methodology and Therapeutic Strategies. Blackwell Science, Oxford, 1996, p. 67.
2. Grace ND, Groszmann RJ, Garcia-Tsao G, et al. Portal hypertension and variceal bleeding: an AASLD single topic symposium. Hepatology 1998;28:868–880.
3. Schepis F, Camma C, Niceforo D, et al. Which patients with cirrhosis should undergo endoscopic screening for esophageal varices detection? Hepatology 2001;33:333–338.
4. D'Amico G, Luca A. Natural history. Clinical-hemodynamic correlations. Prediction of the risk of bleeding. Baillieres Clin Gastroenterol 1997;11:243–256.
5. D'Amico G, García-Tsao G, Calès P, et al. "Diagnosis of portal hypertension. how and when?" portal hypertension III. In: De Franchis R, ed. Proceedings of the Third Baveno International Consensus Workshop on Definitions, Methodology and Therapeutic Strategies. Blackwell Science, Oxford, 2001, pp. 36–63.
6. De Franchis R. Updating consensus in portal hypertension. Report of the Baveno III consensus workshop on definitions, methodology and therapeutic srategies in portal hypertension. J Hepatol 2000;33: 846–852.
7. D'Amico G. The clinical course of portal hypertension in liver cirrhosis. In: Rossi P, ed. Diagnostic Imaging and Imaging Guided Therapy. Springer-Verlag, Berlin, 2000, pp. 15–24.
8. Steinlauf AF, Garcia-Tsao G, Zakko MF, Dickey K, Gupta T, Groszmann RJ. Low-dose midazolam sedation: an option for patients undergoing serial hepatic venous pressure measurements. Hepatology 1999;29:1070–1073.
9. The North Italian Endoscopic Club for the Study and Treatment of Esophageal Varices. Prediction of the first variceal hemorrhage in patients with cirrhosis of the liver and esophageal varices. A prospective multicenter study. N Engl J Med 1988;319:983–989.
10. Merkel C, Zoli M, Siringo S, et al. Prognostic indicators of risk for first variceal bleeding in cirrhosis: a multicenter study in 711 patients to validate and improve the North Italian Endoscopic Club (NIEC) index. Am J Gastroenterol 2000;95:2915–2920.
11. Rigau J, Bosch J, Bordas JM, et al. Endoscopic measurement of variceal pressure in cirrhosis: correlation with portal pressure and variceal hemorrhage. Gastroenterology 1989;96:873–880.
12. Polio J, Groszmann RJ. Hemodynamic factors involved in the development and rupture of esophageal varices: a pathophysiologic approach to treatment. Semin Liver Dis 1986;6:318–331.
13. Nevens F, Bustami R, Scheys I, Lesaffre E, Fevery J. Variceal pressure is a factor predicting the risk of a first variceal bleeding: a prospective cohort study in cirrhotic patients. Hepatology 1998;27:15–19.
14. Caletti GC, Brocchi E, Ferrari A, et al. Value of endoscopic ultrasonography in the management of portal hypertension. Endoscopy 1992;24(Suppl 1):342–346.
15. Zoli M, Merkel C, Magalotti D, Marchesini G, Gatta A, Pisi E. Evaluation of a new endoscopic index to predict first bleeding from the upper gastrointestinal tract in patients with cirrhosis. Hepatology 1996; 24:1047–1052.
16. Nevens F, Bustami R, Scheys I, et al. Variceal pressure is a factor predicting the risk of a first variceal bleeding: a prospective cohort study in cirrhotic patients. Hepatology 1998;27:15–19.
17. El Atti EA, Nevens F, Bogaerts K, Verbeke G, Fevery J. Variceal pressure is a strong predictor of variceal hemorrhage in patients with cirrhosis as well as in patients with non-cirrhotic portal hypertension. Gut 1999;45:618–621.

18. Groszmann RJ. Reassessing portal venous pressure measurements. Gastroenterology 1984;86:1611–1614.
19. Norton ID, Andrews JC, Kamath PS. Management of ectopic varices. Hepatology 1998;28:1154–1158.
20. Escorsell A, Bosch J. The pathophysiology of variceal formation and rupture. In: Arroyo V, Bosch J, Bruguera M, Rodés J, eds. Therapy in Liver Diseases. The Pathophysiological Basis of Therapy. Masson, S.A., Barcelona, 1997, pp. 71–79.
21. Pagliaro L, de Franchis R. Where were we? A summary of the issues where consensus was reached in Baveno I. In: De Franchis, R, ed. Portal Hypertension II: Proceedings of the Second Baveno International Consensus Workshop on Definitions, Methodology and Therapeutic Strategies. Blackwell Science, Oxford, 1996, pp. 1–9.
22. Bosch J, Bordas JM, Rigau J, et al. Noninvasive measurement of the pressure of esophageal varices using an endoscopic gauge: comparison with measurements by variceal puncture in patients undergoing endoscopic sclerotherapy. Hepatology 1986;6:667–672.
23. Mosimann R. Nonaggressive assessment of portal hypertension using endoscopic measurement of variceal pressure. Preliminary report. Am J Surg 1982;143:212–214.
24. Polio J, Hanson J, Sikuler E, et al. Critical evaluation of a pressure-sensitive capsule for measurement of esophageal varix pressure. Studies in vitro and in canine mesenteric vessels. Gastroenterology 1987; 92:1109–1115.
25. Polio J, Leonard R, Groszmann RJ, et al. An improved pressure-sensitive capsule for endoscopic measurement of esophageal variceal pressure. Dig Dis Sci 1988;33:737–740.
26. Feu F, Bordas JM, Garcia-Pagan JC, et al. Double-blind investigation of the effects of propranolol and placebo on the pressure of esophageal varices in patients with portal hypertension. Hepatology 1991; 13:917–922.
27. Escorsell A, Bordas JM, Feu F, et al. Endoscopic assessment of variceal volume and wall tension in cirrhotic patients: effects of pharmacological therapy. Gastroenterology 1997;113:1640–1646.
28. Escorsell A, Feu F, Bordas JM, et al. Effects of isosorbide-5-mononitrate on variceal pressure and systemic and splanchnic hemodynamics in patients with cirrhosis. J Hepatol 1996;24:423–429.
29. Feu F, Bordas JM, Luca A, et al. Reduction of variceal pressure by propranolol: comparison of the effects on portal pressure and azygos blood flow in patients with cirrhosis. Hepatology 1993;18:1082–1089.
30. Nevens F, Lijnen P, VanBilloen H, et al. The effect of long-term treatment with spironolactone on variceal pressure in patients with portal hypertension without ascites. Hepatology 1996;23:1047–1052.
31. Nevens F, Sprengers D, Feu F, et al. Measurement of variceal pressure with an endoscopic pressure sensitive gauge: validation and effect of propranolol therapy in chronic conditions. J Hepatol 1996;24: 66–73.
32. Escorsell A, Bordas JM, Castaneda B, et al. Predictive value of the variceal pressure response to continued pharmacological therapy in patients with cirrhosis and portal hypertension. Hepatology 2000; 31:1061–1067.
33. Brensing KA, Neubrand M, Textor J, et al. Endoscopic manometry of esophageal varices: evaluation of a balloon technique compared with direct portal pressure measurement. J Hepatol 1998;29:94–102.
34. Gertsch P, Fischer G, Kleber G, et al. Manometry of esophageal varices: comparison of an endoscopic balloon technique with needle puncture. Gastroenterology 1993;105:1159–1166.
35. Scheurlen C, Roleff A, Neubrand M, et al. Noninvasive endoscopic determination of intravariceal pressure in patients with portal hypertension: clinical experience with a new balloon technique. Endoscopy 1998;30:326–332.
36. Pontes JM, Leitao MC, Portela F, Nunes A, Freitas D. Endosonographic Doppler-guided manometry of esophageal varices: experimental validation and clinical feasibility. Endoscopy 2002;34:966–972.
37. Miller ES, Kim JK, Gandehok J, et al. A new device for measuring esophageal variceal pressure. Gastrointest Endosc 2002;56:284–291.
38. Ueno K, Hashizume M, Ohta M, et al. Noninvasive variceal pressure measurement may be useful for predicting effects of sclerotherapy for esophageal varices. Dig Dis Sci 1996;41:191–196.
39. Ruiz del Arbol L, Martin de Argila C, Vázquez M, et al. Endoscopic measurement of variceal pressure during hemorrhage from esophageal varices. Hepatology 1992;16:147.
40. Suzuki T, Matsutani S, Umebara K, et al. EUS changes predictive for recurrence of esophageal varices in patients treated by combined endoscopic ligation and sclerotherapy. Gastrointest Endosc 2000;52: 611–617.

41. Koutsomanis D, Papakonstantinou V. Fractal-assisted EUS image-analysis in the evaluation of variceal eradication after elastic band ligation. Hepatogastroenterology 1999;46:3142–3147.
42. Burtin P, Cales P, Oberti F, et al. Endoscopic ultrasonographic signs of portal hypertension in cirrhosis. Gastrointest Endosc 1996;44:257–261.
43. Miller L, Banson FL, Bazir K, et al. Risk of esophageal variceal bleeding based on endoscopic ultrasound evaluation of the sum of esophageal variceal cross-sectional surface area. Am J Gastroenterol 2003;98:454–459.

IV NATURAL HISTORY AND TREATMENT OF ESOPHAGEAL VARICES

12

Clinical Features and Natural History of Variceal Hemorrhage

Implications for Surveillance and Screening

Juan G. Abraldes and Jaime Bosch

CONTENTS

INTRODUCTION
CLINICAL CONSEQUENCES OF PORTAL HYPERTENSION
PATHOPHYSIOLOGY OF VARICEAL FORMATION AND RUPTURE
THE NATURAL HISTORY AND CLINICAL COURSE
   OF VARICEAL BLEEDING
ACKNOWLEDGMENTS
REFERENCES

INTRODUCTION

Variceal bleeding is is one of the more frequent and severe complications of cirrhosis. Mortality of a variceal bleeding episode has decreased in the last two decades from 40% to 20% owing to the implementation of effective treatments and improvement in general medical care. The management of varices includes the screening and surveillance of cirrhotic patients to detect varices and its progression, which allows to establish effective prophylactic treatment, the treatment of the acute bleeding episode, and the prevention of variceal rebleeding. These should be based on the knowledge of the natural history and pathophysiology of variceal formation, progression, and rupture, which is the topic covered in this chapter.

The key factor in the natural history of esophageal varices is the increased portal pressure, which in cirrhosis is caused by the combination of an increased hepatic vascular resistance and an increased portal collateral blood flow. The maintenance and aggravation of this situation owing to progression of the liver disease, together with reiterated bounds of portal pressure and blood flow caused by unavoidable daily activities leads to the progressive dilatation of the varices and thinning of the variceal wall, until the tension exerted by the variceal wall exceeds the elastic limit of the vessel, determining variceal hemorrhage. This explains why detection of large varices, of red color signs on the wall of the varices, of increased portal pressure gradient, and of worsening of the Child–Pugh

From: *Clinical Gastroenterology: Portal Hypertension*
Edited by: A. J. Sanyal and V. H. Shah © Humana Press Inc., Totowa, NJ

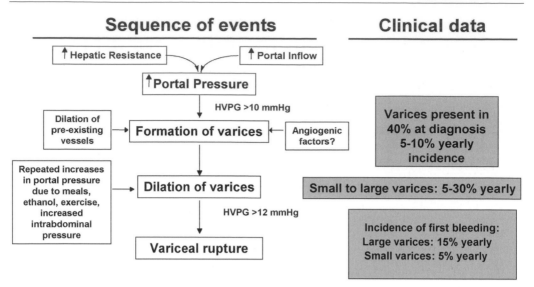

Fig. 1. Variceal bleeding is the last step of a chain of events initiated by an increase in portal pressure, followed by the development and progressive dilation of varices until these finally rupture and bleed. The correlation with clinical data is shown on the left column.

score are associated with an increased risk of bleeding. Prognostic factors in the acute bleeding episode include the above as well as associated complications (hepatocellular carcinoma, portal vein thrombosis, infections, renal failure, shock, and severity of the bleeding).

CLINICAL CONSEQUENCES OF PORTAL HYPERTENSION

The portal hypertensive syndrome is responsible for many of the manifestations of advanced liver disease. Some of these complications are the direct consequences of portal hypertension, such as gastrointestinal bleeding from ruptured gastroesophageal varices and from portal hypertensive gastropathy and colopathy, hyperkinetic circulatory syndrome, ascites and abnormalities of renal function, hypersplenism and increased systemic availability of drugs, and endogenous compounds with rapid hepatic uptake. In other complications, portal hypertension plays a key role, although it is not the only pathophysiological factor in their development. These include spontaneous bacterial peritonitis, hepatopulmonary syndrome, and hepatic encephalopathy *(1)*. In this chapter, we will review the natural history and clinical course of variceal bleeding, which constitutes the basis for a rational management of portal hypertensive patients.

PATHOPHYSIOLOGY OF VARICEAL FORMATION AND RUPTURE

Variceal bleeding is the final step of a chain of events initiated by an increase in portal pressure, followed by the development and progressive dilation of varices until these finally rupture and bleed (Fig. 1). This sequence of events can be reverted by treatments decreasing portal pressure (portocaval shunts, TIPS, drug therapy), underlining the reversibility of the portal hypertension syndrome.

Formation of Varices

ANATOMICAL FACTORS

Available evidence indicates that the most important factor in the formation of the portal-systemic collaterals is the dilatation of preexistent embryonic channels, although an active angiogenic process is also thought to contribute to collateral formation (see Chapter 7). The portal system and the systemic venous circulation are connected at several locations *(2)*. Gastroesophageal collaterals develop from connections between the left gastric (coronary) vein and short gastric veins with the esophageal, azygos, and intercostal veins resulting in the formation of esophageal and gastric varices. These are the most frequent and clinically relevant collaterals. Other collaterals may develop between the superior hemorrhoidal venous plexus and the middle and inferior hemorrhoidal veins, giving rise to anorectal varices; between portal and epigastric veins through the reopening of remnants of the umbilical or paraumbilical veins, forming a vascular net that is at times apparent on the abdominal wall as a *caput medusae* and causing a murmur over the umbilicus (the Cruveilhier–Baumgartner syndrome); between the portal system and the posterior abdominal wall through the liver capsule and diaphragm; and between the portal system and the left renal vein, forming spontaneous spleno-renal shunts. In instances of portal vein thrombosis "hepatopetal" collaterals develop between the splenic vein and the coronary vein via the short gastric veins, giving rise to gastric varices, and from the mesenteric or portal vein and the intrahepatic vena porta through the veins of Sappey, causing pseudocavernomas of the portal vein *(2)*. *Ectopic varices* may develop at other locations depending on local anatomical factors. Most ectopic varices develop in the duodenum (mostly associated with extrahepatic portal hypertension) and in the colon and small intestine, and are far more frequent in patients who have previously undergone abdominal surgery. Overall, these ectopic varices account for between 1% and 5% of all variceal bleeding episodes *(3,4)*.

HEMODYNAMIC FACTORS

Increased portal pressure is the initial and most important factor leading to the development of portal-systemic collaterals. As discussed in a previous chapter, portal hypertension in cirrhosis is initiated by an increased intrahepatic resistance to portal blood flow. When collaterals begin to develop, the portal venous inflow increases because of splanchnic vasodilatation. The increased portal venous inflow (which is equivalent to the sum of the portal and the collateral blood flow) represents an important factor contributing to maintain and worsen the portal pressure elevation. A threshold increase in the portal pressure gradient (most commonly evaluated in clinical practice by its equivalent, the hepatic venous pressure gradient or HVPG) of approx 10 mmHg has been established for the development of esophageal varices *(5–7)*.

However, above this threshold, there is no close correlation between the portal pressure elevation and the risk of formation and rupture of esophageal varices. Therefore, a high-pressure gradient is necessary, but not sufficient for the development of esophageal varices.

The amount of blood flow diverted from portal to systemic circulation through the gastroesophageal collaterals is thought to be another important factor in the formation and progressive dilatation of varices *(8)*. This is suggested by studies evaluating azygos blood flow, an index of blood flow through gastroesophageal collaterals, including esophageal varices, in portal hypertensive patients *(9,10)*. There is an exponential relationship between portal pressure and azygos blood flow, as well as a parallelism between the presence and size of the varices and the increase in azygos blood flow *(10)*. However, about 5% of patients with high azygos blood flow and increased portal pressure do not have gastroesophageal varices, illustrating that formation of collaterals is not always associated with development of varices *(10)*.

Once collateralization is extensive, factors modulating the collateral resistance become important determinants of portal pressure *(11)*. Portosystemic collaterals and varices do have a vascular smooth muscle layer that is able to actively modify vessel diameter and, therefore, collateral resistance. Collateral resistance is influenced by endogenous vasoactive factors, including the adrenergic and serotoninergic tone, nitric oxide (NO), vasopressin, and endothelin *(12,13)*, which are all frequently activated in cirrhosis. Therefore, the pharmacological manipulation of these systems may modify portal pressure and collateral formation *(14,15)*.

Enlargement of Varices

Several factors may contribute to progressive dilation of the varices. The first is the chronic increase in portal pressure and blood flow. On top of this increased portal pressure, cirrhotic patients experience sharp increases in portal pressure and flow associated with meals *(16,17)*, ethanol consumption *(18)*, and circadian rhythms *(19)*. In addition, physical exercise *(20)* and increased intra-abdominal pressure *(21,22)* cause abrupt increases in portal and variceal pressure. Such repeated increases in pressure and blood flow may contribute to progressive dilation of the varices (Fig. 1), and their prevention should be contemplated in the management of portal hypertension.

Variceal Rupture

For many years, it was thought that variceal bleeding was favored by mechanical trauma (caused by swallowing solid food) or external erosion (caused by gastroesophageal reflux) over the thin wall of the varices. However, there is no evidence to substantiate that view because there is no proven relationship between eating and bleeding, neither the incidence of reflux nor esophagitis is greater in patients with bleeding varices than in those without *(23,24)*. Because of that, most authors at present accept the so-called "explosion" hypothesis of variceal rupture in which the main factor implicated is the increased wall tension of the varix. If this wall tension exceeds the elastic limit of the vessel, then variceal rupture occurs. Wall tension (*WT*: the inwardly directed force exerted by the variceal wall against progressive distention) can be defined according to Frank's modification of Laplace's law, by the equation:

$$WT = (Pi - Pe) \times r/w,$$

in which *Pi* is the intravariceal pressure, *Pe* is the pressure in the esophageal lumen, *r* is the radius of the varix, and *w* is the thickness of its wall *(1,23)*. Thus, the three factors that interplay in variceal rupture are variceal pressure, size, and wall thickness (Fig. 2). Variceal pressure is the more important one because it provides the driving force for the dilatation of the varices, and as the varices dilate, their wall becomes thinner, which further contributes to increase wall tension (Fig. 3).

Variceal pressure is a function of portal pressure. Indeed, many studies have shown that variceal bleeding does not occur if the HVPG does not reach a threshold value of 12 mmHg *(5,6,25)*. Conversely, if the HVPG is substantially reduced (by more than 20%

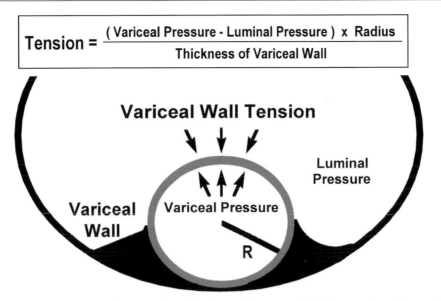

$$\text{Tension} = \frac{(\text{Variceal Pressure} - \text{Luminal Pressure}) \times \text{Radius}}{\text{Thickness of Variceal Wall}}$$

Fig. 2. Laplace's Law applied to esophageal varices allows to explain how different factors interact in the pathophysiology of variceal bleeding.

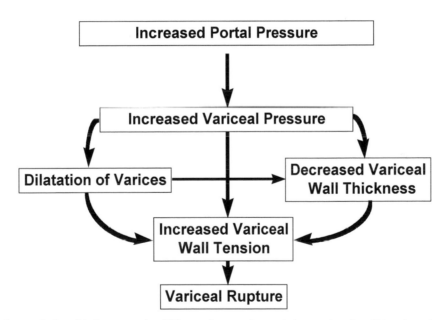

Fig. 3. Interrelationship between the different factors determining variceal wall tension. As shown, the most important factor is the increased portal pressure, which causes the formation, dilatation and rupture of the varix.

of baseline levels or to less than 12 mmHg), there is a marked reduction in the risk of bleeding, a significant increase in survival probability, and a significant decrease in the size of the varices, that can even disappear *(26–29)*. This is of utmost importance, because it demonstrates that the portal hypertension syndrome is reversible by effective pharmacological treatment *(29)*.

The recent introduction of endoscopic techniques for the measurement of variceal pressure (reviewed in Chapter 12) has allowed new observations to support the role of increased intravariceal pressure determining variceal rupture. Variceal pressure measurements have shown that patients with previous bleeding have higher variceal pressures than nonbleeders and that variceal pressure is a better discriminator of the risk of bleeding than HVPG *(7)*. Longitudinal studies have further shown that variceal pressure is a good prognostic indicator of the bleeding risk and of the response to pharmacological therapy *(30,31)*.

The concept of variceal wall tension also explains why esophageal varices are more prone to bleed than other collaterals, either in the thorax (as the periesophageal veins) or in the gut or other abdominal organs (ectopic varices). This is because the transmural pressure is higher at the esophageal varices than in varices of other locations, due to the negative esophageal luminal pressure during inspiration. Furthermore, esophageal varices lack external tissue support, which decreases the elastic limit of the vessel.

Variceal size and wall thickness are the other factors implicated in wall tension (Fig. 2). Frank's equation indicates that a large variceal size multiplies the deleterious effects of a high intravariceal pressure increasing the tension exerted on the wall of the varices; a big varix with thin walls will reach a high wall tension (and risk of bleeding) at much lower variceal pressures than a small varix with thick walls. This is clearly supported by clinical observations. Prospective follow-up studies of large series of patients have shown that the risk of bleeding is directly related to variceal size and inversely to variceal wall thickness (evaluated as the presence of red wale markings, which reflect areas where the wall of the varices is especially thin) *(32)*. Thus, the risk of bleeding in patients with "large" varices is double from that of patients with "small" varices.

The factors determining variceal wall tension are mutually interrelated, increased variceal pressure increasing wall tension directly, but also by increasing the size (radius) of the varix and, by the same mechanism, decreasing wall thickness (Fig. 3).

Natural History of Varices as a Function of Variceal Wall Tension

According to the above considerations, the natural history of portal hypertension can be described as a function of variceal wall tension. Once wall tension increases to values exceeding the elastic limit of the varices, the patient will experience a first bleeding episode. After this, the patient remains at a high risk of rebleeding unless wall tension is decreased. This can be achieved by pharmacological means by decreasing portal pressure and/or collateral blood flow. Similarly, primary prophylaxis protects from the risk of bleeding by preventing or delaying variceal wall tension to reach the rupture point.

In summary, the sequence of events leading to variceal hemorrhage is therefore initiated by a high portal pressure, which promotes the opening of collaterals and the formation of varices. The maintenance of an increased intravascular pressure, together with a high collateral blood flow, cause the dilatation of the varices, and as the varices dilate, their walls become thinner. At this moment, any further increase in variceal pressure or size, or any defect in the variceal wall, will cause rupture of the varices and clinical hemorrhage.

THE NATURAL HISTORY
AND CLINICAL COURSE OF VARICEAL BLEEDING

The information on the natural history and clinical manifestations of portal hypertension is primarily drawn from patients with liver cirrhosis, the best-studied disease causing portal hypertension. It is generally accepted that this information is applicable to most of the other causes of portal hypertension, although some differences may be identified in specific diseases.

Rate and Risk Factors for the Development, Progression, and Rupture of Esophageal Varices The Rationale for Screening and Surveillance

DEVELOPMENT OF ESOPHAGEAL VARICES

When cirrhosis is diagnosed, varices are present in about 30–40% of compensated patients and in 60% of those who present with ascites *(33,34)*. Because portal hypertension develops eventually in almost every patient with cirrhosis, it is thought that if cirrhotic patients are followed long enough, virtually all will develop varices *(35)*.

In those cirrhotic patients that present without varices, the annual incidence of new varices is about 5–10% *(34–37)*. A single report in patients with advanced liver disease showed a much higher incidence *(38)*. An HVPG over 10 mmHg *(39)* is a strong predictor for the development of varices. This is in keeping with the previously discussed role of portal pressure as the driving force for the development of collaterals. No other factors have been associated with the development of varices *(37,40)*.

PROGRESSION OF ESOPHAGEAL VARICES FROM SMALL TO LARGE

Once developed, varices increase in size from small to large before they eventually rupture and bleed. Studies assessing the progression from small to large varices are controversial, showing rates of progression of varices ranging from 5% to 30% per year *(37, 38,41–44)*. The most likely reason for such variability is the different patient selection and follow-up endoscopy schedule across studies *(40)*. The factor that has been most consistently associated with variceal progression is baseline Child–Pugh or its worsening during follow-up *(37,38,43)*. Other reported factors were alcoholic etiology of cirrhosis and the presence of red wale markings *(37)*. It has been shown that changes in HVPG (either "spontaneous" or caused by drug therapy or TIPS) are usually accompanied by parallel variations in the size of the esophageal varices, which are significantly reduced when HVPG decreases below 12 mmHg *(26,45)*. Thus, an increased HVPG plays a key role both in development and progression of the varices.

INCIDENCE AND RISK INDICATORS OF FIRST BLEEDING FROM ESOPHAGEAL VARICES

Once diagnosed, the overall incidence of variceal bleeding is in the order of 25% at 2 yr in nonselected patients *(46)*. Many efforts have been made to define risk criteria for the development of variceal bleeding. The most important predictive factors related to the risk of bleeding are variceal size, severity of liver dysfunction expressed by the Child–Pugh classification and red wale marks *(32)*. As explained above, variceal size and red color signs are associated with increased bleeding risk probably because they contribute to increase variceal wall tension, which is the decisive factor determining variceal rupture *(8)*. These risk indicators have been combined in the NIEC index, which allows to classify patients in different groups with predicted 1-yr bleeding risk ranging from 6 to 76% *(32)*. However, the predictive power of this index is far from satisfactory. In fact, the best operative characteristics of the NIEC index in the prediction of the bleeding risk are 74% sensitivity and 64% specificity with a positive predictive value of 33% and negative of 91% *(47)*. Whether these indexes can be improved by incorporating additional parameters related with portal hypertension (i.e., spleen size, platelet count, HVPG measurement) remains to be determined. Overall, variceal size remains the most useful predictor for variceal bleeding *(47)*, and this is the variable that is used in clinical practice to decide whether a patient should be given prophylactic therapy or not. The risk of bleeding is very low (between 1 and 2%) in patients without varices at the first examination, and increases to about 5% per year in those with small varices and to 15% per year in those with medium or large varices at diagnosis *(1,48)*.

Screening for Esophageal Varices and Subsequent Surveillance

The aim of the screening for esophageal varices is to detect those patients that are going to receive prophylactic treatment, which, according to current recommendations, are those with large varices *(49)*.

Thus, the current consensus is that every cirrhotic patient should be endoscopically screened for varices at time of diagnosis *(49)*. Although several studies indicate that non-invasive tests (particularly platelet count and data obtained from abdominal ultrasound) may have a potential use in selecting a group of patients with a high risk for varices *(4,50–53)*, so far none of these has proved in independent samples to be accurate enough so that endoscopy can be safely omitted in patients with negative noninvasive indicators. Two recently published cost-effectiveness decision analysis have challenged universal endoscopy screening in cirrhosis *(54,55)*. In these reports, it is suggested that empiric β-blocker therapy for all patients without endoscopic screening is more cost-effective than universal screening and primary prophylaxis only in patients with large varices. A third study suggested also that empiric β-blocker therapy is more cost-effective, but only in patients with decompensated cirrhosis *(56)*. However, the major drawbacks of β-blockers are patient adherence and side effects (and, thus, quality of life), which are difficult to fully account for in decision analysis studies. The response to this question can only be answered with a prospective randomized study. However, the lack of effectiveness of β-blockers preventing the development of varices, and the high rate of side effects observed even in well-compensated patients *(39)* questions whether such a trial is worth doing.

In patients without varices on initial endoscopy, a second (follow-up) evaluation should be performed to detect the development of varices before these bleed. The current consensus is that endoscopy should be repeated after 2–3 yr in patients without varices at the first endoscopy *(49)*. The expected incidence of large varices and/or variceal bleeding in these patients (and, thus, the risk of leaving patients without prophylaxis when it was indicated) is less than 10% at 3 yr *(37,40,41)*. In those centers in which hepatic hemodynamic studies are available, it is advisable to measure HVPG. An HVPG over 10 mmHg indicates a more rapid progression to complications of cirrhosis, and calls for shorter surveillance intervals *(39)*.

In patients with small varices on initial endoscopy the aim of subsequent evaluations is to detect the progression of small to large varices because of its important prognostic and therapeutic implications. Based on an expected 10–15% per year rate of progression of variceal size, endoscopy should be repeated every 1–2 yr in patients with small varices *(49)*. In patients with advanced cirrhosis, red wale marks or alcoholic etiology of cirrhosis, a 1-yr interval might be recommended *(37,40)*.

The Course of the Acute Bleeding Episode: Prognostic Factors

Ruptured esophageal varices cause 70% of all upper gastrointestinal bleeding episodes in patients with portal hypertension *(57)*. Thus, in any cirrhotic patient with acute upper gastrointestinal bleeding, a variceal origin should be suspected. Clinical features are those of upper gastrointestinal bleeding (often masive), combined with those of liver cirrhosis. The incidence of variceal bleeding shows a diurnal rhythm, with two peak incidences at 8–10 AM and 8–10 PM *(19,58)*. This rhythmicity is probably explained by circadian variations in portal pressure *(19)*. Variceal bleeding is often intermittent, which should be taken into account in its diagnostic approach. Diagnosis is established at emergency endoscopy based on observing one of the following: (a) active bleeding from a varix (observation of blood spurting or oozing from the varix) (near 20% of patients); (b) white nipple or clot adherent to a varix; (c) presence of varices without other potential sources of bleeding.

Initial control of bleeding. Because variceal bleeding is frequently intermittent, it is difficult to assess when the bleeding stops and when a new hematemesis or melena should be considered an episode of rebleeding. Several consensus conferences have addressed this issue and set definitions for events and timing of events related to episodes of variceal bleeding *(49,59,60)*. According to these definitions, the index bleeding episode is separated from the first episode of rebleeding by at least a 24-h interval without bleeding, during which no new hematemesis and/or melena occurs and all of the following criteria are verified: stable hemoglobin levels, systolic blood pressure above 100 mmHg or a postural change of less than 20 mmHg, and a pulse rate below 100/min. Using these criteria, the median duration of an acute episode of variceal bleeding is approx 10 h *(1)*. Data from placebo-controlled clinical trials have shown that variceal bleeding is spontaneously controlled in 40–50% of patients *(46)*. With currently available treatments control of bleeding increases to about 80–90% of the patients *(57)*.

Early rebleeding. The incidence of early rebleeding ranges between 30% and 40% in the first 6 wk. The risk peaks in the first 5 d with 40% of all rebleeding episodes occurring in this very early period, remain high during the first 2 wk and decline then slowly in the next 4 wk. After 6 wk, the risk of further bleeding becomes virtually equal to that before bleeding *(61)*. A recently published series shows that currently available treatments have reduced 6-wk rebleeding to 20% *(57)*. In this series, only 25% of rebleedings occurred within 5 d, a finding that stresses that elective treatment to prevent rebleeding should be initiated as soon as the patient is stabilized. Early rebleeding is a strong predictor of death within 6 wk, indicating that its prevention should be a priority in the management of variceal bleeding. Prognostic indicators for early rebleeding were assessed in most studies together with initial failure to control bleeding and 5-d risk for death, conforming a composite end-point referred to as "5-d failure." Bacterial infection *(62–64)*, active bleeding at emergency endoscopy *(57,63,65)*, Child–Pugh class or score *(57,63)*, AST levels *(57)*, the presence of portal vein thrombosis *(57)*, and a HVPG > 20 mmHg measured shortly after admission *(66)* (Fig. 4) have been reported as significant predictors of risk for 5-d failure (Table 1).

Mortality. Mortality from variceal bleeding has greatly decreased in the last two decades from a 42% mortality registered in the Graham and Smith study in 1981 *(61)* to the 20% reported by D'Amico in a prospective cohort study in Italian patients carried out between 1997 and 1999 *(57)*. This trend was previously suggested by the analysis of the control groups of successive randomized trials in variceal bleeding *(67)*, and from two retrospective studies from the United States *(68,69)*. This decrease is caused by the implementation of effective treatments, such as endoscopic and pharmacological therapies and TIPS, as well as from improved general medical care (i.e., antibiotic prophylaxis). Because it may be difficult to assess the true cause of death (i.e., bleeding vs liver failure or other

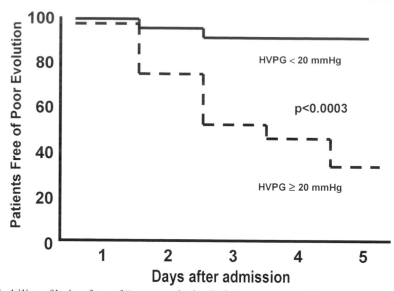

Fig. 4. Probability of being free of "poor evolution" (failure to control bleeding, early rebleeding, or death) in acute variceal bleeding patients according to HVPG. Those patients with an HVGP ≥ 20 had a poorer outcome [unpublished figure elaborated with data from Moitinho et al. *(66)*].

adverse events), the general consensus is that any death occurring within 6 wk from hospital admission for variceal bleeding should be considered as a bleeding-related death *(49)*.

Immediate mortality from uncontrolled bleeding is in the range of 4–8% *(34,36,57)*. The only available study that addresses pre-hospital mortality from variceal bleeding estimated that 3% of the patients with variceal bleeding die before arriving to a hospital *(70)*. Like the risk for rebleeding, the risk for mortality peaks the first days after bleeding, slowly declines thereafter, and after 6 wk becomes constant and virtually equal to that before bleeding *(46,61)*. Nowadays, only 40% of the deaths are directly related to bleeding, whereas 50% are caused by liver failure and hepatorenal syndrome *(57)*. Thus, although there is still room for improving hemostatic treatments, to substantially decrease mortality from variceal bleeding therapies should be able to prevent liver and renal function deterioration.

Accurate indicators of risk for early death, available at hospital admission, could allow selection of patients for more aggressive therapies, such as emergency shunt or TIPS, before their conditions deteriorate hampering further therapy. Unfortunately, the indicators of risk so far identified are also indicators of poor outcomes after derivative treatments and, consequently, are of limited clinical value. On hospital admission, the most consistently reported death risk indicators are Child–Pugh classification or its components, BUN or creatinine, active bleeding on endoscopy, hypovolemic shock, and hepatocellular carcinoma *(57,61,62,71–73)*. Additionally, an HVPG >20 mmHg *(66)* has been reported as strong indicator of treatment failure. Conceivably, it is also associated with a higher risk of death, although its specific prognostic role for 6-wk mortality has not been assessed. Prognostic indicators gathered in the early follow-up are of no help in selecting immediate therapy, but do aid in developing a more focused and rational management of the patient. The most important among late prognostic indicators are early rebleeding *(65,72)*, bacterial infection *(64)*, and renal failure *(72,73)* (Table 2). From these data it is clear that man-

Table 1
Prognostic Indicators, With Their Reported
Odds Ratio/Hazard Ratio, for Early Rebleeding or "5-d Failure"
(Failure To Control Bleeding, Early Rebleeding or Death)

Variable	OR/HR	References
HVPG $\geq$ 20 mmHg	11.4	(66)
Bacterial infection	4.6–9.7	(62–64)
Active bleeding at endoscopy	2.1–3.7	(57,63,65)
Portal vein thrombosis	3.1	(57)
Child–Pugh class	2.7	(57)
Child–Pugh score	1.2	(63)
AST levels (per IU increase)	1.003	(57)

HVPG: hepatic venous pressure gradient.

Table 2
Prognostic Indicators, With Their Reported
Odds Ratio/Hazard Ratio, For Bleeding-Related Death

Variable	OR/HR	References
At admission		
Shock	5.8–9.9	(64,73)
Hepatocellular carcinoma	3.1–7.5	(57,71,72)
Hepatic encephalopathy	2.4–6.9	(57,64,65,72)
Active bleeding	5.4	(61)
Child–Pugh score	4.5	(62)
Prothrombin time, Bilirrubin, Albumin	—	(57,65,71)
Creatinine, Urea	—	(65,71)
Late prognostic indicators		
Renal failure	17.1–52.1	(72,73)
Bacterial infection	12.6	(64)
Early rebleeding	3.2–8.7	(65,72)

agement of bleeding cirrhotic patient should be aimed not only at controlling the bleeding, but also at preventing early rebleeding, infection, and renal failure.

Models to predict treatment failure and mortality. A number of models to predict mortality and/or treatment failure have been proposed in the recent few years *(65,71,74, 75)*. None of them has permeated clinical practice or trial design, where Child–Pugh score is still the leading prognostic tool. The most recent proposal has been that of D'Amico et al. *(57)*, who have developed and validated in a prospective multicenter study prognostic models for 5-d failure and 6-wk morality. These models were found to fare better than Child–Pugh score. However, whether these models really improve other regression models *(65,71,74,75)* and how they might serve to direct clinical practice or to stratify patients in clinical trials is uncertain. Another suggestion has been to apply the APACHE II score (which is used to assess patients in critical care units) to predict prognosis in variceal bleeding. Although this score showed similar theoretical predictive value to Child–Pugh, Gatta's, and Garden's scores, it greatly overestimated mortality

36. de Franchis R, Primignani M. Natural history of portal hypertension in patients with cirrhosis. Clin Liver Dis 2001;5:645–663.
37. Merli M, Nicolini G, Angeloni S, et al. Incidence and natural history of small esophageal varices in cirrhotic patients. J Hepatol 2003;38:266–272.
38. Cales P, Desmorat H, Vinel JP, et al. Incidence of large oesophageal varices in patients with cirrhosis: application to prophylaxis of first bleeding. Gut 1990;31:1298–1302.
39. Groszmann RJ, Garcia-Tsao G, Makuch R, et al. Multicenter, randomized placebo-controlled trial of non-selective beta-blockers in the prevention of the complications of portal hypertension: final results and identification of a predictive factor. Hepatology 2003;38(Suppl 1):206A.
40. De Franchis R. Evaluation and follow-up of patients with cirrhosis and oesophageal varices. J Hepatol 2003;38:361–363.
41. Pagliaro L, D'Amico G, Pasta L, Politi F, Vizzini G, Traina M. Portal hypertension in cirrhosis. Natural history. In: Bosch J, Groszmann RJ, eds. Portal Hypertension, Pathophysiology and Treatment. Blackwell Scientific, Oxford, 1994, pp. 72–92.
42. Cales P, Oberti F, Payen JL, et al. Lack of effect of propranolol in the prevention of large oesophageal varices in patients with cirrhosis: a randomized trial. French-Speaking Club for the Study of Portal Hypertension. Eur J Gastroenterol Hepatol 1999;11:741–745.
43. Zoli M, Merkel C, Magalotti D, et al. Natural history of cirrhotic patients with small esophageal varices: a prospective study. Am J Gastroenterol 2000;95:503–508.
44. Merkel C, Marin R, Angeli P, et al. A placebo-controlled clinical trial of nadolol in the prophylaxis of growth of small esophageal varices in cirrhosis. Gastroenterology 2004;127:476–484.
45. Vorobioff J, Groszmann RJ, Picabea E, et al. Prognostic value of hepatic venous pressure gradient measurements in alcoholic cirrhosis: a 10-year prospective study. Gastroenterology 1996;111:701–709.
46. D'Amico G, Pagliaro L, Bosch J. Pharmacological treatment of portal hypertension: an evidence-based approach. Semin Liver Dis 1999;19:475–505.
47. Merkel C, Zoli M, Siringo S, et al. Prognostic indicators of risk for first variceal bleeding in cirrhosis: a multicenter study in 711 patients to validate and improve the North Italian Endoscopic Club (NIEC) index. Am J Gastroenterol 2000;95:2915–2920.
48. D'Amico G, Pagliaro L. The Clinical Course of portal hypertension in liver cirrhosis. In: Rossi P, ed. Diagnostic Imaging and Imaging Guided Therapy. Springer Verlag, Berlin, 2000, pp. 15–24.
49. de Franchis R. Updating consensus in portal hypertension: report of the Baveno III Consensus Workshop on definitions, methodology and therapeutic strategies in portal hypertension. J Hepatol 2000;33: 846–852.
50. Zaman A, Hapke R, Flora K, Rosen HR, Benner K. Factors predicting the presence of esophageal or gastric varices in patients with advanced liver disease. Am J Gastroenterol 1999;94:3292–3296.
51. Chalasani N, Imperiale TF, Ismail A, et al. Predictors of large esophageal varices in patients with cirrhosis. Am J Gastroenterol 1999;94:3285–3291.
52. Madhotra R, Mulcahy HE, Willner I, Reuben A. Prediction of esophageal varices in patients with cirrhosis. J Clin Gastroenterol 2002;34:81–85.
53. Giannini E, Botta F, Borro P, et al. Platelet count/spleen diameter ratio: proposal and validation of a non-invasive parameter to predict the presence of oesophageal varices in patients with liver cirrhosis. Gut 2003;52:1200–1205.
54. Saab S, DeRosa V, Nieto J, Durazo F, Han S, Roth B. Costs and clinical outcomes of primary prophylaxis of variceal bleeding in patients with hepatic cirrhosis: a decision analytic model. Am J Gastroenterol 2003;98:763–770.
55. Spiegel BM, Targownik L, Dulai GS, Karsan HA, Gralnek IM. Endoscopic screening for esophageal varices in cirrhosis: Is it ever cost effective? Hepatology 2003;37:366–377.
56. Arguedas MR, Heudebert GR, Eloubeidi MA, Abrams GA, Fallon MB. Cost-effectiveness of screening, surveillance, and primary prophylaxis strategies for esophageal varices. Am J Gastroenterol 2002; 97:2441–2452.
57. D'amico G, De Franchis R. Upper digestive bleeding in cirrhosis. Post-therapeutic outcome and prognostic indicators. Hepatology 2003;38:599–612.
58. Merican I, Sprengers D, McCormick PA, Minoli G, McIntyre N, Burroughs AK. Diurnal pattern of variceal bleeding in cirrhotic patients. J Hepatol 1993;19:15–22.

59. de Franchis R, Pascal JP, Ancona E, et al. Definitions, methodology and therapeutic strategies in portal hypertension. A Consensus Development Workshop, Baveno, Lake Maggiore, Italy, April 5 and 6, 1990. J Hepatol 1992;15:256–261.

60. de Franchis R. Developing consensus in portal hypertension. J Hepatol 1996;25:390–394.

61. Graham D, Smith J. The course of patients after variceal hemorrhage. Gastroeneterology 1981;80: 800–806.

62. Bernard B, Cadranel JF, Valla D, Escolano S, Jarlier V, Opolon P. Prognostic significance of bacterial infection in bleeding cirrhotic patients: a prospective study. Gastroenterology 1995;108:1828–1834.

63. Goulis J, Armonis A, Patch D, Sabin C, Greenslade L, Burroughs AK. Bacterial infection is independently associated with failure to control bleeding in cirrhotic patients with gastrointestinal hemorrhage. Hepatology 1998;27:1207–1212.

64. Vivas S, Rodriguez M, Palacio MA, Linares A, Alonso JL, Rodrigo L. Presence of bacterial infection in bleeding cirrhotic patients is independently associated with early mortality and failure to control bleeding. Dig Dis Sci 2001;46:2752–2757.

65. Ben Ari Z, Cardin F, McCormick AP, Wannamethee G, Burroughs AK. A predictive model for failure to control bleeding during acute variceal haemorrhage. J Hepatol 1999;31:443–450.

66. Moitinho E, Escorsell A, Bandi JC, et al. Prognostic value of early measurements of portal pressure in acute variceal bleeding. Gastroenterology 1999;117:626–631.

67. McCormick PA, O'Keefe C. Improving prognosis following a first variceal haemorrhage over four decades. Gut 2001;49:682–685.

68. El Serag HB, Everhart JE. Improved survival after variceal hemorrhage over an 11-year period in the Department of Veterans Affairs. Am J Gastroenterol 2000;95:3566–3573.

69. Chalasani N, Kahi C, Francois F, et al. Improved patient survival after acute variceal bleeding: a multicenter, cohort study. Am J Gastroenterol 2003;98:653–659.

70. Nidegger D, Ragot S, Berthelemy P, et al. Cirrhosis and bleeding: the need for very early management. J Hepatol 2003;39:509–514.

71. Gatta A, Merkel C, Amodio P, et al. Development and validation of a prognostic index predicting death after upper gastrointestinal bleeding in patients with liver cirrhosis: a multicenter study. Am J Gastroenterol 1994;89:1528–1536.

72. del Olmo JA, Pena A, Serra MA, Wassel AH, Benages A, Rodrigo JM. Predictors of morbidity and mortality after the first episode of upper gastrointestinal bleeding in liver cirrhosis. J Hepatol 2000;32: 19–24.

73. Cardenas A, Gines P, Uriz J, et al. Renal failure after upper gastrointestinal bleeding in cirrhosis: incidence, clinical course, predictive factors, and short-term prognosis. Hepatology 2001;34:671–676.

74. Garden OJ, Motyl H, Gilmour WH, Utley RJ, Carter DC. Prediction of outcome following acute variceal haemorrhage. Br J Surg 1985;72:91–95.

75. Ohmann C, Stoltzing H, Wins L, Busch E, Thon K. Prognostic scores in oesophageal or gastric variceal bleeding. Scand J Gastroenterol 1990;25:501–512.

76. Afessa B, Kubilis PS. Upper gastrointestinal bleeding in patients with hepatic cirrhosis: clinical course and mortality prediction. Am J Gastroenterol 2000;95:484–489.

77. Grace ND, Groszmann RJ, Garcia-Tsao G, et al. Portal hypertension and variceal bleeding: an AASLD single topic symposium. Hepatology 1998;28:868–880.

Table 1
Mechanisms of Action of Treatments for Portal Hypertension

			Treatment		
Action on	Vasoconstrictors	Vasodilators	Vasoconstrictors+ vasodilators	Shunts	Endoscopy
Flow	↓↓	—	↓	↑	—
Resistance	↑	↓	↓	↓↓↓	—
Portal pressure	↓	↓	↓↓	↓↓↓	—
Varicose channels	—	—	—	—	+

Variceal bleeding carries a mortality which, in the most recent studies, ranges around 20% *(1,2)*; in addition, a patient surviving a variceal bleed has a risk of rebleeding, if untreated, of about 60% *(3)*. Therefore, therapeutic strategies for portal hypertension must include measures to prevent the first bleed, to treat acute bleeding, and to prevent rebleeding.

To prevent variceal formation, growth, and rupture, several approaches can be considered. Portal pressure may be reduced by drugs that decrease portal venous inflow, such as vasoconstrictors (terlipressin, somatostatin, or its analogs for acute bleeding, nonselective β blockers to prevent first bleeding and rebleeding), or by drugs that decrease intrahepatic resistance, such as vasodilators (isosorbide-5 mononitrate). A greater reduction in portal pressure can be obtained by a combination of vasoconstrictors and vasodilators, which decreases both portal flow and intrahepatic resistance *(4)*. An even greater reduction in portal pressure may be achieved by surgical or radiological shunt interventions, which divert the portal blood into the systemic circulation. Finally, variceal bleeding may be prevented by endoscopic treatments aimed at obliterating the varices, which, although not influencing portal pressure, decrease the risk of bleeding by closing the varicose channels. The mechanisms of action of the different therapeutic means to prevent and treat variceal bleeding are summarized in Table 1.

In this chapter, I will review the possible strategies to prevent and treat esophageal variceal rupture.

PRIMARY PROPHYLAXIS OF PORTAL HYPERTENSION

The prevention of the first variceal bleed (primary prophylaxis) could start at three different points in time:

1. when portal hypertension is present, but varices have not yet appeared, aiming at preventing variceal formation;
2. when small varices are present, aiming at preventing the growth of varices;
3. when large varices are already present, aiming at preventing variceal rupture.

Prevention of Variceal Formation

This approach has been evaluated in two studies, in which β-blockers were used. In the first one *(5)*, 208 patients, of which 38% had no varices at enrolment, were randomized to placebo or propranolol treatment. At 2 yr of follow-up, significantly more patients on propranolol (31%) had developed large varices as compared with patients on placebo (14%; $p < 0.05$). There was no difference in the development of large varices in patients with no varices or with small varices at inclusion. The proportion of patients who bled from varices (2%) was identical in the two groups. This study has been criticized because no measurement of portal pressure was done and there was a 35% overall dropout rate. The second study (6) enrolled 213 patients with no varices and proven portal hypertension (HVPG >6 mmHg), which were randomized to placebo or timolol. At 4 yr of follow-up, 37% of patients developed esophageal varices and 3% bled, with no difference between the study groups. The number of serious adverse events was significantly higher in patients treated with timolol (19% vs 6%; $p < 0.01$).

From the above data, it appears that β-blockers treatment is not effective in preventing the development of varices in patients with portal hypertension.

Prevention of the Growth of Small Varices to Large Ones

This approach has been investigated in two studies, the French one mentioned above (5), in which propranolol was ineffective in preventing the growth of varices in the 62% of patients with small varices at enrolment, and an Italian trial (7), in which 161 patients with small varices were randomized to receive either nadolol or placebo. At 3 yr, the varices had increased in size in 11% of patients in the nadolol group and in 37% of those receiving placebo ($p < 0.01$). Significantly fewer patients bled in the nadolol group (2.4%) than in the placebo group (11.5%; $p = 0.022$). Thus, two studies of similar design gave opposite results. Therefore, no definitive conclusion can be drawn on the efficacy of β-blocker treatment in preventing the enlargement of varices.

Prevention of First Bleeding

Historically, the first treatment used to prevent the first variceal hemorrhage in cirrhotic patients has been the surgical portacaval shunt. However, this form of therapy has been abandoned because shunted patients had a significantly higher mortality than control patients (8). In the 1980s, both nonselective β-blockers and endoscopic sclerotherapy were studied as possible treatments for prevention of first bleeding. Sclerotherapy has subsequently been abandoned because of inconsistency of results across trials (9,10), whereas β-blockers have become the mainstay of prophylaxis (11,12). It is generally agreed that only patients with medium-sized or large varices should be treated prophylactically (12, 13), because the risk of bleeding in patients with small varices is very low (13). A recent meta-analysis (13) of trials comparing β-blockers with placebo showed that β-blockers reduce the mean weighted incidence of bleeding from 25% to 15%, with a relative risk reduction of 40% and an absolute risk reduction of 10% (95% confidence intervals −16% to −5%). This means that 10 patients must be treated with β-blockers to prevent one bleed that would have occurred if all patients had been treated with placebo [number needed to treat (NNT) = 10]. Patients in whom β-blockers decrease the HVPG to below 12 mmHg are completely protected from bleeding (14), whereas a reduction of 20% from baseline values reduces the incidence of bleeding to less than 10% (15). Unfortunately, a reduction below 12 mmHg or a 20% decrease of the HVPG from baseline can only be achieved in about 20% and 35% of patients, respectively. In addition, β-blockers cause side effects in 16–20% of cases, which lead to the withdrawal of 6–12% of patients from therapy (16–18).

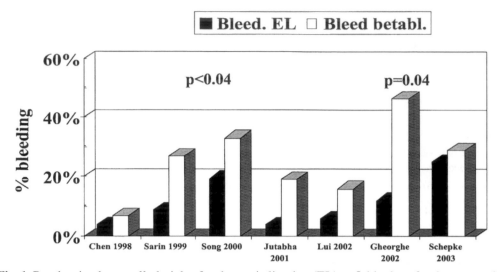

Fig. 1. Randomized controlled trials of endoscopic ligation (EL) vs β-blockers for the prevention of the first variceal bleed.

These facts have stimulated the search for alternative strategies for preventing first bleeding. Nitrovasodilators have been investigated for their ability to decrease portal pressure by decreasing hepatic and portocollateral resistance. In one study *(19)*, isosorbide-5-mononitrate was equivalent to propranolol in preventing bleeding, but, on extended follow-up *(20)*, was associated with a significantly higher mortality in patients over 50 yr of age. In a study in decompensated cirrhotic patients *(21)*, isosorbide-5-mononitrate had significantly fewer side effects as compared to nadolol, but was significantly less effective in preventing bleeding. A third study comparing isosorbide-5 mononitrate with placebo in patients with intolerance or contraindications to β-blockers *(22)* showed no difference between treatments for the prevention of bleeding. Experimentally, combination therapy with isosorbide-5-mononitrate and β-blockers has been shown to enhance the portal pressure lowering effect of β-blockers *(4)*. This combination has been compared with β-blockers alone in three studies *(23–25)*. Meta-analysis of these studies *(13)* showed no significant difference in efficacy between treatments, although side effects were remarkably more frequent with the combination therapy. Thus, isosorbide-5-mononitrate, alone or in combination with β-blockers, does not appear to be a suitable alternative to β-blockers for prevention of the first variceal bleeding.

In recent years, band ligation has been compared with no treatment in five trials *(26–30)*. Meta-analysis of these studies *(31)* has shown that band ligation significantly decreases both the incidence of first bleeding and mortality. A comparison between band ligation and β-blockers has been made in seven trials *(32–38*, Fig. 1), only two of which *(33,36)* are published in full. In all studies, band ligation was more effective than β-blockers in preventing first bleeding, but the difference reached statistical significance only in two *(33, 37)*. Meta-analysis of these trials shows that band ligation reduces the incidence of first bleeding from 23% to 14%, with a relative risk reduction of 39%, an absolute risk reduction of 9% (95% confidence interval: −17% to −3%) and a number needed to treat of 11 (Fig. 2A). Mortality was equal with the two treatments. It has been argued that in the only two trials that showed a significant difference in favor of band ligation *(33,37)*, the per-

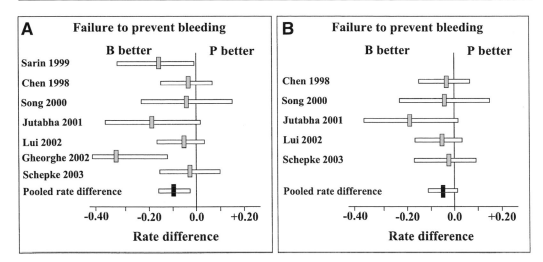

Fig. 2. Meta-analysis of randomized controlled trials of primary prophylaxis of variceal haemorrhage: band ligation (B) vs propranolol (P).

formance of β-blockers was exceedingly poor. In effect, when these two trials are excluded from meta-analysis, the difference disappears [Fig. 2B; bleeding: β-blockers 20%, band ligation 14%, relative risk reduction 30%; absolute risk reduction 6% (95% C.I. −12% to +0.2%; number needed to treat 17)]. At any rate, it appears that band ligation and β-blockers are roughly equivalent in preventing first bleeding.

An attempt at optimizing the pharmacological prevention of variceal bleeding has recently been made by Bureau et al. *(39)*. In this study, the HVPG was measured before starting treatment with propranolol and at a mean of 9 d thereafter. Patients responding to treatment (primary responders, i.e., showing a reduction of the HVPG to below 12 mmHg or by 20% from baseline) continued with propranolol. Nonresponders received additional treatment with I-5MN. In these, a third HVPG measurement was made at a mean of 17 d after starting I-5MN. Both secondary responders and nonresponders continued the combined treatment (Fig. 3). There were 10 primary and 4 secondary responders, none of which bled, whereas 2 of 6 (33%) nonresponders bled.

It appears thus that prevention of first variceal bleeding should start when patients have medium-sized or large varices. β-blockers remain the mainstay of treatment, whereas band ligation should be the first-line treatment for patients with contraindications or intolerance to β-blocker treatment *(12)* (Fig. 4). Cost-effectiveness analyses should be made to clarify whether band ligation can be used as an alternative to β-blockers for all patients. Whether the tailoring of pharmacological treatment based on HVPG monitoring is really worthwhile should be verified in larger patients series.

These recommendations have recently been challenged by a study by Spiegel et al. *(40)*, who evaluated the cost-effectiveness ratio of different strategies for preventing first bleeding by a decision analysis based on the Markov model. The authors conclude that the most cost-saving strategy would be to treat all cirrhotic patients with β-blockers, without any selection based on the endoscopic appearance of the varices. This theoretical study will have to be verified in practice. In this respect, the recent study by Groszmann et al. mentioned above *(7)* goes against the conclusions of Spiegel et al. *(40)*.

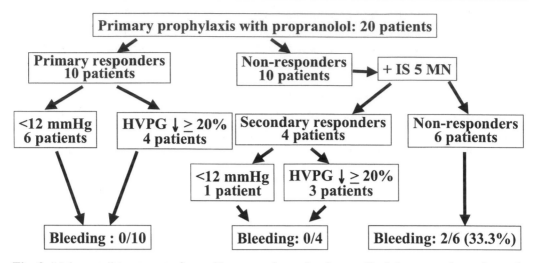

Fig. 3. "A la carte" treatment of portal hypertension: adapting medical therapy to hemodynamic response for the prevention of bleeding (from ref. *39*).

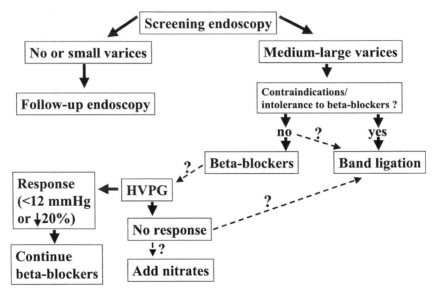

Fig. 4. Algorithm for prevention of first variceal bleeding in cirrhosis. Dotted arrows with question marks denote steps that need to be verified.

CLINICAL MANAGEMENT OF ACTIVE BLEEDING

Variceal bleeding is a life-threatening complication of portal hypertension which, in spite of recent progress *(41)*, still carries a high mortality *(1,2)* and has substantial resource-use implications *(42)*. Mortality is related to several factors such as failure to control bleeding, early rebleeding, the severity of the underlying liver disease, the presence of infection and of disease in other systems. The management of the acute bleed is a multi-step process that includes the initial assessment of the patient, effective resuscitation, timely diagnosis, control of bleeding, and prevention of early rebleeding and complications such as infection, renal failure, or hepatic encephalopathy. It has been recently shown that about two-thirds of deaths in which bleeding is the precipitating cause occur within 24 h of the onset of bleeding, thus emphasizing the need to act fast and decisively as soon as the patient reaches the hospital (43).

Initial Assessment of the Patient

The presence of alcohol abuse, NSAIDs or aspirin consumption, previous bleeding, or previous diagnosis of liver disease should be investigated. Physical examination must include the search for signs of chronic liver disease. The initial examination and investigations should assess the severity of bleeding, the presence of renal dysfunction and of disease in other systems, the severity of liver disease (Child–Pugh score) and the presence of infection (cultures).

Resuscitation

Care must be taken to avoid aspiration, especially in unconscious patients; endotracheal intubation may be necessary. Peripheral and central lines must be inserted, blood gas analysis must be done, and pulse oximetry must be monitored during endoscopy. Volume replacement must be done cautiously and carefully, because it has been demonstrated experimentally that complete volume restitution may result in overshoot in portal pressure, with inherent risk of further bleeding (44,45). Current guidelines suggest to use packed red cells to maintain the hematocrit between 25–30%, and plasma expanders to maintain haemodynamic stability (12).

Diagnosis

Upper GI endoscopy is the mainstay of diagnosis, as it allows the identification of the cause and type of bleeding. It has been recently confirmed (1) that about 25–30% of bleeds in cirrhotic patients are of nonvariceal origin, mainly peptic ulcer and portal hypertensive gastropathy. In addition, when endoscopy is done early, active bleeding is found in only about 39–44% of patients, whereas 33–44% show signs of recent bleeding (clots or "white nipple" on varices) (46), and no sign of active or recent hemorrhage is found in the remaining 12–28% (1,42). This has important implications for both the prognosis and management of patients, because active bleeding at endoscopy is a predictor of early treatment failure. Thus, endoscopy should be performed as soon as possible after admission (within 12 h), especially in patients with clinically significant bleeding or in patients with features suggesting cirrhosis (12).

Control of Bleeding and Prevention of Early Rebleeding

Treatment of acute variceal bleeding should aim both at controlling bleeding and at preventing early rebleeding, which is particularly common within the first week and is associated with increased mortality (47). Both pharmacologic therapy with vasoactive drugs (terlipressin, somatostatin, octreotide) (13) and endoscopic treatment (sclerotherapy and band ligation) (10) have been shown to be effective in controlling acute bleeding. Studies comparing endoscopic sclerotherapy and pharmacologic treatment with vasoactive drugs have shown that the two treatment modalities have similar efficacy, whereas sclerotherapy has a somewhat higher complication rate (48,49). A recent study from Spain (50) compared different schedules of somatostatin administration. A retrospective analysis of the data suggested that a double dose of somatostatin infusion (500 µg/h) may be more

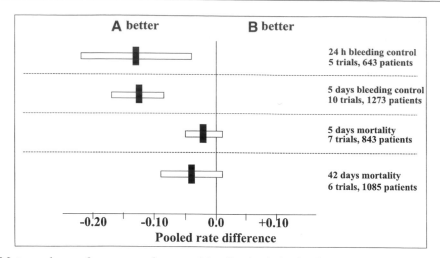

Fig. 5. Meta-analyses of treatments for acute bleeding in cirrhosis: drugs + endoscopic treatments (**A**) vs endoscopic treatments alone (**B**). (10 trials; 1273 patients).

effective than the standard 250 µg/h dose in patients with active bleeding at endoscopy. This finding will have to be confirmed in prospective studies.

Treatment regimens combining the use of a vasoactive drug (terlipressin, somatostatin, or its analog octreotide or vapreotide) with endoscopic therapy (sclerotherapy or band ligation) have received a great deal of attention in recent years. Between 1995 and 2001, 10 studies *(51–60)*, including a total of 1273 patients, have compared combined treatments with endoscopic treatments alone. A recent meta-analysis *(61)* including eight of these trials *(52–55,57–60)* showed that pharmacologic + endoscopic treatment is more effective than endoscopic therapy alone in controlling acute bleeding and preventing 5 d rebleeding, although there was no difference in mortality. Even including the studies that were excluded *(51,56)* or only partly included *(55)* in this meta-analysis, the results do not change [control of acute bleeding: combination 90%, endoscopic treatment alone 76%, relative risk reduction 16%, absolute risk reduction 14% (95% confidence intervals –4 to –23%), NNT = 7; 5-d prevention of rebleeding: combination 72%, endoscopic treatment alone 59%, relative risk reduction 18%, absolute risk reduction 13% (95% confidence intervals –17% to –8%); NNT = 7.7]. There was no difference in 5-d and 42-d mortality figures (combination 7%; endoscopic treatment alone 9% at 5 d; 22 and 27%, respectively, at 42 d) (Fig. 5). The combination of emergency sclerotherapy plus somatostatin or octreotide infusion has been compared with somatostatin or octreotide alone in two trials *(62,63)*. In both, the combined treatment was more effective than drug treatment alone in controlling bleeding and preventing early rebleeding, although statistical significance was only reached in the first one. It appears thus that the combination of endoscopic and pharmacologic treatment can control bleeding in about 90% of patients and prevent early rebleeding in about 80% *(61)*. A recent survey has shown that this combination is widely adopted in the routine management of variceal bleeders *(1)*.

It has recently been shown that the administration of recombinant activated factor VII (rFVIIa) normalizes prothrombin time in bleeding cirrhotics *(64)*. The potential role of rFVIIa has been evaluated in a multicenter European trial *(65)*, including 245 bleeding cirrhotic patients who were randomized to receive eight doses of rFVIIa, 100 µg/kg or placebo in addition to combined endoscopic + pharmacologic treatment. The primary endpoint was a composite including: failure to control bleeding at 24 h, failure to prevent rebleeding between 24 h and 5 d, and death within 5 d. No significant effect was found when analyzing the whole patients population; however, an exploratory analysis showed that, in Child–Pugh B and C variceal bleeders, rFVIIa significantly reduced the occurrence of the primary endpoint (from 23% in patients receiving placebo to 8% in patients receiving rFVIIa, $p = 0.03$), and improved bleeding control at 24 h (from 88% to 100%, $p = 0.03$). These data are encouraging, but require confirmation by studies specifically targeted on the appropriate patients.

Prevention of Complications

Bacterial infection is a serious complication of advanced cirrhosis, particularly in bleeding patients *(66–70)*. The urinary tract, ascites, respiratory tract, or multiple sites may be involved *(68)*, with spontaneous bacterial peritonitis accounting for 7–12% *(67,68)*; the enteric flora accounts for the majority of infections, and *Escherichia coli* is the most frequently involved pathogen. Infections have been reported to occur in more than one-third of bleeding cirrhotic patients *(66)* within 7 d of admission, and are associated with failure to control bleeding *(69)*, early rebleeding *(66)*, and early death *(69)*. It has been postulated that infection may impair coagulation, thus facilitating failure to control bleeding and early rebleeding *(71,72)*. Eight trials have evaluated the efficacy of antibiotic prophylaxis in bleeding cirrhotic patients: two meta-analyses, including 5 *(73)* and 8 *(74)* trials, respectively, have shown that antibiotic prophylaxis is effective in preventing infection and increasing survival. Thus, antibiotic prophylaxis has become an integral part of the management of bleeding cirrhotic patients *(12)*. When different antibiotic regimens were compared, no specific regimen showed a superiority over other regimens in preventing infection or improving survival *(74)*.

Management of Failures of First-Line Treatments

Even in the best situation, the current therapies fail to control bleeding or to prevent early rebleeding in about 8–12% of patients, who should be treated by alternative means. In principle, emergency shunt surgery and the transjugular intrahepatic porto-systemic stent shunt (TIPS) appear as appropriate therapies; however, since the majority of these patients have severe liver insufficiency (Child–Pugh class C), TIPS is probably the best option. To date, TIPS has been used as a salvage treatment in patients failing first-line therapy in 15 studies *(75)*, including 509 patients, 64% of whom were Child–Pugh class C. Overall, immediate control of bleeding was achieved in 94% of patients (range 75–100%); 10 studies give figures for rebleeding, with a mean of 11.4% (range 6–27%) at 7–30 d, whereas 30 d mortality was 31.9% (range 15–75%). Although none of the studies is a randomized trial, and only one is a retrospective comparison with an alternative surgical therapy *(76)*, these results strongly suggest that emergency TIPS is a valid salvage procedure for patients failing first-line endoscopic and pharmacologic treatment *(12)*.

In conclusion, the management of acute bleeding should include a careful assessment of the patient, to evaluate both the severity of the bleeding and of the underlying cirrhosis. Resuscitation should include measures to avoid aspiration, monitoring of blood gases and pulse oximetry; transfusions should be made cautiously to avoid overshoot in portal pressure; antibiotic prophylaxis and treatment with vasoactive drugs should be started early, and the latter should be continued for up to 5 d. Endoscopy should be done as soon

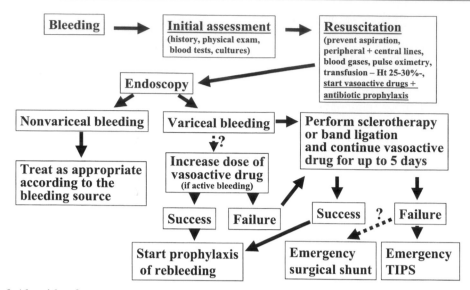

Fig. 6. Algorithm for treatment of acute variceal bleeding in cirrhosis. Dotted arrows with question marks denote steps that need to be verified.

as the patient can tolerate it; either sclerotherapy or band ligation can be used as hemostatic treatments. The value of increasing the dose of vasoactive drugs in active bleeders and of adding rFVIIa in Child–Pugh B and C patients needs further evaluation in appropriately designed trials. For patients failing combined vasoactive and endoscopic therapy, emergency TIPS appears to be an effective salvage therapy; surgical shunts may be indicated in good risk patients, whereas the feasibility of liver transplant should be considered for patients with severe liver failure *(12)*. Figure 6 shows an algorithm for the management of acute variceal bleeding based on the above recommendations.

SECONDARY PROPHYLAXIS OF PORTAL HYPERTENSION

If left untreated, patients surviving a variceal hemorrhage have median risks of rebleeding and of death of 63% and 33%, respectively, *(9)*. Given these figures, the current recommendation is to treat all patients to prevent rebleeding *(46)*. In principle, rebleeding could be prevented by surgical shunts, drugs, endoscopy, and TIPS.

Total shunts have largely been used in the 1960s and 1970s, but have subsequently been almost abandoned because they do not increase survival in comparison to conservative treatment *(77)*. The distal splenorenal shunt (DSRS) has been compared with sclerotherapy in four trials. Meta-analysis of these studies *(78)* showed that the DSRS significantly reduces the incidence of rebleeding and only slightly increases the occurrence of chronic encephalopathy, but does not improve survival. The small diameter prosthetic H-graft portacaval shunt has been compared with TIPS in a large randomized controlled trial *(79)*, showing a significant decrease of rebleeding and a better cost-effectiveness ratio *(80)* in patients undergoing the surgical procedure. In spite of these results, surgical shunt are rarely performed nowadays, and the majority of patients is treated with drugs or by endoscopy.

β-blockers are more effective than placebo in preventing rebleeding and death *(13)* [average rebleeding rate: placebo: 63%, β-blockers 42%, relative risk reduction 33%, absolute risk reduction 21% (95% confidence intervals −30% to −13%) NNT = 4.76; mortality: placebo 27%; β-blockers 20%; relative risk reduction 26%; absolute risk reduction 7% (95% confidence interval −12% to −2%); NNT 14.2]. Endoscopic sclerotherapy is also more effective than conservative treatment *(10)* [rebleeding: conservative treatment: 57%, sclerotherapy: 43%, relative risk reduction 25%, absolute risk reduction 14% (95% confidence intervals −22% to −7%); NNT = 7.14; mortality: conservative treatment 54%, sclerotherapy: 44%, relative risk reduction 19%, absolute risk reduction 10% [95% confidence intervals −18% to −2%), NNT 10]. Comparisons between β-blockers and sclerotherapy have shown a slight advantage for sclerotherapy in preventing rebleeding, with no difference in mortality; however, because there is a marked heterogeneity among trials, this result should be interpreted with caution *(10)*. The same applies for studies comparing sclerotherapy alone with sclerotherapy + β-blockers *(10)*.

With the advent of banding ligation, thirteen studies have been performed comparing ligation with sclerotherapy. Meta-analysis of these trials *(10)* shows that band ligation is significantly more effective than sclerotherapy in preventing rebleeding [banding 22%, sclerotherapy 35%, relative risk reduction 37%, absolute risk reduction 13% (95% confidence intervals −18% to −6%), NNT = 8], whereas there is no difference in mortality (22% vs 25%). As a consequence, band ligation is now the recommended endoscopic therapy to prevent variceal rebleeding *(12)*. Recently, a medical regimen of β-blockers + isosorbide-5-mononitrate has been compared with sclerotherapy in one trial *(81)* and with band ligation in 3 *(82–84)*. The combined medical treatment was superior to sclerotherapy in preventing rebleeding, with no difference in mortality *(81)*, although the three trials in which band ligation was used gave conflicting results: the medical regimen was significantly better than banding in preventing rebleeding in one *(82)*, significantly worse in the second *(83)*, whereas the third showed no difference between treatments *(84)* (Table 2). None of the trials showed a difference in mortality. Meta-analysis of these studies shows no difference between treatments in preventing rebleeding [medical treatment: 37.5%, banding 40%, relative risk reduction 6.25%, absolute risk reduction 2.5% (95% confidence intervals −23% to + 3%), NNT = 40] and death [medical treatment: 26%, banding 34%, relative risk reduction 24%, absolute risk reduction 8% (95% confidence intervals −1% to + 17%), NNT = 12.5] (Table 2). However, this conclusion should be interpreted with caution, since the number of patients included in the trials is relatively small. Therefore, the question whether medical treatment with β-blockers + isosorbide mononitrate is better than band ligation or vice-versa is still open. A single trial *(85)* compared a combination of band ligation, beta blockers and sucralfate with band ligation alone, showing that the combined therapy was better than ligation alone in preventing rebleeding and variceal recurrence. These data need confirmation.

In 11 studies, TIPS has been compared with endoscopic therapy for the prevention of variceal rebleeding. Two meta-analyses *(86,87)* have come to identical results, i.e., that TIPS significantly reduces rebleeding as compared to endoscopic therapy (19 vs 47%, $p < 0.001$), but significantly increases encephalopathy (34 vs 19%, $p < 0.001$), although there is no difference in survival. Recently, two cost-effectiveness analyses comparing TIPS and endoscopic therapy have been made *(88,89)*. The first one *(88)*, based on true patients data, shows that TIPS is not cost-saving in comparison with sclerotherapy; the second one, *(89)* based on theoretical scenarios, suggests that TIPS may be cost-effective compared to endoscopic therapy in the short term. At any rate, TIPS is not considered a first-line therapy to prevent rebleeding *(12)*; conceivably, TIPS can be viewed as a salvage

Table 2
Randomized Controlled Trials Comparing Band Ligation
with β-Blockers + Isosorbide Mononitrate in the Prevention of Variceal Rebleeding

Author	Treatment	No. Pts.	% Rebleeding	% Mortality
Villanueva	Banding/Nadolol + isosorbide mononitrate	72/72	49/33	42/32
Lo	Banding/ Nadolol + isosorbide mononitrate	60/61	20/43	25/13
Patch	Banding/ Propranolol + isosorbide mononitrate	51/51	53/37	33/33
Pooled data		183/184		
P.O.R.			1.13	1.46
(95% C.I.)			(0.74–1.72)	(0.93–2.29)

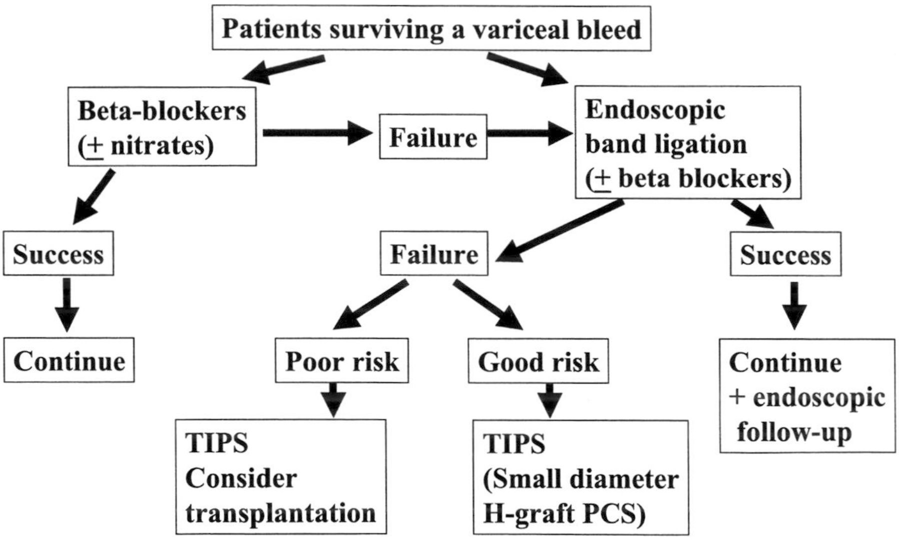

Fig. 7. Algorithm for the prevention of variceal rebleeding in cirrhosis.

treatment in patients who continue to rebleed despite pharmacologic or endoscopic treatment. In this setting, small diameter H-graft portacaval shunt could also be considered for patients who are good surgical risks. For patients with advanced cirrhosis, the feasibility of liver transplantation should also be considered *(12)*.

In conclusion, all patients surviving an episode of variceal bleeding should enter a therapeutic program to prevent rebleeding. β-blockers (with or without nitrates) and endoscopic band ligation (with or without β-blockers) are the first-line treatment options. Patients who continue to rebleed should be treated with TIPS. Depending on local resources, in good surgical risks, a small-diameter H-graft portacaval shunt can also be done, although poor risk patients should be considered for liver transplantation *(12)*. Figure 7 shows an algorithm for prevention of variceal rebleeding.

REFERENCES

1. D'Amico G, de Franchis R, and a cooperative study group. Upper digestive bleeding in cirrhosis. Post-therapeutic outcome and prognostic indicators. Hepatology 2003;38:599–612.
2. Chalasani N, Kahi C, Francois F, et al. Improved patient survival after acute variceal bleeding: a multicenter, cohort study. Am J Gastroenterol 2003;98:653–659.
3. de Franchis R, Primignani M. Natural history of portal hypertension in patients with cirrhosis. In: Sanyal A, ed. Portal Hypertension. Clinics in Liver Disease. Saunders, Philadelphia, 2001, vol. 5, pp. 645–663.
4. Garcia-Pagan JC, Navasa M, Bosch J, Bru C, Pizcueta P, Rodés J. Enhancement of portal pressure reduction by the association of isosorbide-5 mononitrate to propranolol administration in patients with cirrhosis. Hepatology 1990;11:330–338.
5. Calés P, Oberti F, Payen JL, et al. Lack of effect of propranolol in the prevention of large oesophageal varices in patients with cirrhosis: a randomized trial. Eur J Gastroenterol Hepatol 1999;11:741–745.
6. Groszmann R, Garcia-Tsao G, Makuch R, et al. Multicenter randomized trial of non-selective beta-blockers in the prevention of complications of portal hypertension: final results and identification of a predictive factor. Hepatology 2003;38(Suppl 1):206A.
7. Merkel C, Marin R, Angeli P, et al. Beta-blockers in the prevention of the aggravation of esophageal varices in patients with cirrhosis and small varices: a placebo-controlled clinical trial. Hepatology 2003; 38(Suppl 1):217A.
8. Conn HO, Lindenmuth WW, May CJ, Ramsby GR. Prophylactic portacaval anastomosis: a tale of two studies. Medicine 1972;51:27–40.
9. D'Amico G, Pagliaro L, Bosch J. The treatment of portal hypertension: a meta-analytic review. Hepatology 1995;22:332–354.
10. de Franchis R, Primignani M. Endoscopic treatments for portal hypertension. Sem Liver Dis 1999;19: 439–455.
11. de Franchis R. Developing consensus in portal hypertension. J Hepatology 1996;25:390–394.
12. de Franchis R. Updating consensus in portal hypertension: report of the Baveno III consensus workshop on definitions, methodology and therapeutic strategies in portal hypertension. J Hepatol 2000;33: 846–852.
13. D'Amico G, Pagliaro L, Bosch J. Pharmacologic treatment of portal hypertension: an evidence-based approach. Sem Liver Dis 1999;19:475–505.
14. Groszmann R, Bosch J, Grace ND, et al. Hemodynamic events in a prospective randomized trial of propranolol versus placebo in the prevention of a first variceal hemorrhage Gastroenterology 1990;99: 1401–1407.
15. Feu F, Garcia-Pagan JC, Bosch J, et al. Relation between portal pressure response to pharmacotherapy and risk of recurrent variceal hemorrhage in patients with cirrhosis. Lancet 1995;346:1056–1059.
16. Bernard B, Lebrec D, Mathurin P, Opolon P, Poynard T. Propranolol and sclerotherapy in the prevention of gastrointestinal rebleeding in patients with cirrhosis: a meta-analysis. J Hepatol 1997;26:312–324.
17. Bernard B, Lebrec D, Mathurin P, Opolon P, Poynard T. Beta-adrenergic antagonists in the prevention of gastrointestinal rebleeding in patients with cirrhosis: a meta-analysis. Hepatology 197:25:63–70.
18. Bolognesi M, Balducci G, Garcia-Tsao G, et al. Complications of the medical treatment of portal hypertension. In: de Franchis R, ed. Portal Hypertension III. Proceedings of the Third Baveno International Consensus Workshop on Definitions, Methodology and Therapeutic Strategies. Blackwell Science, Oxford, 2001, pp. 180–201.
19. Angelico M, Carli L, Piat C, et al. Isosorbide-5-mononitrate versus propranolol in the prevention of first bleeding in cirrhosis. Gastroenterology 1993;104:1460–1465.
20. Angelico M, Carli L, Piat C, Gentile S, Capocaccia L. Isosorbide-5-mononitrate compared with propranolol on first bleeding and long-term survival in cirrhosis. Gastroenterology 1997;113:1632–1639.
21. Borroni G, Salerno F, Cazzaniga M, et al. Nadolol is superior to isosorbide mononitrate for the prevention of the first variceal bleeding in cirrhotic patients with ascites. J Hepatol 2002;37:315–321.
22. Garcia Pagán JC, Villanueva C, Vila C, et al. Isosorbide-5-mononitrate in the prevention of the first variceal bleed in patients who cannot receive beta-blockers. Gastroenterology 2001;121:908–914.
23. Merkel C, Marin R, Enzo E, et al. Randomised trial of nadolol alone or with isosorbide mononitrate for primary prophylaxis of variceal bleeding in cirrhosis. Lancet 1996;348:1677–1681.

24. Pietrosi G, D'Amico G, Pasta L, et al. Isosorbide mononitrate (IMN) with nadolol compared to nadolol alone for prevention of first bleeding in cirrhosis: a double blind placebo-controlled randomised trial. J Hepatol 1999;30(Suppl 1):66 (abstract).

25. Garcia-Pagán JC Morillas R, Bañares R, et al. Propranolol + placebo vs. propranolol + isosorbide-5-mononitrate in the prevention of the first variceal bleed. A double blind RCT Hepatology 2003;37:1260–1266.

26. Sarin SK, Guptan RKC, Jain AK, Sundaram KR. A randomized controlled trial of endoscopic variceal band ligation for primary prophylaxis of variceal bleeding. Eur J Gastroenterol Hepatol 1996;8:337–342.

27. Lay CS, Tsai YT, Teg CY, et al. Endoscopic variceal ligation in prophylaxis of first variceal bleeding in cirrhotic patients with high-risk esophageal varices. Hepatology 1997;25:1346–1350.

28. Chen CY, Chen CY, Chang TT. Prophylactic endoscopic variceal ligation for esophageal varices. Gastroenterology 1997;112:A1240 (abstract).

29. Gameel K, Waked I, Saleh S, Sallam M, Abdel-Fattah S. Prophylactic endoscopic variceal band ligation (EVL) versus sclerotherapy (EVS) for the prevention of variceal bleeding in high risk varices: a prospective randomized controlled trial. Hepatology 1997;26(Suppl):361A (abstract).

30. Lo GH, Lai KH, Cheng JS, Lin CK, Hau PI, Chiang HT. Prophylactic banding ligation of high-risk esophageal varices in patients with cirrhosis: a prospective randomized trial. J Hepatol 1999;31:451–456.

31. Imperiale TF, Chalasani N. A meta-analysis of endoscopic variceal ligation for primary prophylaxis of esophageal variceal bleeding. Hepatology 2001;33:802–807.

32. Chen CY, Sheu MZ, Su SY. Prophylactic endoscopic variceal ligation (EVL) with multiple band ligator for esophageal varices. Gastroenmterology 1998;114(Suppl):A1224 (abstract).

33. Sarin SK, Lamba GS, Kumar M, Misra A, Murthy NS. Comparison of endoscopic ligation and propranolol for the primary prevention of variceal bleeding. N Engl J Med 1999;340:988–993.

34. Song IH, Shin JW, Kim IH, et al. A prospective randomized trial between the prophylactic endoscopic variceal ligation and propranolol administration for prevention of first bleeding in cirrhotic patients with high-risk esophageal varices. J Hepatol 2000;32(Suppl 2):41(abstract).

35. Jutabha R, Jensen DM, Martin P, et al. A randomized, prospective study of prophylactic rubber band ligation compared to propranolol for prevention of first variceal hemorrhage in cirrhotics with large esophageal varices. Gastrointest Endosc 2001;53:AB70 (abstract).

36. Lui HF, Stanley AJ, Forrest EH, et al. Primary prophylaxis of variceal hemorrhage: a randomized controlled trial comparing band ligation, propranolol, and isosorbide mononitrate. Gastroenterology 2002; 123:735–744.

37. Gheorghe C, Gheorghe L, Vadan R, Hrehoret D, Popescu I. Prophylactic banding ligation of high risk esophageal varices in patients on the waiting list for liver transplantation: an interin analysis. J Hepatol 2002;36(Suppl 1):38 (abstract).

38. Schepke M, Goebel C, Nuernberg D, Willert J, Koch L, Sauerbruch T. Endoscopic banding ligation versus propranolol for the primary prevention of variceal bleeding in cirrhosis: a randomized controlled multicenter trial. Hepatology 2003;38(Suppl 1):218A.

39. Bureau C, Péron JM, Alric L, et al. A la carte treatment of portal hypertension: adapting medical therapy to hemodynamic response for the prevention of bleeding. Hepatology 2002;36:1361–1366.

40. Spiegel BMR, Targownik L, Dulai GS, Karsan HA, Gralnek IM. Endoscopic screening for esophageal varices in cirrhosis: is it ever cost-effective? Hepatology 2003;37:366–377.

41. Pagliaro L, D'Amico G, Pasta L, et al. Efficacy and efficiency of treatments in portal hypertension. In: de Franchis R, ed. Portal Hypertension II. Proceedings of the Second Baveno International Consensus Workshop on Definitions, Methodology and Therapeutic Strategies. Blackwell, Oxford, 1996, pp. 159–179.

42. McCormick PA, Greenslade L, Matheson LA, Matsaganis M, Bosanquet N, Burroughs AK. Vasoconstrictors in the management of bleeding from oesophageal varices. A clinicoeconomical appraisal in the UK. Scand J Gastroenterol 1995;30:377–383.

43. Nidegger D, Ragot S, Berthélemy P, et al. Cirrhosis and bleeding: the need for very early management. J Hepatol 2003;39:509–514.

44. Kravetz D, Bosch J, Arderiu M, Pizcueta P, Rodés J. Hemodynamic effects of blood volume restitution following a hemorrhage in rats with portal hypertension due to cirrhosis of the liver: influence of the extent of portal-systemic shunting. Hepatology 1989;9:808–814.

45. Castañeda B, Morales J, Lionetti R, et al. Effects of blood volume restitution following a portal hypertensive-related bleeding in anesthetized cirrhotic rats. Hepatology 2001;33:821–825.

46. de Franchis R, Pascal JP, Ancona E, et al. Definitions, methodology and therapeutic strategies in portal hypertension. A consensus development wokshop, Baveno, Lake Maggiore, Italy, April 5, 1990. J Hepatol 1992;15:256–261.

47. Ben-Ari Z, Cardin F, McCormick PA, Wannamethee G, Burroughs AK. A predictive model for failure to control bleeding during acute variceal hemorrhage. J Hepatol 1999;31:443–450.

48. Escorsell A, Bordas JM, Ruiz del Arbol L, et al. Randomized controlled trial of sclerotherapy versus somatostatin infusion in the prevention of early rebleeding following acute variceal hemorrhage in patients with cirrhosis. J Hepatol 1998;29:779–788.

49. Escorsell A, Ruiz del Arbol L, Planas R, et al. Multicenter randomized controlled trial of terlipressin versus sclerotherapy in the treatment of acute variceal bleeding: the TEST study. Hepatology 2000;32:471–476.

50. Moitinho E, Planas R, Bañares R, et al. Multicenter randomized controlled trial comparing different schedules of somatostatin in the treatment of acute variceal bleeding. J Hepatol 2001;35:712–718.

51. Levacher S, Letoumelin PH, Paternon D, Blaise M, Lepandry C, Pourriat JL. Early administration of terlipressin plus gliceryltrinitrate for active upper gastrointestinal hemorrhage in cirrhotic patients. Lancet 1995;346:865–868.

52. Besson I, Ingrand P, Person B, et al. Sclerotherapy with or without octreotide for acute variceal bleeding. N Engl J Med 1995;333:555–560.

53. Sung JJ, Chung SCS, Yung MY, et al. Prospective randomised study of effect of octreotide on rebleeding from esophageal varices after endoscopic ligation. Lancet 1995;346:1666–1669.

54. Signorelli S, Negrini F, Paris B, Bonelli M, Girola M. Sclerotherapy with or without somatostatin or octreotide in the treatment of acute variceal hemorrhage: our experience. Gastroenterology 1996;110 (Suppl):A1326 (abstract).

55. Brunati S, Ceriani R, Curioni R, Brunelli L, Repaci G, Morini L. Sclerotherapy alone vs. sclerotherapy plus terlipressin vs. sclerotherapy plus octreotide in the treatment of acute variceal hemorrhage. Hepatology 1996;24(Suppl):207A (abstract).

56. Burroughs AK. Double blind RCT of 5 day octreotide versus placebo, associated with sclerotherapy for trial failures. Hepatology 1996;24(Suppl):352A (abstract).

57. Signorelli S, Paris B, Negrin F, Bonelli M, Auriemma M. Esophageal varices bleeding: comparison between treatment with sclerotherapy alone vs. sclerotherapy plus octreotide. Hepatology 1997;26(Suppl): 137A (abstract).

58. Avgerinos A, Nevens F, Raptis S, Fevery J. Early administration of somatostatin and efficacy of sclerotherapy in acute oesophageal variceal bleeds: The European Acute Bleeding oesophageal variceal episodes (ABOVE) randomised trial. Lancet 1997;350:1495–1499.

59. Zuberi BF, Baloch Q. Comparison of endoscopic variceal sclerotherapy alone and in combination with octreotide in controling acute variceal hemorrhage and early rebleeding in patients with low-risk cirrhosis. Am J Gastroenterol 2000;95:768–771.

60. Calés P, Masliah C, Bernard B, et al. Early administration of vapreotide for variceal bleeding in patients with cirrhosis. N Engl J Med 2001;344:23–28.

61. Bañares R, Albillos A, Rincon D, et al. Endoscopic treatment versus endoscopic plus pharmacologic treatment for acute variceal bleeding: a meta-analysis. Hepatology 2002;35:609–615.

62. Villanueva C, Ortiz J, Sàbat M, et al. Somatostatin alone or combined with emergency sclerotherapy in the treatment of acute esophageal variceal bleeding: a prospective randomized trial. Hepatology 1999; 30:384.389.

63. Novella MT, Villanueva C, Ortiz J, et al. Octreotide vs. sclerotherapy and octreotide for acute variceal bleeding: a pilot study. Hepatology 1996;24(Suppl):207A (abstract).

64. Ejlersen E, Melsen T, Ingerslev J, Andreasen RB, Vilstrup H. Recombinant activated factor VII (rFVIIa) acutely normalizes prothrombin time in patients with cirrhosis during bleeding from oesophageal varices. Scand J Gastroenterol 2001;36:1081–1085.

65. Thabut D, de Franchis R, Bendtsen F, et al. Efficacy of activated recombinant factor VIII (RFVIIa; Novoseven®) in cirrhotic patients with upper gastrointestinal bleeding: a randomised placebo-controlled double-blind multicenter trial. J Hepatol 2003;38(Suppl 2):13 (abstract).

66. Bernard B, Cadranel JF, Valla D, Escolano S, Jarlier V, Opolon P. Prognostic significance of bacterial infection in bleeding cirrhotic patients. Gastroenterology 1995;108:1828–1834.

67. Deschenes M, Villeneuve JP. Risk factors for the development of bacterial infections in hospitalized patients with cirrhosis. Am J Gastroenterol 1999;94:2001–2003.

68. Borzio M, Salerno F, Piantoni L, et al. Bacterial infection in patients with advanced cirrhosis: a multicenter prospective study. Dig Liver Dis 2001;33:41–48.
69. Vivas S, Rodriguez M, Palacio MA, Linares A, Alonso JL, Rodrigo L. Presence of bacterial infection in bleeding cirrhotic patients is independently associated with early mortality and failure to control bleeding. Dig Dis Sci 2001;46:2752–2757.
70. Almeida D, Lopes AA, Santos-Jesus R, Paes I, Bittencourt H, Parana R. Comparative study of bacterial infection prevalence between cirrhotic patients with and without upper gastrointestinal bleeding. Braz J Infect Dis 2001;5:136–142.
71. Goulis J, Patch D, Burroughs AK. Bacterial infection in the pathogenesis of variceal bleeding. Lancet 1999;353:139–142.
72. Montalto P, Vlachogiannakos J, Cox DJ, Pastacaldi S, Patch D, Burroughs AK. Bacterial infection in cirrhosis impairs coagulation by a heparin effect: a prospective study. J Hepatol 2002;37:463–470.
73. Bernard B, Grangé JD, Khac EN, Amiot X, Opolon P, Poynard T. Antibitic prophylaxis for the prevention of bacterial infections in cirrhotic patients with gastrointestinal bleeding: a meta-analysis. Hepatology 1999;29:1655–1661.
74. Soares-Weiser K, Brezis M, Tur-Kaspa R, Leibovici L. Antibiotic prophylaxis for cirrhotic patients with gastrointestinal bleeding. Cochrane Database Syst Rev 2002;(2):CD002907.
75. Vangeli M, Patch D, Burroughs AK. Salvage TIPS for uncontrolled variceal bleeding. J Hepatol 2002; 37:703–704 (letter).
76. Jalan R, John TG, Redhead DN, et al. A comparative study of emergency transjugular intrahepatic portosystemic stent-shunt and esophageal transection in the management of uncontroled variceal hemorrhage, Am J Gastroenterol 1995;90:1932–1937.
77. Pagliaro L, Burroughs AK, Soerensen TIA, et al. Therapeutic controversies and randomised controlled trials (RCTs): prevention of bleeding and rebleeding in cirrhosis. Gastroenterol Int 1989;2:71–84.
78. Spina GP, Henderson JM, Rikkers LF, et al. Distal spleno-renal shunt versus endoscopic sclerotherapy in the prevention of variceal rebleeding. J Hepatol 1992;16:338–345.
79. Rosemurgy AS, Serafini FM, Zweibel BR, et al. Transjugular intrahepatic portosystemic shunt vs. small diameter prosthetic H-graft portacaval shunt: extended follow-up of an expanded randomized prospective trial. J Gastrointest Surg 2000;4:589–597.
80. Rosemurgy AS, Zervos EE, Bloomston M, Durkin AJ, Clark WC, Goff S. Post–shunt resource consumption favors small-diameter prosthetic H-graft portacaval shunt over TIPS for patients with poor hepatic reserve. Ann Surg 2003;237:825–827.
81. Villanueva C, Balanzò J, Novella MT, et al. Nadolol plus isosorbide mononitrate compared with sclerotherapy for the prevention of variceal rebleeding. N Engl J Med 1996;334:1624–1629.
82. Villanueva C, Miñana J, Ortiz J, et al. Endoscopic ligation compared with nadolol and isosorbide mononitrate to prevent recurrent variceal bleeding. N Engl J Med 2002;345:647–655.
83. Lo GH, Chen WC, Chen MH, et al. Banding ligation versus nadolol and isosorbide mononitrate for the prevention of esophageal variceal rebleeding. Gastroenterology 2002;123:728–734.
84. Patch D, Sabin CA, Goulis J, et al. A randomized, controlled trial of medical therapy versus endoscopic ligation for the prevention of variceal rebleeding in patients with cirrhosis. Gastroenterology 2002;123:1013–1019.
85. Lo GH, Lai KH, Cheng JS, et al. Endoscopic variceal ligation plus nadolol and sucralfate compared with ligation alone for he prevention of variceal rebleeding: a prospective, randomized trial. Hepatology 2000;32:461–465.
86. Papatheodoridis GV, Goulis J, Leandro G, Patch D, Burroughs AK. Transjugular intrahepatic portosystemic shunt compared with endoscopic treatment for prevention of variceal rebleeding: a meta-analysis. Hepatology 1999;30:612–622.
87. Luca A, D'Amico G, La Galla R, Midiri M, Morabito A, Pagliaro L. TIPS for prevention of recurrent bleeding in patients with cirrhosis: meta-analysis of randomized clinical trials. Radiology 1999;212:411–421.
88. Meddi P, Merli M, Lionetti R, et al. Cost analysis for the prevention of variceal rebleeding: a comparison between transjugular intrahepatic portosystemic shunt and endoscopic sclerotherapy in a selected group of Italian cirrhotic patients. Hepatology 1999;29:1074–1077.
89. Russo MW, Zacks SL, Sandler RS, Brown RS. Cost-effectiveness analysis of transjugular intrahepatic portosystemic shunt (TIPS) versus endoscopic therapy for the prevention of recurrent esophageal variceal bleeding. Hepatology 2000;31:358–363.

14

Pharmacologic Therapy for Management of Esophageal Varices

Biology and Utility of Available Agents

Norman D. Grace, MD
and Richard S. Tilson, MD

CONTENTS

INTRODUCTION
PREPRIMARY PROPHYLAXIS
PREVENTION OF FIRST VARICEAL HEMORRHAGE
TREATMENT OF ACUTE VARICEAL HEMORRHAGE
SECONDARY PROPHYLAXIS OF VARICEAL HEMORRHAGE
CONCLUSION
REFERENCES

INTRODUCTION

Portal hypertension is responsible for the major complications of cirrhosis including the development of ascites, variceal hemorrhage, portal systemic encephalopathy, and the hepatorenal syndrome. Until the late 1970s, surgically created shunts were the primary treatment for the complications of portal hypertension. Although shunts successfully lowered portal pressure, they were complicated by progressive liver failure, hepatic encephalopathy, and, in the case of primary prophylaxis, an increase in mortality compared to supportive medical treatment *(1)*. Endoscopic sclerotherapy was popularized in the 1970s and 1980s as the primary medical therapy for the control of initial variceal hemorrhage and the prevention of recurrent hemorrhage. Sclerotherapy for primary prophylaxis was extensively studied in randomized controlled trials (RCT) but two very well designed RCTs had to be terminated by the external monitoring committees because of a higher mortality in patients treated with sclerotherapy when compared to a medical control group *(2)*. Most recently, sclerotherapy has essentially been replaced by endoscopic variceal ligation. However, endoscopic therapy does not alter portal pressure and is ineffective for nonesophageal variceal hemorrhage and portal hypertensive gastropathy.

Pharmacologic therapy for the treatment of active variceal hemorrhage was introduced in 1956 by Kehne et al. when they reported on the use of surgical pituitrin for the control

From: *Clinical Gastroenterology: Portal Hypertension*
Edited by: A. J. Sanyal and V. H. Shah © Humana Press Inc., Totowa, NJ

of acute variceal hemorrhage *(3)*. The first controlled trial supporting the use of posterior pituitary extract was reported by Merigan et al. in 1962 *(4)*. Although several RCTs evaluating vasopressin, given both intravenously, by bolus, and by selective intraarterial infusion followed, the modern era of pharmacologic therapy was introduced in 1980 by Lebrec et al. when he described the use of propranolol, a nonselective β adrenergic blocker, for the treatment of portal hypertension in patients with cirrhosis *(5)*. This was followed in 1981 by the publication of the first randomized controlled trial demonstrating the efficacy of propranolol for the prevention of recurrent variceal hemorrhage *(6)*.

Rational for Pharmacologic Therapy

Portal hypertension is defined as an increase in the portal venous pressure gradient (>6 mmHg) and is a function of portal venous blood flow and hepatic and portocollateral resistance (Ohm's law). In patients with cirrhosis there is a hyperdynamic circulation induced by significant peripheral vasodilation, with nitric oxide acting as the primary mediator. Also contributing are increased circulating levels of glucagon, prostaglandins, TNF α, and other cytokines. Both fixed and dynamic factors contribute to the increase in intrahepatic resistance. The early fixed changes include sinusoidal encroachment (i.e., enlarged hepatocytes) and collagen deposition in the presinusoidal region or space of Disse. Later changes include pruning of the vascular tree and development of regenerating nodules causing further obstruction. The dynamic component is governed by an increased endogenous production of endothelin, a potent vasoconstrictor and a decreased intrahepatic production of the vasodilator, NO. The goal of pharmacologic therapy is to decrease either portal venous blood flow by drugs producing splanchnic vasoconstriction or to decrease intrahepatic and portocollateral resistance by drugs inducing intrahepatic vasodilatation. Although a number of pharmacologic agents have been shown to lower portal pressure by either of these above mechanisms in animal models, most have not been well tolerated when given to patients with cirrhosis. Systemic hypotension has been a major drawback to the clinical use of many otherwise promising agents. Therefore, we are confining the discussion to agents that have been shown to be clinically effective and tolerable, based on results of randomized controlled trials.

Agents Producing Vasoconstriction: Nonselective β Adrenergic Blockers (Propranolol, Nadolol, Timolol)

Nonselective β blockers act by decreasing cardiac output via blockade of β1 cardiac receptors and by producing splanchnic vasoconstriction caused by a blockade of β2 receptors, leaving unopposed α adrenergic activity. In a study comparing propranolol with the cardioselective agent, atenolol, propranolol produced a 50% greater reduction in portal venous pressure in spite of a similar reduction in cardiac output, thus clearly demonstrating the importance of the β2 effect *(7)*. However, the decrease in portal pressure produced by β blockers may be offset by an increase in portocollateral resistance *(8,9)*. The variable effect produced by β blockers on portocollateral resistance may account for the failure of some patients with cirrhosis to achieve a reduction in portal pressure despite being adequately β-blocked *(10)*. In a study where the dose of propranolol was determined by the usual standards of a reduction in resting heart rate of 25%, a reduction to 55 BPM, or a systolic blood pressure below 80, only 37% of patients with cirrhosis achieved a >20% decrease in HVPG, a target reduction for the prevention of recurrent variceal hemorrhage *(11)*. The addition of a long acting nitrate, isosorbide-5-mononitrate, has been shown to ameliorate the increased resistance to portal blood flow in most patients, thus converting hemodynamic nonresponders to β blockers to responders with a reduction in HVPG *(10,12)*.

Although the three nonselective β blockers have not been compared directly in clinical trials, there are some theoretical differences. Nadolol is longer acting than propranolol, is not metabolized by the liver, is not lipophilic, and penetrates the blood–brain barrier to a lesser extent *(13)*. In the randomized trials for prevention of initial variceal bleeding, there are fewer reported significant side effects of treatment in patients receiving nadolol compared to those receiving propranolol *(14)*. Timolol probably has a greater hemodynamic effect in patients with cirrhosis because of its enhanced β2 effect, further decreasing splanchnic blood flow.

Approximately 15–20% of patients have contraindications to the use of nonselective β blockers, including congestive heart failure, asthma, heart block, bradycardia, severe chronic obstructive pulmonary disease, significant peripheral vascular disease, and, to a lesser extent, insulin-dependent diabetes mellitus and a history of bronchospasm. In addition, 10–20% of patients with cirrhosis who participated in RCTs of β blocker therapy had to be withdrawn because of severe side effects. Side effects have included depression, development of congestive heart failure, symptomatic bradycardia, worsening of COPD, and generalized asthenia. Although there was some initial concern about development of hepatic encephalopathy or the hepatorenal syndrome, this concern has not been borne out in numerous RCTs testing these drugs. Also, a rebound effect with possible variceal hemorrhage after sudden cessation of treatment has been a very infrequent clinical occurrence *(15)*.

The standard method for determining the dose of a nonselective β blocker has been borrowed from the cardiologists and includes a reduction in resting heart rate of 25%, a reduction in heart rate not to exceed 55 BPM or the development of symptoms. Unfortunately, there is no correlation between β blockade as determined by these clinical parameters and a reduction in portal pressure as determined by measurements of HPVG *(16)*. Measuring the hemodynamic response to a β blocker is the best way to determine a pharmacologic effect on portal hypertension *(10–12,16,17)*.

Vasopressin

Vasopressin, a posterior pituitary hormone, has been used for the treatment of acute variceal hemorrhage for 40 yr. It is a potent vasoconstrictor producing a marked reduction in splanchnic blood flow. After an intravenous infusion of vasopressin, Bosch et al. demonstrated a fall in the HVPG pressure gradient of 23% and a decrease in the intravariceal pressure measured directly of 14% *(18)*. The relatively lower effect on intravariceal pressure suggests less of an effect on the transmural pressure gradient, a key determinant of variceal wall tension that predicts the risk of variceal hemorrhage. Tsai et al. found a diminished reduction in HVPG in patients with active variceal hemorrhage, especially in patients in shock, when compared to stable control patients *(19)*. This decreased hemodynamic efficacy of vasopressin may be caused by the splanchnic vasoconstriction already present during active bleeding and is supported by animal studies which show that vasopressin has little effect on portal hemodynamics during severe hypotensive bleeding *(20)*. Because of its systemic vasoconstrictive and ADH effects, use of vasopressin has been associated with significant complications including myocardial and peripheral vascular ischemia, bradycardia, hypertension, hyponatremia, and fluid retention. The addition of nitroglycerin, given either intravenously, sublingually, or by transdermal patch has been shown to ameliorate many of the side effects of vasopressin and improve the portal hemo-dynamic response to the drug *(21,22)*.

Terlipressin

Terlipressin, or triglycyl-vasopressin, is an analog of vasopressin that, in vivo, is slowly activated by cleavage of the N-terminal glycyl residue, to lysine vasopressin. Because of the slow release with a longer half-life of the drug, blood levels are lower, tissue pene-tration is higher, and clinical trials have documented fewer side effects when compared to vasopressin. A single intravenous injection of 2 mg of terlepressin produced a 21% decrease in HVPG and a 25% reduction in azygous blood flow, a reduction that lasted for up to 4 h *(23)*. Direct measurements of variceal pressure after a 2 mg intravenous (iv) bolus showed a 21% decrease in the intravariceal pressure at 1 h, compared to a 14% decrease in the HVPG during the same time period *(24)*.

Somatostatin

Somatostatin is a biologically active peptide found naturally in many tissues including the brain, pancreas, upper gut, and enteric neurons *(25)*. Intravenous infusion of somato-statin reduces hepatic blood flow and portal pressure in patients with cirrhosis without altering the systemic circulation *(26)*. Because of its short half-life of 2 min, it has to be given by continuous infusion. Clinical trials have shown variable results in the reduction of portal pressure with, at best, half the effect of vasopressin *(26–28)*. Studies in portal hypertensive rats failed to show a direct effect of somatostatin on smooth muscle tone, sug-gesting that the vasoconstriction produced may be mediated by inhibition of circulating vasodilatory substances such as glucagon *(29,30)*. Bolus injections of somatostatin appear to produce a greater reduction of portal pressure than obtained by continuous infusion *(31)*. Although, in clinical trials, somatostatin is safe with very few reported side effects, iv infu-sion of somatostatin has been shown to induce renal vasoconstriction with impairment in glomerular filtration, free water clearance, and sodium excretion in patients with cirrhosis and ascites *(32)*.

Somatostatin Analogs (Octreotide, Lanreotide, Vapreotide)

Octreotide is a synthetic long-acting somatostatin analog with a half-life of 1.5 h. It is more potent than naturally occurring somatostatin in its inhibition of glucagon and growth hormone *(33)*. Octreotide has an affinity for somatostatin receptors 2 and 5. Its reported effects on lowering portal pressure have been variable with a majority of studies reporting little to no effect *(34)*. This may be explained by the development of tachyphy-laxis after repeated bolus injections, negating an initial reduction in portal pressure and azygous blood flow *(35)*. Octreotide, like somatostatin, may act through inhibition of glu-cagon and other intestinal hormones. It may also have an indirect role in producing a local vasoconstrictive effect on vascular smooth muscle of the superior mesenteric artery via interaction with other vasoconstrictors involving activation of protein kinase C *(36)*. How-ever, the primary mechanism for the control of variceal hemorrhage in patients with cir-rhosis may be through inhibition of postprandial hyperemia *(37,38)*. Lanreotide and vapre-otide are additional long-acting analogs of somatostatin with pharmacologic properties similar to octreotide. Long-acting preparations of both octreotide and lanreotide are cur-rently being assessed in the treatment of portal hypertension.

Agents Producing Vasodilitation

Both short-acting nitroglycerin and the longer-acting preparations, isosorbide-5-mononitrate and isosorbide dinitrate, produce vasodilitation by acting as NO donors. Administration of sublingual nitroglycerin in patients with cirrhosis has been shown to lower the HVPG within 2–12 min of administration *(39)*. Two theories have been postulated for the mechanism of action, a reduction in portal blood flow, or development of portocollateral vasodilation. The relative role of these mechanisms may vary and may account for the variable effect on azygous blood flow *(39)*. Isososorbide-5-mononitrate is the long-acting nitrate of choice in patients with cirrhosis because of minimal first pass metabolism *(40)*. Navasa et al. demonstrated an 18% reduction in the HVPG after a 40-mg dose of isosorbide-5-mononitrate which was maintained over the 2-h observation period, but was associated with a 19% decrease in arterial pressure *(41)*. Long-term administration of isosorbide-5-mononitrate produced a significant reduction in HVGP with no change in azygous or portal blood flow, confirming the major mechanism involved is a reduction in hepatic and portocollateral resistance *(42)*. Isosorbide-5-mononitrate has also been shown to reduce variceal pressure as measured directly *(43)*. The addition of isosorbide-5-mononitrate to propranolol has been shown to decrease hepatic and portocollateral resistance induced by the nonselective β blockers *(10,12)*.

Diuretics

Continuous administration of spironolactone plus a low sodium diet produces a modest reduction in HVPG in patients with compensated cirrhosis *(44)*. These changes correlated with a reduction in plasma volume. Patients with compensated cirrhosis who were given spironolactone 100 mg per d over a 6-wk period had a significant reduction in variceal pressure as measured by an endoscopically placed pressure gage *(45)*. This change was associated with a reduction in plasma volume, α natriuretic peptide and plasma renin activity.

PREPRIMARY PROPHYLAXIS

Animal studies have demonstrated that pretreatment with propranolol inhibits the development of portal–systemic shunting in a chronic murine schistosomiasis model of portal hypertension *(46)*. Pretreatment with propranolol reduced the severity of portal hypertension and portal–systemic shunts in portal-vein-ligated rats *(47)*. These observations, in addition to the success achieved with the use of nonselective β adrenergic blockers in RCTs for the prevention of initial and recurrent variceal hemorrhage, have stimulated investigation of very early administration of nonselective β adrenergic blockers to patients with compensated cirrhosis but no evidence of varices or ascites, in an attempt to prevent the development of these complications of portal hypertension.

Preliminary results of a four center, 10-yr randomized, placebo-controlled, double-blind study failed to demonstrated that early treatment with a nonselective β blocker prevented the development of esophageal varices, ascites, or the time to development of these complications *(48)*. In this study, 213 patients with biopsy-proven cirrhosis but no evidence of varices by endoscopy and an HVPG > 6 mmHg were randomly assigned to treatment with timolol or a placebo, the dosage determined by a 25% reduction in resting heart rate from baseline, a heart rate to 55 BPM or a maximum dose of 80 mg per d. Yearly follow-up with endoscopy and portal hemodynamic measurements was performed, with the primary end point, the development of esophageal varices as confirmed by two independent observers. The median follow up was 4.2 yr. Although 78 patients developed varices and six patients presented with a variceal bleed, there was no difference based on treatment assignment. No differences were found, based on treatment, in development of ascites, hepatic encephalopathy, mortality, or need for liver transplantation. There were, however, more serious adverse events in the group of patients receiving timolol. An HVPG > 10 mmHg was predictive of development of the primary and secondary end points.

In a double-blind, placebo-controlled, randomized trial, Cales et al. found that propranolol did not prevent development of varices nor the progression from small to large varices in patients with cirrhosis (49). Patients were randomly assigned to a longer acting propranolol (160 mg per d) or a placebo, and the study included both patients with no varices at entry and patients with small varices. At 2 yr, 31% of patients in the propranolol group had large varices compared to 14% in the placebo group ($p < 0.05$).

In a single-blind, randomized-controlled trial evaluating progression from small to large varices, patients were randomly assigned to nadolol or placebo with endoscopic evaluation at 12-mo intervals (50). After a mean follow-up of 36 mo, 11% of patients receiving nadolol had progressed to large varices compared to 37% receiving a placebo ($p < 0.01$). There was no significant difference in variceal hemorrhage or mortality between the groups. The authors concluded that nadolol prevented the progression from small to medium or large esophageal varices and suggested that preprimary prophylaxis be considered.

These studies differ in patient selection, design, and evaluation of the primary end points. The trial by Groszmann et al. (48) included only patients with no varices, the adjustment of the dose of timololol was blinded, and the primary end point was confirmed by two independent observers. The trial by Cales et al. (49) included both patients with no and small varices, the patients received a standard dose of propranolol and one-third of the patients were lost to follow-up. In the trial by Merkel et al. (50), the inclusion criterion was the presence of small varices and the adjustment of the nadolol dose was not blinded. Two of the three studies have yet to reach full publication. At this time, preprimary prophylaxis with nonselective β blockers cannot be recommended.

PREVENTION OF FIRST VARICEAL HEMORRHAGE

In a prospective study of 321 patients with cirrhosis, esophageal varices, and no prior variceal bleeding, 85 patients (26.5%) bled from varices during a median follow-up of 23 mo, with the majority of patients experiencing the bleeding episode within the first year after the diagnosis of varices (51). An additional prospective study showed 2-yr bleeding incidence of 30% in patients with medium to large varices and 10% in patients with small varices (52). The mortality for each bleeding episode ranges from 15% to 20%, depending on the Child–Pugh status and the severity of the bleeding episode (53). Therefore, therapy to prevent the initial episode of variceal hemorrhage is highly desirable and has been recommended in practice guidelines (54).

Based on the results of 11 well-designed, randomized, controlled trials, nonselective β adrenergic blockers have become the established first line therapy (55,56) (Figs. 1 and 2). Nine of these trials used propranolol and two, nadolol, with a total of 1189 patients entered. A meta-analysis of these trials shows a reduction in bleeding rate from 24% in the treatment group to 15% in the control group ($p < 0.01$) (55) (Tables 1 and 2). If one study that was an outlier is excluded, the absolute risk difference was 10% and the number

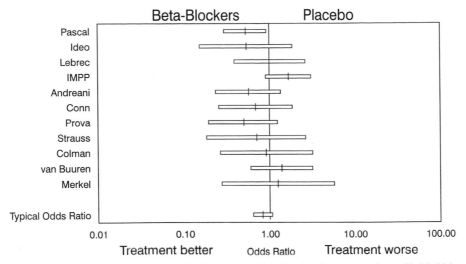

Fig. 1. Randomized controlled trials of β-blockers vs placebo for the prevention of initial bleed-all sites. The odds ratio for the group is 0.55; 95% confidence interval 0.41–0.74 ($p < 0.0001$).

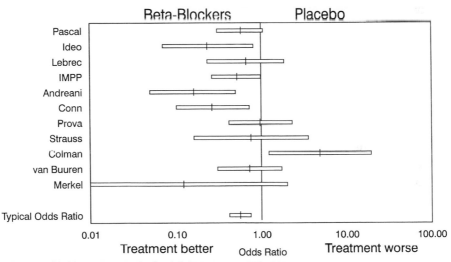

Fig. 2. Randomized controlled trials of β-blockers vs placebo for mortality. The odds ratio for the group is 0.82; 95% confidence interval 0.63–1.07 ($p <$ NS).

needed to treat (NNT) to prevent one episode of variceal hemorrhage was 10. Six of these trials included only patients with medium to large varices. Analysis of these trials shows a reduction in the risk of bleeding from 24% to 8% with an NNT of 6 *(55)*. In patients with ascites, the NNT was 11. Although there is a trend toward improved survival, it does not reach statistical significance (Fig. 2). Only three trials included patients with small varices and the sample size is too small for meaningful analysis. As there are very few Child–Pugh class C patients entered in these trials, treatment should be confined to Child–Pugh class A and B patients *(57)*. Therefore, selection criteria for treatment should include patients with medium to large varices who are deemed compliant in taking medication

Table 1
Prevention of EVH-Efficacy of β-Blockers Subgroup Analysis

	No RCTs	No Pts	Bleeding rate C/T	Mortality C/T (%)	NNT C/T (%)
All RCTs	11	600/590	24/15	27/23	
Colman omitted	10	575/567	25/15		10
Large or Medium EV	8	411/400	30/14	30/28	6
• without ascites	4	146/134	25/12	NR	8
• with ascites	4	156/149	31/22	NR	11
Small Varices	3	100/91	7/2	NR	

From ref. 55.

and without contraindications to the use of β blockers. Treatment should be continued indefinitely as discontinuation of treatment results in a return to pretreatment risk for variceal bleeding (58).

Are there alternative pharmacological agents for patients who have contraindications to or are unable to tolerate nonselective β adrenergic blockers? In an RCT comparing isosorbide-5-mononitrate (ISMN) to propranolol for the prevention of first variceal hemorrhage, Angelico initially reported that the drug had similar efficacy for the prevention of initial variceal hemorrhage with no difference in survival or side effects (59). However, a longer follow-up, extending over 7 yr, showed an increase in mortality in patients taking ISMN who were older than 50 yr of age (60). A meta-analysis of three trials comparing propranolol or nadolol with ISMN comprising 271 patients demonstrated a 28% incidence of variceal hemorrhage in patients receiving ISMN compared to 17% in patients on a nonselective β blocker ($p < 0.05$) (60–62). In a multicenter, double-blind RTC comparing ISMN to a placebo in patients with cirrhosis who either had contraindications to β blocker therapy or had to be withdrawn from treatment because of side effects, the actuarial probability of bleeding at 2 yr was 29% in the patients on ISMN compared to 14% in those on placebo ($p = 0.56$) (63). Therefore, ISMN as monotherapy cannot be recommended as an alternative to nonselective β blockers.

As has been detailed previously in this chapter, long-acting nitrates can increase the portal hemodynamic response to nonselective β blockers. This prompted Merkel et al. to compare the combination of nadolol and ISMN to nadolol alone for the prevention of first variceal hemorrhage (64). Combination therapy resulted in a reduction in the risk of first variceal hemorrhage with a slightly higher incidence of side effects and no survival advantage. A second trial by the Spanish Variceal Bleeding Study Group enrolled 347 cirrhotic patients who were randomized to receive propranolol plus ISMN vs propranolol plus placebo (65). There were no significant differences in the 1- and 2-yr actuarial probability of variceal bleeding, new onset or worsening of ascites, impairment of renal function, or survival. Headache was a more frequent complication in the combination therapy group. In conclusion, combination therapy, although safe, does not offer a significant advantage over monotherapy and should not be considered as first line therapy.

Spironolactone may have a synergestic effect for the reduction of portal pressure when combined with a nonselective β blocker. In a randomized controlled trial, nadolol plus spironolactone was compared with nadolol plus placebo for the prevention of first variceal hemorrhage in cirrhotic patients with medium to large varices and no ascites *(66)*. Cumulative probabilities of remaining free of bleeding and ascites were similar for both groups with no difference in survival. However, clinically significant ascites was higher in the group taking nadolol plus placebo, suggesting that combination therapy may be beneficial for this subgroup.

Assessing the hemodynamic response to pharmacologic therapy is predictive of outcome. In a randomized double-blind placebo-controlled trial, Groszmann et al. demonstrated a reduction in the HVPG to <12 mmHg was associated with an absence of variceal hemorrhage *(67)*. Merkel et al. defined a response to pharmacologic therapy as reduction in the HVPG of >20% or a reduction to <12 mmHg *(68)*. They found a significant reduction in the incidence of bleeding in the responders when compared to the nonresponders and confirmed the absence of variceal bleeding in patients with an HVPG < 12mmHg. Using a Markov decision model, Imperiale et al. found that measuing the hemodynamic response of pharmacological therapy for the prevention of first variceal hemorrhage substantially reduced the number of bleeding episodes and was cost-effective or cost-saving over a wide range of sensitivity analyses *(69)*. For patients who cannot tolerate pharmacologic therapy or who may not be good candidates because of severity of liver disease or noncompliance, esophageal variceal ligation is a good alternative. A detailed discussion of this is in Chapter 15 by Cello. Variceal ligation and nonselective β blockers have comparable efficacy at least over the short term, for the prevention of variceal hemorrhage *(70)*.

A recent decision analysis by Spiegel et al. recommended empiric β blocker therapy in all compensated cirrhotics as the most cost effective approach to management *(71)*. We have significant concerns about this approach as it does not take into account the side effects of treatment. This approach needs to be evaluated in a prospective manner before any consideration of its adoption.

TREATMENT OF ACUTE VARICEAL HEMORRHAGE

The pharmacologic management of acute variceal bleeding began more than 40 yr ago when the vasoconstrictor, vasopressin, was used *(72)*. Since then, there have been 10 RCTs performed with the drug, four of which included a placebo arm with a total of 157 patients *(72)*. In those trials, vasopressin decreased the failure rate of therapy from 82% to 50%, but had no direct effect on mortality, a recurrent theme in the pharmacologic management of variceal bleeding *(55)*. However, unlike the newer compounds, treatment with vasopressin resulted in frequent side effects that mandated cessation of therapy in 25% of the treated patients, and, more troubling, resulted in three treatment-related deaths *(55)*. The most serious of the side effects of vasopressin therapy stem from its systemic vasoconstrictive properties, and include cardiac arrythmias, myocardial infarction, and ischemia of the mesenteric and cerebral vessels. Nitroglycerin has been added to vasopressin to both combat the dangerous cardiac vasoconstriction and augment the decrease in portal venous pressure with moderate effect. The combination has been tested against isolated vasopressin in three RCT with a total of 146 subjects with improvement in the ability to control bleeding but no difference in mortality *(55)*. Currently, isolated use of vasopression cannot be recommended given its high rate of potentially detrimental effects, and combination therapy with nitroglycerin should only be undertaken with great caution.

Terlipressin, a synthetic analogue of vasopression, has both an intrinsic effect as well as the effect of vasporessin after enzymatic cleavage of its triglycyl residues. This permits regular rather than continuous dosing without changing biological half-life. Terlipressin has been evaluated in seven placebo-controlled trials including 443 patients (73). A meta-analysis of the seven trials demonstrated a significant reduction in the ability to control bleeding (RR 0.66, 95% CI 0.53–0.82), and, unique among vasoconstrictive agents, a significant reduction in mortality (RR 0.66, 95% CI 0.49–0.88) (55,73). In trials using terlipressin or placebo as adjunct to sclerotherapy, although the benefit of terlipressin was decreased overall, its use was still associated with beneficial effects that were statistically significant (reduction in failure of hemostasis) or approached statistical significance (mortality) (74). Terlipressin has been compared in one trial of 219 subjects to endoscopic therapy, and showed no significant difference in control of hemorrhage, recurrent hemorrhage, mortality, or transfusion requirement (75). Overall, terlipressin is an effective vasoconstrictive agent with equal efficacy to both sclerotherapy and vasopressin in the acute management of variceal hemorrhage, with fewer side effects than even the vasopressin/nitroglycerin combination. Terlipressin is currently one of the most widely used first line agents for control of acute variceal hemorrhage in Europe, but is unavailable for clinical use in the United States.

Somatostatin reduces splanchnic blood flow, portal pressure, and azygous blood flow in cirrhotic patients, and is therefore well suited as an agent for management of acute variceal bleeding. Bolus injections of somatastatin have more pronounced effects than continuous infusion (31), and should be used as the initial mode of delivery in standard doses of 250 µg, although two studies showed a higher rate of bleeding control, fewer transfusions, and better survival with doses of 500 µg (76,77). There have been three double-blind, randomized-controlled trials comparing somatostatin to placebo and four trials comparing somatostatin with nonactive treatment, including a total of 552 subjects (55). The results of these trials are mixed, with two of the placebo trials showing no benefit, and the remaining showing a trend toward benefit. Whereas a meta-analysis demonstrated significant decrease in failure to control bleeding, there was no significant decrease in mortality and the benefit was less than that seen with terlipressin (54). There have been seven head-to-head trials comparing somatostatin with vasopressin, the pooled results of which demonstrate equal efficacy with significantly fewer side effects in the group receiving somatostatin (55), although only two of the studies used vasopressin in combination with nitroglycerin. There have been three studies comparing somatostatin to terlipressin including a total of 302 subjects that again demonstrated equal efficacy and side effects (55).

Somatostatin has also been shown to have equal efficacy to emergency sclerotherapy in three trials with significantly fewer side effects. In all studies involving somatostatin with sclerotherapy, the use of somatostatin significantly improved visualization of the bleeding varix and overall bleeding control, a fact borne out in a trial by Villanueva et al. of 100 bleeding episodes designed to test whether combination therapy (emergency sclerotherapy plus somatostatin) improved outcome over pharmacologic therapy alone (78). In this trial, therapeutic failure decreased from 24% to 8% and early rebleeding decreased from 24% to 7% (both statistically significant decreases) without a concomitant decrease in mortality. The effect of combined therapy is likely caused by improved visualization of a bleeding varix owing to decreased acute bleeding at the time of endoscopy secondary to drug effect (only 27% compared to historical controls of 50%). Finally, combination therapy with somatostatin plus isosorbide mononitrate has been tested in a randomized placebo-controlled trial, the results of which demonstrated similar outcomes but more frequent side effects in subjects in the combination arm, and led the authors to recommend against the combination in clinical use *(79)*. Currently, somatostatin is a first line agent for the treatment of acute variceal bleeding both alone and in combination with endoscopic therapy in Europe, but is unavailable for clinical use in the United States.

Octreotide is widely used in the acute management of variceal bleeding, although it has not been approved for this use by the United States FDA. Compared with somatostatin, it has a much longer half-life and can potentially be given subcutaneously. A recent study demonstrated that bolus octreotide injection, like somatostatin, causes a marked decrease in portal pressure and azygous blood flow, but that the continuous octreotide infusion neither maintains nor prolongs the effect *(35)*. Despite these results, octreotide given as bolus and subsequent continuous infusion has been compared to terlipressin, vasopressin, somatostatin, and endoscopic therapy in a number of prospective randomized-controlled trials, and reported in a recent meta-analysis *(80)*. This meta-analysis suggests that octreotide is superior to all alternative therapies combined, vasopressin/terlipressin, and placebo (among subjects receiving endoscopic therapy prior to octreotide), with equal efficacy to immediate sclerotherapy regarding control of bleeding. Although flawed, the paper underscores data already published in other meta-analyses, namely that octreotide is equally effective as sclerotherapy and other pharmacologic modalities for the treatment of acute variceal hemorrhage. Finally, there have been several prospective randomized controlled trials and one meta-analysis of octreotide and somatastatin as adjuncts to endoscopic therapy *(81,82)*. Although there was no survival benefit noted for the use of combined therapy, combination of early administration of octreotide and endoscopy has a 33% higher rate of 5-d hemostasis, in part related to an increased visualization of the culprit varices.

The newest agent with potential use in acute variceal bleeding is recombinant activated factor VII. Administration of recombinant factor VII works to augment the initiation of coagulation and intensify the thrombin effect at the site of injury with limited effect on the clotting cascade elsewhere. Its applicability in variceal hemorrhage has been demonstrated in two small trials, one of which was a double-blind, placebo-controlled study *(83)*, although further study is required before the drug can be accepted as standard therapy. Notably, this study demonstrated significant improvement in outcome in patients with Child's B and C disease who had uncontrollable bleeding from varices, implying a possible role in patients with more severe liver disease. There are no demonstrated severe side effects associated with the drug, but its cost ($3000–$4000/dose) and short half life (2.3 h in actively bleeding patients) requiring multiple doses in clinical trials will limit the use of this medication for patients with hemorrhage that can be controlled with standard pharmacologic/endoscopic therapy *(84)*.

SECONDARY PROPHYLAXIS OF VARICEAL HEMORRHAGE

The risk of rebleeding in patients who survive an episode of variceal hemorrhage is very high, with a median incidence of 63% within 1–2 yr among controls of RCTs *(72)*, with a corresponding mortality of 33%. To date, pharmacologic therapy aimed at preventing recurrent bleeding has focused on nonselective β blockers and nitrates, used alone and in combination, and independently or alongside endoscopic therapy. Because of the variability in response to these agents, the potential for intolerable side effects, and inconsistent results among clinical trials, specific drug dosing, and endoscopy schedules cannot be prescribed with a guarantee that a compliant patient will not have further bleed-

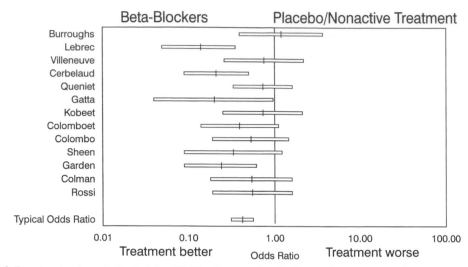

Fig. 3. Randomized controlled trials of β-blockers vs placebo/nonactive treatment for the prevention of rebleeding. The odds ratio for the group is 0.56; 95% confidence interval 0.31–0.42 ($p < 0.0001$).

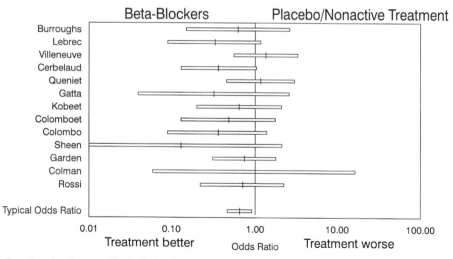

Fig. 4. Randomized controlled trials of β-blockers vs placebo/nonactive treatment for mortality. The odds ratio for the group is 0.91; 95% confidence interval 0.46–0.65 ($p = 0.0177$).

ing episodes. However, given the relative efficacy of current therapy and the clear risk of rebleeding in untreated patients, it has been agreed that all patients who survive a variceal bleed require treatment for prevention of rebleeding *(56)*.

Since their use in prevention of rebleeding was first described in 1980, propanolol and the other nonselective β blockers have been demonstrated effective therapy for secondary prophylaxis. A total of 13 RCTs comparing β blockers with placebo have been reported in two meta-analyses *(55,85)* (Figs. 3 and 4). In both analyses, β blockers effectively decreased variceal rebleeding with a number needed to treat of 5, and mortality from 27% to 20%, with an associated decreased mortality from bleeding from 24% to 16% (Table 2).

Table 2
Prevention of Recurrent EVH Efficacy of β Blockers
(13 RCTs)

	β Blockers	Placebo, NT
No. Patients	410	399
Rebleeding	42%	63%
Mortality	20%	27%
NNT	Rebleeding	5
	Death	14

From ref. 55.

There was a 17% adverse event rate among those trials reporting adverse events, with a concomitant dose reduction or discontinuation of the drug in 6% or subjects. These drugs are therefore effective single agents for secondary prophylaxis of variceal bleeding, and form the cornerstone of therapy for patients who have experienced a variceal bleed. Unless contraindicated, they should be started as soon as patients are hemodynamically stable and titrated to a dose that yields either a 25% reduction in the resting heart rate, a heart rate of 55, or development of side effects.

β-Blockers have been compared to sclerotherapy in 10 trials, a meta-analysis of which demonstrates that no significant difference in survival or rebleeding exists between the two therapies, although β blockers are reported to carry fewer side effects (55,86). In these studies, the mean percentage of patients free of variceal bleeding was significantly higher in the patients treated with sclerotherapy (55%) than with β blockers (39%), although because β blockers decrease portal hypertension and therefore decrease all bleeding events including bleeding from gastropathy and gastric varices, overall bleeding episodes were not significantly different between the two therapies. The increased risk of side effects and relative ease of administration of the drug led the authors of one of the meta-analyses to recommend β blockers as the preferred primary therapy for secondary prophylaxis (86).

Combination β blocker and sclerotherapy has been compared to sclerotherapy alone, using the logic that direct obliteration of varices will decrease immediate risk of variceal bleeding, and that pharmacologic therapy will decrease long-term risk by persistently decompressing the portal system. In several of the trials, β blockers were discontinued after endoscopic eradication of varices, so that the longer-term value of β blockers on preventing variceal bleeding from all sites was not assessed. Two meta-analyses have reported higher rebleeding rates in patients treated with β blockers alone (absolute risk difference 19%), but no significant difference in mortality (55,87). A similar result evaluating esophageal variceal ligation was recently reported by Lo et al. (88), although this study was unblinded, did not use HVPG as a measurement of therapeutic efficacy and used sucralfate in the combination arm which may have decreased the rate of complications in the combined therapy arm (89).

Combined therapy using β-blockers and nitrates has been compared to β-blockers alone in two trials. The combination was initially described in 1991 by Garcia-Pagan et al., where the group noted that after 3 mo, the HVPG decreased by more than 20% from baseline values in 10% of the subjects taking propanolol alone, compared to 50% in patients receiving combination therapy. To date, propanolol has been compared to combined therapy with nitrates in only two trials, one of which has only been reported in abstract *(90,91)* with mixed results. In the trial reported in abstract, a significantly higher mortality with combination therapy was reported, although this was not seen in the second trial. Despite the paucity of head-to-head clinical trials, combination therapy using nitrates has gained acceptance as therapy for secondary prophylaxis against recurrent variceal bleeding, and has been evaluated as maximal pharmacologic therapy versus endoscopic therapy in several trials.

Endoscopic therapy has been compared with combined therapy with β blockers and nitrates in three prospective trials *(92–94)*. All trials except one *(94)* demonstrated that combined pharmacologic therapy was more effective than endoscopic therapy at prevention of bleeding, although none demonstrated a survival advantage for pharmacologic therapy. This trial demonstrated an advantage for endoscopic therapy but used much lower doses of β blocker, had a rebleeding rate similar to the placebo arm of previous trials, and did not use HVPG as a gauge for therapeutic efficacy in the pharmacologic arm. The paper by Patch et al. *(94)* used measurements of HVPG performed at 3 mo after baseline studies to determine pharmacologic efficacy. As a number of the patients in this study had recurrent bleeding before the second measurement of HVPG was obtained, isosorbide-5-mononitrate which as per protocol was given to nonresponders, was never administered to these patients. As a result, many patients in this study were treated only with β-blocker monotherapy. Therefore, despite the higher incidence of side effects limiting tolerability, combination therapy may be a reasonable first line therapy for patients with high risk of rebleeding.

It has been clearly demonstrated that there is no uniform reduction in portal pressure with the use of β blockers among patients with varices, and that easily measured parameters (pulse and blood pressure) are poor surrogates for therapeutic efficacy. The data for the effectiveness of lowering portal pressure in preventing variceal bleeding are clear: variceal rebleeding occurs in less than 6% of patients in whom the HVPG can be lowered below 12, and patients in whom HVPG can be lowered by 20% have improved survival and a significantly lower risk of developing complications of portal hypertension *(95,96)*. As is discussed elsewhere in this text, current techniques for measuring portal pressure are invasive, expensive, and best performed in centers with a significant amount of experience. Although noninvasive methods are in development, currently, none of these have shown the reliability and accuracy necessary to supplant measuring the HVPG. Tailored therapy with a stepwise titration of β-blocker, addition of nitrate, and addition of endoscopy to achieve the threshold goals is a reasonable approach, although it requires accurate measurement *(97)*, and reliably tested end points *(98)* before it will be widely adapted in clinical practice. This approach needs to be tested in RCTs. For now, because of the rarity of complications *(97)* HVPG should be measured and reported in all clinical trials, and deserves a prominent role in the management of variceal bleeding and pharmacological dosing in all centers with expertise in its use.

Promising Compounds

A number of pharmacological agents have been shown to lower portal pressure in both animal models and acute trials in patients with cirrhosis. However, the associated systemic arterial hypotension has precluded their use for long-term treatment. These agents have been recently reviewed by Bosch and Garcia-Pagan and are listed in Table 3 *(99)*.

Table 3
Manipulation of Intrahepatic Circulation

Adrenergic Antagonists
    Prazosin (α-1 antagonist)
    Clonidine (central α-2 agonist)
    Carvedilol (α-1 antagonist and nonselective β-blocker)
Blockade of the Renin-Angiotension System
    Losartin (angiotension-2 antagonist)
Serotonin antagonists
    Ritanserin (selective serotonin-S2 receptor antagonist)
    Ketanserin (5-hydroxytryptamine 2-receptor blocker)

Adapted from ref. 99.

Of these drugs, the two that have drawn the most attention in the last few years are carvedilol and losartin.

Carvedilol has the theoretical advantage of combining a nonselective β adrenergic blocker with an α-1 adrenergic antagonist. In a randomized trial comparing carvedilol with propranolol in a study in which the HVPG was measured at baseline and after 3 mo of treatment, carvedilol produced a 19% reduction in the HVPG compared to 12% for propranolol ($p < 0.001$) (100). Carvedilol was successful in reaching a hemodynamic end point (HVPG reduction $\geq 20\%$ or ≤ 12 mmHg) in 54% of cirrhotic patients compared to 23% for propranolol ($p < 0.05$). There was a significant reduction in mean arterial pressure (11%) with carvedilol compared with no significant change in patients receiving propranolol. There was no difference between the drugs with regards to impairment of renal function or adverse events requiring discontinuation of therapy. The systemic arterial hypotension produced by carvedilol may be especially troublesome in patients with ascites (101). If the effect on systemic arterial pressure can be minimized, carvedilol has significant potential and needs to be assessed in long-term RCTs.

Losartan, an angiotensin II type 1 receptor blocker, generated significant interest when Schneider et al. reported a 45% decrease in HVPG after 1 wk of treatment with 25 mg losartan daily, compared to no change in HVPG in controls (102). They reported a slight decrease in mean arterial pressure but felt the drug was reasonably well tolerated. However, a longer trial (6 wk) by Gonzalez-Abraldes et al. (103) failed to demonstrate any effect of losartan on HVPG but did show a significant systemic arterial hypotensive effect and a deleterious effect on renal function in patients with more advanced cirrhosis.

Based on the hypothesis that statins might increase NO production in the hepatic microcirculation, Zafra et al. (104) evaluated simvastatin in a group of patients with cirrhosis. Although simvastatin did not alter the HVPG, it did produce a 14% decrease in hepatic sinusoidal resistance without any effect on systemic hemodynamics. In a separate study, pretreatment with simvastatin attenuated the postprandial increase in HVPG. If these effects can be verified in a study over a longer time period, statin drugs may play an important role in the treatment of portal hypertension. However, potential adverse effects on liver function will have to be monitored carefully.

Another potential specific intrahepatic NO donor, NCX-1000, derived from ursodeoxycholic acid, has been shown to lower portal pressure (105) and to blunt an increase in portal pressure produced by progressive blood volume expansion (106) in animal models of portal hypertension. Whether this drug will be tolerated in studies in patients with cirrhosis has yet to be determined *(107)*.

In summary, the most exciting new drugs are those that might be specific NO donors to the intrahepatic circulation. In combination with a vasoconstrictor, i.e., a nonselective β adrenergic blocker, the hemodynamic goal of ≥20% decrease in HVPG or a decrease in HVPG ≤12 mmHg might be achievable in patients with cirrhosis and portal hypertension. Like so many other clinical entities, it is likely that a combination of pharmacologic agents will be required to produce maximum benefits.

CONCLUSION

Over the last 25 yr, use of nonselective β adrenergic blockers has become the first line therapy for prevention of first variceal hemorrhage and, along with endoscopic variceal ligation, first line therapy for prevention of recurrent variceal bleeding. However, a hemodynamic response (>20% reduction in HVPG or a reduction to <12 mmHg) is obtained in only one-third of patients. The addition of a long-acting vasodilator such as isosorbide-5-mononitrate has been shown to increase the hemodynamic response, with more than 50% of patients achieving a therapeutic end point. Unfortunately, results from RCTs have yet to establish the clinical superiority of combination pharmacologic therapy for prevention of first variceal hemorrhage. Use of combination therapy for prevention of recurrent variceal hemorrhage is more promising but additional studies are needed to establish clinical efficacy. The use of pharmacologic agents (terlipressin, somatostatin, octreotide, vapreotide), usually in combination with endoscopic therapy, has become the standard of care for control of acute variceal hemorrhage.

Unresolved issues include the value of treating patients with small esophageal varices with β-blockers, the role of portal hemodynamic measurements in the routine care of patients with esophageal varices, and the indications for the use of combined endoscopic and pharmacologic therapy. Future research will assess pharmacologic agents that can either be used as alternatives for patients unable to tolerate nonselective β blockers or as vasodilatory agents that might enhance the efficacy of nonselective β blockers. Currently, the most promising new agents are those that are selective NO donors for the intrahepatic circulation.

REFERENCES

1. Grace ND, Muench H, Chalmers TC. The present status of shunts for portal hypertension in cirrhosis. Gastroenterology 1966;50:684–691.
2. Lopes GM, Grace ND. Gastroesophageal varices: prevention of bleeding and rebleeding. Gastroenterol Clin North Am 1993;22:801–820.
3. Kehne JH, Hughes FA, Gompertz ML. Use of surgical pituitrin in a control of esophageal varix bleeding: experimental study and report of 2 cases. Surgery 1956;39:917–925.
4. Merigan TC, Plotkin GR, Davidson CS. Effect of intravenously administered posterior pituitary extract on hemorrage from bleeding esophageal varices; a controlled trial. N Engl J Med 1962;266:134–135.
5. Lebrec D, Nouel O, Corbic M, Benhamou JP. Propanolol—a medical treatment for portal hypertention? Lancet 1980;2:180–182.
6. Lebrec D, Poynard T, Hillon P, Benhamou JP. Propanolol for prevention of recurrent gastrointestinal bleeding in patients with cirrhosis, a controlled study. N Engl J Med 1981;305:1371–1374.
7. Hillon P, Lebrec D, Munoz C, Jungers M, Goldfarb G, Benhamou JP. Comparison of the effects of a cardioselective and non selective β-blocker in portal hypertension in patients with cirrhosis. Hepatology 1982;5:528–531.

8. Kroeger RJ, Groszmann RJ. Increased portal venous resistance hinders portal pressure reduction during the administration of b-adrenergic blocking agents in a portal hypertensive model. Hepatology 1985;5:97–100.

9. Pizcueta MP, De Lacey AM, Kravitz D, Bosch J, Rodes J. Propranolol decreases portal pressure without changing portocollateral resistance in cirrhosic rats. Hepatology 1989;10:953–957.

10. Merkel C, Sacerdoti D, Bolognesi M, et al. Hemodynamic evaluation of the addition of isosorbide-5-mononitrate to nadolol in cirrhotic patients with insufficient response to the b-blocker alone. Hepatology 1997;26:34–39.

11. Feu F, Garcia-Pagan JC, Bosch J, et al. Relation between portal pressure response to pharmacotherapy and risk of recurrent variceal hemorrage in patients with cirrhosis. Lancet 1995;346:1056–1059.

12. Garcia-Pagan JC, Feu F, Bosch J. Propranolol compared with propranolol plus isosorbide-5-mononitrite for portal hypertension in cirrhosis. A randomized controlled study. Ann Intern Med 1991;114: 869–873.

13. Gatter A, Sacerdoti D, Merkel C, Milani L, Battaglia G, Zuin R. Effects of nadolol treatment on renal and hepatic hemodynamics and function in cirrhotic patients with portal hypertension. Am Heart J 1984;108:1167–1172.

14. Grace ND. Prevention of initial variceal hemorrhage. Gastroenterol Clin North Am 1992;21:149–161.

15. Lebrec D, Bernuau J, Rueff B, Benhamou JP. Gastrointestinal bleeding after abrupt cessation of propranolol administration in cirrhosis. N Engl J Med 1982;307:560.

16. Garcia-Tsao G, Grace ND, Groszmann RJ, et al. Short-term effects of propranolol on portal venous pressure. Hepatology 1986;6:101–106.

17. Groszmann RJ, Bosch J, Grace ND, et al. Hemodynamic events in a prospective randomized trial of propranolol versus placebo in the prevention of a first variceal hemorrhage. Gastroenterology 1990; 99:1401–1407.

18. Bosch J, Bordas JM, Mastai R, et al. Effects of vasopressin on the intravariceal pressure in patients with cirrhosis: comparison with the effects on portal pressure. Hepatology 1988;8:861–865.

19. Tsai YT, Lee FY, Lin HC, et al. Hyposensitivity to vasopressin in patients with hepatitis B-related cirrhosis during acute variceal hemorrhage. Hepatology 1991;13:407–412.

20. Valla D, Girod C, Lee SS, Braillon A, Lebrec D. Lack of vasopressin action on splanchnic hemodynamics during bleeding: a study in conscious, portal hypertensive rats. Hepatology 1988;8:10–15.

21. Bosch J, Groszmann RJ, Garcia-Pagan JC, et al. Association of transdermal nitroglycerin to vasopressin infusion in the treatment of variceal hemorrhage: a placebo-controlled clinical trial. Hepatology 1989;10:962–968.

22. Groszmann RJ, Kravetz D, Bosch J, et al. Nitroglycerin improves the hemodynamic response to vasopressin in portal hypertension. Hepatology 1982;2:757–762.

23. Escorsell A, Bandi JC, Moitinho E, et al. Time profile of the haemodynamic effects of terlipressin in portal hypertension. J Hepatol 1997;621–627.

24. Romero G, Kravetz D, Argonz J, Bildozola M, Suarez A, Terg R. Terlipressin is more effective in decreasing variceal pressure than portal pressure in cirrhotic patients. J Hepatol 2000;32:419–425.

25. Dudley FJ. Somatostatin and portal hypertensive bleeding: a safe therapeutic alternative? Gastroenterology 1992;103:1973–1977.

26. Bosch J, Kravetz D, Rodes J. Effects of somatostatin on hepatic and systemic hemodynamics in patients with cirrhosis of the liver: comparison with vasopressin. Gastroenterology 1981;80:518–525.

27. Eriksson LS, Law DH, Sato Y, Wahren J. Influence of somatostatin on splanchnic haemodynamics in patients with liver cirrhosis. Clin Physiol 1984;4:5–11.

28. Kleber G, Sauerbruch T, Fischer G, Paumgartner G. Somatostatin does not reduce oesophageal variceal pressure in liver cirrhotics. Gut 1988;29:153–156.

29. Sieber CC, Mosca PG, Groszmann RJ. Effect of somatostatin on mesenteric vascular resistance in normal and portal hypertensive rats. Am J Physiol (Gastrointest & Liver Physiol) 1992;25:274–277.

30. Kravetz D, Bosch J, Arderiu MT, et al. Effects of somatostatin on splanchnic hemodynamics and plasma glucagon in portal hypertensive rats. Am J Physiol 1988;254:322–328.

31. Cirera I, Feu F, Luca A, et al. Effects of bolus injections and continuous infusions of somatostatin and placebo in patients with cirrhosis: a double-blind hemodynamic investigation. Hepatology 1995;22: 106–111.

32. Gines A, Salmeron JM, Gines P, et al. Effects of somatostatin on renal function in cirrhosis. Gastroenterology 1992;103:1868–1874.
33. Lamberts SW, van der Lely AJ, de Herder WW, Hofland LJ. Octreotide. N Engl J Med 1996;334:246–254.
34. Lin HC, Tsai YT, Lee FY, et al. Hemodynamic evaluation of octreotide in patients with hepatitis B-related cirrhosis. Gastroenterology 1992;103:229–234.
35. Escorsell A, Bandi JC, Andreu V, et al. Desensitization to the effects of intravenous octreotide in cirrhotic patients with portal hypertension. Gastroenterology 2001;120:161–169.
36. Wiest R, Tsai MH, Groszmann RJ. Octreotide potentiates PKC-dependent vasoconstrictors in portal-hypertensive and control rats. Gastroenterology 2001;120:975–983.
37. Albillos A, Rossi I, Iborra J, et al. Octreotide prevents postprandial splanchnic hyperemia in patients with portal hypertension. J Hepatol 1994;21:88–94.
38. McCormick PA, Biagini MR, Dick R, et al. Octreotide inhibits the meal-induced increases in the portal venous pressure of cirrhotic patients with portal hypertension: a double-blind, placebo-controlled study. Hepatology 1992;16:1180–1186.
39. Garcia-Tsao G, Groszmann RJ. Portal hemodynamics during nitroglycerin administration in cirrhotic patients. Hepatology 1987;7:805–809.
40. Garcia-Pagan JC, Escorsell A, Moitinho E, Bosch J. Influence of pharmacological agents on portal hemodynamics: basis for its use in the treatment of portal hypertension. Seminars Liver Dis 1999;19:427–438.
41. Navasa M, Chesta J, Bosch J, Rodes J. Reduction of portal pressure by isosorbide-5-mononitrate in patients with cirrhosis. Effects on splanchnic and systemic hemodynamics and liver function. Gastroenterology 1989;96:1110–1118.
42. Garcia-Pagan JC, Feu F, Navasa M, et al. Long-term haemodynamic effects of isosorbide 5-mononitrate in patients with cirrhosis and portal hypertension. J Hepatol 1990;11:189–195.
43. Escorsell A, Feu F, Bordas JM, et al. Effects of isosorbide-5-mononitrate on variceal pressure and systemic and splanchnic haemodynamics in patients with cirrhosis. J Hepatol 1996;24:423–429.
44. Garcia-Pagan JC, Salmeron JM, Feu F, et al. Effects of low-sodium diet and spironolactone on portal pressure in patients with compensated cirrhosis. Hepatology 1994;19:1095–1099.
45. Nevens F, Lijnen P, VanBilloen H, Fevery J. The effect of long-term treatment with spironolactone on variceal pressure in patients with portal hypertension without ascites. Hepatology 1996;23:1047–1052.
46. Sarin SK, Groszmann RJ, Mosca PG, et al. Propranolol ameliorates the development of portal-systemic shunting in a chronic murine schistosomiasis model of portal hypertension. J Clin Invest 1991;87:1032–1036.
47. Lin HC, Soubrane O, Cailmail S, Lebrec D. Early chronic administration of propranolol reduces the severity of portal hypertension and portal-systemic shunts in conscious portal vein stenosed rats. J Hepatol 1991;13:213–219.
48. Groszmann RJ, Garcia-Tsao G, Makuch R, et al. Multicenter randomized placebo-controlled trial of non selective beta-blockers in the prevention of the complications of portal hypertension: final results and identification of predictive factors. Hepatology 2003;38:206A.
49. Cales P, Oberti F, Payen JL, et al. Lack of effect of propranolol in the prevention of large oesophageal varices in patients with cirrhosis: a randomized trial. French-Speaking Club for the Study of Portal Hypertension. Eur J Gastroenterol Hepatol 1999;11:741–745.
50. Merkel C, Angeli P, Zanella P, et al. Beta-blockers in the prevention of aggravation of esophageal varices in patients with cirrhosis and small varices: a placebo controlled clinical trial. Hepatology 2003;38:217A.
51. A prospective multicenter study The North Italian Endoscopic Club for the Study and Treatment of Esophageal Varices. Prediction of the first variceal hemorrhage in patients with cirrhosis of the liver and esophageal varices. N Engl J Med 1988;319:983–989.
52. Pagliaro L, D'Amico G, Pasta L, et al. Portal hypertension in cirrhosis: natural history. In: Bosch J, Groszmann, RJ, eds. Portal Hypertension: Pathphysiology and Treatment. MA Blackwell Scientific, Cambridge, 1994, pp. 72–92.
53. D'Amico G, De Franchis R. Upper digestive bleeding in cirrhosis. Post-therapeutic outcome and prognostic indicators. Hepatology 2003;38:599–612.

54. Grace ND. Diagnosis and treatment of gastrointestinal bleeding secondary to portal hypertension. American College of Gastroenterology Practice Parameters Committee. Am J Gastroenterol 1997;92: 1081–1091.

55. D'Amico G, Pagliaro L, Bosch J. Pharmacological treatment of portal hypertension: an evidence-based approach. Semin Liver Dis 1999;19:475–503.

56. Grace ND, Groszmann RJ, Garcia-Tsao G, et al. Portal hypertension and variceal bleeding: an AASLD single topic symposium. Hepatology 1998;28:868–880.

57. Lopes GM, Grace ND. Gastroesophageal varices. Prevention of bleeding and rebeeding. Gastroenterol Clin North Am 1993;22:801–820.

58. Abraczinskas DR, Ookubo R, Grace ND, et al. Propranolol for the prevention of first esophageal variceal hemorrhage: a lifetime commitment? Hepatology 2001;34:1096–1102.

59. Angelico M, Carli L, Piat C, et al. Isosorbide-5-mononitrate versus propranolol in the prevention of first bleeding in cirrhosis. Gastroenterology 1993;104:1460–1465.

60. Angelico M, Carli L, Piat C, Gentile S, Capocaccia L. Effects of isosorbide-5-mononitrate compared with propranolol on first variceal bleed and long term survival in cirrhosis. Gastroenterology 1997; 113:1632–1639.

61. Borroni G, Salerno F, Cazzaniga M, et al. Nadolol is superior to isosorbide mononitrate for the prevention of the first variceal bleeding in cirrhotic patients with ascites. J Hepatol 2002;37:315–321.

62. Lui HF, Stanley AJ, Forrest EH, et al. Primary prophylaxis of variceal hemorrhage: a randomized controlled trial comparing band ligation, propranolol, and isosorbide mononitrate. Gastroenterology 2002;123:735–744.

63. Garcia-Pagan JC, Villanueva C, Vila MC, et al. MOVE Group. Mononitrato Varices Esofagicas. Isosorbide mononitrate in the prevention of first variceal bleed in patients who cannot receive beta-blockers. Gastroenterology 2001;121:908–914.

64. Merkel C, Marin R, Sacerdoti D, et al. Long-term results of a clinical trial of nadolol with or without isosorbide mononitrate for primary prophylaxis of variceal bleeding in cirrhosis. Hepatology 2000; 31:324–329.

65. Garcia-Pagan JC, Morillas R, Banares R, et al. Spanish Variceal Bleeding Study Group. Propranolol plus placebo versus propranolol plus isosorbide-5-mononitrate in the prevention of a first variceal bleed: a double-blind RCT. Hepatology 2003;37:1260–1266.

66. Abecasis R, Kravetz D, Fassio E, et al. Nadolol plus spironolactone in the prophylaxis of first variceal bleed in nonascitic cirrhotic patients: a preliminary study. Hepatology 2003;37:359–365.

67. Groszmann RJ, Bosch J, Grace ND, et al. Hemodynamic events in a prospective randomized trial of propranolol vs. placebo in the prevention of the first variceal hemorrhage. Hepatology 1990;99: 1401–1407.

68. Merkel C, Bolognesi M, Sacerdoti D, et al. The hemodynamic response to medical treatment of portal hypertension as a predictor of clinical effectiveness in the primary prophylaxis of variceal bleeding in cirrhosis. Hepatology 2000;32:930–934.

69. Imperiale TF, Chalasani N, Klein RW. Measuring the hemodynamic response to primary pharmacoprophylaxis of variceal bleeding: a cost-effectiveness analysis. Am J Gastroenterol 2003;98:2742–2750.

70. Imperiale TF, Chalasani N. A meta-analysis of endoscopic variceal ligation for primary prophylaxis of esophageal variceal bleeding. Hepatology 2001;33:802–807.

71. Spiegel BM, Targownik L, Dulai GS, Karsan HA, Gralnek IM. Endoscopic screening for esophageal varices in cirrhosis: is it ever cost effective? Hepatology 2003;37:366–377.

72. D'Amico G, Pagliaro L, Bosch J. The treatment of portal hypertension: a meta-analytic review. Hepatology 1995;22:332–354.

73. Ioannou GN, Doust J, Rockey DC. Systematic review: terlipressin in acute oesophageal variceal haemorhage. Aliment Pharmacol Ther 2003;17:53–64.

74. D'Amico G, Criscuoli V, Fili D, Pagliaro L. Meta-analysis of trials for variceal bleeding. Hepatology 2002;36:1023–1024.

75. Escorsell A, Ruiz del Arbol L, Planas R, Albillos A, Banares R, Bosch J. Multicenter randomized controlled trial of terlipressin versus sclerotherapy in the treatment of acute variceal bleeding: the TEST study. Hepatology 2000;32:471–476.

76. Avgerinos A, Viazis N, Vlachogiannakos J, et al. Two different doses and duration schedules of somatostatin–14 in the treatment of patients with bleeding oesophageal varices: a non-randomised controlled study. J Hepatol 2000;32:171–174.

77. Moitinho E, Planas R, Banares R, et al. Muticenter randomized controlled trial comparing different schedules of somatostatin in the treatment of acute variceal bleeding. J Hepatol 2001;35:712–718.

78. Villanueva C, Ortiz J, Sabat M, et al. Somatostatin alone or combined with emergency sclerotherapy in the treatment of acute esophageal variceal bleeding: a prospective randomized controlled trial. Hepatology 1999;30:384–389.

79. Junquera F, Loperz-Talavera JC, Mearin F, et al. Somatostatin plus isosorbide 5-mononitrate versus somatostatin in the control of acute gastro-esophageal variceal bleeding: a double blind, randomized, placebo controlled clinical trial. Gut 2000;46:127–132.

80. Corley DA, Cello JP, Adkisson W, Ko WF, Kerlilowske K. Octreotide for acute esophageal variceal bleeding: a meta-analysis. Gastroenterology 2001;120:946–954.

81. Banares R, Albillos A, Rincon D, et al. Endoscopic treatment versus endoscopic treatment plus pharmacologic treatment for acute variceal bleeding: a meta analysis. Hepatology 2002;35:609–615.

82. D'Amico G, Criscuoli V, Fili D, Mocciaro F, Pagliaro L. Meta-analysis of trials for variceal bleeding. Hepatology 2002;36:1023–1024.

83. Thabut D, De Franchis R, Bendtsen F, et al. Efficacy of activated recombinant factor VII in cirrhotic patients with upper GI bleeding: a randomized placebo-controlled double blind multi-center trial. Gastroenterology 2003;124:A697.

84. Caldwell SH, Chang C, Macik BG. Recombinant Activated Factor VII (rfVIIa) as a hemostatic agent in liver disease: a break from convention of controlled trials. Hepatology 2004:3;592–598.

85. Bernard B, Lebrec D, Mathurin P, Opolon P, Poynard T. Propanolol and sclerotherapy in the prevention of gastrointestinal rebleeding in patients with cirrhosis: a meta-analysis. J Hepatol 1997;26: 312–324.

86. Bernard B, Lebrec D, Mathurin P, Opolon P, Poynard T. Beta-adrenergic antagonists in the prevention of gastrointestinal rebleeding in patients with cirrhosis: a meta-analysis. Hepatology 1997;25:63–70.

87. DeFranchis, Primignani M. Endoscopic treatments for portal hypertension. Semin Liver Dis 1999;19: 475–505.

88. Lo GH, Lai KH, Cheng JS, et al. Endoscopic variceal ligation plus nadolol and sucralfate compared with ligation alone for the prevention of variceal rebleeding: a prospective randomized trial. Hepatology 2000;32:461–465.

89. Bosch J. Prevention of variceal rebleeding: endoscopes, drugs, and more. Hepatology 2000;32:660–662.

90. Gournay J, Masliah C, Martin T, Perrin D, Galmiche JP. Isosorbide mononitrate and propanolol compared to propanolol alone for the prevention of variceal rebleeding. Hepatology 2000;31:1239–1245.

91. Patti R, Pasta L, D'Amico G, et al. Isorbide Mononitrate with nadolol compared to nadolol alone for prevention of recurrent bleeding in cirrhosis. A double blind placebo controlled randomized trial. Final report. J Hepatol 2002;(S1):63.

92. Lo GH, Chen WC, Chen MH, et al. Banding ligation versus nadolol and isosorbide mononitrate for the prevention of esophageal variceal rebleeding. Gastroenterology 2002;123:728–734.

93. Villanueva C, Minana J, Ortiz J, et al. Endoscopic ligation compared with combined treatment with nadolol and isosorbide mononitrate to prevent recurrent variceal bleeding. NEJM 2001;345:647–655.

94. Patch D, Sabin A, Goulis J, et al. A randomized controlled trial of medical therapy versus endoscopic ligation for the prevention of variceal rebleeding in patients with cirrhosis. Gastroenterology 2002; 123:1013–1019.

95. Abraldes JG, Tarantino I, Turnes J, Garcia-Pagan JC, Rodes J, Bosch J. Hemodynamic response to pharmacological treatment of portal hypertension and long-term prognosis of cirrhosis. Hepatology 2003;37:902–908.

96. Bureau C, Peron JM, Alric L, et al. "A la Carte" treatment of portal hypertension: adapting medical therapy to hemodynamic response for the prevention of bleeding. Hepatology 2002;36:1361–1366.

97. Groszmann RJ, Wongcharatrawee S. The hepatic venous pressure gradient: anything worth doing should be done right. Hepatology 2004;39:280–282.

98. Thalheimer U, Mela M, Patch D, Burroughs AK. Targeting portal pressure measurementsL a critical reappraisal. Hepatology 39:286–290.

99. Bosch J, Garcia-Pagan JC. Complications of cirrhosis. I. Portal hypertension. J Hepatol 2000;32: 141–156.
100. Banares R, Moitinho E, Matilla A, et al. Randomized comparison of long-term carvedilol and pro-pranolol administration in the treatment of portal hypertension in cirrhosis. Hepatology 2002;36: 1367–1373.
101. Forrest EH, Bouchier IA, Hayes PC. Acute haemodynamic changes after oral carvedilol, a vaso-dilating beta-blocker, in patients with cirrhosis. J Hepatol 1996;25:909–915.
102. Schneider AW, Kalk JF, Klein CP. Effect of losartan, an angiotensin II receptor antagonist, on portal pressure in cirrhosis. Hepatology 1999;29:334–339.
103. Gonzalez-Abraldes J, Albilos A, Banares R, et al. Randomized comparison of long-term losartan versus propranolol in lowering portal pressure in cirrhosis. Gastroenterology 2001;121:382–388.
104. Zafra C, Abraldes JG, Turnes J, et al. Simvastatin enhances hepatic nitric oxide production and decreases the hepatic vascular tone in patients with cirrhosis. Gastroenterology 2004;126:749–755.
105. Fiorucci S, Antonelli E, Brancaleone V, et al. NCX-1000, a nitric oxide-releasing derivative of urso-deoxycholic acid, ameliorates portal hypertension and lowers norepinephrine-induced intrahepatic resistance in the isolated and perfused rat liver. J Hepatol 2003;39:932–939.
106. Loureiro-Silva MR, Cadelina GW, Iwakiri Y, Groszmann RJ. A liver-specific nitric oxide donor improves the intra-hepatic vascular response to both portal blood flow increase and methoxamine in cirrhotic rats. J Hepatol 2003;39:940–946.
107. Bosch J. Decreasing hepatic vascular tone by liver-specific NO donors: wishful thinking or a prom-ising reality? J Hepatol 2003;39:1072–1075.

15 Endoscopic Treatment for Bleeding Esophageal Varices

John P. Cello, MD

CONTENTS

INTRODUCTION
PATHOPHYSIOLOGY OF VARICEAL HEMORRHAGE
ENDOSCOPIC SCLEROTHERAPY
ENDOSCOPIC ESOPHAGEAL VARIX LIGATION
REFERENCES

INTRODUCTION

John Brown, Royal Physician at Saint Thomas Hospital in London, was the first clinician to describe the gross appearance of the liver in a patient with cirrhosis, portal hypertension, and ascites. He noted marked ascites in his patient, a soldier of the King's Guard. Following multiple unsuccessful paracenteses, the solider expired. At autopsy, a nodular liver was observed by Dr. Brown. It was left, however, to Rene Laennec to first use the term "cirrhosis" to describe a shrunken tawny-colored liver with a nodular granular consistency.

Esophageal variceal hemorrhage is a significant cause of morbidity and mortality around the world. Among patients admitted to acute-care urban hospitals or medical centers, variceal hemorrhage is documented in 10–20% of patients admitted with significant upper gastrointestinal tract bleeding. Patients with hemorrhage from esophageal varices still have substantial mortality despite the dramatic recent advances in care. In one of the earliest studies of the natural history of esophageal varices, Olsen from Sahlgrenska Hospital in Gothenburg, Sweden, noted the prevalence of esophageal varices among 224 postmortem documented cirrhotics *(1)*. Only 150 of the 224 cirrhotic patients (61% of the total) were actually found to have esophageal varices at autopsy. In a retrospective chart review, only 100 of the 150 patients with documented varices at autopsy had a history of bleeding varices. However, 87 of the 100 patients who had a history of variceal bleeding died directly or indirectly related to variceal bleeding. Thus, 39% of all cirrhotics, in this early study from Sweden, expired related to a variceal bleed.

There have been reports of recent substantial improvements in survival following an initial variceal bleed. One of the earlier publications by Graham and Smith in *Gastroenterology* (1981) studied 85 patients at a Veterans Administration Hospital who were admitted for their initial variceal hemorrhage *(2)*. Seventy percent of these patients were

From: *Clinical Gastroenterology: Portal Hypertension*
Edited by: A. J. Sanyal and V. H. Shah © Humana Press Inc., Totowa, NJ

Child's class C. The authors noted that 31% of the patients rebled within 6 wk and 41% of the patients died within 6 wk following the onset of variceal bleeding. Furthermore, 27% of their patients expired within the first week following the index variceal hemorrhage. Overall, mortality statistics in the Graham and Smith publication were staggering with two-thirds of the patients dead within 12 mo and 75% dead within 2 yr.

The mortality of variceal hemorrhage is clearly related in great measure to the severity of the underling liver disease. Kleber in 1991 identified prospectively several important risk factors for death following a variceal hemorrhage (3). These included: Child's B or C designation, presence of significant ascites, encephalopathy, a serum bilirubin level over 3 mg per dL, an albumin less than 2.5 g per dL, and age over 50 yr. These patients had been followed prospectively for a mean of 20 mo following the identification of nonbleeding varices.

There has been significant recent improvement in survival following variceal hemorrhage. El-Serag et al. in 2000 reviewed retrospectively a large group of patients who had variceal hemorrhage (4). They identified a cohort of 1300 patients who had a variceal bleed during 1981–1982 and compared their survival to that of a cohort of 3600 patients with variceal hemorrhage from 1988 to 1991. The 30-d mortality dropped significantly from 1981–1982 to 1988–1991 (30% vs 21%, $p = 0.0001$). In addition, the 6-yr survival had improved significantly. In the initial 1981–1982 cohort, 75% of patients were dead within 6 yr vs 70% mortality among the 1988–1991 cohort. They noted, however, that for patients surviving the first 30 d, there was no difference in 6-yr survival between the two cohorts. Nonetheless, there have been dramatic improvements in survival following variceal hemorrhage. Many factors have played a role in enhancing survival including better resuscitation techniques, the use of pharmacologic therapy and, not to an inconsiderable degree, the improvement in survival related to nonoperative endoscopic treatment of variceal hemorrhage.

PATHOPHYSIOLOGY OF VARICEAL HEMORRHAGE

Multiple postulates have been proposed to explain the actual onset of variceal hemorrhage in patients with cirrhosis of the liver (5–8). Many of these theories such as reflux esophagitis, acid peptic ulcerations, and Mallory–Weiss tears of the gastroesophageal junction have been dismissed long ago as not fitting either histopathologic or endoscopic findings. Our understanding of endoscopic treatment has also gained considerably from a better clarification of the mechanism of the variceal bleed in patients with established cirrhosis and esophageal varices. The major risk factors for variceal hemorrhage appeared to be a portal venous pressure higher than 11.5 mmHg above IVC pressure, large varices, and the presence of unique variceal findings called collectively "red color signs." It is clear that a certain level of portal hypertension is necessary but not sufficient to explain the development of the actual variceal bleed. Many investigators have demonstrated that a portal pressure above 11.5 mmHg is the baseline elevated pressure above which variceal hemorrhage may occur. Clearly, however, many patients with markedly elevated portal pressures do not bleed from varices. The presence of giant varices was first demonstrated by Lebrec as being a major risk factor for the development of variceal hemorrhage (8). He noted that among patients with nearly identical portal hypertension, the likelihood of variceal hemorrhage was markedly increased for patients with large varices. In addition to the size of varices and elevation of portal pressure, a number of investigators have demonstrated the importance of "red color signs." Beppu et al. in 1991 demonstrated that certain endoscopic findings were important features associated with variceal bleeding *(6)*. These included the presence of red color signs such as red wale markings, cherry red spots, and hematocystic spots. They also noted that blue varices, giant coiled varices, and panoesophageal varicies were all individually associated with an increased risk of variceal hemorrhage. Snady et al. in 1988 prospectively evaluated the endoscopic prediction of variceal hemorrhage employing a grading system, which scored size of varices, color of varices, location of varices, and intensity of the red color signs *(7)*. They noted prospectively that those patients who had "low-grade risk" varices had a 29% chance of bleeding over a 1-yr period of follow-up compared to a 91% risk of variceal hemorrhage in the inpatients who had a high score for varices. Thus, in Snady's study, giant varices, panesophageal varices, varices with prominent red color signs in patients who have a baseline portal pressure above 11.5 mmHg are at risk for development of variceal hemorrhage. Yet another feature, namely the intravarix pressure, has also been identified as a risk factor for variceal hemorrhage. Rigau et al. in 1989 noted in a group of patients who had the same portal hypertension that those patients who bled from varices had a significantly elevated varices pressure and elevated esophageal varix wall tension when compared to those patients who had not bled from varices *(9)*.

ENDOSCOPIC SCLEROTHERAPY

From 1940 to 1980, the routine approach to patients with documented variceal hemorrhage was surgical portacaval shunting. The endoscopic treatment of variceal hemorrhage was first reported from Stockholm, Sweden, in 1938 by Crafford and Frenckner *(10)*. They described endoscopic sclerotherapy using rigid operative esophagoscopes with patients under general anesthesia. Treatment was repeated monthly until all varices were obliterated. During the era of portacaval shunting, very little endoscopic sclerotherapy was performed other than in children with congenital hepatic fibrosis and portal hypertension. The first publications of extensive experience with endoscopic sclerotherapy came from Johnston and Rodgers in 1973 who reported on 117 patients who received 217 injections for 194 episodes of acute variceal hemorrhage *(11)*. This report covered their treatment experience from the years 1958 through 1972. All patients were treated using rigid esophagoscopes under general anesthesia employing intravariceal injections of ethanolamine oleate. The authors reported a 90% success rate in the control of acute variceal hemorrhage. However, 29% of their patients expired in the hospital, including 10% of the patients expiring from uncontrollable variceal hemorrhage. Terblanche and Northover in 1979 reported on rigid esophagoscopy in 51 episodes of endoscopically proven acute variceal hemorrhage in 22 patients *(12)*. They reported 92% definitive control of acute variceal hemorrhage during the index hospitalization. However, 28% of their patients expired during the hospitalization. Over a 25-mo period, 41% of the patients expired with the majority of deaths related to progressive hepatic failure. Fleig in 1982 likewise reported on 25 patients with acute variceal hemorrhage not controlled by balloon tamponade who were treated using rigid esophagoscopy *(13)*. They injected 1% polydocanol "paravariceally" (i.e., into the submucosa superficial to the varices) repeating treatment every 4–7 d. Acute variceal hemorrhage was controlled in more than 90% of the patients. Once again, a hospital mortality rate of 40% was reported with an additional 20% of patients rebleeding following discharge from the index hospitalization.

Table 2
Total Mortality in Trials of Serial Endoscopic Variceal Sclerotherapy

Trial	Follow-up (mo)	Withdrawals (total/randomized)	Dead/total %		Risk difference	Two-tailed p value
			Experimental	Control		
Barsoum	12–48	0/100	15/50 (30)	26/50 (52)	-0.22 (-0.41 to -0.03)	0.03
Terblanche	12–60	0/75	23/37 (62)	28/38 (63)	-0.01 (0.23 to $+0.21$)	0.94
Copenhagen	9–52	0/187[b]	60/93 (65)	74/94 (79)	-0.14 (-0.27 to -0.01)	0.03
Paquet	36[c]	4/43	7/21 (33)	17/22 (77)	-0.44 (-0.71 to -0.17)	0.01
Korula	13.6[c]	26/120	21/63 (33)	19/57 (33)	0.00 (-0.17 to $+0.17$)	1.00
Westaby	19–68	26/116	18/56 (32)	32/60 (53)	-0.21 (-0.39 to -0.04)	0.02
Soderlund	22[c]	0/117	32/57 (56)	35/50 (70)	-0.14 (-0.32 to $+0.04$)	0.14
Total		55/748	176/377 (47)	227/371 (61)	-0.15 (-0.08 to -0.04)[d]	<0.0005[e]

[a]Values in parentheses are 95% confidence limits.
[b]This total excludes 29 patients withdrawn because of violation of eligibility criteria.
[c]Median or mean follow-up.
[d]Overall risk difference estimated by a weighted average of individual risk differences Mantel–Haenszel $\chi^2 = 16.81$; test of homogeneity; $Q_w = 10.14$ ($p = 0.12$).

226

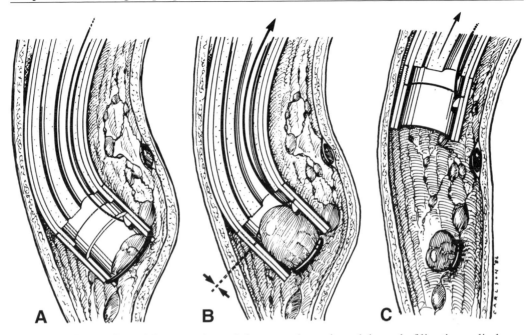

Fig. 1. (**A**) Circumferential contact is made between the varix and the end of ligating cylinder on the tip of the endoscope. (**B**) Suction is engaged drawing in the varix entirely inside the cylinder. The trip wire is then pulled releasing the elastic ring around the neck of the entrapped varix. (**C**) The ligated varix is withdrawn from the cylinder the endoscopic moving while insulfating air *(26)*.

Although the most common sclerosant in North America for patients undergoing endoscopic sclerotherapy is ethanolamine oleate, others have used a polymer glue, cyanoacrylate, and have demonstrated a superior control of hemorrhage and a reduction in the number of treatment sessions occasioned by the use of cyanoacrylate . This agent is not however routinely available in the United States and does have significant problems with respect to costs, administration, and endoscopic equipment damage.

A general consensus concerning endoscopic sclerotherapy can be reached. Endoscopic treatment should be done in the vast majority of patients employing conscious sedation with flexible fiberoptic or video-optic endoscopy without overtubes. The most commonly used sclerosants are ethanolamine oleate or sodium tetradecyl sulfate injected intravariceally in volumes of 1–2 mL per site up to a maximum or 20–30 mL total per treatment session. Treatment sessions should be repeated at least every 2–3 wk until all visible varices are obliterated. Some additional medical therapy should be given to decrease the risk of interval rebleeding, including β-blockers with or without long-acting nitrates.

ENDOSCOPIC ESOPHAGEAL VARIX LIGATION

Although banding of external hemorrhoids had been reported for a decade or more, the adaptation of the "rubber band" technique for hemorrhoids to esophageal varix band ligation was first developed in the late 1980s (Figs. 1 and 2). The first reports of endoscopic varix ligation appeared in 1988 and 1989 *(24,25)*. Stiegmann and Goff first reported successful varix ligation in 14 consecutive patients who had recently bled from esophageal varices *(25)*. In their seminal publication in *Gastrointestinal Endoscopy*, they reported

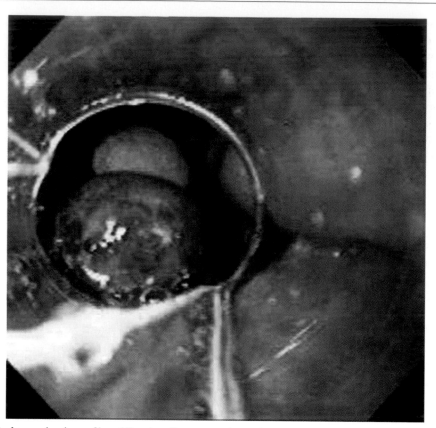

Fig. 2. Endoscopic view of band ligation. Large esophageal varices are noted, two of which have had bands applied to them. Following ligation, the banded varices have dusky in color.

on 132 individual varix ligations performed during 44 separate ligation sessions *(25)*. The ligation device that they developed placed a single "O" ring before requiring removal of the endoscope and replacing the ring. To facilitate passage of the scope with the varix ligation device on it, an overtube was used in the initial studies similar to that described for endoscopic sclerotherapy. Ten of the fourteen consecutive patients treated by Stiegman and Goff had complete varix eradication following a mean of 3.9 treatment sessions. No major complications occurred and there were no treatment failures. In a follow-up to their original study, Stiegmann and Goff describe varix ligation in 68 consecutive patients treated over a 16-mo period of time. Fourteen patients died within a mean of 12.5 d after the initial ligation session. Overall success in controlling acute variceal hemorrhage was noted in 88% of patients who were actively bleeding at the time of the initial treatment session. Thirty-five of sixty-eight consecutive patients had all visible varices eradicated or reduced to small size with a mean of five treatment sessions. Once again, they reported no significant treatment-related complications during the course of 265 sessions.

In a landmark publication in the *New England Journal of Medicine* in 1982, Stiegmann, Goff, and colleagues randomized 129 cirrhotics with documented bleeding esophageal varices *(26)*. Sixty-five patients were treated with endoscopic sclerotherapy, whereas 64 were treated with esophageal varix ligation. The initial treatment for the acute bleeding was followed by repeat sessions to eradicate varices. Patients were followed for a mean of 10 mo during which time the number of episodes of rebleeding, number of treatment sessions, complications, and survival were tabulated. Active bleeding from varices was controlled by sclerotherapy in 77% of patients and by ligation in 86%. More sclerotherapy-treated patients had recurrent bleeding during the study compared to ligation-treated patients (48% vs 36%, $p = 0.072$). The number of treatment sessions needed to obliterate varices was less with ligation when compared to sclerotherapy (4 ± 2 vs 5 ± 2, $p = 0.056$). Most importantly, there was significantly higher morbidity among sclerotherapy-treated patients predominantly from esophageal strictures, pneumonias, and other infections. The mortality rate was likewise significantly higher in the sclerotherapy-treated group when compared to the group treated by endoscopic ligation (45% vs 28%, $p = 0.041$).

The histological effects within the esophageal wall of endoscopic sclerotherapy had been extensively described and reported over many years. The effects of endoscopic varix ligation are however less well understood. Polski et al. described the changes in autopsy specimens from six patients who underwent esophageal varix ligation ranging from 9 h–22 mo before death *(27)*. Soon after ligation, the banded varix had the histologic appearance of a polyp with its base, of course, tightly compressed by the band. Thrombosis of the varix was noted by the second day following ligation. Ischemic necrosis of the "polyp" occurred anywhere from the day of banding to 5 d following ligation. Superficial ulceration of the overlying mucosa was noted well into the third week following band ligation of esophageal varices. Following complete healing of the superficial ulceration, submucosal fibrosis was noted.

Rebleeding from esophageal varices occurs in between 5% and 35% of patients during the treatment period invariably before variceal obliteration is achieved. The factors related to rebleeding are unknown. Wipassakornwarawugh et al. studied the risk factors associated with rebleeding in patients who were treated endosopically by band ligation *(28)*. All patients received regular EVL until varix disappearance. Whereas no major complication occurred, rebleeding was documented in 26% of patients. The vast majority of these episodes of rebleeding were related to portal hypertension but not to varix rebleeding. Patient platelet count and prothrombin time were not related to rebleeding ($p = 0.79$). However, Child's–Pugh C patients had a significantly higher rebleeding rate when compared to those that were Child's A or B ($p = 0.047$). Rebleeding was associated with significant mortality and a significant number of these patients experienced exsanguination.

Endoscopic varix ligation can be associated with a worsening of and/or appearance of portal hypertensive gastropathy. Pereira-Lima studied the impact of endoscopic ligation on portal pressure *(29)*. Twenty-two cirrhotic patients with variceal bleeding underwent hepatic venous pressure gradient studies before and following successful varix ligation therapy. The mean hepatic venous pressure gradient before varix ligation was 14.1 and 13.5 mmHg following eradication. After successful eradication of varices by endoscopic ligation, 12 of 22 patients experienced a reduction in portal pressure, whereas 10 were noted to have an elevation in portal pressure. Three of the twenty-two patients developed new gastric fundal varices. There was no significant difference in the hepatic venous pressure gradient before and after successful varix ligation. Portal hypertensive gastropathy worsened in nine patients. However, the increase in pressure gradient was not significantly different between those patients who developed portal hypertensive gastropathy and those who did not. Thus, esophageal varix ligation does not significantly alter the hepatic venous pressure gradient.

Table 3
Results of Ligation Compared
with Sclerotherapy for Treatment of Bleeding Esophageal Varices

Variable	Trials (Patients), n(n)	Odds Ratio (95% CI)*
Hemostasis for active bleeding	5 (106)	1.14 (0.44 to 2.90)
Variceal Obliteration	7 (547)	1.24 (0.87 to 1.76)
Rebleeding	7 (547)	0.52 (0.37 to 0.74)
—Rebleeding caused by varices	5 (315)	0.47 (0.29 to 0.78)
Mortality	7 (547)	0.67 (0.46 to 0.98)
—Mortality caused by bleeding	5 (368)	0.49 (0.24 to 0.996)
Complications[I]		
—Esophageal stricture	7 (547)	0.10 (0.03 to 0.29)
—Bleeding caused by treatment-induced ulcerations	7 (547)	0.56 (0.28 to 1.15)
Pulmonary infection	6 (524)	0.52 (0.21 to 1.34)
Bacterial peritonitis	5 (421)	0.74 (0.34 to 1.62)
Complications leading to death	5 (421)	0.47 (0.15 to 1.48)

*Odds ratios for ligation compared with sclerotherapy; all odds ratios favor ligation.
[I]Refers to number of patients with complications rather than to number of events.

Multiple studies have compared banding to endoscopic sclerotherapy *(30–38)*. A classic publication by Lane and Cook in *Gastroenterology* (1996) describes a meta-analysis of multiple controlled clinical trials *(33)* (Table 3). Control of variceal bleeding was not significantly different between banding and endoscopic sclerotherapy. Likewise, there was no significant difference in ultimate variceal obliteration. Rebleeding from esophageal varices, mortality, and development of esophageal strictures, however, were significantly decreased in patients receiving band ligation compared to those receiving endoscopic sclerotherapy. In addition to the efficacy of endoscopic banding versus sclerotherapy, Lane and Cook noted a significant reduction in number of treatment sessions required for variceal obliteration (Table 4). In four of seven studies reviewed, they noted a reduction in the number of treatment sessions varying from one to two sessions less for patients undergoing band ligation when compared to those undergoing endoscopic sclerotherapy *(33)*.

Others have looked at combining band ligation and sclerotherapy. A meta-analysis by Singh in 2002 noted no statistical difference between the two treatment programs. Thus, the addition of sclerotherapy to band ligation does not appear to enhance the overall efficacy of endoscopic band treatment *(33)*. They noted no significant difference in either the control of hemorrhage or in the long-term and short-term survival. D'Amico also performed a meta-analysis comparing a wide range of nonsurgical treatments for the prevention of rebleeding of esophageal varices *(16)*. He noted that endoscopic sclerotherapy was significantly better than β-blockers in the prevention of bleeding but not mortality. Endoscopic sclerotherapy plus β blockade was likewise significantly better at reducing bleeding when compared to sclerotherapy alone. Once again, however, there was no significant improvement in overall mortality.

Table 4
Banding vs Sclerotherapy Treatment Sessions needed for Obliteration of Varices

Study	No. sessions-ligation	No. sessions-sclerotherapy	p value
Jensen et al.	3.1	2.9	>0.20
Laine et al.	4.1	6.2	<0.001
Lo et al.	3.8	6.5	<0.001
Stiegman	4	5	0.056
Gimson et al.	3.4	4.9	0.006
Young et al.	3.6	6.2	<0.001
Mundo et al.	3.5	6.5	Not stated

Adapted from Laine L and Cook D *(33)*.

Recently, we published the results of a randomized controlled trial of endoscopic sclerotherapy versus transjugular intrahepatic portasystemic shunting. Among patients who were largely alcoholic cirrhotics with endoscopically documented variceal hemorrhage, we demonstrated a decrease in variceal hemorrhage in patients undergoing TIPS vs those undergoing endoscopic sclerotherapy. However, there was no significant difference in total duration of hospitalization or in health care costs. Overall mortality when followed for a mean of 850 d was not significantly different between the groups. Others have also looked at endoscopic varix ligation compared to TIPS and have also not demonstrated any significant difference in gastrointestinal tract bleeding following successful varix ligation when compared to TIPS. Gulberg et al. likewise demonstrated neither significant difference in bleeding nor improvements in survival when comparing TIPS to endoscopic varix ligation *(39)*.

Dhiman and Chawla reported on the new technique of combining endoscopic sclerotherapy and varix ligation during the same treatment session *(40)*. They placed a single band at 5–10 cm proximal to the gastroesophageal junction over each varix. This was followed by an intravariceal injection of 1.5% ethoxyscleorol (4 mL each) at 2–3 cm proximal to the gastroesophageal junction on the ligated varices. The injections were made distal to the initially deployed band. Immediately following sclerotherapy; varix ligation was performed at the injection site. All other varices were injected and ligated distal to proximally. This technique was performed successfully in all patients and was associated with a mean number of treatment sessions of only three (range one to four sessions). This appears to be a substantially less number of treatment sessions than with either varix ligation or sclerotherapy alone. However, randomized control trials are required to find out its relative efficacy and impact on the recurrence of esophageal varices.

Whereas successful eradication of varices by varix ligation can be accomplished in virtually all patients, a recurrence of varices clearly occur in a substantial number of patients. The possibility exists that thermal treatment of the distal esophageal mucosa may prevent recurrence of varices previously treated by sclerotherapy or band ligation. Cipolletta et al. from Italy investigated the use of argon plasma coagulation in reducing variceal recurrence following successful endoscopic varix ligation *(41)*. They randomized thirty patients who had undergone successful eradication of varices by endoscopic ligation to either argon plasma coagulation (APC) or expectant management. In the APC group, the entire esophageal mucosa 4–5 cm proximal to the gastroesophageal junction was coagulated circumferentially in from one to three sessions performed at weekly intervals. Endoscopy was performed routinely every 3 mo to check for recurrence of varices in both groups. Following APC, no recurrence of varices was observed. Over the same mean 16-mo follow-up, varices recurred in 43% of patients in the control group. Thus, both recurrence of varices and rebleeding from varices was significantly more common in the observation group when compared to the APC group. Thus, argon plasma coagulation of the distal esophageal mucosa following successful eradication of varices by varix ligation appears to be safe and is possibly effective at reducing the rate of varix recurrence.

The impact of endoscopic treatment of esophageal varices on esophageal motility and gastroesophageal reflux has not been extensively investigated. Older studies did suggest that esophageal dysmotility could occur following endoscopic sclerotherapy principally hypotension of the lower esophageal sphincter. Viazis et al. from Athens studied 60 patients with variceal bleeding who where randomized to receive either sclerotherapy or ligation until varix eradication 42). These 60 patients underwent esophageal manometry and 24-h esophageal pH studies at inclusion and at 1-mo following varix eradication. Following varix eradication by sclerotherapy, peristaltic wave amplitude significantly decreased. There was a corresponding increase in the number of simultaneous contractions and the percentage of time with the pH less than 4.0. There was also an increase in the reflux time from 1.60 ± 0.25 to $4.91 \pm 1.16\%$ in the proximal port and from 1.82 ± 0.27 to $5.69 \pm 1.37\%$ in the most distal channel. In contrast, neither esophageal manometric findings nor 24-h esophageal pH studies were significantly different following endoscopic band ligation. Thus, there is a significantly different outcome with respect to esophageal function in patients following endoscopic sclerotherapy when compared to those treated by endoscopic varix ligation.

Can a consensus be reached with respect to endoscopic treatment of patients bleeding from esophageal varices? Whereas both endoscopic sclerotherapy and band ligation are equally effective in the acute control of hemorrhage, where practical and available, the modality of first choice should be band ligation. The exception to this clearly appears to be in treating patients with exsanginating variceal hemorrhage when there is marked difficulty in visualizing the mucosa. It is nigh to impossible to place endoscopic bands in this situation, so the use of emergency endoscopic sclerotherapy is preferable. Toward the end of intended treatment sessions, the smaller varices may be difficult to band simply because their small size does not allow suctioning into the banding chamber. In this instance, the endoscopist may choose to obliterate these small residual varices by sclerotherapy.

REFERENCES

1. Olsson R. The natural history of esophageal varices. Digestion 1972;6:65–74.
2. Graham DY, Smith JL. The course of patients after variceal hemorrhage. Gastroenterology 1981;80: 800–809.
3. Kleber G, Sauerbruch T, Ansari H, Paumgartner G. Prediction of variceal hemorrhage in cirrhosis: a prospective follow-up study. Gastroenterology 1991;100:1332–1337.
4. El-Serag HB, Everhart JE. Improved survival after variceal hemorrhage over an 11-year period in the Department of Veterans Affairs. Am J Gastroenterol 2000;95:3566–3573.
5. Eckardt VF, Grace ND. Gastroesophageal reflux and bleeding esophageal varices. Gastroenterology 1979;76:39–42.
6. Beppu K, Inokuchi K, Koyanagi N, et al. Prediction of variceal hemorrhage by esophageal endoscopy. Gastrointestinal Endoscopy 1981;27:213–218.

7. Snady H, Feinman L. Prediction of variceal hemorrhage: a prospective study. Am J Gastroenterol 1988; 83:519–525.
8. Lebrec D, De Fleury P, Rueff B, Nahum H, Benhamou JP. Portal hypertension, size of esophageal varices, and risk of gastrointestinal bleeding in alcoholic cirrhosis. Gastroenterology 1980;79:1139–1144.
9. Rigau J, Bosh J, Bordas JM, et al. Endoscopic measurement of variceal pressure in cirrhosis: correlation with portal pressure and variceal hemorrhage. Gastroenterology 1989;96:873–880.
10. Crafford C, Freckner P. New surgical treatment of varicose veins of the esophagus. Acta Otolar 1939; 27:422.
11. Johnson GW, Rodgers HW. A review of 15 years' experience in the use of sclerotherapy in the control of acute haemorrhage from oesophageal varices. Br J Surg 1973;60(10):797–800.
12. Terblanche J, Northover J, Northover M, et al. A prospective controlled trial of sclerotherapy in the long-term managmento of patients after esophageal variceal bleeding. Surg Gynecol Obst 1979;148: 323–333.
13. Fleig WE, Stange EF, Ruettenauer K, Ditschuneit H. Emergency endoscopic sclerotherapy for bleeding esophageal varices: a prospective study in patients not responding to balloon tamponade. Gastrointest Endosc 1983;29:8–14.
14. Sivak M, Stout DJ, Skipper G. Endoscopic injection sclerosis (EIS) of esophageal varices. Gastrointestinal Endoscopy 1981;27:52–58.
15. Infante-Rivard C, Esnaola S, Villeneuve JP. Role of endoscopic variceal sclerotherapy in the long-term management of variceal bleeding: a meta-analysis. Gastroenterology 1989;96:1087–1092.
16. D'Amico G, Pietrosi G, Tarantino I, Pagliaro L. Emergency sclerotherapy versus vasoactive drugs for variceal bleeding in cirrhosis: a Cochrane meta-analysis. Gastroenterology 2003;124:1277–1291.
17. Goodale RL, Silvis SE, O'Leary JF, et al. Early survival after sclerotherapy for bleeding esophageal varices. Surg Gynecol Obstet 1982;155:523–528.
18. Paquet K-J, Feussner H. Endoscopic sclerosis and esophageal balloon tamponade in acute hemorrhage from esophagogastric varices. Hepatology 1985;5:580–583.
19. Cello JP, Grendell JG, Crass RA, Weber TE, Trunkey DD. Endoscopic sclerotherapy vs. portacaval shunt in patients with severe cirrhosis and acute variceal hemorrhage: long-term follow-up. N Engl J Med 1987;316:11–15.
20. Westaby D, Macdougall BR, Melia W, Theodossi A, Williams R. A prospective randomized study of two sclerotherapy techniques for esophageal varices. Hepatology 1983;3(5):681–684.
21. Kitano S, Iso Y, Yamaga H, Hashizume M, Higashi H, Sugimachi K. Trial of sclerosing agents in patients with oesophageal varices. Br J Surg 1988;75(8):751–753.
22. Sarin SK, Mishra SP, Sachdev GK, Thorat V, Dalal L, Broor SL. Ethanolamine oleate versus absolute alcohol as a variceal sclerosant: a prospective, randomized, controlled trial. Am J Gastroenterol 1988; 83:526–530.
23. Kochhar R, Goenka MK, Mehta S, Mehta SK. A comparative evaluation of sclerosants for esophageal varices: a prospective randomized controlled study. Gastrointest Endosc 1990;36:127–130.
24. Goff JS, Reveille RM, Van Stiegmann G. Endoscopic sclerotherapy versus endoscopic variceal ligation: esophageal symptoms, complications, and motility. Am J Gastroenterol 1988;83:1240–1244.
25. Stiegmann GV, Goff JS, Sun JH, Davis D, Bozdech J. Endoscopic variceal ligation: an alternative to sclerotherapy. Gastrointest Endosc 1989;35:431–434.
26. Stiegmann GV, Goff JS, Michaeletz-Onody PA, Korula J, Lieberman D, Saeed ZA. Endoscopic sclerotherapy as compared with endoscopic ligation for bleeding esophageal varices. N Engl J Med 1992; 326:1527–1532.
27. Polski JM, Brunt EM, Saeed ZA. Chronology of histological changes after band ligation of esophageal varices in humans. Endoscopy 2001;33:443–447.
28. Wipassakornwarawuth S, Opasoh M, Ammaranun K, Janthawanit P. Rate and associated risk factors of rebleeding after endoscopic variceal band ligation. J Med Assoc Thai 2002;85:698–702.
29. Pereira-Lima JC, Zanette M, Lopes CV, de Mattos AA. The influence of endoscopic variceal ligation on the portal pressure gradient in cirrhotics. Hepatogastroenterology 2003;50:102–106.
30. Lo GH, Lai KH, Cheng JS, et al. A prospective, randomized trial of sclerotherapy versus ligation in the management of bleeding esophageal varices. Hepatology 1995;22:466–471.
31. Gimson AE, Ramage JK, Panos MZ, et al. Randomised trial of variceal banding ligation versus injection sclerotherapy for bleeding oesophageal varices. Lancet 1993;342:391–394.

32. Laine L, El-Newihi HM, Migikovsky B, Sloane R, Garcia F. Endoscopic ligation compared with sclerotherapy for the treatment of bleeding esophageal varices. Ann Intern Med 1993;119:1–7.
33. Laine L, Cook D. Endoscopic ligation compared with sclerotherapy for treatment of esophageal variceal bleeding. Ann Intern Med 1995;123:280–287.
34. Baroncini D, Milandri GL, Borioni D, et al. A prospective randomized trial of sclerotheraphy versus ligation in the elective treatment of bleeding esophageal varices. Endoscopy 1997;29:235–240.
35. Masci E, Stigliano R, Mariana A, et al. Prospective Multicenter randomized trial comparing banding ligation with sclerotherapy of esophageal varices. Hepato-Gastroenterology 1999;46:1769–1773.
36. De la Pena J, Rivero M, Sanchez E, Fabrega E, Crespo J, Romero FP. Variceal ligation compared with Endoscopic sclerotherapy for variceal hemorrhage: prospective randomized trial. Gastrointest Endosc 1999;49:417–423.
37. Shafqat F, Khan A, Alam A, Butt AK, Shah SWH, Naqvi AB. Band ligation vs. endoscopic sclerotherapy in esophageal varices: a prospective randomized comparison. JPMA 1998;48:192–196.
38. Singh P, Pooran N, Indaram A, Bank S. Combined ligation and sclerotherapy versus ligation alone for secondary prophylaxis of esophageal variceal bleeding: a meta-analysis. Am J Gastroenterol 2000;97: 623–629.
39. Gulberg V, Schepke M, Geigenberger G, et al. Transjugular intrahepatic portosystemic shunting is not superior to endoscopic variceal band ligation for prevention of variceal rebleeding in cirrhotic patients: a randomized, controlled trial. Scan J Gastroenterol 2002;37:338–343.
40. Dhiman RK, Chawla YK. A new technique of combined endoscopic sclerotherapy and ligation for variceal bleeding. World J Gastroenterol 2003;5:1090–1093.
41. Cipolletta L, Bianco MA, Rotondano G, Marmo R, Meucci C, Piscopo R. Argon plasma coagulation prevents variceal recurrence after band ligation of esophageal varices: preliminarly results of a prospective randomized trial. Gastrointest Endosc 2002;56:600–603.
42. Viazis N, Armonis A, Vlachogiannakos J, Rekoumis G, Stefanidis G. Effects of endoscopic variceal treatment on oesophageal function a prospective, randomized study. Eur J Gastroenterol Hepatol 2002; 14:263–269.

16 Surgical Therapies for Management

Surgical Shunts and Liver Transplantation

J. Michael Henderson, MD

HISTORY

Surgeons have played a role in the management of portal hypertension since Eck performed the first end-to-side portacaval shunt (the Eck fistula) in dogs at the end of the 19th century (1). Several surgeons in the early 1900s attempted to manage variceal bleeding with various procedures, but it was in the 1940s that there was the first systematic use of surgical shunts to control variceal bleeding by the Columbia Presbyterian Group in New York.

Surgeons have played a key role in randomized trials for the management of variceal bleeding with the use of prophylactic shunts, therapeutic shunts, the different types of shunt, and comparison of surgical shunts to other newer treatments of variceal bleeding. Many contributions to the understanding of the pathophysiology of portal hypertension came from these surgical studies. The most significant contribution from surgeons to management of portal hypertension has been liver transplant, which has become a widespread clinical reality in the last two decades.

The diminishing use of nontransplant surgery to treat portal hypertension has in part been a result of the introduction of liver transplantation, but also to the wider use of other new therapies. Pharmacologic therapy reduces portal hypertension; endoscopic therapy has evolved to the point of playing a major role in first line treatment of patients who have

From: *Clinical Gastroenterology: Portal Hypertension*
Edited by: A. J. Sanyal and V. H. Shah © Humana Press Inc., Totowa, NJ

bled from varices. Radiologic therapy with transjugular intrahepatic portal systemic shunt has provided a less invasive way of decompressing portal hypertension. All of these alternative approaches to managing variceal bleeding are addressed elsewhere in this book and the role of this chapter is to show where other surgical therapies fit relative to these.

SURGICAL ANATOMY

Knowledge of the surgical anatomy, and the ability to study it accurately are important to the surgeon managing portal hypertension (2). The portal venous system developmentally is formed from the vitelline and umbilical veins, with the hepatic sinusoids developing from the septum transversum. The portal vein is formed behind the neck of the pancreas as the junction of the superior mesenteric and splenic veins. It runs for approx 6–8 cm and is 1–1.2 cm in diameter. With respect to portal hypertension, it is the entering tributaries that are important, but they are also very variable. The splenic vein is usually consistent and runs in the posterior surface of the pancreas. The inferior mesenteric vein is variable, entering either into the superior mesenteric or the splenic vein. The left gastric (coronary vein) is also variable coming off either the splenic or the portal vein and being one of the major feeding vessels for gastroesophageal varices. The surgical venous anatomy at the gastroesophageal junction has been extensively studied, and the zones of venous drainage have been clarified at, above, and below the gastroesophageal junction. The submucosal zone shunts large volumes of blood in this plane just above the gastroesophageal junction with significant perforating veins feeding the intercommunicating plexuses.

PATHOPHYSIOLOGY

This is dealt with in detail elsewhere in this text, but from the surgeon's perspective, the two important changes are: (i) the change in the portal circulation and (ii) the change in the systemic circulation. The high pressure in the portal system is associated with the development of significant collaterals with the gastroesophageal varices being most important clinically. These are primarily fed off the left gastric vein and the short gastric veins from the spleen. In conjunction with the development of portal hypertension and collateral development, there are also systemic hemodynamic changes. Increased plasma volume is associated with decreased total vascular resistance and the development of a hyperdynamic systemic circulation. These hemodynamic changes have implications to the surgeon managing these patients, particularly in the patients' response to surgical procedures.

EVALUATION

The surgeon plays a role in overall evaluation of patients with variceal bleeding and portal hypertension. Most patients will be seen by a surgeon if they are having recurrent bleeding episodes through first line treatment. The essential components of evaluation to the surgeon are endoscopy, vascular imaging, and assessment of liver function.

Endoscopy defines the site, size, and bleeding risk factors for gastroesophageal varices. Persistent high-risk varices with clinically recurrent bleeding through first line treatment may well be an indication for surgical intervention.

Vascular imaging is primarily done with ultrasound, but may require angiography. Doppler ultrasound will allow screening of the major vessels for patency and directional flow. When surgical decompression is being considered, angiography is usually required

Table 1
Child–Pugh Score

Parameter	1 Point	2 Points	3 Points
Serum bilirubin (mg/dL)	<2	2–3	<3
Albumin (g/dL)	>3.5	2.8–3.5	<2.8
Prothrombin time ($\uparrow$, S)	1–3	4–6	>6
Ascites	None	Slight	Moderate
Encephalopathy	None	1–2	3–4

Grades: A, 5–6 points; B, 7–9 points; C, 10–15 points.

Table 2
MELD Score

$$\text{Score} = 0.957 \times \log_e \text{creatinine (mg/dL)} + 0.378 \times \log_{e\ \text{bilirubin (mg/dL)}} + 1.120 \log_{e\ \text{INR}}$$

for more accurate definition of the major vessels and the feeding tributaries. The second component of imaging is looking at liver morphology. This should always be a component of assessment of patients with cirrhosis and chronic liver disease, particularly to exclude focal lesions that are potentially hepatomas.

Liver function is assessed by a combination of clinical and laboratory measurements. Childs–Pugh classification is the standard for evaluating these patients (Table 1). In the last several years, the Model for End-stage Liver Disease (MELD) score is receiving increasing attention and use (Table 2). The Childs–Pugh classification has stood the test of time and is valuable in assessing surgical risk for patients being considered for shunt surgery. The MELD score was initially developed for predicting outcome in patients receiving TIPS, and has become widely used for assessing liver disease severity for transplant listing and organ allocation. Its role in defining risk for patients with variceal bleeding continues to be evaluated.

Liver biopsy is occasionally indicated in the patient being considered for surgical decompression. This may be done either by a blind percutaneous biopsy or by transjugular biopsy. The indications for a preoperative biopsy are when there is doubt as to the diagnosis and the need for confirmation for cirrhosis, or for assessment of degree of disease activity.

Quantitative tests to assess liver function have received considerable attention but have not come to wide clinical use. Indocyamine green clearance, galactose elimination capacity, or MGEX formation have been the main tests studied. They do provide information as to functional capacity of the liver, measuring, predominantly, flow, hepatocyte function, or a combination of the two. They are more cumbersome to perform and do not significantly alter treatment decisions.

TREATMENT

First-line treatment for variceal bleeding is with pharmacologic and endoscopic therapy. These topics are dealt with elsewhere in this text: these should be used initially in all patients, and it is only the 25–30% of patients who rebleed significantly through such therapy that are candidates for surgical intervention.

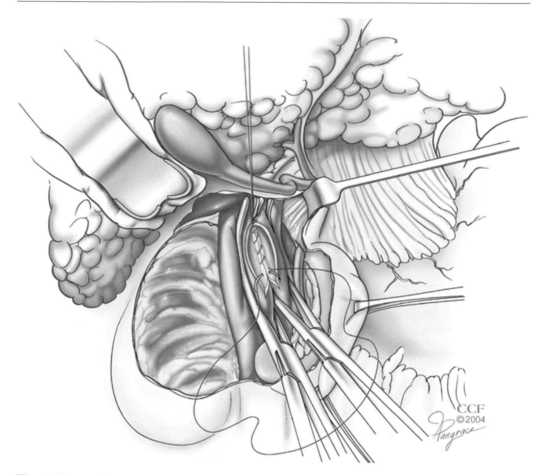

Fig. 1. Side-to-side portacaval shunt. When >10 mm diameter, this shunt is a total shunt, diverting all portal flow and decompressing the liver sinusoids.

Surgical options in treating portal hypertension are: (1) decompressive shunts; (2) devascularization procedures; and (3) liver transplantation. These three operative approaches all have a role in the management of patients with portal hypertension with specific indications that are complimentary rather than competitive. Each of these approaches will be discussed.

DECOMPRESSIVE SURGICAL SHUNTS

The surgical shunts fall into three distinct groups: (1) total portal systemic shunts that decompress all portal hypertension; (2) partial portal systemic shunts that reduce portal pressure to 12 mmHg or less, but permit some ongoing portal flow; (3) selective shunts that decompress gastroesophageal varices and the spleen but maintain portal hypertension and portal flow to the liver.

Total portal systemic shunts are any shunt >10 mm in diameter between the portal vein or one of its main tributaries and the inferior vena cava or one of its main feeding vessels. The most commonly used total portal systemic shunt is a side-to-side portacaval shunt that directly anastomoses the portal vein to the infrahepatic inferior vena cava (IVC) (Fig. 1) *(3,4)*. This shunt not only decompresses all the portal hypertension with excel-

Table 3
Total Shunt (>10 mm PCS)—Outcomes

	1	2
Rebleeding	1%	7.6%
Encephalopathy	9%	50%
Op Mortality	15%	6.4%
Late Survival	71% (10 yr)	31% (10 yr)

[1]Orloff et al., J Am Coll Surg 1995.
[2]Stipa et al., W J Surg 1994.

lent control of variceal bleeding, but also decompresses the hepatic sinusoids and relieves ascites. The portal vein acts as an outflow tract from the liver in this operation, giving total diversion of portal flow and potential adverse effects on liver function. Alternative operations which are total portal systemic shunts are mesocaval or mesorenal shunts >10 mm in diameter.

The outcome for total portal systemic shunts is excellent control of bleeding and ascites in more than 90% of patients. The risks following total portal systemic shunt are progressive liver failure and encephalopathy. Encephalopathy rates of 40–50% are reported by most, although Orloff's experience has been a significantly lower rate. Results from two series reported in the 1990s are shown in Table 3.

The main indications for a side-to-side portacaval shunt at the present time are limited. It may be used in the patient with massive bleeding who also has ascites, but TIPS has largely replaced this indication. Second, the patient with acute Budd–Chiari syndrome with ongoing hepatocyte necrosis can be treated by a side-to-side portacaval shunt that decompresses the sinusoids and halts this ongoing liver damage (5).

Partial portal systemic shunts are achieved by reducing the size of the anastomosis of a side-to-side shunt to 8 mm diameter. Sarfeh et al. documented that progressive reduction of graft size down to 8 mm allowed a maintenance of portal perfusion in 80% of patients, with reduction of portal pressure to ≤12 mmHg (6). This shunt requires a similar operative approach as the side-to-side portacaval shunt, except for the interposition graft as shown in Fig. 2.

Data on partial shunts indicate equivalent control of bleeding to total portal systemic shunts and better control of bleeding than with TIPS. The ability to maintain some portal flow with these shunts results in a lower incidence of encephalopathy and liver failure compared to total portal systemic shunts. Data from recent series of partial shunts are given in Table 4 (7,8).

Other groups have advocated the use of limited-sized interposition grafts in the mesocaval position in a similar manner (9). The longer length of these grafts, which are of small diameter, does make them more prone to thrombosis. No randomized data are available on such interposition mesocaval small-bore shunts.

Selective shunts decompress gastroesophageal varices, but maintain portal perfusion of the liver. The most commonly performed selective shunt is the distal splenorenal shunt (10), but the coronary caval shunt has also been used primarily in Japan (11). The distal splenorenal shunt anastomoses the superior mesenteric end of the splenic vein to the left renal vein, thus, decompressing the spleen, gastric fundus, and lower esophagus to control

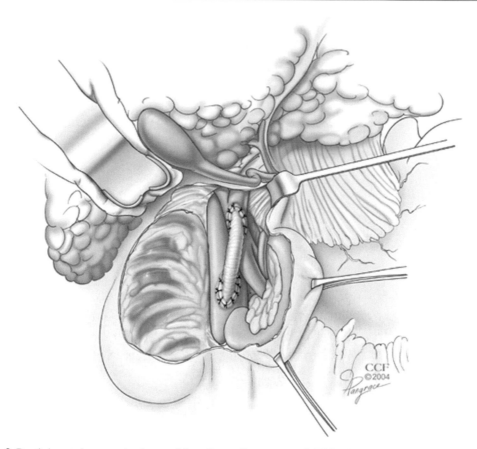

Fig. 2. Partial portal systemic shunt with an 8mm diameter graft. This shunt reduced portal pressure to ≤12 mmHg and maintains same prograde portal flow.

Table 4
8 mm H-graft—Outcomes

	1	2
Child's A/B/C	52/38/10 (%)	14/36/50 (%)
Rebleeding	8%	3%
Encephalopathy	20%	3% (early)
Op Mortality	8%	20%
Late Survival	54% (7 yr)	70% (4 yr)

[1]Sarfeh et al., Arch Surg 1998.
[2]Rosemurgy et al., J G I Surg 2000.

variceal bleeding. Portal hypertension is maintained in the splanchnic and portal venous system to maintain portal flow to the cirrhotic liver (Fig. 3).

The outcome following distal splenorenal shunt gives a >90% control of variceal bleeding with initial excellent maintenance of portal perfusion. Patients with nonalcoholic liver disease maintain portal perfusion well, whereas 50% of patients with alcoholic liver disease will lose portal perfusion over time. The incidence of encephalopathy

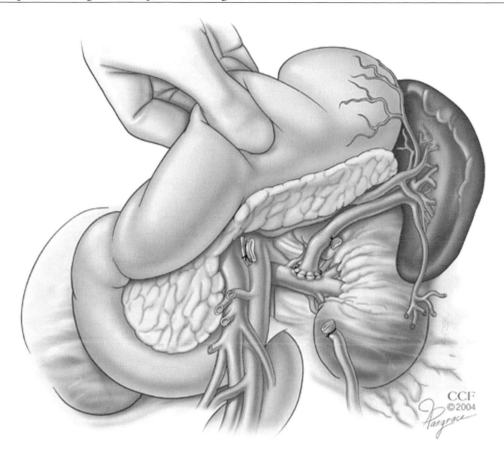

Fig. 3. Distal splenorenal shunt decompresses the spleen and gastroesophageal varices, while maintaining portal hypertension and flow to the liver in the portal vein.

Table 5
DSRS—Outcomes (Child's A/B)

	1	2	3	4
Rebleeding	6.3%	6.8%	6%	11%
Encephalopathy	12%	15%	5%	9%
Op Mortality	0	6%	5%	2.7%
Late Survival	86% (3 yr)	74% (5 yr)	85% (5 yr)	76% (5 yr)

[1]Henderson et al., Surgery 2000.
[2]Jenkins et al., Arch Surgery 1999.
[3]Orozco et al., LTS 1997.
[4]Rikkers, Ann Surg 1998.

is lower with distal splenorenal shunt than total shunts in four of the seven randomized trials comparing the two approaches *(12)*. The incidence of encephalopathy after distal splenorenal shunt is the same as the incidence of encephalopathy following endoscopic therapy in randomized trials *(13)*.

Results from some more contemporary series of distal splenorenal shunt are given in Table 5. It can be seen that the majority of these more recent series have been in Child's

TIPS, if correctly placed, has no adverse effect on the transplant operation. Placing a TIPS stent too high so that it impedes upper IVC cross-clamping, or too low in the portal vein to jeopardize its safe use, are potential technical problems. Close communication with the interventional radiologists who place TIPS is important in overall management strategy. The concept that TIPS placed prior to transplant to relieve the portal hypertension would make transplant technically easier has not been supported by data *(26)*.

Prior surgical shunts do make transplant procedures more difficult with longer operative times and higher blood loss *(27)*. Shunts close to the liver hilus make for more complex transplants than "remote" shunts. Clear visualization of vessels, probably using angiography, prior to transplant is helpful in operative planning: this helps decide how and if venovenous bypass may be used, and the need for venous grafts. Specific to transplant in patients with prior DSRS, angiography will define the degree of collateralization that has occurred between the portal vein and the shunt, and dictate the need for splenectomy and shunt ligation. If there are large siphoning collaterals from the portal vein to the splenic vein seen on venous phase superior mesenteric study, then splenectomy and shunt ligation are required. If collaterals are not present, then the spleen and shunt can be left undisturbed.

REFERENCES

1. Donovan AJ, Covey PC. Early history of the portacaval shunt in humans. Surgery Gynecol Obstet 1978; 147:423–430.
2. Henderson JM. Anatomy of the portal venous system in portal hypertension. In: Bircher, Benhamaou, McIntyre, Rizzetto, Rodes, eds. Oxford Textbook of Clinical Hepatology. Oxford Univ Press, U.K., 1999, pp. 645–651.
3. Orloff MJ, Orloff MS, Orloff SL, Rambotti M, Girard B. Three decades of experience with emergency portacaval shunt for acutely bleeding esophageal varices in 400 unselected patients with cirrhosis of the liver [see comments]. J Am Coll Surg 1995;180:257–272.
4. Stipa S, Balducci G, Ziparo V, Stipa F, Lucandri G. Total shunting and elective management of variceal bleeding. World J Surg 1994;18:200–204.
5. Henderson JM, Warren WD, Millikan WJ Jr, et al. Surgical options, hematologic evaluation, and pathologic changes in Budd-Chiari syndrome. Am J Surg 1990;159:41–48; discussion 48–50.
6. Sarfeh IJ, Rypins EB, Mason GR. A systematic appraisal of portacaval H-graft diameters. Clinical and hemodynamic perspectives. Ann Surg 1986;204:356–363.
7. Collins JC, Ong MJ, Rypins EB, Sarfeh IJ. Partial portacaval shunt for variceal hemorrhage: longitudinal analysis of effectiveness. Arch Surg 133(6):590–592.
8. Rosemurgy AS, Serofini FM, Zweibal BR, et al. TIPS versus small diameter prosthetic H-graft portacaval shunt: extended follow-up of an expanded randomized prospective trial. J Gastrointest Surg 2000; 4:589–597.
9. Mercado MA, Orozco H, Guillen-Novarro E, et al. Small diameter mesocaval shunts: a 10 year evaluation. J Gastrointest Surg 2000;4:453–457.
10. Warren WD, Zeppa R, Fomon JJ. Selective trans-splenic decompression of gastroesophageal varices by distal splenorenal shunt. Ann Surg 1967;166:437–455.
11. Inokuchi K. A selective portacaval shunt. Lancet 1968;2:51–52.
12. Henderson JM. Role of distal splenorenal shunt for long-term management of variceal bleeding. World J Surg 1994;18:205–210.
13. Spina GP, Henderson JM, Rikkers LF, et al. Distal spleno-renal shunt versus endoscopic sclerotherapy in the prevention of variceal rebleeding. A meta-analysis of 4 randomized clinical trials. J Hepatol 1992; 16:338–345.
14. Henderson JM, Nagle A, Curtas S, Geisinger MA, Barnes D. Surgical Shunts and TIPS for variceal decompression in the 1990's. Surgery 2000;128:540–547.
15. Jenkins RL, Gedaly R, Pomposelli JJ, et al. Distal splenorenal shunt: role, indications, and utility in the era of liver transplantation. Arch Surg 1999;134:416–420.

16. Orozco H, Mercado MA, Garcia JG, et al. Selective shunts for portal hypertension current role of a 21 year experience. Liver Transplant Surg 1997;3:475–480.

17. Rikkers LF, Jin G, Langnas AN, Shaw BW Jr. Shunt surgery during the era of liver transplantation. Ann Surg 1997;226:51–57.

18. Sugiura M, Futagawa S. Esophageal transection with paraesophagogastric devascularizations (the Sugiura procedure) in the treatment of esophageal varices. World J Surg 1984;8:673–679.

19. Idezuki Y, Kokudo N, Sanjo K, Bandai Y. Sugiura procedure for management of variceal bleeding in Japan. World J Surg 1994;18:216–221.

20. Orozco H, Mercado MA, Takahashi T, et al. Elective treatment of bleeding varices with the Sugiura operation over 10 years. Am J Surg 1992;163:585–589.

21. Dagenais M, Langer B, Taylor BR, Greig PD. Experience with radical esophagogastric devascularization procedures (Sugiura) for variceal bleeding outside Japan. World J Surg 1994;18:222–228.

22. Henderson JM. Liver transplantation for portal hypertension. Gastroenterol Clin North Am 1992;21:197.

23. Bismuth H, Adam R, Mathur S, Sherlock D. Options for elective treatment of portal hypertension in cirrhotic patients in the transplantation era. Am J Surg 1990;160:105.

24. Ringe B, Lang H, Tusch G, Pichlmayr R. Role of liver transplantation in management of esophageal variceal hemorrhage. 1994;18:233.

25. Abu-Elmagd K, Iwatsuki S. Portal hypertension: role of liver transplantation. In: Cameron J, ed. Current Surgical Therapy: 7th ed. Mosby, St. Louis, 2001, pp. 406–413.

26. Roberts JP, Ring E, Lake JR, Sterneck M, Ascher NL. Intrahepatic portocaval shunt for variceal hemorrhage prior to liver transplantation. Transplantation 1991;52:160–162.

27. Mazzaferro V, Todo S, Tzakis AG, Stieber AC, Makowka L, Starzl TE. Liver transplantation in patients with previous portasystemic shunt. Am J Surg 1990;160:111–116.

succeeded in entering the portal vein through the hepatic parenchyma, and this led to the idea of creating a fistula between the hepatic and portal veins giving rise to a portosystemic shunt. Initial attempts at creating a TIPSS in animal models using nonexpandable tubing (3), drilling (4), and cryoprobe freezing (5) were hampered by shunt dysfunction, with primary patency limited to a maximum of 2 wk.

The introduction of balloon angioplasty catheters in the latter half of the 1970s was the key to the successful creation of TIPSS. Animal models demonstrated the potential for TIPSS to be kept patent for up to 1 yr by regular dilatations, despite the high early occlusion rate (6). The first clinical application of TIPSS was by Colapinto et al. in 1982, who used a 9-mm catheter to significantly reduce portal pressure (7). Further studies were performed in patients with cirrhosis and variceal bleeding, where despite a significant reduction in the portal pressure, most patients rebled and died or required surgery. The fact that most of the fistulas were patent at autopsy suggested that further measures were necessary to maintain portal decompression.

The use of expandable metal stents in the mid-1980s led to the development of 10-mm Palmaz stents, which were initially used in animal models (8,9). The patency of these shunts was much better in patients with chronic rather than acute portal hypertension, lasting for up to 48 wk. These experiments led to the first clinical application of expandable metal stents involving the use of two Palmaz stents, resulting in both hemodynamic and clinical improvement in portal hypertension (10). The patient unfortunately died at d 12 from adult respiratory distress syndrome, although the shunt was noted to be patent at autopsy. These early experiences stimulated enormous interest among interventional radiologists and gastroenterologists, resulting in many centers using TIPSS and further refining the technique and expanding its use for other indications.

HEMODYNAMIC EFFECTS OF TIPSS

Cirrhosis and portal hypertension results in the hyperdynamic circulation first described by Kowalski and Abelmann (11), and later validated by others (12). The characteristic features are increased cardiac output and decreased systemic vascular resistance. Heart rate and stroke volume are also increased and directly proportional to cardiac output. The arterial pressure in patients with portal hypertension is normal or lower than in controls (13,14). In addition, the severity of liver disease is inversely proportional to the arterial pressure (15). The effects of TIPSS on this hyperdynamic circulation have been well studied.

Portal Circulation

Successful TIPSS results in immediate reduction of portal pressure. Traditionally, the portal pressure gradient is utilized [portal pressure gradient (PPG): portal pressure – inferior vena cava (IVC) pressure]. It was widely believed that variceal bleeding was very unlikely below a threshold hepatic venous pressure gradient (HVPG) of 12 mmHg (16), leading to this being adopted as a therapeutic goal following TIPSS insertion, and is achieved for most patients in our and others' series. The ideal target PPG following insertion of TIPSS remains undefined. The lower the PPG after TIPSS, the greater is the likelihood of control of variceal bleeding and prevention of rebleeding. This has to be balanced against the risk of encephalopathy and reduction of liver blood flow, which are likely to be compounded by larger shunt sizes.

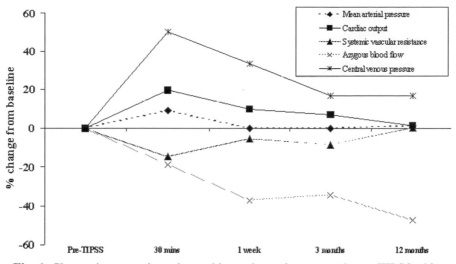

Fig. 1. Change in systemic and portal hemodynamics pre- and post-TIPSS *(18)*.

The insertion of TIPSS diverts the portal blood from the liver directly into the systemic circulation thereby reducing hepatic perfusion through the portal vein. The larger the shunt, the greater is the degree of shunting. TIPSS has been shown to reduce liver blood flow, which is most marked acutely, but is restored 3-mo afterward *(17,18)*. This restoration of liver blood flow is thought to be caused by compensatory increase in liver blood flow, possibly mediated by the hepatic arterial buffer response. The degree of restoration of liver blood flow is thought to depend upon the severity of the underlying liver disease. In the more advanced stages of cirrhosis, the reduction in liver blood flow after TIPSS insertion is more marked probably because of reduced hepatic arterial buffer response *(19,20)*.

The azygous blood flow, which is a measure of the collateral blood flow, decreases acutely following TIPSS insertion, with a maximum decrease of 30% of baseline values 1 yr following TIPSS insertion. This study also identified a correlation between the change in PPG following TIPSS insertion and the azygous blood flow.

Systemic Circulation

The potential for a TIPSS to aggravate an already hyperdynamic circulation was demonstrated in several studies *(21)*. The acute effect at 30 min post-TIPSS insertion is an increase in cardiac output (CO), right atrial pressure (RAP), and pulmonary artery and pulmonary wedge pressure, with a fall in systemic vascular resistance (SVR). No change was observed in heart rate (HR) or mean arterial pressure (MAP). The fall in the portoatrial pressure gradient correlated with the rise in CO and drop in SVR. These changes were confirmed in a recent study of a larger population over a 1-yr period following TIPSS insertion *(18)*. In addition to the acute effects, there was an increase in MAP and HR. The acute increase in CO persisted for up to 3 mo, although the SVR started to increase after 1 wk (Fig. 1). Other parameters of the systemic circulation returned to normal after a year.

Therefore, the acute detrimental hemodynamic effect of TIPSS insertion is not maintained in the long term. The acute increase in the cardiac output and increase in venous return may result in acute pulmonary edema or unmask preexisting cardiomyopathy.

Caution is needed in patients with pulmonary hypertension or known cardiac dysfunction. The mechanism by which TIPSS produces detrimental effects on the circulation is not clear but recent studies suggest that TIPSS induced increase in nitric oxide production may underlie these pathophysiological effects.

COMPLICATIONS OF TIPSS

The complications relate to the procedure itself, the underlying liver disease, and the function of the shunt.

Procedural

The overall rate of procedure-related mortality in our unit of almost 500 consecutive TIPSS over a 10-yr period is 1.2% *(22)*. Direct complications of the TIPSS included gallbladder perforation and intraperitoneal hemorrhage. There are also other rare nonfatal procedure-related complications such as portal vein to bile duct fistula, localized collection between gallbladder and liver, shunt migration, pneumothorax, and neck hematoma. An unusual complication was the presence of a right atrial clot noted at routine portography resulting in shunt insufficiency. This was successfully removed under ultrasound guidance.

Patients with liver disease are immunosuppressed, and the insertion of a TIPSS does not appear to increase the risk of infection, although an unusual type of infection can occur in the presence of a thrombus or vegetation in the TIPSS known as "endotipsitis" *(23)*. The patient presents with fever, hepatomegaly, and positive blood cultures. Prolonged antibiotic therapy is required. As in the case of infective endocarditis, there is usually one organism isolated. We have a policy of administering intravenous third-generation cephalosporins pre- and for 48 h post-TIPSS insertion. Nevertheless, TIPSS infection has to be considered when no other source of sepsis can be identified. In around 13% of patients, there may be clinically significant hemolysis, which may manifest as jaundice or anemia *(24)*. This usually resolves within 3–4 wk as the TIPSS becomes covered with a neointimal layer.

Hepatic Encephalopathy

One of the principal concerns of TIPSS has been the increased risk of hepatic encephalopathy, and this is confirmed with the current studies. The overall risk of hepatic encephalopathy following TIPSS of 34% compares with 19% following endoscopic therapy, resulting in one episode of *de novo* or worsening hepatic encephalopathy for one in eight patients treated with a TIPSS *(25)*. This obviously has major implications on the quality of life of patients, and the resources needed to manage encephalopathy including shunt occlusion in up to 5% *(22)*. Selecting patients free from hepatic encephalopathy prior to TIPSS insertion may reduce the incidence of post-TIPSS encephalopathy *(26)*. However, in clinical practice this is difficult to accomplish particularly where TIPSS is used to rescue those who have failed endoscopic therapy because these individuals are likely to be encephalopathic from recurrent bleeding and/or have limited alternative treatment options.

However, it must be appreciated that TIPSS is often performed as a rescue procedure in patients with advanced liver disease who have already failed other pharmacological interventions. They may have an element of ischemic liver damage, sepsis, and deranged electrolyte status related to the bleeding and/or resuscitation. In this sort of environment,

Table 1
Shunt Insufficiency: Portographic Appearances

Abnormality on portography	Frequency (%)
Intimal hyperplasia	60
Hepatic vein stenosis	21
Thrombosis within shunt	6
Occluded shunt	12
Portal vein thrombosis	<1%

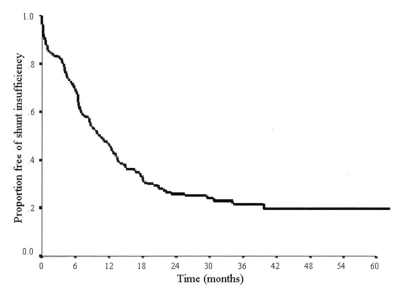

Fig. 2. Kaplan Meier graph of primary patency of standard stents used for TIPSS (22).

introduction of TIPSS can result in catastrophic brain edema and death from cerebral herniation. In our case series of the first 80 TIPSS procedures, we have observed five such cases (27). The mechanism by which TIPSS induces brain swelling is not clear but likely to be multifactorial related to ischemic liver injury, hyperammonemia, sepsis, electrolyte disturbances, and as we have recently shown, a TIPSS induced increase in cerebral blood flow (27).

Shunt Insufficiency

Shunt insufficiency is a significant limitation of TIPSS. Fifty percent of shunts will become insufficient, i.e., significantly stenosed or blocked within a year of TIPSS insertion (Table 1, Fig. 2) (28), with most episodes resulting from acute thrombosis and leading to variceal rebleeding, probably as a result of thrombogenic biliary material entering the shunt (29,30). Early controlled studies revealed a lower incidence of complete occlusion after heparin with no reduction in the reintervention rate (31). A recent study suggested that heparin combined with antiplatelet drugs reduces the risk of stenosis of the hepatic vein and variceal rebleeding, although no effect was seen for stenosis within the stent (32).

Later episodes of shunt dysfunction result from pseudointimal hyperplasia. Regular invasive portographic surveillance, which is essential for maintaining shunt patency is not available in all centers, and places an additional burden on resources. Noninvasive methods of assessing TIPSS patency such as Doppler ultrasound are not as sensitive as regular portography (33), and studies which used this method had a higher rebleeding rate (1). In any case, Doppler ultrasound does not allow for interventions, such as balloon angioplasty and restenting nor the measurement of portal pressure.

Variables identified as predicting shunt insufficiency include PPG pre-TIPSS of >18 mmHg (26), and the presence of diabetes has been shown to be associated with delayed shunt occlusion (34). A recent study published in abstract form identified stent diameter, distance of shunt through IVC, duration of the procedure, and portal pressure gradient post-TIPSS as independent predictors of early shunt insufficiency (35).

The observations that variceal bleeding occurs rarely at PPG < 12 mmHg (36) or if there is a >25% reduction in the PPG, has led to shunt insufficiency being defined as an increase in the PPG to >12 mmHg or an increase in the PPG of more than 20% of the immediate post-TIPSS value if the pre-TIPSS PPG was ≤12 mmHg (27). Primary patency is defined as patency without intervention. Secondary or assisted patency, defined as patency with intervention, is more than 70% during a follow-up period of 20 mo in our series (22).

An interesting observation in our experience is that the risk of variceal rebleeding 2 yr post-TIPSS is very low, even in the presence of shunt insufficiency (22,37). This may reflect the fact that patients who survive this long post-TIPSS are usually in the better prognostic group, and therefore have a lower risk of variceal bleeding. This finding brings into question the need for continued portographic surveillance 2 yr post-TIPSS insertion, and merits further study.

THE ROLE OF TIPSS IN THE MANAGEMENT OF VARICEAL HEMORRHAGE

Variceal hemorrhage is a life-threatening complication of portal hypertension with an in-hospital mortality between 30% and 60%, depending on severity of liver disease (38). There has been much research in recent years aimed at finding the best therapy to prevent and treat variceal hemorrhage. In most centers, endoscopic therapy is instituted as first-line therapy, with pharmacological therapy such as terlipressin having an important role (37). Broad spectrum antibiotics should be administered to all patients with cirrhosis following gastrointestinal hemorrhage, as this has been shown to improve survival (37). In refractory cases or where the risk of variceal rebleeding is high, TIPSS is utilized (Fig. 3). It terminates variceal hemorrhage in more than 90% of patients, and prevents rebleeding in 80–90% of patients (39). The availability of TIPSS still remains restricted to the more established units but its availability is increasing. Despite the increasing use of TIPSS, the number of controlled studies involving the use of TIPSS in the management of variceal hemorrhage is rather limited. At the present time, there is no evidence to support the use of TIPSS in the prevention of the first variceal bleed, so TIPSS cannot be recommended for primary prophylaxis.

Management of Acute Variceal Bleeding

The role of TIPSS in the management of acute variceal hemorrhage as "salvage" therapy is well established. In such cases, patients have been treated with endoscopic methods

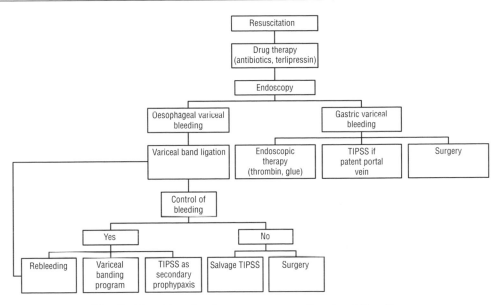

Fig. 3. Algorithm for the management of variceal bleeding.

and/or pharmacological therapies without success. Many clinicians would attempt a second endoscopic procedure prior to referring the patient to specialized centers for a TIPSS, but this will depend on the severity of the acute bleed. In severe cases where balloon tamponade is needed to control bleeding, a TIPSS may be indicated at an earlier stage. Prior to the introduction of TIPSS, patients would have been referred for a surgical procedure such as esophageal transection, which is associated with a high mortality in this setting *(40)*. Studies indicate that TIPSS results in control of acute variceal bleeding in more than 90% of cases *(40–54)* (Table 2). However, the mortality is high and reflects the severity of liver disease at the time of TIPSS insertion. In the setting of uncontrolled variceal bleeding, the rebleeding rate is 18% and mortality is 38%, with most deaths occurring early *(55)*.

The rather dismal statistics prompted investigators to identify clinical and hemodynamic variables that could predict poor outcome. Early studies from our unit identified Child–Pugh score, hyponatremia, pre-TIPSS encephalopathy, and pre-TIPSS PPG > 16 (in alcoholic cirrhotics) to predict mortality post TIPSS *(26,56)*. The role of portal pressure as a predictor of mortality was reinforced by recent studies *(57,58)*. Others have suggested a greater role of the model of end stage liver disease (MELD) as a predictor of early mortality *(59)*. There still remains some controversy regarding the best prognostic model following a recent study which failed to identify any single variable to predict mortality following salvage TIPSS *(54)*. The clinical utility of such models is limited as many clinicians even knowing the likely poor outcome would proceed with "salvage" therapy.

Prevention of Variceal Rebleeding

ENDOSCOPIC THERAPIES VS TIPSS

There are 13 trials comparing endoscopic therapies (usually injection sclerotherapy) with TIPSS for the management of variceal bleeding and especially rebleeding (Table 3) *(60–72)*. One of these studies has been published in abstract form *(72)*. In most trials,

Table 2
Studies Utilizing TIPSS as "Rescue" Therapy for Variceal Bleeding

Author	No. Patients	% patients with Pugh class C disease	Previous endoscopic treatment	Initial hemostasis (%)	Rebleeding (%)	Mortality (%)
LaBerge et al. (43)	32	N/a	ES	97	N/a	N/a
Haag et al. (107)	19	68	N/a	100	11	26 (30 d)
Helton et al. (44)	23	78	ES	N/a	N/a	56 (in hospital)
Le Moine et al. (108)	4	N/a	ES	N/a	N/a	75 (30 d)
Rubin et al. (109)	12	N/a	ES/VBL	75	N/a	N/a
Jalan et al. (40)	19	68	ES	100	16	42 (30 d)
Jabbour et al. (48)	25	48	ES	96	N/a	44 (30 d)
Sanyal et al. (49)	30	73	ES	100	7	40 (6 wk)
Perarnau et al. (50)	48	56	ES	92	9	25 (30 d)
Banares et al. (51)	56	41	ES	95	14	15 (30 d)
Gerbes et al. (52)	11	64	ES/VBL	91	27	27 (30 d)
Chau et al. (41)	112 (OV 84, GV 28) (OV 75, GV 61)	71	ES	96	OV 13 GV 14	37 (30 d) (OV 34, GV 42)
Barange et al. (42)	32	47	ES	90	14	25 (30 d)
Bizollon et al. (53)	28	61	ES/VBL	96	8	25 (40 d)
Azoulay et al. (54)	58	81	ES	90	6	29 (30 d)

ES, endoscopic sclerotherapy; VBL, variceal band ligation; OV, oesophageal varices; GV, gastric varices.

Table 3
Studies Comparing TIPSS vs Endoscopic Therapy for the Prevention of Variceal Rebleeding

First author	Number of patients (TIPSS/ET)	ET arm	Variceal rebleeding (%)		Mortality (%)		Encephalopathy (%)	
			TIPSS	ET	TIPSS	ET	TIPSS	ET
Cabrera et al. (71)	31/32	Sclerotherapy	23	50	19	16	32	13
Rossle et al. (69)	61/65	Sclerotherapy or VBL + propranolol	15	45	13	12	13	14
Sanyal et al. (70)	41/39	Sclerotherapy	22	21	29	18	29	13
Cello et al. (67)	24/25	Sclerotherapy	13	48	33	32	50	44
Sauer et al. (63)	42/41	Sclerotherapy + propranolol	14	51	29	27	33	7
Jalan et al. (68)	31/27	VBL	10	56	42	37	16	11
Merli et al. (65)	38/43	Sclerotherapy	18	40	24	19	55	23
Garcia-Villareal et al. (64)	22/24	Sclerotherapy	9	50	14	33	23	25
GEAIH (72)	32/33	Sclerotherapy + propranolol	41	61	50	42	N/a	
Pomier-Layrargues et al. (61)	41/39	VBL	20	56	41	41	37	41
Gulberg et al. (60)	28/26	VBL	25	27	14	15	7	4
Narahara et al. (62)	38/40	Sclerotherapy	18	33	29	18	34	15
Sauer et al. (110)	43/42	VBL	16	43	26	29	37	21

ET, Endoscopic therapy; VBL, variceal band ligation.

255

TIPSS was also used to rescue refractory bleeders in the endoscopic therapy arm *(60–62,64–71)*. The variceal rebleeding rate of 19% in the TIPSS arm compares favorably with 47% in the endoscopic therapy arm *(1)*. Taking all the 13 trials together, the number needed to prevent one variceal rebleeding episode is 4 *(25)*. A reduced rate of rebleeding is demonstrated by all but two studies which showed similar efficacy of TIPSS and endoscopic therapy *(60,70)*. The rate of rebleeding appears to be related to the Pugh score, although the results with surgical shunts are better *(73)*. The majority of rebleeding episodes are related to shunt insufficiency, which is reflected in the high early rebleeding rates reported in most trials.

However, there appears to be no benefit of TIPSS over endoscopic therapy in overall rates of mortality (27.3% vs 26.5%, respectively) *(1)*. The risk of rebleeding and death was highest in the trials with $\geq$40% patients in Pugh class C. A recent retrospective study over an 11-yr period in our unit identified this group to have a lower mortality than those treated with endoscopic therapy for variceal hemorrhage *(74)*. The cost of endoscopic therapy and TIPSS is similar because TIPSS is so much more effective in reducing rebleeding and the potential need for very expensive ITU care.

PHARMACOLOGICAL AGENTS COMPARED WITH TIPSS

The only publication is a study recently published, that randomized patients to either TIPSS alone ($n = 47$) or propranolol and isosorbide-5-mononitrate combination therapy ($n = 44$) *(75)*. The TIPSS arm had significantly fewer episodes of rebleeding (13% vs 39%, $p = 0.007$), but encephalopathy was significantly higher in the shunted group (38% vs 14%, $p = 0.007$). Mortality was similar in both groups. The cost of TIPSS was more than twice that of drug therapy. Interestingly the drug-treated arm has more frequent improvement in the Pugh score during follow-up. This finding is not fully explained by the authors, and it would have been useful to know how many of the patients with alcoholic liver disease remained abstinent in each arm.

It should be emphasized that the addition of propranolol to endoscopic therapy does not confer any benefit over endoscopic therapy alone, although the incidence of encephalopathy is less *(63,69,76)*. However, outside of clinical trials it is unlikely that most patients will comply fully with follow up banding sessions and drug therapy particularly those patients that have alcoholic cirrhosis.

TIPSS VS SURGERY

The use of surgical shunts is limited by the very high mortality rates in patients with advanced liver disease. Early experience strongly favored the use of TIPSS over esophageal transection, with the latter associated with a higher mortality and rate of infection *(40)*, despite similar efficacy as TIPSS in the prevention of variceal rebleeding. This probably reflects the fact that most patients referred for a TIPSS had advanced liver disease, thus making such major surgery particularly hazardous. The only randomized controlled study comparing shunt surgery using a portocaval H-graft with TIPSS revealed more episodes of variceal rebleeding in the TIPSS arm (11% vs 0%), although the technical success of the TIPSS procedure was poorer than with most other series *(73)*. It is also noteworthy that the average portal pressure following TIPSS insertion was high at 25 ± 7.5 mmHg. Others have looked at distal splenorenal shunt (DSRS) surgery vs TIPSS in a nonrandomized study of cirrhotic patients in Pugh class A and B *(77)*. The results were in favor of surgery with lower rates of rebleeding (6.3% vs 25.7%), encephalopathy (18.8% vs 42.9%), and shunt dysfunction (6.3% vs 68.6%). There was no difference in survival (6.2% vs 5.7%).

From the limited data it appears that surgery may be better suited to patients in Pugh class A to B, with TIPSS being used in patients with more severe liver disease who would not normally be candidates for shunt surgery.

TIPSS FOR THE MANAGEMENT OF GASTRIC VARICEAL BLEEDING

The management of bleeding gastric varices has been a particular challenge to clinicians. The risk of bleeding from gastric varices but is less than that of esophageal varices, the outcome once bleeding has occurred is worse, particularly for isolated gastric varices (IGV) *(78)*.

Historically, the management of gastric variceal bleeding has been suboptimal. Endoscopic measures have met with varying degrees of success *(79,80,38)*. Iatrogenic complications such as embolic phenomena and the potential for equipment damage may limit the use of tissue adhesives *(81,82)*. Thrombin seems to be promising *(83)*, but large multicenter controlled trials have yet to emerge *(84,85)*. Two of the previous studies have used bovine thrombin, which has the potential risk of prion transmission *(83,84)*. Surgical shunts may be of value in patients with early liver disease *(86)*, but have the disadvantage of high mortality in patients with advanced liver disease particularly in the emergency setting.

Owing to gastric variceal hemorrhage being relatively uncommon, there are no controlled trials and only few studies assessing the efficacy of TIPSS in bleeding gastric varices. The complications of TIPSS such as encephalopathy and shunt dysfunction are also similar. TIPSS has recently been studied in the management of refractory bleeding from gastric varices and results suggest that TIPSS is effective in the arresting hemorrhage from and prevention of rebleeding from gastric varices *(42,87)*. In a retrospective study we found that TIPSS had similar efficacy in the prevention rebleeding irrespective of whether they were from esophageal or gastric varices *(17)*. Like others we found that the PPG pre-TIPSS was significantly lower for patients who bled from gastric varices compared with esophageal varices (15.8 ± 0.8 vs 21.4 ± 0.5 mmHg, $p < 0.001$). This may be as a result of the development of gastrorenal portosystemic shunts *(88)*. This study also highlighted the significant number of patients who bled at PPG < 12 mmHg, particularly from gastric varices. It may be that factors other than portal pressure such as variceal size and variceal wall tension *(89)* play an important part in the risk of variceal bleeding in patients with PPG of < 12 mmHg. It is also true that portal pressure directly affects the variceal wall tension, and attempts to reduce the portal pressure by a TIPSS will be beneficial. Interestingly, there was a significant difference ($p < 0.05$) in favor of the gastric varices group in the 1-yr mortality (30.7% vs 38.7%) and 5-yr mortality (49.5% vs 74.9%), particularly in those patients that bled at PPG > 12 mmHg. This chapter emphasizes the influence of portal pressure on mortality as discussed above.

NEW DEVELOPMENTS

TIPSS in Combination with Other Therapies

One of the limitations of TIPSS is the high incidence of shunt insufficiency and the need for lifelong invasive portography and intervention. There have been two recent studies investigating the effect of adjuvant drug therapy in patients with an insufficient TIPSS *(90,91)*. The administration of intravenous propranolol in the presence of an insufficient TIPSS resulted in a significant reduction in the PPG of 30%, although the effect was not so pronounced in those patients with severe shunt insufficiency. A second study confirmed these finding with propranolol, although no effect was seen with nitrates. Both these studies were uncontrolled, and no data were available on the incidence of variceal bleeding. If controlled studies are favorable, the addition of drug therapy to reduce the need for shunt surveillance sounds attractive. However, it is likely only to be of temporary benefit. In addition, the side effect profile of propranolol is not favorable in our experience, and compliance could be a major problem *(92)*.

The alternative strategy is to combine variceal banding ligation (VBL) with TIPSS. VBL is associated with a high rate of rebleeding particularly in the month following the index variceal bleed *(68)*. However, once the varices have been eradicated, VBL may be as effective as a patent TIPSS in preventing variceal rebleeding. Thus, following variceal eradication in a patient with a TIPSS, it may not be necessary to continue TIPSS surveillance to maintain TIPSS patency and may potentially reduce the risk of hepatic encephalopathy. This hypothesis was tested in a recent randomized controlled trial comparing long-term portographic follow-up vs VBL following TIPSS for preventing esophageal variceal rebleeding *(93)*. It was found that terminating TIPSS surveillance following eradication of esophageal varices did not increase the rebleeding rate or mortality, but has the potential to reduce the risk of hepatic encephalopathy. The combination of VBL and short-term TIPSS surveillance is therefore an attractive alterative to standard TIPSS surveillance for patients who present with an esophageal variceal bleed, particularly where facilities for TIPSS portography are limited or if patients are encephalopathic prior to TIPSS.

Covered Stents

The idea of covering the stent to reduce clotting and intimal hyperplasia, comes from cardiovascular medicine where it has been successful. Early results with covered TIPSS using Dacron were rather disappointing, possibly owing to its nonbiocompatible nature *(94)*. Subsequent studies using polytetrafluoroethylene (PTFE) have been more successful. The Viatorr endoprosthesis is made of titanium, which supports a reduced permeability expanded PTFE graft with a bile resistant membrane. It comprises a 2-cm unlined distal section, and a lined section available in 4–8-cm lengths, separated by a radio opaque marker (Fig. 4A). It is available in 8, 10, and 12-mm diameters. Unlike uncovered stents (Fig. 4B), the length of the tract is determined prior to stent deployment. This is measured using a catheter with markings at 1-cm intervals. The aim is to cover the entire tract from the portal vein entry point to the IVC (Fig. 5A,B). This is likely to favor the patency of the Viatorr stents by reducing the risk of hepatic vein stenosis. Encouraging results in animals *(95,96)* have been reproduced in humans in small uncontrolled studies *(97–104)*. Overall, the results are impressive, with primary patency rates between 80% and 100%. Our results on 100 patients with the Viatorr endoprosthesis showed a primary patency of 92% (Fig. 6), and variceal rebleeding rate of 9.5% over an average follow-up period of 10 mo. The rates of encephalopathy were comparable to standard uncovered TIPSS. The main reasons for shunt insufficiency seem to be inadequate covering of the tract in the hepatic vein, resulting in hepatic vein stenosis. In some cases, we had to use an uncovered stent to extend the tract to the hepatic vein, and this was another source of shunt insufficiency. However, the absence of shunt thrombosis in our series is remarkable. Interim results of a randomized controlled trial also show excellent shunt patency *(105)*. Clearly, if in the final analysis the results are favorable, there may be much reduced need for long-term portographic surveillance.

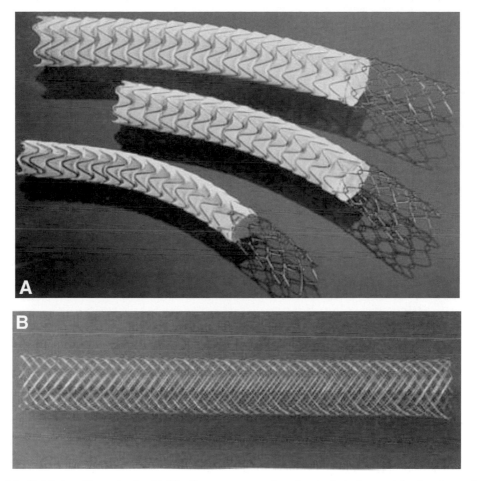

Fig. 4A–B. Viatorr Gore stents (**A**). The 2-cm uncovered end extends to the portal vein. A standard Wallstent is shown for comparison (**B**).

A potential complication of PTFE-covered stents is the development of segmental hepatic ischemia, which has been reported in a small number of patients *(106,107)*. This arises from extending the tract to the hepatic vein almost as far the IVC, resulting in a partial Budd–Chiari-like syndrome. Some patients reported abdominal pain, and were found to have abnormalities on the CT scan. In all cases, patients were managed conservatively, and did not have long-term complications. We have had experience of one asymptomatic patient who was noted to have an abnormal area of low attenuation in a CT scan. These changes resolved on further scanning 3 mo later, probably as a result of collaterals. It is, therefore, important to bear in mind this complication, particularly because there is the need to extend the tract to the hepatic vein to ensure good patency.

CONCLUSION

The ideal management of acute variceal bleeding is still unclear and is affected by the availability of local facilities and expertise. In addition to pharmacological and endosco-

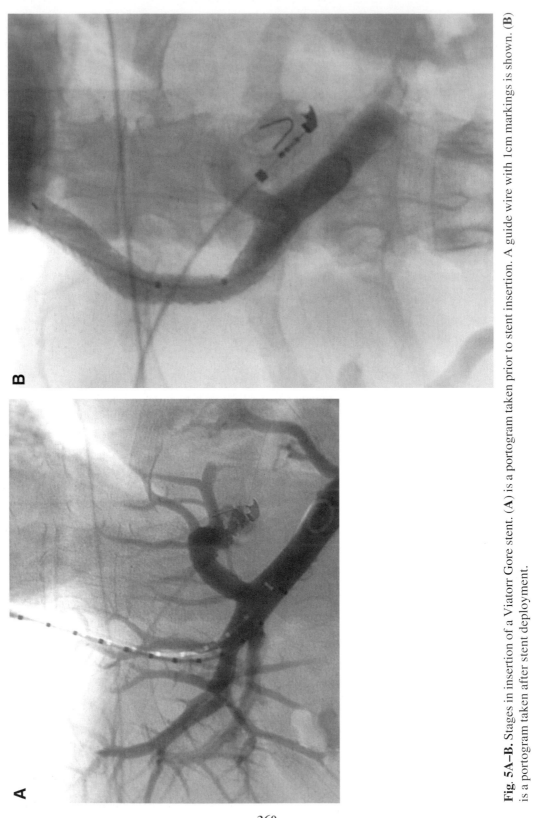

Fig. 5A–B. Stages in insertion of a Viatorr Gore stent. (**A**) is a portogram taken prior to stent insertion. A guide wire with 1cm markings is shown. (**B**) is a portogram taken after stent deployment.

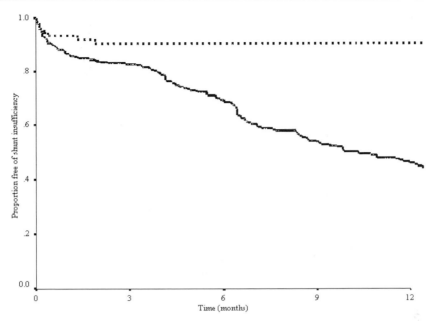

Fig. 6. Kaplan–Meier graph of 12-mo shunt patency. The Viatorr Gore covered stent (----) has significantly better primary patency than the standard uncovered stents (—).

pic therapies, TIPSS has an important role for managing esophageal variceal bleeding, both as salvage therapy and as secondary prophylaxis. However, the evidence surrounding the treatment of gastric varices is poor with little consensus on the best treatment. The lack of controlled trials reflects the much lower incidence of gastric variceal bleeding. Our experience is favorable, and we would recommend TIPSS for patients who present with bleeding gastric varices and a patent portal vein. The problems of increased encephalopathy and invasive portographic surveillance could be potentially overcome by the combination of short-term TIPSS surveillance and VBL. The latest PTFE covered stents promise superior patency, although controlled studies comparing these shunt with uncovered stents are lacking. In the future, it is likely that TIPSS insertion will be "prescribed," in terms of target pressure, type of stent to be used, TIPSS with or without portographic surveillance, and whether or not ancillary measures such as the need for adjuvant endoscopic or pharmacological therapies.

REFERENCES

1. Papatheodoridis GV, Goulis J, Leandro G, Patch D, Burroughs AK. Transjugular intrahepatic portosystemic shunt compared with endoscopic treatment for prevention of variceal rebleeding: a meta-analysis. Hepatology 1999;30(3):612–622.
2. Rosch J, Hanafee WN, Snow H. Transjugular portal venography and radiologic portacaval shunt: an experimental study. Radiology 1969;92(5):1112–1114.
3. Rosch J, Hanafee W, Snow H, Barenfus M, Gray R. Transjugular intrahepatic portacaval shunt. An experimental work. Am J Surg 1971;121(5):588–592.
4. Koch G, Rigler B, Tentzeris M, Schuy S, Sakulin M, Schmidt-Kloiber H. The intrahepatic portocaval shunt. Langenbecks Arch Chir 1973;333(3):237–244.
5. Reich M, Olumide F, Jorgensen E, Eiseman B. Experimental cryoprobe production of intrahepatic portocaval shunt. J Surg Res 1977;23(1):14–18.

6. Burgener FA, Gutierrez OH. Experimental intrahepatic portocaval shunts created in portal hypertension by balloon angioplasty catheters. Invest Radiol 1988;23(1):24–29.

7. Colapinto RF, Stronell RD, Birch SJ, et al. Creation of an intrahepatic portosystemic shunt with a Gruntzig balloon catheter. Can Med Assoc J 1982;126(3):267–268.

8. Palmaz JC, Sibbitt RR, Reuter SR, Garcia F, Tio FO. Expandable intrahepatic portacaval shunt stents: early experience in the dog. AJR Am J Roentgenol 1985;145(4):821–825.

9. Palmaz JC, Garcia F, Sibbitt RR, et al. Expandable intrahepatic portacaval shunt stents in dogs with chronic portal hypertension. AJR Am J Roentgenol 1986;147(6):1251–1254.

10. Rockey DC. Vasoactive agents in intrahepatic portal hypertension and fibrogenesis: implications for therapy. Gastroenterology 2000;118(6):1261–1265.

11. Kowalaski B, Abelmann WH. The cardiac output at rest in Laennec's cirrhosis. J Clin Invest 1953;32: 1025–1033.

12. Murray JF, Dawson AM, Sherlock S. Circulatory changes in chronic liver disease. Am J Med 1958; 32:358–367.

13. Lowke HF. Reduction of hypertension after liver disease. Arch Intern Med 1962;110:45–52.

14. Mashford ML, Mahow WA, Chalmers TC. Studies of the cariovascular system in the hypotension of liver failure. N Engl J Med 1962;267:1071–1074.

15. Plevris JN, Hauer JL, Hayes PC, Bouchier IA. Blood pressure and liver cirrhosis. J Hum Hypertens 1990;4(6):725–726.

16. D'Amico G, Pagliaro L, Bosch J. The treatment of portal hypertension: a meta-analytic review. Hepatology 1995;22(1):332–354.

17. Tripathi D, Therapondos G, Jackson E, Redhead DN, Hayes PC. The role of the transjugular intrahepatic portosystemic stent shunt (TIPSS) in the management of bleeding gastric varices: clinical and haemodynamic correlations. Gut 2002;51(2):270–274.

18. Lotterer E, Wengert A, Fleig WE. Transjugular intrahepatic portosystemic shunt: short-term and long-term effects on hepatic and systemic hemodynamics in patients with cirrhosis. Hepatology 1999; 29(3):632–639.

19. Kleber G, Steudel N, Behrmann C, et al. Hepatic arterial flow volume and reserve in patients with cirrhosis: use of intra-arterial Doppler and adenosine infusion. Gastroenterology 1999;116:906–914.

20. Zipprich A, Steudel N, Behrmann C, et al. Functional significance of hepatic arterial flow reserve in patients with cirrhosis. Hepatology 2003;37:385–392.

21. Azoulay D, Castaing D, Dennison A, Martino W, Eyraud D, Bismuth H. Transjugular intrahepatic portosystemic shunt worsens the hyperdynamic circulatory state of the cirrhotic patient: preliminary report of a prospective study. Hepatology 1994;19:129–132.

22. Tripathi D, Helmy A, Macbeth K, et al. Ten years' follow-up of 472 patients following transjugular intrahepatic portosystemic stent-shunt insertion at a single centre. Eur J Gastroenterol Hepatol 2004; 19:9–18.

23. Sanyal AJ, Reddy KR. Vegetative infection of transjugular intrahepatic portosystemic shunts. Gastroenterology 1998;115(1):110–115.

24. Jalan R, Redhead DN, Allan PL, Hayes PC. Prospective evaluation of haematological alterations following the transjugular intrahepatic portosystemic stent-shunt (TIPSS). Eur J Gastroenterol Hepatol 1996;8(4):381–385.

25. Burroughs AK, Vangeli M. Transjugular intrahepatic portosystemic shunt versus endoscopic therapy: randomized trials for secondary prophylaxis of variceal bleeding: an updated meta-analysis. Scand J Gastroenterol 2002;37(3):249–252.

26. Jalan R, Elton RA, Redhead DN, Finlayson ND, Hayes PC. Analysis of prognostic variables in the prediction of mortality, shunt failure, variceal rebleeding and encephalopathy following the transjugular intrahepatic portosystemic stent-shunt for variceal haemorrhage. J Hepatol 1995;23(2):123–128.

27. Jalan R, Stanley AJ, Redhead DN, Hayes PC. Shunt insufficiency after transjugular intrahepatic portosystemic stent- shunt: the whens, whys, hows and what should we do about it? [editorial]. Clin Radiol 1997;52(5):329–331.

28. Jalan R, Dabos K, Redhead DN, Lee A, Hayes PC. Elevation of intracranial pressure following transjugular intrahepatic portosystemic stent-shunt for variceal haemorrhage. J Hepatol 1997;27:928–933.

29. Sze DY, Vestring T, Liddell RP, et al. Recurrent TIPS failure associated with biliary fistulae: treatment with PTFE-covered stents. Cardiovasc Intervent Radiol 1999;22(4):298–304.

30. Jalan R, Harrison DJ, Redhead DN, Hayes PC. Transjugular intrahepatic portosystemic stent-shunt (TIPSS) occlusion and the role of biliary venous fistulae. J Hepatol 1996;24(2):169–176.

31. Sauer P, Theilmann L, Herrmann S, et al. Phenprocoumon for prevention of shunt occlusion after transjugular intrahepatic portosystemic stent shunt: a randomized trial. Hepatology 1996;24(6):1433–1436.

32. Siegerstetter V, Huber M, Ochs A, Blum HE, Rossle M. Platelet aggregation and platelet-derived growth factor inhibition for prevention of insufficiency of the transjugular intrahepatic portosystemic shunt: a randomized study comparing trapidil plus ticlopidine with heparin treatment. Hepatology 1999;29(1):33–38.

33. Ferguson JM, Jalan R, Redhead DN, Hayes PC, Allan PL. The role of duplex and colour Doppler ultrasound in the follow-up evaluation of transjugular intrahepatic portosystemic stent shunt (TIPSS). Br J Radiol 1995;68(810):587–589.

34. Shah SH, Lui HF, Helmy A, Redhead DN, Penny K, Hayes PC. Transjugular intrahepatic portosystemic stent-shunt insufficiency and the role of diabetes mellitus. Eur J Gastroenterol Hepatol 2001; 13(3):257–261.

35. Balata S, Lui HF, Helmy A, Tripathi D, Redhead DN, Hayes PC. Role of technical variables in early shunt insufficiency following TIPSS for the treatment of portal hypertension. Gut 2002;50:427.

36. Groszmann RJ, Bosch J, Grace ND, et al. Hemodynamic events in a prospective randomized trial of propranolol versus placebo in the prevention of a first variceal hemorrhage. Gastroenterology 1990; 99(5):1401–1407.

37. Ferguson JW, Tripathi D, Hayes PC. Review article: the management of acute variceal bleeding. Aliment Pharmacol Ther 2003;18(3):253–262.

38. Jalan R, Hayes PC. UK guidelines on the management of variceal haemorrhage in cirrhotic patients. British Society of Gastroenterology. Gut 2000;46(Suppl 3-4):III1–III15.

39. Stanley AJ, Jalan R, Forrest EH, Redhead DN, Hayes PC. Longterm follow up of transjugular intrahepatic portosystemic stent shunt (TIPSS) for the treatment of portal hypertension: results in 130 patients. Gut 1996;39(3):479–485.

40. Jalan R, John TG, Redhead DN, et al. A comparative study of emergency transjugular intrahepatic portosystemic stent-shunt and esophageal transection in the management of uncontrolled variceal hemorrhage. Am J Gastroenterol 1995;90(11):1932–1937.

41. Chau TN, Patch D, Chan YW, Nagral A, Dick R, Burroughs AK. "Salvage" transjugular intrahepatic portosystemic shunts: gastric fundal compared with esophageal variceal bleeding. Gastroenterology 1998;114(5):981–987.

42. Barange K, Peron JM, Imani K, et al. Transjugular intrahepatic portosystemic shunt in the treatment of refractory bleeding from ruptured gastric varices. Hepatology 1999;30(5):1139–1143.

43. Laberge JM, Ring EJ, Gordon RL, et al. Creation of transjugular intrahepatic portosystemic shunts with the wallstent endoprosthesis: results in 100 patients. Radiology 1993;187(2):413–420.

44. Helton WS, Belshaw A, Althaus S, Park S, Coldwell D, Johansen K. Critical appraisal of the angiographic portacaval shunt (TIPS). Am J Surg 1993;165(5):566–571.

45. Haag K, Rossle M, Hauenstein KH, Sellingwer M, Ochs A, Blum U. Der transjugulare intrahepatische portosystemischhe Stent-Shunt (TIPS) in der Notfallbehandlung der portalen Hypertension. Intensivmed 1993;30:479–483.

46. Le Moine O, Deviere J, Ghysels M, Francois E, Rypens F, VanGansbeke D. Transjugular intrahepatic portosystemic stent shunt as a rescue treatment after sclerotherapy failure in variceal bleeding. Scand J Gastroenterol 1994;207(Suppl):23–28.

47. Rubin RA, Haskal ZJ, O'Brien CB, Cope C, Brass CA. Transjugular intrahepatic portosystemic shunting: decreased survival for patients with high APACHE II scores. Am J Gastroenterol 1995;90(4): 556–563.

48. Jabbour N, Zajko AB, Orons PD, et al. Transjugular intrahepatic portosystemic shunt in patients with end-stage liver disease: results in 85 patients. Liver Transpl Surg 1996;2(2):139–147.

49. Sanyal AJ, Freedman AM, Luketic VA, et al. Transjugular intrahepatic portosystemic shunts for patients with active variceal hemorrhage unresponsive to sclerotherapy. Gastroenterology 1996;111 (1):138–146.

50. Perarnau JM. Le shunt intra-hepatique (TIPS): 5 ans apres. Act Med Int Gastroenterol 1997;111:278–285.

51. Banares R, Casado M, Rodriguez-Laiz JM, et al. Urgent transjugular intrahepatic portosystemic shunt for control of acute variceal bleeding. Am J Gastroenterol 1998;93(1):75–79.

52. Gerbes AL, Gulberg V, Waggershauser T, Holl J, Reiser M. Transjugular intrahepatic portosystemic shunt (TIPS) for variceal bleeding in portal hypertension: comparison of emergency and elective interventions. Dig Dis Sci 1998;43(11):2463–2469.

53. Bizollon T, Dumortier J, Jouisse C, et al. Transjugular intra-hepatic portosystemic shunt for refractory variceal bleeding. Eur J Gastroenterol Hepatol 2001;13(4):369–375.

54. Azoulay D, Castaing D, Majno P, et al. Salvage transjugular intrahepatic portosystemic shunt for uncontrolled variceal bleeding in patients with decompensated cirrhosis. J Hepatol 2001;35(5):590–597.

55. Burroughs AK, Patch D. Transjugular intrahepatic portosystemic shunt. Semin Liver Dis 1999;19(4): 457–473.

56. Stanley AJ, Robinson I, Forrest EH, Jones AL, Hayes PC. Haemodynamic parameters predicting variceal haemorrhage and survival in alcoholic cirrhosis. QJM 1998;91(1):19–25.

57. Moitinho E, Escorsell A, Bandi JC, et al. Prognostic value of early measurements of portal pressure in acute variceal bleeding. Gastroenterology 1999;117(3):626–631.

58. Patch D, Armonis A, Sabin C, et al. Single portal pressure measurement predicts survival in cirrhotic patients with recent bleeding. Gut 1999;44(2):264–269.

59. Salerno F, Merli M, Cazzaniga M, et al. MELD score is better than Child-Pugh score in predicting 3-month survival of patients undergoing transjugular intrahepatic portosystemic shunt. J Hepatol 2002; 36(4):494–500.

60. Gulberg V, Schepke M, Geigenberger G, et al. Transjugular intrahepatic portosystemic shunting is not superior to endoscopic variceal band ligation for prevention of variceal rebleeding in cirrhotic patients: a randomized, controlled trial. Scand J Gastroenterol 2002;37(3):338–343.

61. Pomier-Layrargues G, Villeneuve JP, Deschenes M, et al. Transjugular intrahepatic portosystemic shunt (TIPS) versus endoscopic variceal ligation in the prevention of variceal rebleeding in patients with cirrhosis: a randomised trial. Gut 2001;48(3):390–396.

62. Narahara Y, Kanazawa H, Kawamata H, et al. A randomized clinical trial comparing transjugular intrahepatic portosystemic shunt with endoscopic sclerotherapy in the long-term management of patients with cirrhosis after recent variceal hemorrhage. Hepatol Res 2001;21(3):189–198.

63. Sauer P, Theilmann L, Stremmel W, Benz C, Richter GM, Stiehl A. Transjugular intrahepatic portosystemic stent shunt versus sclerotherapy plus propranolol for variceal rebleeding. Gastroenterology 1997;113(5):1623–1631.

64. Garcia-Villarreal L, Martinez-Lagares F, Sierra A, et al. Transjugular intrahepatic portosystemic shunt versus endoscopic sclerotherapy for the prevention of variceal rebleeding after recent variceal hemorrhage. Hepatology 1999;29(1):27–32.

65. Merli M, Salerno F, Riggio O, et al. Transjugular intrahepatic portosystemic shunt versus endoscopic sclerotherapy for the prevention of variceal bleeding in cirrhosis: a randomized multicenter trial. Gruppo Italiano Studio TIPS (G.I.S.T.). Hepatology 1998;27(1):48–53.

66. Sauer P, Hansmann J, Richter GM, Stremmel W, Stiehl A. Transjugular intrahepatic portosystemic stent shunt (TIPS) vs. endoscopic banding in the prevention of variceal rebleeding: a long-term randomized trial. Gastroenterology 2000;118(4):6723.

67. Cello JP, Ring EJ, Olcott EW, et al. Endoscopic sclerotherapy compared with percutaneous transjugular intrahepatic portosystemic shunt after initial sclerotherapy in patients with acute variceal hemorrhage. A randomized, controlled trial. Ann Intern Med 1997;126(11):858–865.

68. Jalan R, Forrest EH, Stanley AJ, et al. A randomized trial comparing transjugular intrahepatic portosystemic stent-shunt with variceal band ligation in the prevention of rebleeding from esophageal varices. Hepatology 1997;26(5):1115–1122.

69. Rossle M, Deibert P, Haag K, et al. Randomised trial of transjugular-intrahepatic-portosystemic shunt versus endoscopy plus propranolol for prevention of variceal rebleeding. Lancet 1997;349(9058): 1043–1049.

70. Sanyal AJ, Freedman AM, Luketic VA, et al. Transjugular intrahepatic portosystemic shunts compared with endoscopic sclerotherapy for the prevention of recurrent variceal hemorrhage. A randomized, controlled trial. Ann Intern Med 1997;126(11):849–857.

71. Cabrera J, Maynar M, Granados R, et al. Transjugular intrahepatic portosystemic shunt versus sclerotherapy in the elective treatment of variceal hemorrhage. Gastroenterology 1996;110(3):832–839.

72. GEAIH. Tips vs sclerotherapy plus propranolol in the prevention of variceal rebleeding—preliminary-results of a multicenter randomized trial. Hepatology 1995;22(4):761.

73. Rosemurgy AS, Goode SE, Zwiebel BR, Black TJ, Brady PG. A prospective trial of transjugular intrahepatic portasystemic stent shunts versus small-diameter prosthetic H-graft portacaval shunts in the treatment of bleeding varices. Ann Surg 1996;224(3):378–384.

74. Jalan R, Bzeizi KI, Tripathi D, Lui HF, Redhead DN, Hayes PC. Impact of transjugular intrahepatic portosystemic stent-shunt for secondary prophylaxis of oesophageal variceal haemorrhage: a single-centre study over an 11-year period. Eur J Gastroenterol Hepatol 2002;14(6):615–626.

75. Escorsell A, Banares R, Garcia-Pagan JC, et al. TIPS versus drug therapy in preventing variceal rebleeding in advanced cirrhosis: a randomized controlled trial. Hepatology 2002;35(2):385–392.

76. Sauer P, Hansmann J, Richter GM, Stremmel W, Stiehl A. Endoscopic variceal ligation plus propranolol vs. transjugular intrahepatic portosystemic stent shunt: a long-term randomized trial. Endoscopy 2002;34(9):690–697.

77. Khaitiyar JS, Luthra SK, Prasad N, Ratnakar N, Daruwala DK. Transjugular intrahepatic portosystemic shunt versus distal splenorenal shunt—a comparative study. Hepatogastroenterology 2000; 47(32):492–497.

78. Sarin SK, Lahoti D, Saxena SP, Murthy NS, Makwana UK. Prevalence, classification and natural history of gastric varices: a long-term follow-up study in 568 portal hypertension patients. Hepatology 1992;16(6):1343–1349.

79. Gimson AE, Westaby D, Williams R. Endoscopic sclerotherapy in the management of gastric variceal haemorrhage. J Hepatol 1991;13(3):274–278.

80. Ramond MJ, Valla D, Gotlib JP, Rueff B, Benhamou JP. Endoscopic obturation of esophagogastric varices with bucrylate. I. Clinical study of 49 patients. Gastroenterol Clin Biol 1986;10(8–9):575–579.

81. Lee GH, Kim JH, Lee KJ, et al. Life-threatening intraabdominal arterial embolization after histoacryl injection for bleeding gastric ulcer. Endoscopy 2000;32(5):422–424.

82. See A, Florent C, Lamy P, Levy VG, Bouvry M. Cerebrovascular accidents after endoscopic obturation of esophageal varices with isobutyl-2-cyanoacrylate in 2 patients. Gastroenterol Clin Biol 1986;10 (8–9):604–607.

83. Przemioslo RT, McNair A, Williams R. Thrombin is effective in arresting bleeding from gastric variceal hemorrhage. Dig Dis Sci 1999;44(4):778–781.

84. Williams SG, Peters RA, Westaby D. Thrombin—an effective treatment for gastric variceal haemorrhage. Gut 1994;35(9):1287–1289.

85. Yang WL, Tripathi D, Therapondos G, Todd A, Hayes PC. Endoscopic use of human thrombin in bleeding gastric varices. Am J Gastroenterol 2002;97(6):1381–1385.

86. Thomas PG, D'Cruz AJ. Distal splenorenal shunting for bleeding gastric varices. Br J Surg 1994;81(2): 241–244.

87. Stanley AJ, Jalan R, Ireland HM, Redhead DN, Bouchier IA, Hayes PC. A comparison between gastric and oesophageal variceal haemorrhage treated with transjugular intrahepatic portosystemic stent shunt (TIPSS). Aliment Pharmacol Ther 1997;11(1):171–176.

88. Watanabe K, Kimura K, Matsutani S, Ohto M, Okuda K. Portal hemodynamics in patients with gastric varices. A study in 230 patients with esophageal and/or gastric varices using portal vein catheterization. Gastroenterology 1988;95(2):434–440.

89. Polio J, Groszmann RJ. Hemodynamic factors involved in the development and rupture of esophageal varices: a pathophysiologic approach to treatment. Semin Liver Dis 1986;6(4):318–331.

90. Bellis L, Moitinho E, Abraldes JG, et al. Acute propranolol administration effectively decreases portal pressure in patients with TIPS dysfunction. Transjugular intrahepatic portosystemic shunt. Gut 2003; 52(1):130–133.

91. Brensing KA, Horsch M, Textor J, et al. Hemodynamic effects of propranolol and nitrates in cirrhotics with transjugular intrahepatic portosystemic stent-shunt. Scand J Gastroenterol 2002;37(9):1070–1076.

92. Luo B, Abrams GA, Fallon MB. Endothelin-1 in the rat bile duct ligation model of hepatopulmonary syndrome: correlation with pulmonary dysfunction. J Hepatol 1998;29(4):571–578.

93. Tripathi D, Lui HF, Helmy A, et al. Randomized controlled trial of long term portographic follow up versus variceal band ligation following transjugular intrahepatic portosystemic stent shunt for preventing oesophageal variceal rebleeding. Gut 2004;53:431–437.

94. Otal P, Rousseau H, Vinel JP, Ducoin H, Hassissene S, Joffre F. High occlusion rate in experimental transjugular intrahepatic portosystemic shunt created with a Dacron-covered nitinol stent. J Vasc Interv Radiol 1999;10(2 Pt 1):183–188.
95. Nishimine K, Saxon RR, Kichikawa K, et al. Improved transjugular intrahepatic portosystemic shunt patency with PTFE-covered stent-grafts: experimental results in swine. Radiology 1995;196(2):341–347.
96. Haskal ZJ, Davis A, McAllister A, Furth EE. PTFE-encapsulated endovascular stent-graft for transjugular intrahepatic portosystemic shunts: experimental evaluation. Radiology 1997;205(3):682–688.
97. Otal P, Smayra T, Bureau C, et al. Preliminary results of a new expanded-polytetrafluoroethylene-covered stent-graft for transjugular intrahepatic portosystemic shunt procedures. AJR Am J Roentgenol 2002;178(1):141–147.
98. Rose JD, Pimpalwar S, Jackson RW. A new stent-graft for transjugular intrahepatic portosystemic shunts. Br J Radiol 2001;74(886):908–912.
99. Andrews RT, Saxon RR, Bloch RD, et al. Stent-grafts for de novo TIPS: technique and early results. J Vasc Interv Radiol 1999;10(10):1371–1378.
100. Cejna M, Thurnher S, Pidlich J, Kaserer K, Schoder M, Lammer J. Primary implantation of polyester-covered stent-grafts for transjugular intrahepatic portosystemic stent shunts (TIPSS): a pilot study. Cardiovasc Intervent Radiol 1999;22(4):305–310.
101. Haskal ZJ. Improved patency of transjugular intrahepatic portosystemic shunts in humans: creation and revision with PTFE stent-grafts. Radiology 1999;213(3):759–766.
102. Saxon RR, Timmermans HA, Uchida BT, et al. Stent-grafts for revision of TIPS stenoses and occlusions: a clinical pilot study. J Vasc Interv Radiol 1997;8(4):539–548.
103. Cejna M, Peck-Radosavljevic M, Thurnher S, et al. ePTFE-covered stent-grafts for revision of obstructed transjugular intrahepatic portosystemic shunt. Cardiovasc Intervent Radiol 2002;25(5):365–372.
104. Otal P, Smayra T, Bureau C, et al. Preliminary results of a new expanded-polytetrafluoroethylene-covered stent-graft for transjugular intrahepatic portosystemic shunt procedures. AJR Am J Roentgenol 2002;178(1):141–147.
105. Bureau C, Pagan JCG, Layrargues GP, et al. The use of polytetrafluoroethylene (PTFE) covered stents improves the patency of tips: results of a randomized study. Hepatology 2002;36(4):525.
106. Bureau C, Otal P, Chabbert V, Peron JM, Rousseau H, Vinel JP. Segmental liver ischemia after TIPS procedure using a new PTFE-covered stent. Hepatology 2002;36(6):1554.
107. Laberge JM, Kerlan RK. Liver infarction following TIPS with a PTFE-covered stent: is the covering the cause? Hepatology 2003;38(3):778–779.
108. Haag K, Rossle M, Hauenstein KH, et al. Der transjugulare intrahepatische portosystemischhe Stent-Shunt (TIPS) in der Notfallbehandlung der portalen Hypertension. Intensivmed 1993;30:479–483.
109. Le Moine O, Deviere J, Ghysels M, Francois E, Rypens F, VanGansbeke D. Transjugular intrahepatic portosystemic stent shunt as a rescue treatment after sclerotherapy failure in variceal bleeding. Scand J Gastroenterol 1994;207(Suppl):23–28.
110. Rubin RA, Haskal ZJ, O'Brien CB, Cope C, Brass CA. Transjugular intrahepatic portosystemic shunting: decreased survival for patients with high APACHE II scores. Am J Gastroenterol 1995;90(4):556–563.
111. Sauer P, Benz C, Theilmann L, Richter GM, Stremmel W, Stiehl A. Transjugular intrahepatic portosystemic stent shunt (TIPS) vs. endoscopic banding in the prevention of variceal rebleeding: final results of a randomized study [Abstract]. Gastroenterology 1998;114:A1334.

18

Clinical Features and Management of Gastric Varices, Portal Hypertensive Gastropathy, and Ectopic Varices

Charmaine A. Stewart, MD
and Patrick S. Kamath, MD

CONTENTS

INTRODUCTION
GASTRIC VARICES
PORTAL HYPERTENSIVE GASTROPATHY AND GASTRIC VASCULAR ECTASIA
ECTOPIC VARICES
SUMMARY
REFERENCES

INTRODUCTION

Approximately 10% of portal hypertension-related gastrointestinal hemorrhage occurs from lesions in the stomach. These lesions are mainly gastric varices and, less commonly, portal hypertensive gastropathy and gastric vascular ectasia. Bleeding from varices other than esophageal or gastric, termed ectopic varices, is infrequent and accounts for fewer than 5% of all portal hypertension-related bleeding.

In this chapter, we review the clinical features and management of gastric varices, portal hypertensive gastropathy, gastric vascular ectasia, and ectopic varices.

GASTRIC VARICES

Gastric varices may form as a result of portal hypertension from intrahepatic disease or from extrahepatic portal venous thrombosis. The fundus of the stomach drains via short gastric veins into the splenic vein. Splenic vein thrombosis, also called sinistral portal hypertension, results in isolated gastric varices, that is, gastric varices without esophageal varices. On the other hand, gastric veins may connect to the esophageal submucosal veins leading to the formation of gastroesophageal varices with shunting into the azygous venous system.

From: *Clinical Gastroenterology: Portal Hypertension*
Edited by: A. J. Sanyal and V. H. Shah © Humana Press Inc., Totowa, NJ

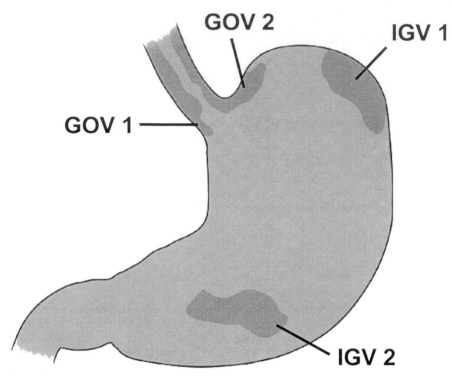

Fig. 1. Classification of gastric varices. GOV1 denotes varices type 1 located in the cardia are an extension of esophageal varices that extend 20–50 mm below the gastroesophageal junction. GOV2 denotes gastric varices type 2, are located in the fundus, and are present in association with esophageal varices. IGV1 denotes isolated gastric varices located in the fundus without association with esophageal varices. IGV2 denotes isolated gastric varices or ectopic gastric varices and may occur in the body, antrum, pylorus, or upper duodenum.

Gastric varices are classified according to location and relationship to esophageal varices. According to Sarin's classification of gastric varices *(1)* (Fig. 1): gastroesophageal varices type 1 (GOV1) are contiguous with esophageal varices and extend 20–50 mm below the gastroesophageal junction; gastroesophageal varices type 2 (GOV 2) occur in the fundus of the stomach, contiguous with esophageal varices; isolated gastric varices type 1 (IGV 1) occur in the fundus of the stomach in the absence of esophageal varices; and isolated gastric varices type 2 (IGV2) or ectopic gastric varices may be found in the gastric body, antrum or pylorus; or in the proximal duodenum.

Causes of Gastric Varices

Gastric varices may be primary or secondary. If diagnosed on initial diagnostic endoscopy, gastric varices are termed primary; if found after treatment with sclerotherapy or band ligation of esophageal varices, they are termed secondary. The prevalence of gastric varices in patients with portal hypertension is approx 25% (range 7–57%), and the most common type is GOV 1. Both GOV 1 and GOV 2 are seen most commonly with intrahepatic causes of portal hypertension, whereas splenic vein thrombosis usually results in isolated gastric fundal varices (IGV1). The most common cause of IGV1 is actually intrahepatic portal hypertension, as in cirrhosis of the liver. IGV2, or ectopic gastric varices, are most commonly seen in the antrum alone or with varices in the duodenum, fundus or body of the stomach *(1)*.

Natural History of Gastric Varices

Gastric varices (GV) occur later in the course of portal hypertension and most often after the appearance of esophageal varices *(1)*. The most common type of GV is GOV1 (70%), which occurs concurrently with large esophageal varices. Bleeding is more common from GOV2 and IGV 1, that is, fundic varices, than from GOV1 or IGV2 *(1–3)*. Bleeding rates from gastric and esophageal varices are probably comparable *(1)*. In most cases of GOV1, once esophageal varices are obliterated, contiguous GV also disappear. Mortality is higher if GV persist in spite of obliteration of esophageal varices. Six times as many subjects with secondary GOV2 die compared to primary GOV2. This may be a reflection of more advanced liver disease and portal hypertension of long-standing patients with secondary GOV 2. Bleeding from isolated fundal gastric varices (IGV1) is usually massive. Ectopic gastric varices are rarely primary and seldom bleed.

Management of Gastric Varices

The management of patients with gastric varices has not been well defined. Hence, there is much variability in how patients are treated.

Control of Acute Gastric Variceal Hemorrhage

The goals of therapy should be to control acute bleeding and prevent early rebleeding, which is associated with high mortality. Prompt volume resuscitation is critical because gastric variceal hemorrhage may be profuse and associated with hemodynamic instability. Overtransfusion should, however, be avoided because of the risk of rebound portal hypertension that could result in early rebleeding. Antibiotic prophylaxis with norfloxacin is recommended because variceal hemorrhage is associated with a risk of bacterial infection. Endoscopic diagnosis of acute gastric variceal bleeding may be difficult because of poor visualization from active bleeding or pooled blood. However, the diagnosis should be based on visualization of bleeding from a gastric varix, the appearance of blood at the esophagogastric junction or in the gastric fundus, in the presence of gastric varices, or the presence of the "white nipple sign" on gastric varices in the absence of other sources of bleeding in a patient with upper gastrointestinal bleeding, and gastric varices in the absence of other lesions *(4)*. Medical management with vasoactive agents and endoscopic therapy may be beneficial in these patients. In cases where there is failure to control bleeding using endoscopic therapy, balloon tamponade may occasionally be helpful to control bleeding *(5)*.

Current vasoactive agents in use are vasopressin, terlipressin, somatostatin, and its analogs. Vasopressin, a potent vasoconstrictor that acts on the splanchnic and systemic circulation, has fallen out of favor because of association with cerebral and cardiac ischemia. When vasopressin is used concomitantly with nitroglycerine, there is additional reduction in portal pressure. Terlipressin, an inactive pro-drug not available in the United States, is converted by the liver to lypressin, which has actions similar to vasopressin. The slower release results in fewer cardiac and vascular ischemic events. Because of the beneficial effects of terlipressin in the control of acute esophageal variceal hemorrhage, this drug may be recommended in the management of gastric variceal bleeding. The recommended dose is 2 mg intravenously every 4–6 h *(6,7)*. Both somatostatin and octreotide reduce portal pressure by causing splanchnic vasoconstriction, thereby reducing portal flow. However, their effectiveness in controlling acute gastric variceal hemorrhage is unknown. Octreotide has a longer duration of action than somatostatin and is available for clinical use in the United States. The dose of octreotide is 50 µg as a continuous infusion for up to 5 d. Octreotide is safe and selective in its vasoconstricting properties, and has essentially replaced less-favorable vasoconstricting agents, such as vasopressin in the United States. Vasoactive agents ideally should be started at least 30 min before the onset of upper gastrointestinal endoscopy.

Endoscopic Therapy

The preferred endoscopic therapy for gastric variceal bleeding is injection of tissue adhesives (polymers of cyanoacrylate) into the gastric varices *(8–13)*. Unfortunately, such tissue adhesives ("glue") are not available in the United States. Injection of tissue glues into the varix is hampered by pooling of blood in the gastric fundus that obscures proper visualization. Immediate obliteration of varices occurs after injection of the adhesive that hardens on contact with blood. The overlying mucosa eventually sloughs off, occasionally causing an ulcer. Compared to endoscopic sclerotherapy-related ulcers, these ulcers occur later and the risk of bleeding is lower. Hemostasis is achieved in approx 90% cases; early rebleeding is lower in comparison with other endoscopic treatment modalities, and the number of endoscopy sessions to achieve obliteration is fewer *(8–10)*.

In the management of bleeding gastric varices, a higher mortality and more complications have been found with band ligation compared with butyl cyanoacrylate injection *(12)*. There is no difference in rebleeding, obliteration rate or number of sessions needed for obliteration. These results are similar to findings obtained by earlier investigators *(14)*. Although cyanoacrylate injections have been shown to be safe and effective in the control of acute bleeding *(8,12,14)*, there are complications associated with the procedure, namely bacteremia, variceal ulcers leading to rebleeding, and dysphagia. There have also been reports of cerebral and pulmonary embolism. In addition, damage to the endoscope by the glue may occur, but this is less if silicone gel or lipiodol are used and suction is avoided for 10–20 s after injection. In a recent study, cyanoacrylate and alcohol sclerotherapy were found to have similar initial arrest of gastric variceal bleeding and mortality *(13)*.

Sclerotherapy is performed with a flexible endoscope in the straight-end-on technique for GOV1 or in retroflexion for the GOV2 or IGV 1, using intravariceal methods of injection. The traditionally used sclerosants for the treatment of esophageal varices, such as sodium tetradecyl sulfate, ethanolamine oleate, and sodium morrhuate have not been proven to be effective in the management of gastric variceal hemorrhage *(15)*. The success of sclerotherapy in controlling bleeding is mixed, and appears to be dependent on the location of the gastric varices. Some investigators have reported bleeding is easier to control when due to GOV 1 as compared to GOV2 *(17)*. Others conclude that bleeding from both GOV1 and GOV2 are controlled equally well with endoscopic sclerotherapy *(14,17)*. The variable results probably reflect varying degrees of expertise. Sclerotherapy of gastric varices is limited by the development of ulcers at the site of injection. These ulcers usually occur before obliteration is attained and are deep, consequently resulting in rebleeding that is difficult to control *(15,17)*.

It is difficult to assess the efficacy of band ligation for gastric varices because most studies have been performed with small sample sizes. Band ligation to control active gastric variceal bleeding may be successful in up to 90% of subjects *(14)*. In cases of acute bleeding from gastric varices, approx 50% of GOV1 disappear when esophageal varices are obliterated with banding ligation or sclerotherapy *(16)*.

Transjugular Intrahepatic Portosystemic Shunt (TIPS)

TIPS has been shown to be effective in the management of acute gastric variceal hemorrhage *(19–22)*. TIPS may be used during the acute setting if endoscopic therapy has failed or is not feasible either due to profuse bleeding or location of varices. In such settings, balloon tamponade may be used as a temporizing measure to prevent exsanguination until TIPS can be arranged on an emergency basis. TIPS is safer in patients with advanced liver disease than emergency decompressive surgery, which is associated with a high mortality rate of 70–90%. It is, however, well worth noting that patients with high MELD scores that reflect high bilirubin, creatinine, and prothrombin time are associated with increased mortality *(23)*. Hence, TIPS should be inserted in patients as a bridge to transplantation, or in selected subjects with advanced liver disease who are not transplant candidates but in whom the benefit of the procedure exceeds the risk of acute liver failure.

A recent study has compared the cost-effectiveness of endoscopic therapy and TIPS *(24)*. However, it is difficult to draw conclusions because of the retrospective nature of the study and the fact that patients were not randomized to the different therapies.

Prevention of Gastric Variceal Rebleeding

There are no large, well-conducted studies on the ability of pharmacological therapy or endoscopic therapy to prevent rebleeding. Analyses of studies, largely retrospective, on the use of cyanoacrylate glue in the prevention of gastric variceal bleeding demonstrate efficacy of the procedure in the obliteration of gastric varices. However, in the absence of a control group, no conclusions can be drawn regarding efficacy in reducing rebleeding or reducing mortality. Within the United States, the preferred modality for prevention of rebleeding from gastric varices is a portosystemic shunt, either surgical or TIPS. This is because of the lack of availability of cyanoacrylate glue, the lack of evidence supporting the efficacy of pharmacological therapy such as nonselective β-adrenergic blockers *(25)*, and the high mortality and morbidity associated with rebleeding.

Cyanoacrylate may be used to obliterate gastric varices after the index episode of bleeding *(26)*. An average of three sessions are required for obliteration of gastric varices with low rebleeding rates and 1-yr survival of 77%. Small studies have been performed using detachable snares and a combination of gastric variceal band ligation with transvenous occlusion of gastric varices *(29–31)*. The high success rate of these studies may reflect reporting bias. Such therapies cannot be recommended outside of clinical trials.

Splenectomy is curative in patients with isolated splenic vein thrombosis. The most popular surgical shunts are the distal splenorenal shunt and the calibrated portocaval shunt *(27,28)*. Surgical shunts should be carried out in patients with Child–Pugh class A status. TIPS is inserted in patients with more advanced liver disease (Child's class B or C) as a bridge to transplantation and also in patients with advanced liver disease who are not liver transplant candidates. Following TIPS, there is a reduction in episodes of gastric variceal bleeding even though the varices may continue to be visualized on endoscopy. If the patient is not a suitable candidate for portosystemic shunting, then nonselective β-adrenergic blockers may be used.

In general, there is a pressing need for more appropriate randomized, controlled trials to assess the efficacy of glue injection, TIPS, and surgical shunts for the management of gastric varices *(32)*.

PORTAL HYPERTENSIVE GASTROPATHY AND GASTRIC VASCULAR ECTASIA

The mucosal changes in the stomach of patients with portal hypertension include portal hypertensive gastropathy (PHG) and gastric vascular ectasia. It is not clear whether these lesions are related to portal hypertension *per se*, the hyperdynamic circulation, liver dysfunction, or a combination of factors. Response to TIPS and liver transplantation would suggest that portal hypertensive gastropathy is more related to portal hypertension, whereas vascular ectasia is related to liver failure.

The underlying mechanism of portal hypertensive gastropathy is unclear. PHG is more prevalent with longer duration of cirrhosis but does not correlate with the degree of hepatic synthetic dysfunction. It has been postulated that there is increased permeability of the gastric mucosal microvessels mediated by endothelin-1 *(33)*, overexpression of nitric oxide synthase *(34)*, and by increased oxidative stress in the gastric mucosa of cirrhotics *(35)*. Nitric oxide (NO) inhibition, in experimentally induced portal hypertension, has been associated with decreased gastric mucosal blood flow. NO overproduction in cirrhosis may then predispose the gastric mucosa to injury by free radicals *(36)*.

PHG is primarily an endoscopic diagnosis based on the presence of a mucosal mosaic-like pattern (MLP) and red-point lesions (RPLs). MLP is described as the presence of small polygonal areas with surrounding whitish-yellow depressed border. RPLs are round lesions usually > 2 mm in diameter that protrude slightly into the lumen of the stomach. Brown spots are irregularly shaped spots that persist even after washing but are not specific for PHG.

PHG may be graded according to the types of endoscopic lesions that are present. PHG is considered mild when only MLP of any degree is present (Fig. 2). Severe PHG is characterized by discrete red spots in association with a mosaic appearance of the background mucosa (Fig. 3) *(37–40)*. It is also worth noting that PHG is a dynamic process that may endoscopically progress or regress over time *(41,42)*. The presence of red spots on a background of mosaic pattern and in a predominantly proximal distribution favors PHG. In gastric vascular ectasia (GVE), there is no background mosaic pattern and the distribution is largely antral, though lesions may be present in the proximal stomach. Whether sclerotherapy results in an increased risk of bleeding from PHG is unclear. The presence of gastric varices has been inconsistently shown to be protective *(41,42)* of PHG-related bleeding.

GVE is a unique clinical entity with distinct endoscopic and histological features *(43, 44)*. It may be associated with PHG *(42)*. Endoscopically, GVE appear as aggregates of ectatic vessels confined to the antrum of the stomach [gastric vascular antral ectasia or (GAVE)], or diffusely distributed in the antrum or proximal stomach. When the aggregates are in a linear pattern in the gastric antrum they are also termed the watermelon stomach (Fig. 4). The histological presence of dilated mucosal capillaries with focal areas of fibrin thrombi or ectasia in conjunction with spindle cell proliferation favors a diagnosis of GVE. It should be noted that the endoscopic features correlate well with histology and, therefore, a biopsy is only needed if the endoscopic diagnosis is unclear.

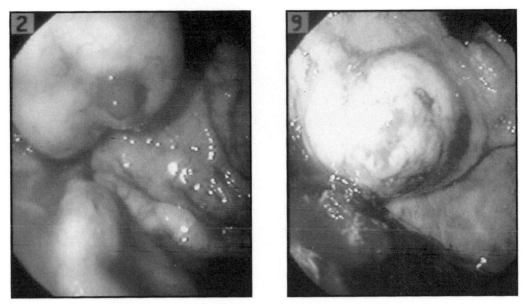

Fig. 2. Gastric varices. Actively bleeding gastric varix (left panel); the same gastric varix after injection of cyanoacrylate (right panel). (Illustration appears in color following p. 112.)

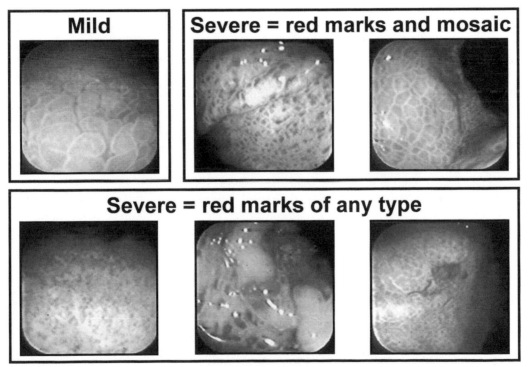

Fig. 3. Severity of portal hypertensive gastropathy. Mild portal hypertensive gastropathy represents endoscopic features of a mosaic-patterned mucosa in a patient with portal hypertension. Severe portal hypertensive gastropathy represents red marks on mucosa with a mosaic background, or red marks of any type. (Illustration appears in color following p. 112.)

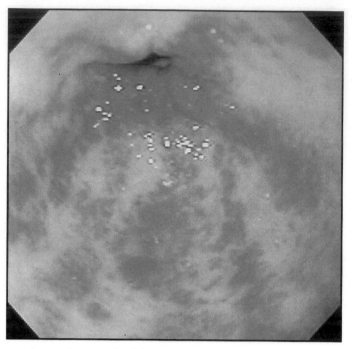

Fig. 4. Gastric antral vascular ectasia. Linear aggregates of ectatic vessels in the antrum of the stomach. (Illustration appears in color following p. 112.)

Management of Portal Hypertensive Gastropathy

The largest prospective study suggests that PHG accounts for 25.8% of all bleeding and for 9.8 % of all acute bleeding *(41)*. The prevalence of acute PHG-related bleeding may, however, be even higher *(42,45)*.

Octreotide has been used in the management of acute gastrointestinal bleeding related to PHG *(46)*. Iron therapy and β-adrenergic blockers are the initial therapies to control chronic blood loss in patients with severe PHG. β-Adrenergic blockers reduce gastric mucosal perfusion, in addition to reducing portal pressures and, therefore, probably decrease bleeding risk of PHG *(47)*. However, this has not been consistently shown by others *(41, 42,48–50)*. In contrast, TIPS, by effectively decompressing the portal system, has been shown to correct bleeding and cause regression of endoscopic changes associated with PHG *(51)*. TIPS should be considered for those patients who are transfusion dependent in spite of therapy with β-adrenergic blockers.

Management of Gastric Vascular Ectasia (Fig. 5)

The management of gastric vascular ectasia is more problematic. Iron replacement and blood transfusions are required for patients who become symptomatic from anemia. When the lesion is localized, the platelet count is greater than $45,000/\mu L$ and the INR < 1.4, and local thermoablative procedures, such as argon plasma coagulation (APC) may be helpful. APC is used at a setting of 65 W at 0.9 L/min gas flow. When neodymium: yttrium-aluminum-garnet (Nd:YAG) lasers are used, the setting is 50–60 W. If this fails, or if the lesion is diffuse, estrogen–progesterone combination therapy may be beneficial. Estrogen–progesterone combination has been shown to stop bleeding and reduce the

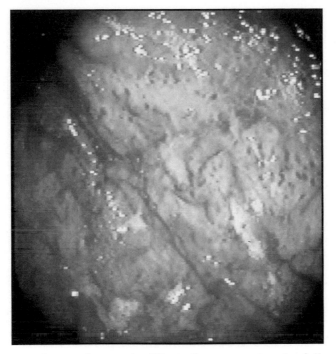

Fig. 5. Diffuse gastric vascular ectasia. (Illustration appears in color following p. 112.)

transfusion requirements in selected cirrhotic patients with GAVE *(52)*. Thermocoagulation is, unfortunately, associated with mucosal bleeding in many patients. Antral resection is carried out in patients with preserved hepatic synthetic function who are transfusion dependent and who have continued bleeding, in spite of thermal ablation therapy and estrogen–progesterone combination. TIPS does not reduce the bleeding risk in patients with GVE and is associated with a high risk of encephalopathy. Therefore, TIPS cannot be recommended as therapy for GVE. Reversal of GVE with liver transplantation even in the presence of persistent portal hypertension strongly suggests that GVE is related to liver failure *(53,54)*.

ECTOPIC VARICES

Ectopic varices refer to portosystemic venous collaterals that are located outside the esophagus and stomach. Ectopic varices account for 1–5% of all variceal related bleeding. Manifestation may be unusual, and include, hemoperitoneum, hemobilia, or hematuria. Collaterals are more apt to form in the duodenum and colon. The distribution of ectopic varies depend, in part, on the etiology of portal hypertension. Duodenal varices are more prevalent in cases of extrahepatic portal hypertension except in the western hemisphere where intrahepatic portal hypertension is a more common cause of duodenal varices. In addition, in the presence of intrahepatic portal hypertension, the most common site of bleeding from ectopic varices is duodenal varices. Duodenal varices form as a result of dilated pancreaticoduodenal veins which connect with retroduodenal veins draining into the inferior vena cava *(55,56)*. The clinical presentation is melena, hematochezia, or hematemesis in patients with portal hypertension in whom endoscopy has not

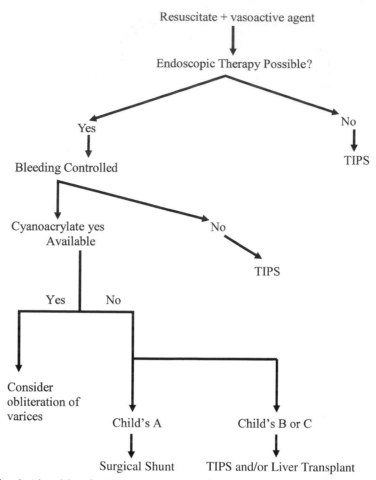

Fig. 6. Algorithm for the management of acute gastric variceal bleeding.

revealed a source of bleeding in the esophagus or stomach. Diagnosis is usually accomplished with endoscopy, but the problems with diagnosis arise from the concomitant presence of esophagogastric varices to which the bleeding may be erroneously attributed. Stomal varices represent collaterals around the bowel stoma in patients with portal hypertension *(57).* These varices result from venous–venous collaterals that form between the high-pressure portal system and the systemic circulation and usually develop at the level of the mucocutaneous border of the stoma. In addition to the obvious oozing of blood from the stoma, there is usually a bluish halo surrounding it.

Management of Bleeding from Ectopic Varices

There have been few studies done on the management of patients with ectopic variceal hemorrhage. The approach to management depends on the anatomic location of the source of bleeding.

Somatostatin and its analog, octreotide, may be used in the acute setting, as in cases of esophagogastric variceal hemorrhage. If a bleeding site is identified by endoscopy, then endoscopic management may be attempted. The results of treatment with sclerosants in

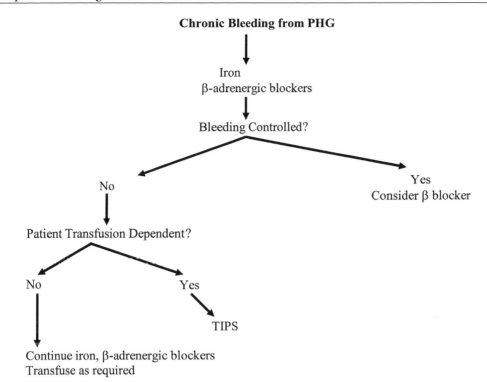

Fig. 7. Algorithm for the management of chronic bleeding from portal hypertensive gastropathy.

the duodenum have been varied, and this is most probably a result of the large varices in this area that dilute the sclerosants, thereby diminishing the obliterative effects. Obliteration with tissue adhesives has been successfully achieved by using cyanoacrylate or thrombin/sclerosant (55,58,59). Patients with bleeding stomal varices are easily managed with local compression if the site of bleeding is apparent by examining the stoma. The mortality rate from bleeding from stomal varices is low, 3–4%, compared with other types of varices (60). If local therapy fails, then transhepatic obliteration of the bleeding stomal varices or TIPS placement (61) may be undertaken.

There are limited data on the use of nonselective β-blockers for prevention of rebleeding from peristomal varices (62–65). Another approach to control bleeding is embolotherapy (65), but only when the portal venous system is patent. Embolization involves occlusion of the varices using a transhepatic approach to the portal venous system, and is able to control bleeding in most cases. Rebleeding is high because the portal system has not been decompressed. During embolotherapy the feeding vein is occluded by steel coils, thereby diverting blood into the systemic system. TIPS is also an option in these patients, if embolization fails to prevent rebleeding. Portosystemic shunting with surgery is the preferred route for patients with Childs–Pugh class A cirrhosis, and in those with portal hypertension from extrahepatic portal vein thrombosis who have a suitable vein for use in a portosystemic shunt. Only nonselective portosystemic shunting using portocaval, mesocaval or central splenorenal shunts will adequately decompress stomal varices.

The outcome of patients who bleed from intraabdominal varices has been dismal. These collaterals may bleed into the peritoneal cavity, mimicking worsening ascites. Diagno-

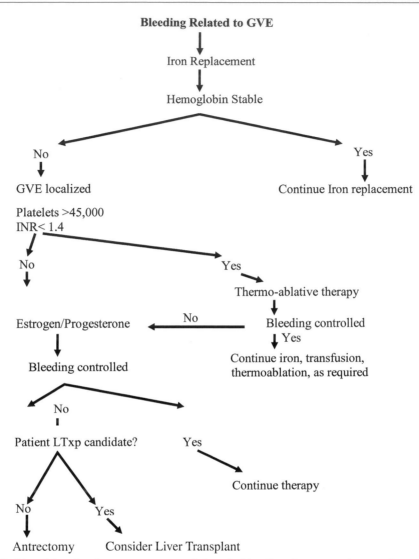

Fig. 8. Algorithm for the management of chronic bleeding from gastric vascular ectasia.

sis can be confirmed by paracentesis or cross-sectional imaging. Management of these patients is difficult and further compounded by the presence of cirrhosis. The aim of treatment is control of the acutely bleeding site by transhepatic obliteration of the varices, angiographic embolization, or surgical ligation of the bleeding varix. The latter procedure, however, has a high associated mortality and TIPS may then be an alternative.

SUMMARY

Management of bleeding from gastric varices, PHG, GVE, and ectopic varices has not been adequately addressed in randomized controlled trials. Our recommendations are summarized in Figs. 6–9. The management of bleeding gastric varices poses a dilemma for most clinicians since the armamentarium for treatment is limited. It appears that obliteration of gastric varices with tissue adhesives is safe and efficacious in the acute man-

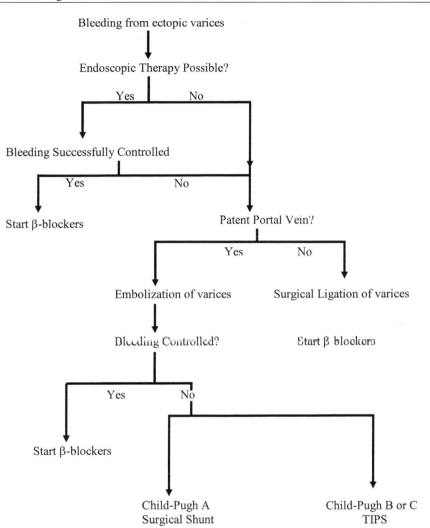

Fig. 9. Algorithm for the management of bleeding ectopic varices.

agement of gastric variceal hemorrhage. Prevention of rebleeding from gastric varices is best carried out with portosystemic shunts. PHG and GVE are in all likelihood distinct lesions, with only PHG responding to portal decompressive measures.

Although there are few studies done in the management of ectopic varices, recognition of this complication in patients who have portal hypertension is important, because this facilitates prompt therapy.

REFERENCES

1. Sarin SK, Lahoti D, Saxena SP, Murthi NS, Makwane UK. Revalence, classification and natural history of gastric varices: a long-term follow-up study in 568 portal hypertension patients. Hepatology 1992;16:1343–1349.
2. Hashizume M, Kitano S, Yamaga H, Koyanagi, Sugimachi K. Endoscopic classification and natural history of gastric varices: a long-term follow-up study in 568 portal hypertension patients. Hepatology 1992;16:1343–1349.

3. Korula J, Chink K, Ko Y, Yamada S. Demonstration of two distinct subsets of gastric varices. Observations during a seven-year study of endoscopic sclerotherapy. Dig Dis Sci 1991;36:303–309.

4. Siringo S, McCormick PA, Mistry P, et al. Prognostic significance of the white nipple sign in variceal bleeding. Gastrointest Endosc 1991;37:51–55.

5. Vlavianos P, Gimson AE, Westaby D, Williams R. Balloon tamponade in variceal bleeding: use and misuse. Br Med J 1989; 298:1158.

6. Soderlund C, et al. Terlipressin (triglycyl-lysine vasopressin) controls acute bleeding oesophageal varices. A double-blind, randomized, placebo-controlled trial. Scan J Gastroenterol 1990;25:622–630.

7. Levacher S, Letoumelin P, Pateron D, et al. Early administration of Terlipressin plus glyceryl trinitrate to control active upper gastrointestinal bleeding in cirrhotic patients. Lancet 1995;346:865–868.

8. Soehendra N, Grimm H, Nam VC, Berger B. N-butyl-2-cyanoacrylate: a supplement to endoscopic sclerotherapy. Endoscopy 1987;19(6):221–224.

9. Grimm H, Maydeo A, Noar M, et al. Bleeding esophagogastric varices: is endoscopic treatment with cyanoacrylate the final answer? Gastrointest Endosc 1991;37:275.

10. Ogawa K, Shinya I, Shimakawa T, Wagatsuma Y, Katsube A, Kajiwara T. Endoscopic variceal ligation and sclerotherapy. Clinical evaluation of endoscopic injection sclerotherapy using n-butyl-2-cyanoacrylate for gastric variceal bleeding. J Gastroenterol Hepatol 1999;14:245–250.

11. Dhiman R, Chawla Y, Taneja S, Biswas R, Sharma T, Dilawari J. Endoscopic sclerotherapy of gastric variceal bleeding with N-butyl-2-cyanoacrylate. J Clin Gastroenterol 2002;35:222–227.

12. Lo G, Lai K, Cheng J, Chen M, Chiang HT. A prospective, randomized trial of butyl cyanoacrylate injection versus band ligation in the management of bleeding gastric varices. Hepatology 2001;33: 1060–1064.

13. Sarin S, Jain AK, Jain M, Gupta R. A randomized controlled trial of cyanoacrylate versus alcohol injection in patients with isolated fundic varices. Am J Gastroenterol 2002;97:1010–1015.

14. Sarin S, Govil A, Jain A, et al. Prospective randomized trial of endoscopic sclerotherapy versus variceal band ligation for esophageal varices: influence on gastropathy, gastric varices and variceal hemorrhage. J Hepatol 1997;26:826–832.

15. Trudeau W, Prindville T. Endoscopic injection sclerosis in bleeding gastric varices. Gastrointest Endosc 1986;32:264–268.

16. Gimson AES, Westaby D, Williams R. Endoscopic sclerotherapy in the management of gastric variceal haemorrhage. J Hepatol 1991;13:274–278.

17. Chang KY, Wu CS, Chen PC. Prospective, randomized trial of hypertonic glucose water and sodium tetradecyl sulfate for gastric variceal bleeding in patients with advanced liver cirrhosis. Endoscopy 1996; 28:481–486.

18. Shiha G, El-Sayed SS. Gastric variceal ligation: a new technique. Gastrointest Endosc 1999;49:437–441.

19. Tripathi D, Therapondos G, Redhead DN, Madhavan KK, Hayes PC. The role of the transjugular intrahepatic portosystemic shunt (TIPSS) in the management of bleeding gastric varices: clinical and haemodynamic correlations. Gut 2002;51:270–274.

20. Barange K, Peron JM, Imani K, et al. Transjugular intrahepatic portosystemic shunt in the treatment of refractory bleeding from ruptured gastric varices. Hepatology 1999;30(5):1139–1143.

21. Stanley AJ, Jalan R, Ireland HM, Redhead DN, Bouchier IA, Hayes PC. A comparison between gastric and oesophageal variceal haemorrhage treated with transjugular intrahepatic portosystemic stent shunt (TIPSS). Aliment Pharmacol Ther 1997;11(1):171–176.

22. Chau T, Patch D, Chan YW, Nagral A, Dick R, Burroughs A. "Salvage" transjugular intrahepatic portosystemic shunts: gastric fundal compared with esophageal variceal bleeding. Gastroenterology 1998; 114:981–987.

23. Malinchoc M, Kamath PS, Gordon FD, Peine CJ, Rank J, ter Borg PCJ. A model to predict poor survival in patients undergoing transjugular intrahepatic portosystemic shunts. Hepatology 2000; 31:864–871.

24. Mahadeva S, Bellamy MC, Kessel D, Davies MH, Millson CE. Cost-effectiveness of N-butyl-2-cyanoacrylate (Histoacryl) glue injections versus transjugular intrahepatic portosystemic shunt in the management of acute gastric variceal bleeding. Am J Gastroenterol 2003;98:2688–2693.

25. Wu C-Y, Yeh H-Z, Chen G-H. Pharmacological efficacy in gastric variceal rebleeding and survival. J Clin Gastroenterol 2002;35 (2):127–132.

26. Greenwald B, Caldwell SH, Hespenheide E, et al. N-2-butyl-cyanoacrylate for bleeding gastric varices: a United States pilot study and cost analysis. Am J Gastroenterol 2003;98:1982–1988.

27. Sarfeh IJ, Rypins EB, Raiszadeh M, Milne N, Conroy R, Lyons KP. Serial measurement of portal hemodynamics after partial portal decompression. Surgery 1986;100:52–57.
28. Rypins E, Mason R, Conroy R, Sarfeh J. Predictability and maintenance of portal flow patterns after small-diameter portacaval H-grafts in man. Surgery 1986;200:706–710.
29. Lee MS, Cho JY, Cheon YK, et al. Use of detachable snares and elastic bands for endoscopic control of bleeding from large gastric varices. Gastrointest Endosc 2002;56(1):83–88.
30. Yoshida T, Harada T, Shigemitsu T, Takeo Y, Miyazaki S, Okita K. Endoscopic management of gastric varices using a detachable snare and simultaneous endoscopic sclerotherapy and O-ring ligation. J Gastroenterol Hepatol 1999;14:730–735.
31. Yoshida T, Hayashi N, Miyazaki S, et al. Endoscopic Ligation of gastric varices using a detachable snare. Endoscopy 1994;26:502–505.
32. de Franchis R. Updating consensus in portal hypertension: Report of the Baveno III Consensus Workshop on definitions, methodology and therapeutic strategies in portal hypertension. J Hepatol 2000;33: 846–852.
33. Migoh S, Hashizume M, Tsugawa K, Tanoue K, Sugimachi K. Mechanism and control of gastric mucosal injury and bleeding. J Gastroenterol Hepatol 2000;15:142–147.
34. Ohta M, Tanoue K, Tarnawski A, et al. Overexpressed nitric oxide synthase in portal hypertensive stomach of rat: a key to increased susceptibility to damage? Gastroenterology 1997;112:1920–1930.
35. Kawanaka H, Tomikawa M, Jones M, et al. Defective mitogen-activated protein kinase (ERK2) signalling in gastric mucosa of portal hypertensive rats: potential therapeutic implications. Hepatology 2001; 34:990–999.
36. Lemarque D, Whittle BJR. Role of oxygen-derived metabolites in the rat gastric mucosal injury induced by nitric oxide donors. Eur J Pharmacol 1995;277:187–194.
37. McCormack TT, Sims J, Eyre-Brook I, et al. Gastric lesion in portal hypertension: inflammatory gastritis or congestive gastropathy. Gut 1985;26:1226–1232.
38. Hashizume M, Sugimachi K. Classification of gastric lesions associated with portal hypertension. J Gastroenterol Hepatol 1995;10:339–343.
39. Spina GP, Arcidiacono R, Bosch J, et al. Gastric endoscopic features in portal hypertension: final report of a consensus conference, Milan, Italy, Sept. 19, 1992. J Hepatol 1994;21:461–467.
40. Sarin SK. Diagnostic issues: portal hypertensive gastropathy and gastric varices. In: DeFranchis R, ed. Portal Hypertension II. Proceedings of the Second Baveno International Consensus Workshop on Definitions, Methodology and Therapeutic Strategies. Blackwell Science, Oxford, UK, 1996, pp. 30–55.
41. Primignani M, Materia M, Preatoni P, et al. Natural history of portal hypertensive gastropathy in patients with liver cirrhosis. Gastroenterology 2000;119:181–187.
42. Stewart C, Sanyal A. Grading portal gastropathy: validation of a gastropathy scoring system. Am J Gastroenterol 2003;98:1758–1765.
43. Jabbari M, Cherry R, Lough JO, et al. Gastric antral vascular ectasia: the watermelon stomach. Gastroenterology 1984;87:1165–1170.
44. Payen JL, Cales P, Voigt JJ, et al. Severe portal hypertensive gastropathy and antral vascular ectasia are distinct entities in patients with cirrhosis. Gastroenterology 1995;108:138–144.
45. D'Amico G, Montalbano L, Traina M, et al. Natural history of congestive gastropathy in cirrhosis. Gastroenterology 1990;99:1558–1564.
46. Zhou Y, Qiao L, Wu J, Hu H, Xu C. Control of bleeding in portal hypertensive gastropathy. Comparison of the efficacy of octreotide, vasopressin, and omeprazole in the control of acute bleeding in patients with portal hypertensive gastropathy: a controlled study. J Gastroenterol Hepatol 2002;17:973–979.
47. Panes J, Bordas J, Pique J, et al. Effects of propranolol on gastric mucosal perfusion in cirrhotic patients with portal hypertensive gastropathy. Hepatology 1993;17:213–218.
48. Perez-Ayuso R, Pique J, Bosch J, et al. Propranolol in prevention of recurrent bleeding from severe portal hypertensive gastropathy in cirrhosis. Lancet 1991;337:1431–1434.
49. Sarin SK, Shahi H, Jain M, Jain A, Issar S, Murthy N. The natural history of portal hypertensive gastropathy: influence of variceal eradication. Am J Gastroenterol 2000;95:2888–2893.
50. Sarin SK, Sreenivas DV, Lahoti D, Saraya A. Factors influencing development of portal hypertensive gastropathy in patients with portal hypertension. Gastroenterology 1992;102:994–999.
51. Kamath PS, Lacerda M, Ahlquist D, McKusick M, Andrews J, Nagorney D. Gastric mucosal responses to intrahepatic portosystemic shunting in patients with cirrhosis. Gastroenterology 2000;118:905–911.

52. Tran A, Villeneuve J-P, Bilodeau M, et al. Treatment of chronic bleeding from gastric antral vascular ectasia (GAVE) with estrogen-progesterone in cirrhotic patients: an open pilot study. Am J Gastroenterol 1999;94:2909–2911.

53. Spahr L, Villeneuve JP, Dufresne MP, et al. Gastric antral ectasia in cirrhotic patients: absence of relation with portal hypertension. Gut 1999;44:739–742.

54. Vincent C, Pomier-Layrargues G, Dagenais M, et al. Cure of gastric antral vascular ectasia by liver transplantation despite persistent portal hypertension: a clue for pathogenesis. Liver Transplant 2002; 8(8):717–720.

55. Perchik L, Max TC. Massive hemorrhage from varices of the duodenal loop in a cirrhotic patient. Radiology 1963;80:641–644.

56. Itzchak Y, Glickman MG. Duodenal varices in extrahepatic portal obstruction. Radiology 1977;124: 619–624.

57. Weisner RH, LaRusso N, Dozois RR. Peristomal varices after proctocolectomy in patients with primary sclerosing cholangitis. Gastroenterology 1986;90:316–322.

58. Smith-Lang G, Scott J, Long RG, Sherlock S. Role of percutaneous transhepatic obliteration of varices in the management of hemorrhage from gastroesophageal varices. Gastroenterology 1981;80:1031–1036.

59. Vlamonte M, Pereiras R, Russel E, LePlage J, White P, Hudson D. Transhepatic obliteration of gastroesophageal varices in acute and non-acute bleeders. Am J Roentgenol 1977:129:237–241.

60. Ackerman NB, Graeber GM, Fey J. Enterostomal varices secondary to portal hypertension: progression of disease in conservatively managed cases. Arch Surg 1980;115:1454–145.

61. Ryu R, Nemack A, Chrisman H, Saker M, Blei A. Treatment of stomal variceal hemorrhage with TIPS: case report and review of the literature. Cardiovasc Intervent Radiol 2000; 23(4):301–303.

62. Burroughs AK, Jenkins WJ, Sherlock S, et al. Controlled trial of propranolol for the prevention of recurrent variceal hemorrhage in patients with cirrhosis. N Engl J Med 1983;309:1539–1542.

63. Lebrec D, Poynard T, Bernuau J, et al. A randomized controlled study of propranolol for prevention of recurrent gastrointestinal bleeding in patients with cirrhosis: a final report. Hepatology 1984;4:355–358.

64. Bernard B, Lebrec D, Mathurin P, Opolon P, Poynard T. Beta-adrenergic antagonists in the prevention of gastrointestinal re-bleeding in patients with cirrhosis: a meta-analysis. Hepatology 1997;25:63–70.

65. Widrich WC, Robbins AH, Nabseth DC. Transhepatic embolization of varices. Cardiovasc Intervent Radiol 1980;3:298–307.

V

NATURAL HISTORY AND TREATMENT OF ASCITES AND HEPATORENAL SYNDROME

Umbilical hernias develop in about 20% of cirrhotic patients with ascites (a rate significantly greater than 3% in patients without ascites) and may increase to up to 70% in patients with long-standing recurrent tense ascites *(6)*. The main risks of these hernias are rupture *(7)* and incarceration, a complication that has been observed mostly in patients in whom ascites is resolved after paracentesis or peritoneovenous shunt *(8)* or after transjugular intrahepatic portosystemic shunt *(9)*.

Pleural effusion (hepatic hydrothorax) develops in about 5% of patients with cirrhosis *(10)* and although it usually develops in patients with ascites, hepatic hydrothorax may develop in patients without detectable ascites *(11)*. Pleural effusion is right-sided in 85%, left-sided in 13%, and bilateral in 2% of the cases *(12)*.

In addition to symptoms associated to the presence of ascites, patients should be questioned regarding risk factors for cirrhosis, including alcohol consumption, risk factors for viral hepatitis C and B, family history of liver disease, risk factors for nonalcoholic steatohepatitis, and a previously diagnosed liver disease.

In patients who do not appear to have cirrhosis as the cause for ascites, history should be elicited to look for other causes. It is important to keep in mind that approx 5% of patients will have more than one cause of ascites, such as cirrhosis and heart failure, tuberculous peritonitis, or malignancy *(13)*.

Physical Examination

Patients in whom ascites is suspected based on their history should be examined to determine whether peritoneal fluid is, in fact, present and, if so, to determine the etiology of ascites.

FINDINGS DEPENDENT ON THE PRESENCE OF ASCITES

Physical examination is relatively insensitive for detecting ascitic fluid, particularly when the amount is small and/or the patient is obese. It is generally stated that patients must have at least 1500 mL of fluid to be detected reliably on physical examination. In a prospective study, ultrasound confirmed the presence of ascites in 82% (9/11) of cases in which physicians had determined that ascites was present and confirmed the absence of ascites in 94% (33/35) of cases in which physicians had determined that ascites was not present *(5)*. In 16 equivocal cases (26% of total), ascites was absent on ultrasound in 13 (81%), a rate that is similar to the one obtained in another small study of 21 patients with questionable ascites, 15 (71%) of whom did not have ascites on ultrasound *(14)*. Therefore, the clinical diagnosis of ascites will be questionable or incorrect in roughly a third of the cases.

INSPECTION

Ascites induces abdominal distention but this sign in itself has a poor specificity *(15)* because other conditions, including obesity, gas, tumors, and pregnancy will also induce abdominal distention. In cirrhosis, gaseous distention may occur as a result of the use of lactulose. When present in smaller amounts, ascites can be identified by bulging flanks. There is often diastasis of the abdominal recti muscles and/or umbilical hernia, indicative of the presence or history of tense ascites.

PALPATION

The fluid wave sign has the poorest sensitivity in the diagnosis of peritoneal fluid, even though its specificity is high *(5,14,15)*. By the time a fluid wave can be elicited, ascites is usually massive and its presence is obvious. Identification of organomegaly or a mass within the ascitic abdomen can be difficult and should be explored by using the balloting method, by which one bounces ones fingers over the abdominal surface with a brief jabbing movement directly over the anticipated structure (e.g., if one is looking for hepatomegaly, balloting should be performed over the right upper quadrant). The presence of a ballotable liver is a good indicator of the presence of ascites *(5)*.

PERCUSSION

In the presence of bulging flanks, flank dullness should be elicited by percussing outward in several directions from a tympanitic area with the patient supine. The presence of flank dullness is one of the most sensitive physical maneuvers in the diagnosis of ascites, and its absence can rule out ascites with more than 90% accuracy *(14)*. When flank dullness is detected, it is useful to see whether it shifts with rotation of the patient (shifting dullness). In a large prospective study, shifting dullness was found to be the most sensitive finding (compared to abdominal distension, bulging flanks, and fluid wave) *(15)*. The puddle sign had been reported to detect as little as 120 mL of peritoneal fluid, however, it is cumbersome, patients find it uncomfortable, and its practice is no longer recommended *(16)*. In cases of abdominal distension from causes other than ascites, percussion will facilitate the differential diagnosis. When it is caused by gaseous distention, the abdomen will be tympanitic, in obesity percussion will be normal, a large solid tumor and pregnancy will yield a dull percussion in the center and tympany in the periphery (reverse of ascites).

AUSCULTATION

In a recent pilot study, bowel sound recordings through an electronic stethoscope showed that the bowel sound pattern distinctly separated patients with a small amount of ascites and patients without ascites, proposing this method as a diagnostic bedside method for the diagnosis of small volume ascites *(17)*. However, these preliminary results require validation and implementation of the method.

Findings Dependent on the Etiology of Ascites

The presence of ascites in a cirrhotic patient denotes a decompensated, more advanced cirrhosis; therefore, patients with ascites resulting from cirrhosis will usually have stigmata of cirrhosis on physical examination. These include spider angiomas (rare below the umbilicus), palmar erythema (most prominent on hypothenar and thenar eminence with sparing of center of palms), and muscle wasting (thenar, hypothenar, and bitemporal regions). There may also be jaundice and signs of portal hypertension such as splenomegaly and abdominal wall collaterals. Finding a palpable (or ballotable) left lobe of the liver (in the epigastric area) is almost pathognomonic of cirrhosis, whereas percussion of the right lobe of the liver usually shows a small liver span.

The neck veins should always be examined for jugular venous distention in patients with ascites to look for cardiac dysfunction as a cause (or at least one cause) of ascites. Presence of a small nodule at umbilicus (Sister Joseph Mary nodule) suggests peritoneal carcinomatosis and an enlarged supraclavicular lymph node (Virchow's node) also suggests malignancy. Large veins on the patients' back with an upward flow suggests inferior vena cava (IVC) blockage. Peripheral edema owing to liver disease is usually confined to lower extremities. Anasarca may be noted in nephritic and cardiac patients.

DIAGNOSIS

Diagnostic tests can be divided into those that have the objective of confirming a clinical suspicion of ascites and tests that look for the etiology of ascites.

Confirmation of the Presence of Ascites by Imaging Techniques

The initial, most cost effective, and least invasive method to confirm the presence of ascites is *abdominal ultrasonography*. It is considered the gold standard for diagnosing ascites as it can detect amounts as small as 100 mL *(18)* and even as small as 1–2 mL when Morison's pouch and the pelvic cul-de-sac are scanned *(19)*. Abdominal ultrasound is useful in determining the best site to perform a diagnostic or therapeutic paracentesis, particularly in patients with a small amount of ascites or in those with loculated ascites. Additionally, although not very sensitive in the diagnosis of cirrhosis, ultrasound is the most useful initial test to investigate the presence of hepatic vein obstruction, an important and frequently overlooked cause of ascites *(19)*. Therefore, in patients with new ascites, abdominal ultrasound should always include Doppler examination of the hepatic veins.

Abdominal *computed tomography (CAT) scan* is also highly sensitive and specific in diagnosing the presence of intraabdominal fluid; however, its cost precludes it as a first diagnostic method to confirm the presence of ascites. Abdominal CAT scan is more sensitive than ultrasonography in determining the presence of cirrhosis. Finding a small, nodular liver, splenomegaly, and collaterals on CAT scan establishes the diagnosis of cirrhosis.

Although not a confirmatory test for the presence of ascites, *diagnostic radionuclide ascites scan* is useful in the diagnosis of hepatic hydrothorax, particularly in cases in which ascites is absent *(20)*. It consists of the injection of Tc-99m-labeled sulfur colloid *(21)* or macroaggregated serum albumin *(20)* into the peritoneal cavity followed by chest imaging every 15–30 min. Transdiaphragmatic movement of ascites into the pleural space is demonstrated generally within 2 h of intraperitoneal injection of the radiotracer.

Determination of the Etiology of Ascites

Although the above-mentioned imaging studies, in addition to confirming the presence of ascites, may help determine the cause of ascites, the simplest and most inexpensive way to orient the diagnostic workup of a patient with ascites is by the analysis of the fluid. Therefore, a diagnostic paracentesis should be the first test performed in the diagnostic workup of a patient with ascites.

DIAGNOSTIC PARACENTESIS

Performed for two purposes: (a) to help determine the most likely source of ascites and (b) to make the diagnosis of spontaneous bacterial peritonitis (SBP), the most lethal complication of cirrhotic ascites.

Indications. In accordance to the Ascites Club consensus recommendations *(22)*, a diagnostic paracentesis should be performed in

- all patients with new onset or worsening ascites;
- all patients with known ascites who are admitted to the hospital (to exclude a subclinical infection of ascites);
- patients showing clinical features or laboratory abnormalities suggestive of infection (fever, abdominal pain, abdominal tenderness, altered mental status, renal failure, peripheral leucocytosis, or acidosis).

Complications. Diagnostic paracentesis is a safe procedure with a very low incidence of serious complications. In a large prospective study of 229 diagnostic paracenteses performed using a 22-gauge needle, the most serious complication was transfusion-requiring wall hematoma that occurred in only two paracenteses (0.9%) performed in a single patient who had a prolonged prothrombin time (>6 s) and a creatinine of 2.3 mg/dL *(23)*. In addition, there were two nontransfusion-requiring hematomas and 22 instances of blood-tinged fluid. No paracentesis led to infection or death. In another large retrospective study, including 391 paracentesis (using 18–20-gauge needles), 3% of the cases had a postprocedure drop in hemoglobin ≥2 g/dL but only 0.2% required blood transfusion and none died *(24)*. Interestingly, this study showed that elevated creatinine levels were associated with a significantly greater hemoglobin drop.

Contraindications. Coagulopathy is not a contraindication to perform a diagnostic paracentesis. In the above-mentioned studies, there were no differences in prothrombin time or in platelet count between patients whose paracentesis resulted in bloody ascites or hematomas and those that did not *(23)*. Conversely, postprocedure changes in hemoglobin were comparable among patients with differing degrees of abnormality in prothrombin time (from normal to >2 s prolonged) and in platelet count (from >100,000 to <20,000/mm^3); however, patients with creatinine levels ≥6 mg/dL had a significantly greater postprocedure drop in hemoglobin level compared to those with lower levels *(24)*.

Paracentesis should probably be avoided in patients with clinically evident severe coagulopathy and renal failure. Because bleeding is the only complication of paracentesis, care should be taken to identify venous structures at the time of the performance of the procedure, irrespective of site. Care should always be taken to avoid abdominal wall collaterals and to avoid the area of the inferior hypogastric artery, which lies midway between anterior superior iliac spine and pubic tubercle. Technically, the midline below the umbilicus is often recommended as a site for paracentesis because of its presumed avascularity. However, a laparoscopic study in 20 patients with cirrhosis demonstrated that, in patients with portal hypertension, this area is commonly vascular *(25)*.

ASCITIC FLUID ANALYSIS

For diagnostic paracentesis, 20–50 cm^3 of ascitic fluid is obtained. In patients with new onset ascites, the fluid should be routinely be evaluated for

- gross appearance;
- albumin (with simultaneous estimation of serum albumin);
- total protein;
- white blood cell count and differential;
- cultures.

The following tests should be performed depending on individual circumstances

- glucose and lactic dehydrogenase (if secondary peritonitis is suspected) *(26)*;
- amylase (if pancreatic ascites is suspected);
- cytology (to exclude malignant ascites);
- acid-fast bacilli smear and culture and adenosine deaminase determination *(27)* (to exclude peritoneal tuberculosis);
- triglycerides (if the fluid has a milky appearance, i.e., chylous ascites);
- red blood cell count in cases in which the appearance of the fluid is unusually bloody.

Measurement of ascites lactate and pH were thought to be useful in the rapid diagnosis of SBP, however, several studies have demonstrated that these tests are not more useful than the ascites polymorphonuclear cell count (PMN) *(28)* and should therefore not be performed.

Gross Appearance. Uncomplicated "normal" ascitic fluid is transparent, straw colored to slightly yellow. It has been stated that fluids with PMN >5000/mm^3 appear cloudy *(3)*. Ascitic fluid with a red blood cell count of >10,000/mm^3 appears pink whereas fluid with red cell count >20,000/mm^3 appears frankly bloody *(3)*. Whereas blood in the fluid resulting from a traumatic tap will clot, nontraumatic bloody fluid will not clot as the blood has already clotted (intraperitoneally) and the clot has lysed. The presence of blood in a nontraumatic tap may indicate malignancy. Milky fluid is indicative of chylous ascites and its presence should be confirmed by measuring triglyceride levels in the fluid (a triglyceride level >200 mg/dL establishes the diagnosis of chylous ascites). An easier way to do this is to place a tube of ascites in the refrigerator, and in case of chylous ascites, it will layer out. Although the most common cause of chylous ascites is postsurgical disruption of lymphatics, the most common cause of nonsurgical chylous ascites is cirrhosis *(29,30)*.

Ascites Total Protein and Serum Ascites Albumin Gradient (SAAG). These two inexpensive tests taken *together* are the most useful in determining the etiology of ascites and, thereby, in further directing the workup of patients with ascites.

Conventionally, ascites had been divided into exudative and transudative based on its *total protein content*, using a cutoff protein of 2.5 g/dL *(31)*. It was considered that ascites secondary to peritoneal processes (malignancy, tuberculosis) would be exudates (protein >2.5 g/dL) whereas ascites secondary to nonperitoneal infiltration, that is, ascites associated with portal hypertension, would be transudates (ascites protein <2.5 g/dL). The characteristic ascitic fluid in patients with peritoneal neoplasms or tuberculous peritonitis is high in protein (exudative) and probably arises from leakage of high protein mesenteric lymph from obliterated lymphatics and perhaps also from surrounding inflamed peritoneal surface *(32)*. However, a high protein fluid can also result from hepatic sinusoidal hypertension when sinusoids are normal. Normal hepatic sinusoids are uniquely permeable ("leaky") and many human and experimental studies have shown that hepatic congestion secondary to hepatic vein or inferior vena caval obstruction or cardiac failure leads to profuse outpouring of protein-rich lymph into the peritoneal cavity *(33,34)*. In hepatic cirrhosis, an abnormally low protein content of liver lymph has been demonstrated as an effect of deposition of fibrous tissue in the sinusoids ("capillarization of the sinusoid") that renders the sinusoid less leaky to macromolecules *(35,36)*. However, it has been shown that, in early cirrhosis, ascitic fluid is high in protein, whereas in advanced cirrhosis, protein content decreases progressively *(37)*, perhaps as the result of progressive sinusoidal alteration. This could explain high protein ascites observed in 15–20% of cirrhotic patients. Additionally, ascites protein content has been shown to increase to exudative values after diuresis and a decrease in ascites volume *(38)*.

The *SAAG* is based on the fact that, per Starling forces, oncotic-hydrostatic balance is the major controlling force determining the protein concentration of fluid in the peritoneal cavity. Calculating the SAAG involves measuring the albumin concentration of serum and ascitic fluid specimens and subtracting the ascitic fluid value from the serum value. Two studies have demonstrated that SAAG is a reflection of the hepatic sinusoidal pressure. In one study, performed in 56 patients with chronic liver disease, a significant correlation ($r = 0.73$) was found between SAAG and the hepatic venous pressure gradient (HVPG) (a measure of sinusoidal hydrostatic pressure) *(39)*. In another study, a significant correlation ($r = 0.88$) was once more reported between the HVPG and the difference between plasma colloidosmotic pressure and ascites colloidosmotic pressure in 20 patients with cirrhosis *(40)*. As colloidosmotic pressure is mostly the result of albumin content, this could be translated as the SAAG. In a subsequent study, the cutoff value that best distinguished patients in whom ascites was secondary to liver disease and those with malignant neoplasm was a SAAG of 1.1 g/dL *(41)*. Interestingly, the SAAG value of 1.1 g/dL roughly corresponds to an HVPG of 11–12 mmHg *(39)*, the threshold pressure that has been described as being necessary for the development of ascites in cirrhotic patients (see below).

Several studies have demonstrated that the SAAG has a greater diagnostic accuracy than ascites protein levels in distinguishing cirrhotic ascites from ascites secondary to peritoneal carcinomatosis *(13,42,43)*. In patients with mixed ascites (e.g., cirrhosis with superimposed peritoneal malignancy), the SAAG is high and the ascites protein is low, that is, the findings of ascites due to cirrhosis predominate *(13)*. Of note, massive hepatic metastasis can lead to the development of ascites but because the mechanism of ascites formation is sinusoidal hypertension, these cases of "malignant ascites" will have a high SAAG *(43)*.

The SAAG, however, does not allow to distinguish intrahepatic causes (e.g., cirrhosis) from posthepatic causes of ascites (e.g., heart failure, Budd–Chiari) because, in both instances, SAAG will be high *(13)*. This differential is extremely important as constrictive pericarditis is one of the few curable causes of ascites and the distinction between cardiac or hepatic origin of ascites is especially important in alcoholic patients, with significant management implications. The ascites total protein content can make this distinction because, unlike the "capillarized" sinusoids of intrahepatic portal hypertension, the sinusoids of posthepatic obstruction are normal ("leaky" to protein). In the largest study comparing total protein and SAAG, all 24 samples obtained from patients with cardiac ascites had a SAAG > 1.1 g/dL (indicative of portal hypertensive type of ascites) and an ascites protein >2.5 g/dL (indicative of a normal "leaky" hepatic sinusoid) *(13)*.

Therefore, as shown in the Fig. 1, the three main causes of ascites—cirrhosis, peritoneal pathology (malignancy or tuberculosis), and heart failure—can be easily distinguished by combining the results of both the SAAG and ascites total protein content.

The accuracy of SAAG is reduced if samples are not obtained simultaneously or if serum albumin levels are very low. Serum hyperglobulinemia (>5 g/dL) leads to a high ascitic fluid globulin concentration and can narrow the albumin gradient by contributing to the oncotic forces. To correct the SAAG in the setting of a high serum globulin level, the uncorrected SAAG should be multiplied by $(0.16) \times$ (serum globulin [in g/dL] + 2.5) *(44)*.

Cell Count and Differential. Spontaneous bacterial peritonitis (SBP) is the most common infection in cirrhosis. Peritoneal infection leads to an inflammatory reaction that results in increased ascites PMN. Despite the use of sensitive methods, ascites culture is negative in approx 40% of patients with clinical manifestations suggestive of SBP and increased ascites PMN *(22)*. Therefore, the diagnosis of SBP is established when objective evidence of a local inflammatory reaction is present, i.e., an elevated ascites PMN count. A PMN count of more than 250/mm^3 is diagnostic of SBP and constitutes an indication to empirically initiate antibiotic treatment. Although an ascitic fluid PMN count greater than 500/mm^3 is more specific for the diagnosis of SBP *(28)*, the risk of not treating the few patients with SBP who have an ascites PMN count between 250 and

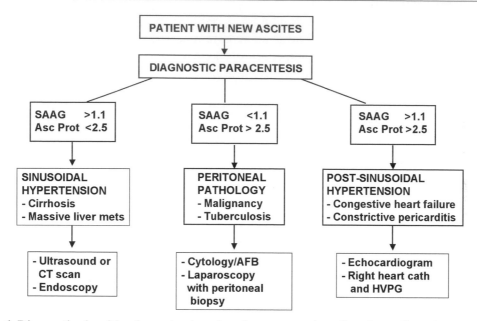

Fig. 1. Diagnostic algorithm for ascites based on the serum-ascites albumin gradient (SAAG) and the ascites total protein (Asc Prot). The most common cause of ascites is cirrhosis that will result in a high SAAG and a low ascites protein. Further workup in these patients will be an ultrasound or CAT scan (to confirm the diagnosis of cirrhosis and to screen for liver tumors) and an endoscopy (to screen for varices). Peritoneal malignancy or tuberculosis will result in a low SAAG and a high ascites protein. While awaiting for cytology and/or AFB results, a laparoscopy would be the next diagnostic procedure. Posthepatic obstruction (as would be seen in heart failure, constrictive pericarditis, posttransplant ascites) will result in a high SAAG and a high ascites protein. The workup will commonly include right heart catheterization and HVPG measurements, which is the ultimate test to determine the source of ascites.

$500/mm^3$ is unacceptable. An ascites PMN count of less than $250/mm^3$ excludes the diagnosis of SBP. In patients with hemorrhagic ascites (i.e., ascites RBC count >10,000/mm^3), a subtraction of one PMN per 250 red blood cells should be made to adjust for the presence of blood in ascites.

PMN count is performed manually in most laboratories and may not be available in all hospitals after hours. An alternative to manual counting proposed recently is the use of reactive strips for leukocyte esterase (45). A reagent strip result of 3 or 4 had a sensitivity of 89% (it correctly identified 51 of 57 fluids with PMN > 250, therefore, six patients with SBP would have not been treated) and a specificity of 99% (it correctly identified 170 of 171 fluids with PMN < 250, therefore, one patient not requiring therapy would have been treated). Importantly, a reagent strip of 3+ or 4+ had a positive predictive value of 98% (46/47 cases had a PMN > 250). Unfortunately, United States regulations mandate that only authorized, credentialed personnel can perform this test, and therefore a clinician at the bedside cannot currently perform this test (46).

Bacteriological Culture. Ascites samples for culture should be collected at the bedside and inoculated into blood culture bottles, including both aerobic and anaerobic media as this method is more likely to yield an infecting organism compared to samples that are centrifuged and plated *(47,48)*. The minimum amount of ascitic fluid inoculated in each bottle should be 10 mL. Because bacteremia occurs in half of the patients with SBP *(28)*, blood cultures should be obtained concomitant to ascites cultures in patients in whom SBP is suspected and before initiating antibiotic administration.

HVPG MEASUREMENT

Similar to the development of gastroesophageal varices, in which a minimal portal pressure gradient of 12 mmHg is necessary *(49)*, the development of ascites also requires surpassing a threshold HVPG. In one study, every patient with ascites had an HVPG (a measure of sinusoidal pressure) of at least 12 mmHg *(50)*. Another study showed that in most patients that developed ascites as the result of TIPS dysfunction, the portal pressure gradient had risen to levels ≥ 12 mmHg *(51)*. Importantly, studies in which the HVPG is reduced below 12 mmHg or at least 20% from baseline values, show a decrease in the development of ascites *(52,53)*. In the early stages of cirrhosis, there may not be sinusoidal hypertension (i.e., the HVPG is normal at 3–6 mmHg) or there may not be a "clinically" significant portal hypertension, i.e., the sinusoidal pressure may not have reached the threshold level of 12 mmHg, and, therefore, ascites would not be formed.

Therefore, the ultimate test to determine whether ascites is the result of sinusoidal hypertension, is to actually perform measurements of HVPG. In cases of cirrhotic ascites, the HVPG will be ≥ 12 mmHg. In cases of cardiac ascites, both the wedged hepatic vein pressure (WHVP) and the free hepatic vein pressure (FHVP) will be elevated (reflecting elevated systemic pressures) and, therefore, the HVPG which is obtained by subtracting the FHVP from the WHVP will be normal *(54)*. In cases of peritoneal ascites (i.e., malignancy or tuberculosis), all hepatic venous pressure measurements (WHVP, FHVP, and HVPG) will be normal, unless the patient has coexisting cirrhosis or heart failure. When performed properly, HVPG measurements are reproducible and safe *(55)*, in fact, hepatic vein catheterization for measurement of hepatic vein pressures allows for the performance, in the same procedure, of a transjugular liver biopsy which will further define the etiology of ascites *(56,57)*.

NATURAL HISTORY

Patients with compensated cirrhosis, that is, those without ascites, variceal hemorrhage, hepatic encephalopathy, or jaundice develop features of decompensation during follow-up at a rate of 7–10% per year, and ascites is the first sign of decompensation in most cases *(1,2)*. Ascites that marks the transition to decompensation refers to ascites that is clinically detectable. With the routine use of abdominal ultrasound in cirrhosis, ascites has been detected at an earlier stage. In fact, a current consensus document classifies ascites in three grades *(58)*:

- *Grade 1*: mild ascites only detectable by ultrasound examination.
- *Grade 2*: moderate ascites manifested by moderate symmetrical distension of abdomen.
- *Grade 3*: large or gross ascites with marked abdominal distension.

Most patients have "uncomplicated" ascites, that is, ascites that is not infected, is not associated with renal dysfunction and responds to diuretic therapy. Around 5–10% of patients with ascites develop refractory ascites, defined as ascites that cannot be mobilized or the early recurrence of which cannot be satisfactorily prevented by medical therapy *(59)*. Refractory ascites assumes either diuretic-resistant ascites (ascites not eliminated even with maximal diuretic therapy) or diuretic-intractable ascites (ascites not eliminated because maximal doses of diuretics cannot be reached given the development of renal and/or electrolyte abnormalities) *(59)*. The hepatorenal syndrome (HRS) is considered part of the clinical spectrum of the cirrhotic patient with ascites because it represents the result of extreme hemodynamic alterations that lead to sodium retention and ascites *(60)*. HRS generally occurs in patients with cirrhosis and ascites and is defined as renal failure occurring in the setting of severe liver disease after exclusion of potentially reversible causes of renal failure (sepsis, hypovolemia, nephrotoxicity) and that does not reverse after volume expansion. HRS may be classified on a clinical basis into two types: HRS type 1, characterized by rapidly progressive deterioration in renal function (doubling in serum creatinine to a level >2.5 g/dL in < 2 wk) and HRS type 2 in which renal failure does not have a rapidly progressive course *(59)*. Patients usually go through a sequence of uncomplicated ascites → refractory ascites → HRS type 2 → HRS type 1, each representing a more advanced stage with a worse prognosis.

Although median survival in patients with compensated cirrhosis is around 9 yr *(2)*, once decompensation occurs, median survival decreases to 1.6–1.8 yr *(1,2)*. In cirrhotic patients with moderate to tense ascites, four parameters have been found to be independent predictors of survival: impaired water excretion, mean arterial pressure, Child–Pugh class, and serum creatinine *(61)*. Except for the Child–Pugh score, which is indicative of a poor liver function, all other parameters indicate a worsened hemodynamic status (that is a more vasodilated state) and are consistent with other studies that have shown that hyponatremia and renal dysfunction are predictors of a poor survival in cirrhosis *(62,63)*.

Prognosis is worse in patients who develop refractory ascites. In a study of 134 outpatients with cirrhosis, the median survival of patients with refractory ascites was 12 mo, significantly lower than 52 mo in patients with uncomplicated ascites *(64)*. In two large prospective studies of different therapies for refractory ascites, median survival was 9 *(65)* and 12 mo *(66)*. Oddly, a higher median survival of around 40 mo was shown in another prospective trial of refractory ascites that included patients with a seemingly more preserved renal function *(67)*. Child–Pugh score is consistently a poor prognostic factor in patients with refractory ascites *(64,65,68)*. Although different therapies for refractory ascites have not been shown to have an effect on survival *(65–67)*, a factor that has been associated with a poorer survival is the development of the "postparacentesis circulatory dysfunction" (PCD), an entity associated with the performance of large-volume paracentesis, the recommended treatment for refractory ascites, particularly when plasma expansion with albumin does not accompany the procedure. Patients with refractory ascites who develop PCD have a median survival of 9 mo compared to 17 mo in patients who do not develop it *(69,70)*.

Of all the complications of cirrhosis, HRS has the worst prognosis. The main determinant of survival is the type of HRS. In type 1, hospital survival is less than 10% and the expected median survival time is only 2 wk *(71)*. In contrast, patients with HRS type 2 have a longer median survival of around 6 mo *(72)*, although still lower than that for refractory ascites.

ASCITES AFTER LIVER TRANSPLANTATION

The presence of self-limited ascites in small to moderate amounts is common in the early postoperative period of liver transplantation and is probably the result of surgical manipulation *(73)*. In contrast, large, persistent ascites, although uncommon after liver transplantation, usually represents a serious complication.

The incidence of significant posttransplantation ascites ranges from 2% *(74)* to 7% *(75)*.

A large study comparing 25 patients who developed significant ascites (defined as production of >500 mL/d lasting for >10 d after transplant) vs 353 patients who did not develop this complication, revealed no differences in the etiology of liver disease that led to transplantation nor in preoperative presence of ascites or SBP, there were also no differences in donor age or cold ischemia time. The factors that differed between groups were recipient gender (88 male vs 60% female) and surgical technique (IVC preservation with piggyback technique, 72 vs 41%) *(75)*.

In the majority of cases of significant posttransplant ascites, a high-pressure gradient between the right atrial pressure and: (a) the WHVP *(75)*; (b) the FHVP *(75)*; and (c) the PVP *(76)* have been described. Given the presence of a normal HVPG *(75)*, this gradient indicates the presence of a postsinusoidal hypertension secondary to hepatic vein outflow obstruction as the cause of ascites. Accordingly, ascitic fluid findings have been shown to be consistent with a posthepatic cause of ascites, that is, with a high total protein (>2.5 g/dL) *(75)* and a high SAAG (mean 2.8 g/dL) *(76)*.

Ascites occurs more frequently in patients in whom liver transplantion is performed preserving the retrohepatic IVC, the so-called piggyback technique, that is becoming more frequently used because it avoids caval cross-clamping during the anhepatic phase of surgery but can lead more frequently to anastomotic stenosis *(75,77,78)*. Modification of the technique utilizing the recipient's three hepatic veins (rather than two), stenting of the hepatic venous outflow tract and transjugular intrahepatic portosystemic shunt have been used to overcome outflow drainage difficulties and improve ascites in the majority of cases *(75,78,79)*.

Other less common causes of significant posttransplant ascites are reduced grafts (in pediatric transplantation) *(80)*, lymphatic leak after surgical dissection resulting in chylous ascites *(81,82)* that has been shown to respond to octreotide and total parenteral nutrition *(82)*, and venoocclusive disease probably resulting from acute rejection *(83–85)* that has been shown to respond to defibrotide *(86)*.

The development of significant posttransplant ascites has been associated with renal impairment, increased incidence of abdominal infection, prolonged hospitalization, and a tendency toward reduced survival *(75,87)*.

Therefore, significant posttransplant ascites is associated with increased morbidity and mortality. Because it is predominantly related to difficulties of hepatic venous drainage, measurement of hepatic vein and atrial pressures to detect a significant gradient and correct possible alterations in hepatic vein outflow should be the first approach in the management of these patients *(75)*.

REFERENCES

1. D'Amico G, Morabito A, Pagliaro L, Marubini E. Survival and prognostic indicators in compensated and decompensated cirrhosis. Dig Dis Sci 1986;31(5):468–475.
2. Gines P, Quintero E, Arroyo V. Compensated cirrhosis: natural history and prognosis. Hepatology 1987; 7:122–128.
3. Runyon BA. Ascites. In: Schiff L, Schiff ER, eds. Diseases of the Liver. Lippincott, Philadelphia, PA, 1993, pp. 990–1015.
4. Fabregues F, Balasch J, Gines P, et al. Ascites and liver test abnormalities during severe ovarian hyperstimulation syndrome. Am J Gastroenterol 1999;94(4):994–999.
5. Simel DL, Halvorsen RA Jr, Feussner JR. Quantitating bedside diagnosis: clinical evaluation of ascites. J Gen Intern Med 1988;3(5):423–428.

6. Belghiti J, Durand F. Abdominal wall hernias in the setting of cirrhosis. Semin Liver Dis 1997;17(3): 219–226.

7. Kirkpatrick S, Schubert T. Umbilical hernia rupture in cirrhotics with ascites. Dig Dis Sci 1988;33(6): 762–765.

8. Lemmer JH, Strodel WE, Eckhauser FE. Umbilical hernia incarceration: a complication of medical therapy of ascites. Am J Gastroenterol 1983;78(5):295–296.

9. Trotter JF, Suhocki PV. Incarceration of umbilical hernia following transjugular intrahepatic porto-systemic shunt for the treatment of ascites. Liver Transpl Surg 1999;5(3):209–210.

10. Lieberman FL, Hidemura R, Peters RL, Reynolds TB. Pathogenesis and treatment of hydrothorax complicating cirrhosis with ascites. Ann Intern Med 1966;64(2):341–351.

11. Rubinstein D, McInnes IE, Dudley FJ. Hepatic hydrothorax in the absence of clinical ascites: diagnosis and management. Gastroenterology 1985;88(1 Pt 1):188–191.

12. Strauss RM, Boyer TD. Hepatic hydrothorax. Sem Liv Dis 1997;17:227–232.

13. Runyon BA, Montano AA, Akriviadis EA, Antillon MR, Irving MA, McHutchison JG. The serum-ascites albumin gradient is superior to the exudate-transudate concept in the differential diagnosis of ascites. Ann Intern Med 1992;117:215–220.

14. Cattau EL Jr, Benjamin SB, Knuff TE, Castell DO. The accuracy of the physical examination in the diagnosis of suspected ascites. JAMA 1982;247(8):1164–1166.

15. Cummings S, Papadakis M, Melnick J, Gooding GA, Tierney LM, Jr. The predictive value of physical examinations for ascites. West J Med 1985;142(5):633–636.

16. Williams JW Jr, Simel DL. The rational clinical examination. Does this patient have ascites? How to divine fluid in the abdomen. JAMA 1992;267(19):2645–2648.

17. Liatsos C, Hadjileontiadis LJ, Mavrogiannis C, Patch D, Panas SM, Burroughs AK. Bowel sounds analysis: a novel noninvasive method for diagnosis of small-volume ascites. Dig Dis Sci 2003;48(8): 1630–1636.

18. Goldberg BB, Goodman GA, Clearfield HR. Evaluation of ascites by ultrasound. Radiology 1970;96 (1):15–22.

19. Black M, Friedman AC. Ultrasound examination in the patient with ascites. Ann Intern Med 1989;110 (4):253–255.

20. Schuster DM, Mukundan S Jr, Small W, Fajman WA. The use of the diagnostic radionuclide ascites scan to facilitate treatment decisions for hepatic hydrothorax. Clin Nucl Med 1998;23(1):16–18.

21. Bhattacharya A, Mittal BR, Biswas T, et al. Radioisotope scintigraphy in the diagnosis of hepatic hydrothorax. J Gastroenterol Hepatol 2001;16(3):317–321.

22. Rimola A, Garcia-Tsao G, Navasa M, et al. Diagnosis, treatment and prophylaxis of spontaneous bacterial peritonitis: a consensus document. J Hepatol 2000;32:142–153.

23. Runyon BA. Management of adult patients with ascites caused by cirrhosis. Hepatology 1998;27(1): 264–272.

24. McVay PA, Toy PT. Lack of increased bleeding after paracentesis and thoracentesis in patients with mild coagulation abnormalities. Transfusion 1991;31(2):164–171.

25. Oelsner DH, Caldwell SH, Coles M, Driscoll CJ. Subumbilical midline vascularity of the abdominal wall in portal hypertension observed at laparoscopy. Gastrointest Endosc 1998;47(5):388–390.

26. Akriviadis EA, Runyon BA. Utility of an algorithm in differentiating spontaneous from secondary bacterial peritonitis. Gastroenterology 1990;98(1):127–133.

27. Dwivedi M, Misra SP, Misra V, Kumar R. Value of adenosine deaminase estimation in the diagnosis of tuberculous ascites. Am J Gastroenterol 1990;85(9):1123–1125.

28. Garcia-Tsao G. Spontaneous bacterial peritonitis. Gastro Clin North Am 1992;21(1):257–275.

29. Runyon BA, Akriviadis EA, Keyser AJ. The opacity of portal hypertension-related ascites correlates with the fluid's triglyceride concentration. Am J Clin Pathol 1991;96(1):142–143.

30. Rector WG Jr. Spontaneous chylous ascites of cirrhosis. J Clin Gastroenterol 1984;6(4):369–372.

31. Rovelstad RA, Bartholomew LG, Cain JC, McKenzie BF, Soule EH. Ascites. I. The value of examination of ascitic fluid and blood for lipids and for proteins by electrophoresis. Gastroenterology 1958; 34(3):436–451.

32. Hirabayashi K, Graham J. Genesis of ascites in ovarian cancer. Am J Obstet Gynecol 1970;106(4): 492–497.

33. Witte CL, Witte MH, Dumont AE, Frist J, Cole WR. Lymph protein in hepatic cirrhosis and experimental hepatic and portal venous hypertension. Ann Surg 1968;168(4):567–577.

34. Witte CL, Witte MH. The congested liver. In: Lautt WW, ed. Hepatic Circulation in Health and Disease. Raven, New York, 1981, pp. 307–323.

35. Dumont AE, Witte CL, Witte MH. Protein content of liver lymph in patients with portal hypertension secondary to hepatic cirrhosis. Lymphology 1975;8(4):111–113.

36. Henriksen JH, Horn T, Christoffersen P. The blood-lymph barrier in the liver. A review based on morphological and functional concepts of normal and cirrhotic liver. Liver 1984;4(4):221–232.

37. Witte CL, Witte MH, Cole WR, Chung YC, Bleisch VR, Dumont AE. Dual origin of ascites in hepatic cirrhosis. Surg Gynecol Obstet 1969;129(5):1027–1033.

38. Hoefs JC. Increase in ascites white blood cell and protein concentrations during diuresis in patients with chronic liver disease. Hepatology 1981;1(3):249–254.

39. Hoefs JC. Serum protein concentration and portal pressure determine the ascitic fluid protein concentration in patients with chronic liver disease. J Lab Clin Med 1983;102:260–273.

40. Henriksen JH. Colloid osmotic pressure in decompensated cirrhosis. A 'mirror image' of portal venous hypertension. Scand J Gastroenterol 1985;20(2):170–174.

41. Pare P, Talbot J, Hoefs JC. Serum-ascites albumin concentration gradient: a physiologic approach to the differential diagnosis of ascites. Gastroenterology 1983;85:240–244.

42. Rector WG Jr, Reynolds TB. Superiority of the serum-ascites albumin difference over the ascites total protein concentration in separation of "transudative" and "exudative" ascites. Am J Med 1984;77(1):83–85.

43. Albillos A, Cuervas-Mons V, Millan I, et al. Ascitic fluid polymorphonuclear cell count and serum to ascites albumin gradient in the diagnosis of bacterial peritonitis. Gastroenterology 1990;98(1):134–140.

44. Hoefs JC. Globulin correction of the albumin gradient: correlation with measured serum to ascites colloid osmotic pressure gradients. Hepatology 1992;16(2):396–403.

45. Castellote J, Lopez C, Gornals J, et al. Rapid diagnosis of spontaneous bacterial peritonitis by use of reagent strips. Hepatology 2003;37(4):893–896.

46. Runyon BA. Strips and tubes: improving the diagnosis of spontaneous bacterial peritonitis. Hepatology 2003;37:745–747.

47. Runyon BA, Canawati HN, Akriviadis EA. Optimization of ascitic fluid culture technique. Gastroenterology 1988;95(5):1351–1355.

48. Bobadilla M, Sifuentes J, Garcia-Tsao G. Improved method for bacteriological diagnosis of spontaneous bacterial peritonitis. J Clin Microbiol 1989;27:2145–2147.

49. Garcia-Tsao G, Groszmann RJ, Fisher RL, Conn HO, Atterbury CE, Glickman M. Portal pressure, presence of gastroesophageal varices and variceal bleeding. Hepatology 1985;5(3):419–424.

50. Morali GA, Sniderman KW, Deitel KM, et al. Is sinusoidal portal hypertension a necessary factor for the development of hepatic ascites? J Hepatol 1992;16:249–250.

51. Casado M, Bosch J, Garcia-Pagan JC, et al. Clinical events after transjugular intrahepatic portosystemic shunt: correlation with hemodynamic findings. Gastroenterology 1998;114:1296–1303.

52. Villanueva C, Minana J, Ortiz J, et al. Endoscopic ligation compared with combined treatment with nadolol and isosorbide mononitrate to prevent recurrent variceal bleeding. N Engl J Med 2001;345:647–655.

53. Abraldes JG, Tarantino I, Turnes J, Garcia-Pagan JC, Rodes J, Bosch J. Hemodynamic response to pharmacological treatment of portal hypertension and long-term prognosis of cirrhosis. Hepatology 2003;37(4):902–908.

54. Myers RP, Cerini R, Sayegh R, et al. Cardiac hepatopathy: clinical, hemodynamic, and histologic characteristics and correlations. Hepatology 2003;37(2):393–400.

55. Groszmann RJ, Wongcharatrawee S. The hepatic venous pressure gradient: anything worth doing should be done right. Hepatology 2004;39(2):280–283.

56. Colapinto RF. Transjugular biopsy of the liver. Clin Gastroenterol 1985;14:451–467.

57. Trejo R, Alvarez W, Garcia-Pagan JC, et al. The applicability and diagnostic effectiveness of transjugular liver biopsy. Medicina Clinica 1996;107:521–523.

58. Moore KP, Wong F, Gines P, et al. The management of ascites in cirrhosis: report on the consensus conference of the International Ascites Club. Hepatology 2003;38(1):258–266.

59. Arroyo V, Gines P, Gerbes AL, et al. Definition and diagnostic criteria of refractory ascites and hepatorenal syndrome in cirrhosis. Hepatology 1996;23:164–176.

60. Schrier RW, Arroyo V, Bernardi M, Epstein M, Henriksen JH, Rodes J. Peripheral arterial vasodilation hypothesis—A proposal for the initiation of renal sodium and water retention in cirrhosis. Hepatology 1988;8:1151–1157.

61. Fernandez-Esparrach G, Sanchez-Fueyo A, Gines P, et al. A prognostic model for predicting survival in cirrhosis with ascites. J Hepatol 2001;34(1):46–52.

62. Arroyo V, Rodes J, Gutierrez Lizarraga MA, Revert L. Prognostic value of spontaneous hyponatremia in cirrhosis with ascites. Am J Dig Dis 1976;21:249–256.

63. Llach J, Gines P, Arroyo V, et al. Prognostic value of arterial pressure, endogenous vasoactive systems, and renal function in cirrhotic patients admitted to the hospital for the treatment of ascites. Gastroenterology 1988;94:482–487.

64. Salerno F, Borroni G, Moser P, et al. Survival and prognostic factors of cirrhotic patients with ascites: a study of 134 outpatients. Am J Gastroenterol 1993;88:514–519.

65. Gines P, Uriz J, Calahorra B, et al. Transjugular intrahepatic portosystemic shunting versus repeated paracentesis plus intravenous albumin for refractory ascites in cirrhosis: a multicenter randomized comparative study. Gastroenterology 2002;123:1839–1847.

66. Gines P, Arroyo V, Vargas V, et al. Paracentesis with intravenous infusion of albumin as compared with peritoneovenous shunting in cirrhosis with refractory ascites. N Engl J Med 1991;325:829–835.

67. Sanyal AJ, Genning C, Reddy KR, et al. The North American Study for the Treatment of Refractory Ascites. Gastroenterology 2003;124:634–641.

68. Guardiola J, Baliellas C, Xiol X, et al. External validation of a prognostic model for predicting survival of cirrhotic patients with refractory ascites. Am J Gastroenterol 2002;97(9):2374–2378.

69. Gines A, Fernandez-Esparrach G, Monescillo A, et al. Randomized trial comparing albumin, dextran-70 and polygeline in cirrhotic patients with ascites treated by paracentesis. Gastroenterology 1996;111: 1002–1010.

70. Ruiz del Arbol L, Monescillo A, Jimenez W, Garcia-Plaza A, Arroyo V, Rodes J. Paracentesis-induced circulatory dysfunction: mechanism and effect on hepatic hemodynamics in cirrhosis. Gastroenterology 1997;113:579–586.

71. Gines A, Escorsell A, Gines P, et al. Incidence, predictive factors, and prognosis of the hepatorenal syndrome in cirrhosis with ascites. Gastroenterology 1993;105:229–236.

72. Gines P, Guevara M, Arroyo V, Rodes J. Hepatorenal syndrome. Lancet 2003;362(9398):1819–1827.

73. Howard TK. Postoperative intensive care management of the adult. In: Bussutil BW, Klintmalm GB, eds. Transplantation of the Liver. Saunders, Philadelphia, PA, 1996, pp. 551–563.

74. Urbani L, Catalano G, Cioni R, et al. Management of massive and persistent ascites and/or hydrothorax after liver transplantation. Transpl Proc 2003;35(4):1473–1475.

75. Cirera I, Navasa M, Rimola A, et al. Ascites after liver transplantation. Liver Transpl 2000;6(2): 157–162.

76. Urbani L, Catalano G, Biancofiore G, et al. Surgical complications after liver transplantation. Minerva Chir 2003;58(5):675–692.

77. Leonardi LS, Boin IF, Leonardi MI, Tercioti V Jr. Ascites after liver transplantation and inferior vena cava reconstruction in the piggyback technique. Transpl Proc 2002;34(8):3336–3338.

78. Bilbao JI, Herrero JI, Martinez-Cuesta A, et al. Ascites due to anastomotic stenosis after liver transplantation using the piggyback technique: treatment with endovascular prosthesis. Cardiovasc Intervent Radiol 2000;23(2):149–151.

79. Urbani L, Catalano G, Cioni R, et al. Management of massive and persistent ascites and/or hydrothorax after liver transplantation. Transpl Proc 2003;35(4):1473–1475.

80. Adetiloye VA, John PR. Intervention for pleural effusions and ascites following liver transplantation. Pediatr Radiol 1998;28(7):539–543.

81. Asfar S, Lowndes R, Wall WJ. Chylous ascites after liver transplantation. Transplantation 1994;58(3): 368–369.

82. Shapiro AM, Bain VG, Sigalet DL, Kneteman NM. Rapid resolution of chylous ascites after liver transplantation using somatostatin analog and total parenteral nutrition. Transplantation 1996;61(9): 1410–1411.

83. Gane E, Langley P, Williams R. Massive ascitic fluid loss and coagulation disturbances after liver transplantation. Gastroenterology 1995;109(5):1631–1638.
84. Sebagh M, Blakolmer K, Falissard B, et al. Accuracy of bile duct changes for the diagnosis of chronic liver allograft rejection: reliability of the 1999 Banff schema. Hepatology 2002;35(1):117–125.
85. Nakazawa Y, Chisuwa H, Mita A, et al. Life-threatening veno-occlusive disease after living-related liver transplantation. Transplantation 2003;75(5):727–730.
86. Mor E, Pappo O, Bar-Nathan N, et al. Defibrotide for the treatment of veno-occlusive disease after liver transplantation. Transplantation 2001;72(7):1237–1240.
87. Starzl TE, Demetris AJ, Van Thiel D. Liver transplantation (2). N Engl J Med 1989;321:1092–1099.

20 Management of Ascites

Florence Wong, MD

CONTENTS

INTRODUCTION
TREATMENT OF REVERSIBLE UNDERLYING CAUSES
BED REST
DIETARY SODIUM RESTRICTION
WATER RESTRICTION
DIURETICS
REFRACTORY ASCITES
LARGE-VOLUME PARACENTESIS
TRANSJUGULAR INTRAHEPATIC PORTOSYSTEMIC STENT SHUNT (TIPS)
LIVER TRANSPLANTATION
SUMMARY
REFERENCES

INTRODUCTION

Abnormal renal sodium handling is an early and common complication of liver cirrhosis and eventually results in ascites formation. At least 50% of patients will develop ascites within 10 yr of diagnosis of cirrhosis (1). The presence of ascites predisposes the cirrhotic patients to further complications such as the development of spontaneous bacterial peritonitis and renal impairment, which significantly worsens the prognosis of these patients. The presence of ascites is also an indication for liver transplantation. Therefore, effective management of ascites is essential for improving the well being and survival of these patients.

TREATMENT OF REVERSIBLE UNDERLYING CAUSES

Alcoholic liver disease is a common cause of cirrhosis. Ascites complicates acute alcoholic hepatitis, and total abstinence of alcohol has been associated with a reduction of portal pressure and either resolution of ascites or improved responsiveness to diuretic therapy (2). The consumption of alcohol can also worsen the clinical course of viral hepatitis (3). Therefore, it is imperative that all patients with ascites are advised to stop alcohol, including "low-alcohol" beers, irrespective of whether alcohol is the primary cause of cirrhosis. The treatment of viral hepatitis B with lamivudine in decompensated

From: *Clinical Gastroenterology: Portal Hypertension*
Edited by: A. J. Sanyal and V. H. Shah © Humana Press Inc., Totowa, NJ

cirrhosis can result in the reduction or resolution of ascites *(4)*. Likewise, weight reduction or better control of diabetes in decompensated ascitic cirrhotic patients who have steato-hepatitis as an underlying cause of their cirrhosis should lead to an improved control of their ascites, although this has not been formally studied.

BED REST

Erect posture with activation of the renin–angiotensin–aldosterone system has been shown to be associated with sodium retention in cirrhosis *(5,6)*. The assumption of the supine posture results in increases in venous return and effective arterial blood volume, with reduction in renin–angiotensin–aldosterone levels and natriuresis *(6)*. Therefore, it is only logical to recommend bed rest for cirrhotic patients to mobilize the ascites. However, to date, there are no clinical trials to support the notion that enforced bed rest actually improves the outcome of medical therapies. In the current climate of economic constraints, it is not feasible to recommend bed rest as a treatment for cirrhotic ascites.

DIETARY SODIUM RESTRICTION

Because sodium retention is central to the development of ascites in cirrhosis, it is recommended that cirrhotic patients with ascites should limit their sodium intake *(7)*. The extent to which ascitic cirrhotic patients need to restrict their sodium intake depends on the ability of their kidneys to excrete sodium. For example, patients whose daily urinary sodium excretion is 100 mmol will not decrease their ascites if they consumes a normal North American diet, which contains 200–300 mmol of sodium. However, similar patients will be in negative sodium balance and start to reduce their ascites if their daily sodium intake is restricted to 50 mmol/d. Therefore, it is important to assess 24-h urinary sodium excretion at first presentation, and whenever ascites increases, to calculate the sodium balance and prescribe the appropriate sodium intake *(7)*. Spot urinary sodium estimations are less accurate, because sodium excretion is not uniform during the day. However, in some patients, it may not be practical to perform a 24-h urine collection. In these instances, a random urine sample with urinary Na/K ratio of greater than 1 will indicate a urinary sodium excretion of more than 78 mmol/d in 95% of patients *(7)*.

Most patients with ascites are prescribed a daily sodium intake of 2 g or 88 mmol *(8)*. This amount of sodium is less than what is contained in a no-added-salt diet of 100–130 mmol. It is not uncommon for patients who have never had sodium restriction to lose weight when sodium restriction is initiated, as their restricted sodium intake may well fall below the renal threshold for sodium excretion and the patient goes into negative sodium balance. Compliance with sodium restriction is best monitored by daily weights, and frequent 24-h sodium excretion measurements. A patient who consumes 88 mmol, and excretes 20 mmol of sodium per day will be in positive sodium balance of 68 mmol/d. Such a patient should gain 3.4 kg of weight in 2 wk (68 mmol/d × 14 d ÷ 140 mmol/L = 3.4 L). Therefore, more rapid weight gain would suggest noncompliance with dietary sodium restriction.

As many patients are unaccustomed to dietary sodium restrictions, all patients with ascites should receive counseling regarding the importance of a low sodium diet, and advice on where to purchase low sodium items. Low sodium items can be unpalatable and are frequently not well tolerated. The introduction of spices and low sodium recipes could make a difference in the acceptance of sodium restriction, and the use of a dietitian is invaluable. The use of salt substitutes should be discouraged, as many of these contain potassium, and can lead to hyperkalemia, especially in patients who are also taking potassium-sparing diuretics.

Despite the widespread use of sodium restriction in the management of ascites in cirrhosis, there is no evidence that sodium restriction has any survival benefits for these patients (9). However, compliance with sodium restriction can significantly reduce diuretic requirement and decrease the time to complete resolution of ascites (10). In a European survey on the management of ascites in cirrhosis, most respondents used a low sodium diet as part of the therapeutic regimen (11). In a more recent survey conducted by the International Ascites Club, 85% of respondents apply sodium restriction to their patients, and 64% do not relax sodium restriction even after ascites has been completely eliminated (8).

WATER RESTRICTION

In cirrhotic patients with ascites, water loss usually follows sodium loss. Therefore, there is usually no need to enforce fluid restriction. However, in patients with hyponatremia of <120 mmol/L, some fluid restriction is recommended (7). Fluid restriction that is too severe is unpleasant, and can only further exaggerate the intravascular depletion that is already present in these patients.

DIURETICS

Sodium restriction alone can only eliminate ascites in about 10% of patients (12). Diuretics are usually required in addition to sodium restriction to mobilize the ascites. Diuretics act on different nephron sites to block sodium reabsorption, thereby increasing renal sodium excretion.

Aldosterone Antagonists

Because hyperaldosteronism is a major factor in promoting renal sodium retention in cirrhosis (13), aldosterone antagonists are the drugs of choice as the initial therapy for the treatment of ascites. Spironolactone, starting at a dose of 100 mg/d, can be titrated up to a maximum of 400 mg/d (7–9,14,15). The absorption of spironolactone is better with food, but the diuretic effects are not observed until 48 h later. The metabolism of spironolactone is impaired in cirrhosis, leading to a very prolonged half-life of up to 35 h. Therefore, the peak effects of spironolactone can be delayed for up to 7–10 d (15), and dose adjustments of spironolactone should not be made more often than every 7–10 d. Similarly, there is a delay in the offset of action when spironolactone is discontinued. Its major side effect is painful gynecomastia. Canrenoate is a metabolite of spironolactone. Its starting dose is 100 mg/d. It is only available in certain parts of Europe and is often used because it is less likely to cause painful gynecomastia (16). Amiloride, another distal diuretic, starting at 5 mg/d and titrating up to 30 mg/d, may be preferred, as it has a quicker onset and offset of action than spironolactone. It also does not produce painful gynecomastia. However, it is weaker than spironolactone and is more expensive (17). All of the distal diuretics can cause hyperkalemia.

Loop Diuretics

A loop diuretic such as furosemide is often added to a spironolactone to produce an earlier natriuresis. Loop diuretics are potent diuretics. They block the reabsorption of sodium in the loop of Henle, and increase the distal delivery of sodium to the distal renal tubule. Loop diuretics should not be used alone because the increased sodium delivered to the distal tubule will be rapidly reabsorbed due to unopposed action of aldosterone *(18)*.

Furosemide has a very quick onset of action. After oral administration, diuresis begins within 30 min, peaks at 1–2 h, and is completed after 3–4 h. The initial oral dose of furosemide is 20–40 mg/d, and the dose can be increased up to a maximum of 160 mg/d to improve the diuretic response *(7–9)*. The dose response curve of furosemide is sigmoidal, that is, once a maximal response is reached, higher doses will not increase the diuresis *(19)*. Rather, high doses of furosemide can predispose the patient to the side effects of hypokalemia, hyponatremia, intravascular volume depletion, and the development of hepatorenal syndrome *(20,21)*. High doses of furosemide can also increase renal ammonia production and predispose the patient to the development of hepatic encephalopathy. The combination of furosemide and spironolactone in the ratio of 40 mg:100 mg usually maintains normokalemia, and, therefore, stepwise increases of both diuretics should maintain this ratio.

Torasemide, another loop diuretic, has been shown to be more effective and better tolerated than furosemide in cirrhosis *(22)*. Its duration of action is also longer. However, it is not universally available and this limits its usefulness in the management of patients with ascites.

Other Diuretics

Diuretics that work on the proximal renal tubule are usually very potent. Mannitol is an osmotic diuretic, which prevents sodium reabsorption in the proximal renal tubule. It is not very effective because the increased sodium delivered to the distal tubule can be reabsorbed distally. In cirrhotic patients with refractory ascites (see below), it is this improved sodium delivery to the distal renal tubule that restores responsiveness to the natriuretic effects of atrial natriuretic peptide *(23,24)*. However, because of its potent diuretic effects, it should not be used as a diuretic in cirrhosis as it can lead to severe dehydration and renal failure.

Metolazone is a thiazide-type diuretic. It inhibits sodium reabsorption at the cortical diluting site, and to a lesser extent, the proximal convoluted tubule. Metolazone has been used in combination with both loop and distal diuretics in patients with ascites. However, the use of metolazone in cirrhosis should be discouraged, as intravascular volume depletion, leading to renal dysfunction is a common complication *(25)*.

Other Adjunctive Therapy

In a recent study, cirrhotic patients with ascites were randomized to receive diuretics with or without weekly 25 g of albumin infusions while inpatients. This was continued after discharge from hospital for approx 20 mo. The albumin-plus-diuretic group had significantly better diuretic response, shorter hospital stays, lower probability of reaccumulation of ascites, and lower likelihood of readmission to hospital *(26)*. The results have since been confirmed *(27)*. However, survival was not affected. The rationale for using albumin was to improve the filling of the effective arterial blood volume, thereby improving renal perfusion. Despite the fact that this makes physiological sense, the practice was not shown to be cost effective, and, therefore, cannot be recommended as the standard of care for these patients.

Spironolactone (mg)	100	200	300	400
Furosemide (mg)	40	80	120	160
Amiloride (mg)	5	10	15	20

Fig. 1. Recommended step-care approach to the use of diuretic therapy. Increase to the next step if the patient has lost <1.5 kg in 1 wk, if the patient has been compliant with Na restriction, and if there are no complications.

Managing Diuretic Therapy

The International Ascites Club recommends that diuretic therapy should be started with spironolactone 100–200 mg/d (8), preferably given with food. However, given the fact that the onset of action of spironolactone is very slow in cirrhotic patients with ascites, many physicians prefer to initiate diuretic therapy with a combination of a loop diuretic and spironolactone. This has the advantage of encouraging compliance because the patient will experience an earlier positive diuretic response when compared to spironolactone alone. The combination approach also is less likely to result in hyperkalemia. Patients on diuretic therapy should have their weight monitored daily. If the diuretic therapy results in a negative sodium balance, the patient should start losing weight. The ideal weight loss should be approx 1/2 kg/d. Too rapid weight loss will result in intravascular volume contraction and predispose the patient to the development of renal failure.

If the response to diuretic therapy is not adequate after 1 wk, and the patient has been compliant with dietary sodium restriction, and there are no other complications, the diuretic doses can be increased in a stepwise fashion (Fig. 1). Patients on spironolactone alone can have a loop diuretic added, whereas those on a combination of a furosemide and spironolactone can have the doses increased by 40 and 100 mg, respectively. Diuretic adjustments can be made weekly until maximum doses of 160 mg for furosemide and 400 mg of spironolactone are reached (28). Periodic assessments of dietary sodium intake should be made to ensure that patients are adhering to dietary sodium restriction, as dietary indiscretions can result in loss of response.

Diuretic therapy can cause electrolyte imbalance, intravascular volume depletion, renal impairment, and precipitate hepatic encephalopathy. Therefore, patients on diuretic therapy should have their serum electrolytes and renal function monitored regularly. In addition, patients should be reviewed on a regular basis to assess for the development of hepatic encephalopathy. Diuretics should be stopped temporarily if the patient develops hyponatremia with serum sodium of <130 mmol/L or permanently if the serum sodium falls below 125 mmol/L (29). Likewise, hyperkalemia of >5.5 mmol/L warrants the permanent discontinuation of diuretic therapy (8). Patients with hyponatremia or hyperkalemia usually have significant intravascular depletion, and infusion of colloid solutions may correct the electrolyte abnormalities. Overzealous use of diuretics can also lead to the development of renal dysfunction. The serum creatinine in cirrhotic patients with ascites is usually falsely low despite the presence of moderate to severe renal impairment (30,31). This is attributed to decreased hepatic creatinine synthesis, increased tubular creatinine secretion, and decreased skeletal mass. Therefore, a rise in serum creatinine is more important than the absolute serum creatinine level in the monitoring of renal function in cirrhotic patients with ascites treated with diuretic therapy. Diuretics should be stopped when the serum creatinine has either doubled or reached an absolute value of >135 mmol/L. The development of muscle cramps or grade 1 hepatic encephalopathy should be treated conventionally with quinine and lactulose, respectively.

The Management of Hyponatremia

Hyponatremia develops when the kidneys are unable to excrete free water. It occurs in about 30% of cirrhotic patients with ascites (32). It is a reflection of the severe reduction of the effective arterial blood volume in these patients and water retention is a compensatory mechanism to increase the intravascular volume (33). The underlying pathophysiology is a nonosmotically stimulated secretion of vasopressin (34). It is exacerbated by diuretics, which reduce the intravascular volume further. The traditional treatment is water restriction. This is unpalatable and is unenforceable, as these patients are usually very thirsty owing to the contracted intravascular volume. Furthermore, water restriction may reduce the intravascular volume further and significantly worsen the renal function. The infusion of colloid volume expanders such as albumin can reduce the water retention and improve the serum sodium. The administration of hypertonic saline is contraindicated, as this carries the potential risk of precipitating central pontine myelinolysis (35) and worsens the sodium retention.

Recent studies have assessed vasopressin antagonism as a means of improving free water excretion in cirrhosis. Reducing vasopressin secretion from the hypothalamus with opioid agonists is associated with too many neurological side effects and, therefore, is of limited use (36). The recent development of vasopressin receptor antagonists which specifically block the V2 receptors in the renal collecting tubule hold much promise. In the recently published randomized placebo-controlled studies using these agents such as VPA985 (37,38), there was a dose-related increase in free water clearance, serum sodium and serum osmolality, and a decrease in urinary osmolality. No orthostatic hypotension or change in serum creatinine levels was observed, although at higher doses, there were some overt and subtle signs of mild dehydration (37). However, both of these studies were of very short duration. Whether these agents can maintain their efficacy with long-term administration remains to be seen.

REFRACTORY ASCITES

The combination of sodium restriction, and combination diuretic therapy is usually effective in eliminating ascites in approx 90% of cirrhotic patients with ascites (19,29). In the remaining 10% of patients, this approach is either ineffective or the patient is intolerant of diuretic therapy. In 1996, the International Ascites Club defined refractory ascites as ascites that cannot be mobilized or the early recurrence of which cannot be satisfactorily prevented by medical therapy (39). These were further divided into diuretic resistant (nonresponsiveness to sodium restriction of 50 mmol/d and 160 mg of furosemide and 400 mg of spironolactone with a weight loss of <1.5 kg/wk for 2 wk), and diuretic-intractable ascites (inability to tolerate maximal doses of diuretics because of complications such as severe electrolyte disturbances and renal failure) *(39)*. Therefore, these patients require second line therapy such as large-volume paracentesis, transjugular intrahepatic portosystemic shunts, or liver transplantation.

LARGE-VOLUME PARACENTESIS

Large-volume paracentesis of 4–6 L has been shown to be safe and effective in the management of ascites in cirrhosis *(40–42)*. In a randomized controlled trial, Gines et al. reported that cirrhotic patients with ascites treated with large volume paracentesis and albumin (8 g/L of ascitic fluid removed) had lower incidence of systemic and hemodynamic disturbance, electrolyte abnormalities, renal impairment, and encephalopathy when compared to patients treated with diuretics *(40)*. Furthermore, patients in the paracentesis group had a shorter initial hospital stay. However, there was no difference in terms of readmission rate, reason for readmission, and survival *(40)*. These results have since been confirmed *(43)*. Therefore, large-volume paracentesis has become a standard treatment for cirrhotic patients with refractory ascites. For a patient who is compliant with dietary sodium restriction, paracentesis should only be required no more often than every 2–3 wk, even if the patient is excreting no urinary sodium. A 6-L paracentesis removes 840 mmol of sodium (140 mmol/L × 6 L), and if the patient has been compliant with a 50 mmol sodium/d intake, it should take 17 d to accumulate 850 mmol of sodium or 6 L of ascitic fluid even with a urinary sodium of 0 mmol. For patients who are actually excreting urinary sodium, the period between paracentesis should be longer. Therefore, any patients who require more frequent paracentesis should have their 3-d food records checked, and receive further dietary counseling.

Myths About Large-Volume Paracentesis

FREQUENT LARGE VOLUME PARACENTESES CAN INCREASE THE RISK OF PERITONITIS

In a prospective study on 29 asymptomatic patients with decompensated cirrhosis (Child–Pugh class B = 11 patients, class C = 18 patients) who underwent repeat large-volume paracentesis as outpatients, with ascitic fluid culture and ascitic fluid cell count performed on all occasions, there was an incidence of 2.5% (3 out of 118 episodes) of spontaneous bacterial peritonitis *(44)*. The infrequent occurrence of spontaneous bacterial peritonitis with repeat large-volume paracentesis has been confirmed in several other studies *(45–47)*. Therefore, it is safe to repeat large-volume paracentesis without the fear of introducing infection provided the procedure is done with strict sterile techniques.

COAGULOPATHY IS A CONTRAINDICATION TO PARACENTESIS

Significant bleeding occurs in approx 1% of cirrhotic patients with ascites who undergo paracentesis *(48)*. Bleeding following paracentesis can occur at the puncture site or intraperitoneally *(49)*. Puncture site hematomas are usually due to bleeding from abdominal wall vessels, and avoidance of the vascular midline area can reduce the incidence *(50)*. Intraperitoneal hemorrhage following paracentesis can be delayed for several days *(51)*, and is usually caused by rapid reduction of intraperitoneal pressure, leading to distension of hypertensive intraabdominal collaterals and their eventual rupture *(52,53)*. To date, there are no data to support a correlation between the extent of coagulopathy and the risk of bleeding after paracentesis, and the correction of coagulopathy has not been shown to reduce the incidence of bleeding *(50,54)*.

LEAKAGE FROM THE PUNCTURE SITE AFTER PARACENTESIS

Leakage of ascitic fluid following paracentesis occasionally occurs, particularly if the patient starts ambulating immediately after completion of paracentesis. This can be managed by placing a purse-string suture around the puncture site and have the patient lie with the puncture site uppermost for a few minutes (8,30). The placement of a colostomy bag over the leaking puncture site to contain the ascitic fluid is to be discouraged, as this allows a direct communication between the sterile peritoneal cavity and the nonsterile external environment, and predisposes the patient to the risk of infection, although to date, there have been no studies to address this issue.

The Controversy of Albumin Replacement

Paracentesis-induced circulatory dysfunction is a pathophysiological state characterized by intravascular volume depletion, elevated renin, and aldosterone levels. It can develop following large-volume paracentesis (43) and is clinically recognized as renal impairment and electrolyte imbalance, particularly hyponatremia. In the only randomized controlled trial comparing albumin infusion (10 g/L of ascitic fluid removed) vs no albumin with paracentesis, the incidence of circulatory dysfunction is significantly decreased in the albumin group (30%) compared to the no albumin group (16%) (43). Albumin seems to be most appropriate solution to prevent this complication of paracentesis, when compared to other colloid solutions (55–59) or saline (60).

The use of albumin with every paracentesis has been challenged, as albumin is very expensive, and carries the risk of transmitting unknown viruses or prion-related diseases (7). This is based on the fact that the use of albumin did not affect either the morbidity or mortality of the ascitic cirrhotic patients in the original study (43). Although a later study showed that patients with postparacentesis circulatory dysfunction had significantly decreased rates of survival at 1 yr, there has been no evidence that plasma expansion can improve the outcome (55). A further study assessing the circulatory changes following a 5-L paracentesis could not confirm any changes in central blood volume, serum sodium levels, or renal function when albumin was not infused with the paracentesis (61). This may be related to the fact that patients in the last study had refractory ascites, and are supposedly more resistant to the paracentesis-induced volume depletion (62), vs the very initial study, which consisted of 30% of patients who were still diuretic sensitive (43). Therefore, the most recent American Association for the Study of Liver Disease practice guideline did not recommend the routine use of albumin with therapeutic paracentesis, especially because a large proportion of the infused albumin is being degraded at an accelerated rate following the infusion (63). Of course, the practice guidelines have been counter-challenged (64). It is clear that further studies are needed. The International Ascites Club recommends that until further results are available, the infusion of albumin of 6–8 g is to be given per liter of ascitic fluid removed for paracentesis of greater than 5–6 L (8). To date, the predictive factors for the development of postparacentesis circulatory dysfunction have yet to be determined.

Single Total Paracentesis vs Repeat Large-Volume Paracenteses

Total paracentesis with albumin infusion has been shown to be as safe as repeat large volume paracentesis in patients with tense ascites (65), including those with hyponatremia (66). Total paracentesis without albumin infusion is associated with the development of effective hypovolumia in at least 40% of patients, mainly owing to the exacerbation of the arterial vasodilatation *(67,68)* followed by the activation of vasoconstrictor systems. Albumin infusion was able to prevent the development of these deleterious hemodynamic changes *(69)*. Therefore, it is reasonable to perform a total paracentesis together with albumin infusion in patients with tense ascites to reduce the frequency of paracenteses.

Patients who are treated with repeat large-volume paracenteses usually have refractory ascites, and by definition are either resistant or unresponsive to diuretic therapy. Therefore, they should not be placed on diuretic therapy after paracentesis. However, they have to remain on sodium restriction to reduce the frequency of paracentesis. The "downside" to a total paracentesis is that it may encourage noncompliance with sodium restriction, as patients can get a quick relief from their rapidly accumulating ascites by requesting a total paracentesis.

TRANSJUGULAR INTRAHEPATIC PORTOSYSTEMIC STENT SHUNT (TIPS)

Because one of the pathogenetic mechanisms of sodium retention and ascites formation in cirrhosis is sinusoidal portal hypertension *(70–72)*, it stands to reason that reduction of portal hypertension should result in increased sodium retention and eventual elimination of ascites. Indeed, surgical portosystemic shunting, which lowers portal pressure, was used several decades ago to treat intractable ascites *(73)*. The advanced state of their liver disease meant that many of the patients were unable to tolerate the surgery and mortality was high. The advent of the nonsurgical portosystemic shunt within the liver, created radiologically through the internal jugular vein, allowed the patients to undergo portal pressure reduction without the attendant surgical risks *(74)*. The addition of a metallic stent improved the patency of the intrahepatic portosystemic shunt *(75)* and widened its clinical applications. The TIPS shunt, as it is now known, functions like a side-to-side portocaval shunt, and connects a branch of the hepatic vein to a branch of the portal vein, thereby allowing decompression of the portal venous system (Fig. 2). It was first used to treat refractory variceal bleeds *(76)*. It was soon realized that in those patients who had concomitant ascites, the ascites was either much reduced or became more responsive to diuretic therapy. There followed a flurry of studies, assessing the use of TIPS as a treatment for ascites. The overall results were very encouraging, with reduction of ascites or elimination of ascites occurring in approximately two-thirds of the patients *(77)*. But the natriuretic response to TIPS, in the absence of diuretics, is not immediate. Rather, natriuresis is delayed for 1–2 wk post-TIPS *(78)*, despite the fact the TIPS returns a significant portion of the splanchnic volume to the systemic circulation and improves the filling of the effective arterial circulation *(78)*. This onset of natriuresis is related to the pre-TIPS renal function and inversely to the patient's age *(78)*. Once natriuresis begins, it continues to improve, so that at 6 mo after TIPS insertion, most patients are in a negative sodium balance on a 22 mmol sodium/d diet, allowing elimination of ascites *(79)*. Once ascites disappears, renal function improves *(80)*; patients achieve positive nitrogen balance *(81)* and report an improved sense of well being *(82,83)*. During long-term follow-up, sodium loading results in sodium retention in some, but not all, of these patients *(80)*. Because the factors involved in sodium retention post-TIPS are unknown, it is advisable for patients to maintain some form of sodium restriction to prevent the recurrence of ascites.

The first randomized controlled trial comparing TIPS vs large-volume paracenteses as a treatment for refractory ascites was reported in 1996 *(84)*. The TIPS patients had significantly higher mortality than those who received repeat large-volume paracentesis *(84)*.

TIPS

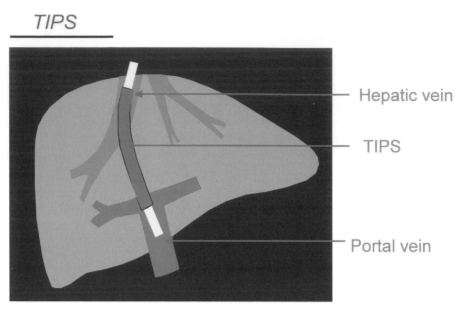

Hepatic vein

TIPS

Portal vein

Fig. 2. TIPS.

It soon became obvious that the patients in Child–Pugh class C with advanced liver dysfunction did not survive beyond 6 mo, whereas those in Child–Pugh class B fared better *(84)*. Since then, there have been four other similar randomized controlled trials published *(85–88)*. All showed that TIPS was superior to repeat large-volume paracentesis as a treatment for refractory ascites. In two of the published studies *(88)*, there was a survival benefit in the TIPS group without liver transplantation. However, this could not be confirmed in the other two published randomized controlled studies *(86,87)*. Meta-analysis of all the studies should provide the answer to the survival advantage of TIPS in ascites patients.

Irrespective of whether TIPS provides a survival benefit or not, appropriate patients with refractory ascites should be considered for this procedure, but TIPS is not the panacea for every cirrhotic patient with ascites. There is sufficient evidence in the literature to support that Child–Pugh class C patients fare poorly after TIPS insertion *(77)*. This may be related to the shunting of blood through the TIPS away from the sinusoids, thus making the liver relatively ischemic after TIPS insertion *(89)*. This could tip the patient into liver failure if the pre-TIPS liver function is already borderline as in Child–Pugh class C patients. In fact, one of the risk factors for mortality after TIPS insertion relates to the severity liver dysfunction (bilirubin >51 µmol/L) *(77)*. Pooled data from published literature also suggest that patients who are elderly *(77,78)* or with pre-TIPS renal impairment *(77,90)* do not respond well to TIPS placement, and, therefore, should not be offered TIPS, although TIPS has been reported to be effective in the management of hepatorenal syndrome *(91)*. Other contraindications to TIPS insertion include intrinsic renal disease with urine protein >500 mg/24 h or active urinary sediment, grade III or IV hepatic encephalopathy, cardiopulmonary disease, portal vein thrombosis, noncompliance with sodium restriction, or the presence of carcinoma that is likely to limit patient's life-span to <1 yr *(92)*. The insertion of TIPS increases the right atrial pressure and the pulmonary

Table 1
Patient Selection Criteria for TIPS Insertion

Age <65 yr
Normal cardiac and renal function
No prior history of encephalopathy
INR <2
Bilirubin <85 µmol/L
Child–Pugh score of <12
Absence of active infection
Patent portal vein

artery pressure by twofold (93). This can precipitate cardiac failure in patients with preexisting cardiopulmonary disease. A thrombosed portal vein makes it technically difficult to insert a TIPS and predisposes the patient to TIPS thrombosis. Noncompliance with sodium restriction delays the elimination of ascites, whereas the insertion of TIPS in someone with a known hepatoma may disseminate the tumor. Other relative contraindications include dental sepsis, spontaneous bacterial peritonitis, and active infection (pneumonia or urinary tract infection). This is to reduce the risks of infection in the TIPS, as TIPS infection is very difficult to eradicate. Table 1 lists the selection criteria for TIPS insertion.

Complications of TIPS Insertion

The TIPS procedure itself is associated with its unique complications. Procedure-related morbidity is 10% and procedure-related mortality is 2% (94). Early complications include neck hematoma, hemobilia, puncture of the liver capsule causing intraabdominal bleeding, and TIPS thrombosis (94). These complications should reduce with the experience of the procedurist. In the early post-TIPS period, deterioration of liver function may occur as blood flow is shunted away from the liver. Deterioration in renal function may occur in those with prior renal dysfunction (creatinine >2.5X upper limit of normal) and may be exacerbated by exposure to radiographic dye. Cardiac failure can occur in patients with unrecognized preexisting cardiac dysfunction. Late TIPS complications include encephalopathy in 30% (77), endothelial hyperplasia causing shunt stenosis in up to 80% of cases, shunt-related foreign-body type hemolysis (95), and reappearance of ascites in noncompliant patients. Elderly patients (>60 yr) and those with pre-TIPS spontaneous hepatic encephalopathy are more susceptible to post-TIPS encephalopathy (96). In most cases, encephalopathy can be managed medically with lactulose or by reduction in shunt size (97); however, refractory cases of encephalopathy were associated with 100% mortality in most studies (77). Shunt stenosis is related to endothelial overgrowth. It is recommended that patients with TIPS should undergo regular ultrasound examinations at three monthly intervals in the first year, and thereafter at six monthly intervals (98). TIPS stenosis can be managed by either balloon dilatation or insertion of a new stent. The use of covered stents has been shown to improve TIPS patency rate (99).

LIVER TRANSPLANTATION

The prognosis of cirrhotic patients with refractory ascites is poor, with 50% survival at 6 mo (100). Therefore, all patients with ascites should be referred for consideration

28. Gatta A, Angeli P, Caregaro L, Menon F, Sacerdoti D, Merkel C. A pathophysiological interpretation of unresponsiveness to spironolactone in a stepped-care approach to the diuretic treatment of ascites in nonazotemic cirrhotic patients. Hepatology 1991;14:231–236.

29. Yeung E, Wong F. The management of cirrhotic ascites. Medscape Gastroenterology eJournal 2002;4:8.

30. Sherman DS, Fish DN, Teitelbaum I. Assessing renal function in cirrhotic patients: problems and pitfalls. Am J Kidney Dis 2003;41:269–278.

31. Caregaro L, Menon F, Angeli P, et al. Limitations of serum creatinine level and creatinine clearance as filtration markers in cirrhosis. Arch Intern Med 1994;154:201–205.

32. Arroyo V, Rodes J, Gutierrez-Lizarraga MA, Revert L. Prognostic value of spontaneous hyponatremia in cirrhosis with ascites. Am J Dig Dis 1976;21:249–256.

33. Schrier RW, Arroyo V, Bernardi M, Epstein M, Henriksen JH, Rodes J. Peripheral arterial vasodilation hypothesis: a proposal for the initiation of renal sodium and water retention in cirrhosis. Hepatology 1988;8:1151–1157.

34. Gines P, Bernardi M, Bichet DG, et al. Hyponatremia in cirrhosis: from pathogenesis to treatment. Hepatology 1998;28:851–864.

35. Laureno R, Karp BI. Myelinolysis after correction of hyponatremia. Ann Intern Med 1997;126:57–62.

36. Gadano A, Moreau R, Pessione F, et al. Aquaretic effects of niravoline, a k-opioid agonist, in patients with cirrhosis. J Hepatology 2000;32:38–42.

37. Wong F, Blei AT, Blendis L, Thuluvath P. A vasopressin receptor antagonist (VPA-985) improves serum sodium concentration in patients with hyponatremia: a multicenter, randomized, placebo-controlled trial. Hepatology 2003;37:182–191.

38. Gerbes AL, Gulberg V, Gines P, et al. VPA Study Group. Therapy of hyponatremia in cirrhosis with a vasopressin receptor antagonist: a randomized double-blind multicenter trial. Gastroenterology 2003; 124:933–939.

39. Arroyo V, Gines P, Gerbes AL, et al. Definition and diagnostic criteria of refractory ascites and hepatorenal syndrome in cirrhosis. International Ascites Club. Hepatology 1996;23:164–176.

40. Gines P, Arroyo V, Quintero E, et al. Comparison of paracentesis and diuretics in the treatment of cirrhosis with tense ascites: results of a randomized study. Gastroenterology 1987;93:234–241.

41. Salerno F, Badalamenti S, Incerti P, et al. Repeated paracentesis and i.v. albumin infusion to treat 'tense' ascites in ascitic patients: a safe alternative therapy. J Hepatol 1987;5:102–108.

42. Pinto PC, Amerian J, Reynolds TB. Large volume paracentesis in non-edematous patients with tense ascites: its effect on intravascular volume. Hepatology 1988;8:207–210.

43. Gines P, Tito L, Arroyo V, et al. Randomized comparative study of therapeutic parcentesis with and without intravenous albumin in cirrhosis. Gastroenterology 1988;94:1493–1502.

44. Jeffries MA, Stern MA, Gunaratnam NT, Fontana RJ. Unsuspected infection is infrequent in asymptomatic outpatients with refractory ascites undergoing therapeutic paracentesis. Am J Gastroenterol 1999;94:2972–2976.

45. Pascual S, Such J, Perez-Mateo M. Spontaneous bacterial peritonitis and refractory ascites. Am J Gastroenterol 2000;95:3686–3687.

46. Evans LT, Kim WR, Poterucha JJ, Kamath PS. Spontaneous bacterial peritonitis in asymptomatic outpatients with cirrhotic ascites. Hepatology 2003;37:897–901.

47. Sola R, Andreu M, Coll S, Vila MC, Oliver MI, Arroyo V. Spontaneous bacterial peritonitis in cirrhotic patients treated using paracentesis or diuretics: results of a randomized study. Hepatology 1995; 21:340–344.

48. Runyon BA. Paracentesis of ascitic fluid. Arch Intern Med 1986;146:2259–2261.

49. Webster ST, Brown KL, Lucey MR, Nostrant TT. Hemorrhagic complications of large volume abdominal paracentesis. Am J Gastroenterol 1996;91:366–368.

50. Oelsner DH, Caldweel SH, Coles M, Driscoll CJ. Subumbilical midline vascularity of the abdominal wall in portal hypertension observed at laparoscopy. Gastrointest Endosc 1998;47:388–390.

51. Martinet O, Reis ED, Mosimann F. Delayed hemoperitoneum following large-volume paracentesis in a patient with cirrhosis and ascites. Digest Dis Sci 2000;45:357–358.

52. Kravetz D, Romero G, Argonz J, et al. Total volume paracentesis decreases variceal pressure, size, and variceal wall tension in cirrhotic patients. Hepatology 1997;25:59–62.

53. Luca A, Feu F, Garcia-Pagan JC, et al. Favorable effects of total paracentesis on splanchnic hemo-dynamics in cirrhotic patients with tense ascites. Hepatology 1994;20:30–33.

54. McVay PA, Toy PT. Lack of increased bleeding after paracentesis and thoracentesis in patients with mild coagulation abnormalities. Transfusion 1991;31:164–171.

55. Ginès A, Fernandez-Esparrach G, Monescillo A, et al. Randomized trial comparing albumin, dextran 70, and polygeline in cirrhotic patients with ascites treated by paracentesis. Gastroenterology 1996; 111:1002–1010.

56. Altman C, Bernard B, Roulot D, Vitte RL, Ink O. Randomized comparative multicenter study of hydroxyethyl starch versus albumin as a plasma expander in cirrhotic patients with tense ascites treated with paracentesis. Eur J Gastroenterol Hepatol 1998;10:5–10.

57. Planas R, Ginès P, Arroyo V, et al. Dextran-70 versus albumin as plasma expanders in cirrhotic patients with ascites treated with total paracentesis. Results of a randomized study. Gastroenterology 1990;99:1736–1744.

58. Salerno F, Badalamenti S, Lorenzano E, Moser P, Incerti P. Randomized comparative study of hemaccel vs albumin infusion after total paracentesis in cirrhotic patients with refractory ascites. Hepatology 1991;13:707–713.

59. Fassio E, Terg R, Landeira G, et al. Paracentesis with dextran 70 vs paracentesis with albumin in cir-rhosis with tense ascites. Results of a randomized study. J Hepatol 1992;14:310–316.

60. Sola-Vera J, Minana J, Ricart E, et al. Randomized trial comparing albumin and saline in the pre-vention of paracentesis-induced circulatory dysfunction in cirrhotic patients with ascites. Hepatology 2003;37:1147–1153.

61. Peltekian K, Wong F, Liu P, Allidina Y, Sherman M, Blendis LM. The effect of large volume para-centesis on total central blood volume, systemic and renal hemodynamics and renal sodium handling in cirrhosis. Am J Gastroenterology 1997;92:394–399.

62. Moller S, Bendtsen F, Henriksen JH. Effect of volume expansion on systemic hemodynamics and central and arterial blood volume in cirrhosis. Gastreonterology 1995;109:1917–1925.

63. Rothschild M, Oratz M, Evans C, Schreiber SS. Alterations in albumin metabolism after serum and albumin infusions. J Clin Invest 1964;43:1874–1880.

64. Arroyo V, Colmenero J. Use of albumin in the management of patients with decompensated cirrho-sis. An independent verdict. Dig Liver Dis 2003;35:668–672.

65. Tito L, Gines P, Arroyo V, et al. Total paracentesis associated with intravenous albumin management of patients with cirrhosis and ascites. Gastroenterology 1990;98:146–151.

66. Vila MC, Coll S, Sola R, Andreu M, Gana J, Marquez J. Total paracentesis in cirrhotic patients with tense ascites and dilutional hyponatremia. Am J Gastroenterol 1999;94:2219–2223.

67. Vila MC, Sola R, Molina L, et al. Hemodynamic changes in patients developing effective hypovole-mia after total paracentesis. J Hepatol 1998;28:639–645.

68. Ruiz-del-Arbol L, Monescillo A, Jimenez W, Garcia Plaza A, Arroyo V, Rodes J. Paracentesis-induced circulatory dysfunction: mechanism and effect on hepatic hemodynamics in cirrhosis. Gastro-enterology 1997;113:579–586.

69. Luca A, Garcia-Pagan JC, Bosch J, et al. Beneficial effects of intravenous albumin infusion on the hemodynamic and humoral changes after total paracentesis. Hepatology 1995;22:753–758.

70. Morali GA, Sniderman KW, Deitel KM, et al. Is sinusoidal portal hypertension a necessary factor for the development of hepatic ascites. J Hepatology 1992;16:249–250.

71. Jalan R, Hayes PC. Sodium handling in patients with well compensated cirrhosis is dependent on the severity of liver disease and portal pressure. Gut 2000;46:527–533.

72. Jalan R, Forrest EH, Redhead DN, Dillon JF, Hayes PC. Reduction in renal blood flow following acute increase in the portal pressure: evidence for the existence of a hepatorenal reflex in man? Gut 1997;40:664–670.

73. Orloff MJ. Surgical treatment of intractable cirrhotic ascites. Ann Surg 1966;164:69–80.

74. Colapinto RF, Stronell RD, Birch SJ, et al. Creation of an intrahepatic portosystemic shunt with a Gruntzig balloon catheter. Can Med Assoc J 1982;126:267–268.

75. Richter GM, Noeldge G, Palmaz JC, Roessle M. The transjugular intrahepatic portosystemic stent-shunt (TIPSS): results of a pilot study. Cardiovasc Intervent Radiol 1990;13:200–207.

Mucosal and Epithelial Barrier Dysfunction: Bacterial Translocation

Most of the organisms that cause SBP are of enteric origin; the remaining bacteria are respiratory or skin flora. An important question is to know how these bacteria may invade mucosal or epithelial barriers, and enter the peritoneum. Bacterial translocation, a phenomenon defined as the passage of viable microorganisms from the gastrointestinal lumen to mesenteric lymph nodes and other extragastrointestinal sites *(4)*, has been postulated as one of the main mechanisms, and probably one of the first steps in the pathogenesis of SBP. In fact, the rat models of Runyon and of Planas and their coworkers virtually duplicate every detail of SBP in humans *(6,7)*.

The normal gut mucosa functions as a selective filter; Gram-negative aerobic bacteria translocate more readily than Gram-positive aerobic bacteria, which, in turn, translocate more readily than anaerobes *(5)*. In cirrhotic rats with ascites, there is an increased passage of bacteria from the gastrointestinal lumen to gastroextraintestinal sites, including mesenteric lymph nodes and the systemic circulation, much more commonly than normal rats; the gut mucosa in the setting of cirrhosis is "leakier" than normal *(6,7)*. Causes for bacterial translocation are a disruption of the intestinal permeability barrier, bacterial overgrowth, and/or decrease in host immune defense mechanism. In patients with cirrhosis, increased permeability of the gut has been shown to correlate with a poor prognosis *(8)*. It is of interest that gut permeability increases with exposure to alcohol and aspirin, and decreases with portacaval shunting *(9–11)*. The decrease in permeability with shunting may explain the decrease in risk of SBP in patients after portacaval shunts. The submucosa of the cecum of cirrhotic rats with ascites becomes markedly edematous and inflamed, suggesting that portal hypertension could produce a rupture in the intestinal permeability barrier in these animals and thus favor bacterial translocation *(7)*. Changes in the permeability of the intestinal mucosa have also been seen in hemorrhagic shock *(12)*, sepsis, injury, or administration of endotoxin.

Even prior to translocation, pathological processes develop in the setting of cirrhosis that would predictably lead to an increased risk of translocation. One of the most important risk factors for translocation is overgrowth of gut flora; 100% of normal mice will translocate if given a large oral dose of *Escheridia coli (13)*. A normal human was documented to translocate *Candida albicans* and develop fungemia and funguria after drinking a large oral inoculum *(14)*. Overgrowth of gut Gram-negative bacterias with subsequent translocation of the overgrowing flora has been documented in an animal model of cirrhosis *(15)*, and Gram-negative bacilli have been found to be significantly increased in the jejunal flora of many cirrhotic patients. In turn, the overgrowth of indigenous flora may be due to the altered bowel motility that has been documented to occur in patients with cirrhosis *(16)*. The change in the intestinal flora caused by the abnormal small bowel colonization in cirrhosis may increase the chance of aerobic Gram-negative bacteria invading the boodstream and cause infections of enteric origin in these patients. In fact, in two different experimental studies performed in ascitic cirrhotic rats, bacterial overgrown and bacterial translocation decreased by accelerating intestinal transit, either with propranolol or with cisapride *(17,18)*.

Bile acids can also be involved in the pathogenesis of bacterial translocation. In cirrhotic patients, bile acid secretion is markedly diminished *(19)*. Such decreased secretion should result in a lowered intraluminal concentration of conjugated bile acids. Because bile acids are bacteriostatic, their decreased intraluminal concentration might well promote bacterial growth, leading to still more deconjugation, and initiating a vicious cycle. The final result of this vicious cycle would be bacterial translocation and endotoxemia. Recently, it has been demonstrated that the administration of conjugated bile acids (cholylsarcosine and cholylglycine) to ascitic cirrhotic rats caused increased bile secretion and led to inhibition of bacterial proliferation in the small intestine, decreased bacterial translocation, decreased endotoxemia, and increased survival (20).

The exact route by which bacteria translocate and the site in the gut where the process is most common are not yet clear. The colon is more permeable than the small bowel and the bacterial load of the colon is many logs greater than that of the small bowel. Clearly, bacteria may leave the intestinal lumen by passing between the tight junctions of mucosal cells or via transcellular passage directly through intact mucosal cells. The gut edema that has been documented in patients with cirrhosis may lead to leaky tight junctions between colonocytes and paracellular passage of bacteria (21). Alternatively, bacteria may pass intracellularly (22). Some bacteria may pass by one route and other bacteria by another route, depending on bacterial virulence factors and local mucosal defense mechanisms.

Several abnormalities peculiar to decompensated cirrhosis may decrease local resistance of the intestinal mucosa to bacterial invasion. First, in patients with decompensated portal hypertension, the splanchnic veins and lymphatics are congested and edema of all splanchnic tissues may exist, thus affecting adversely the mucosal barrier to bacterial invasion. Consequently, the bowel wall is edematous and often inflamed, and the intestinal mucosa is frequently severely degenerated. This underlying mucosal inflammation or secondary irritation may increase the permeability of the mucosal barrier. Finally, qualitative and quantitative abnormalities in the distribution of intestinal bacteria have been demonstrated in cirrhosis, with Gram-negative bacilli significantly increased in the jejunal flora.

When bacteria penetrate the intestinal mucosa into the submucosal tissues, the intestinal lymphatics carry them to the major lymphatic channels and eventually via the thoracic duct into the systemic circulation causing a bacteremia. This bacteremia delivers the organism to the ascitic fluid. This hematogenous route appears to be the most reasonable mechanism to explain the spontaneous bacterial contamination of ascites. Moreover, the depression of the hepatic reticuloendothelial system activity, which causes failure of the liver in "filtering" these bacteria, may allow passage of microorganisms from the bowel lumen to the systemic circulation via the portal vein.

Complement Deficiency and Phagocyte Dysfunction

In general, bacteria causing systemic infection cannot be killed by humoral factors (complement) alone. Coating of bacteria with complement renders them more easily recognizable as foreign and digestible by phagocytes. For optimal killing of bacteria, adequate levels of complement are required, as well as optimally functional phagocytes. Unfortunately, cirrhosis is probably the most common form of acquired complement deficiency (23,24) and dysfunction of both motile phagocytes (neutrophils) and stationary phagocytes (Kupffer cells) is common in the setting of severe liver disease (25–28).

For translocation to become clinically significant, i.e., for it to lead to SBP, bacteremia, or postoperative infection, a failure of local and systemic immune defenses should also be present. That is, in a healthy, nonimmunocompromised host, translocated bacteria may

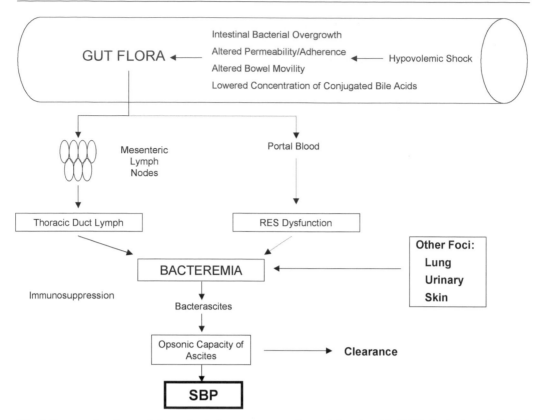

Fig. 1. Proposed pathogenic hypothesis for spontaneous bacterial peritonitis. RES: Reticuloendothelial system.

reach MLN but these will usually be phagocytosed prior to multiplication and seeding of blood and other sites. The majority of patients with cirrhosis and ascites have deficient serum complement levels; some have levels low enough to be comparable to those of patients with congenital complement deficiency. Because complement is required for the opsonization of most virulent organisms, complement deficiency would be expected to predispose to bacterial infections, including bacteremia. The ascitic fluid in patients with advanced cirrhosis is characterized by deficient complement and albumin, which reduce the opsonozing capacity of the ascitic fluid. The concentration of the third and fourth components of complement in low-protein ascitic fluid can be very low, even undetectable.

Neutrophils are attracted to areas of bacterial invasion by bacterial activation of complement. If complement is not activated adequately or neutrophils do not respond appropriately, neutrophil-mediated killing of bacteria does not occur. Kupffer cells extract bacteria from the blood to minimize the duration and severity of bacteremia. If the portal blood bypasses the Kupffer cells and flows through collaterals instead, or if there is a qualitative defect in Kupffer cell function, bacteremia would be expected to be frequent and prolonged.

In summary, the infectious process probably starts by colonization of the gut, urinary bladder, pharynx, or skin by supranormal numbers of bacteria (Fig. 1). Intestinal bacterial overgrowth has been documented in patients and rats with cirrhosis (15,29,30). In the gut, bacterial overgrowth predictably leads to extragastrointestinal dissemination of bacteria with colonization of mesenteric lymph nodes by these bacteria (6,15). Mesenteric lymphatics are under high pressure with high flow rates in the setting of cirrhosis. It is possible that bacteria-laden lymph could leak directly into ascitic fluid from lymphatics that have ruptured under pression, thereby colonizing the ascitic fluid. Alternatively, the bacteria could enter the systemic circulation and then leak across Glisson's capsule into ascitic fluid as contaminated lymph. The portal route could be another less-frequent alternative way of bacterial entrance. Defective neutrophils and poor Kupffer cell function would permit this bacteremia. Spontaneous bacteremia has then occurred. By either the direct lymphatic leak route or the circuitous bacteremia route, bacterascites can develop. Now a battle between the organisms' virulence factors and host's defenses begins. The first lines of defense are ascitic fluid complement and peritoneal macrophages. If the peritoneal macrophages together with complement are unsuccessful in eradicating the colonization, complement is activated and neutrophils are attracted into the ascitic fluid. SBP has then occurred. Although fewer data are available to help explain the pathogenesis of spontaneous bacteremia caused by pneumonia, urinary tract infection, or cellulites, the basic mechanisms are probably similar to those of SBP, that is, multiple defects in host defense.

DIAGNOSIS OF SBP

The high prevalence of immunodeficiency among patients with severe acute or chronic liver disease combined with the high prevalence of bacterial infection should lead to a high index of suspicion of bacterial infection on the part of the physicians caring for these patients. All cirrhotic patients with ascites can develop SBP. Although 87% of patients with SBP have signs or symptoms of infection (including 68% with fever, 49% with abdominal pain, and 54% with mental status change), 13% have no such findings and the change in mental status may be very subtle or misinterpreted as a manifestation of something other than an infection. Bacterial infection may be manifested only by acidosis, azotemia, peripheral leukocytosis, or hypotension or by impairment of liver function or renal failure as the predominant or only features. Moreover, SBP may be asymptomatic or there may be minor symptoms only, particularly when the diagnosis of the infection is made at hospital admission. Therefore, a high index of suspicion of infection is required for early detection and early treatment of the infection and maximum survival of the patient.

A diagnostic paracentesis should be performed on hospital admission in all cirrhotic patients with ascites to investigate the presence of SBP, even in patients admitted for reasons other than ascites. A diagnostic tap should also be performed in hospitalized patients with ascites if and when they develop any of the following: (a) local symptoms or signs suggestive of peritoneal infection, such as abdominal pain, rebound tenderness, or clinically relevant alterations of gastrointestinal motility (i.e., vomiting, diarrhea, ileus); (b) systemic signs of infection, such as fever, leukocytosis, or septic shock; (c) hepatic encephalopathy or rapid impairment in renal function without any clear precipitating factor; and (d) in patients with ascites and gastrointestinal hemorrhage before the administration of prophylactic antibiotics (31) (Table 1).

On the basis of currently available data, the greatest sensitivity for the diagnosis of SBP is reached with a cutoff polymorphonuclear leukocytes (PMN) count of 250/mm^3,

Table 1
Recommendations on Diagnosis of Spontaneous Bacterial Peritonitis

1. Diagnostic parecentesis in cirrhosis with ascites:
   At hospital admission for the study/treatment of an episode of ascites
   Whenever a cirrhotic patient develops any of the following:
   — Local signs of peritonitis (pain, diarrhea, ileus, vomiting)
   — Systemic signs of infection (fever, leukocytosis, septic shock)
   — Hepatic encephalopathy without any clear precipitating factor
   — Rapid renal function impairment without an apparent cause
   Prior to antibiotic prophylaxis, if gastrointestinal bleeding
2. Diagnosis of spontaneous bacterial peritonitis based on ascitic fluid PMN count $>250/mm^3$
3. Cultures:
   Ascitic fluid culture: bedside inoculation into blood culture bottles (minimum amount: 10 mL)
   Blood cultures simultaneous to ascitic fluid cultures

although the greatest specificity is reached with a cutoff of 500 PMN/mm^3. In patients with bloody ascitic fluid, a correction factor of 1 PMN per 250 red blood cells (RBC) has been proposed because this is the maximum expected ratio of PMN to RBCs normally present in peripheral blood.

A PMN count of more than $250/mm^3$ is highly suspicious of SBP and constitutes an indication to empirically initiate antibiotic treatment prior to and independent of ascites bacteriological culture results. Although an ascitic fluid PMN count greater than $500/mm^3$ is more specific for the diagnosis of SBP, the risk of not treating the few patients with SBP who have an ascites PMN between 250 and $500/mm^3$ is unacceptable. An ascitic fluid PMN count of less than $250/mm^3$ excludes the diagnosis of SBP.

The use of reagent strips for leukocyte esterase designed for testing of urine has recently shown to be useful in the diagnosis of SBP; only 1 of 52 cases with reagent strip result of 3+ to 4+ was misclassified (i.e., did not have SBP) (32). However, reagent strip results of 1+ and 2+ (indicative of 25 and 75 PMN/mL, respectively), which constituted the majority of the cases, would have misclassified 6 of 57 cases of SBP (i.e., these patients would have not been treated), although five of them had PMN counts $>250/mm^3$ but $<500/mm^3$.

Culture of ascitic fluid should be performed at the bedside using blood culture bottles, including both aerobic and anaerobic media, and blood cultures should also be obtained before initiating antibiotic administration. The minimum amount of ascitic fluid inoculated in each bottle should be 10 mL. However, even using the method of inoculating ascites into blood culture bottles, cultures are still negative in approx 30–50% of patients with an increased ascites PMN count. This low proportion of positive ascitic fluid cultures is probably a result of the relatively low concentration of bacteria in ascitic fluid compared to infections in other organic fluids, such as urine. In a significant proportion of patients with SBP, blood cultures are positive, in these cases, bacteria isolated from peripheral blood are presumably the same bacteria causing SBP. Despite negative ascitic and blood cultures, patients with an increased ascites PMN count should be considered as having SBP. At present, the Gram stain of a smear of sediment of ascetic fluid is positive

Table 2
Suspicion of Secondary Peritonitis

— Lack of response to antibiotic treatment
— Two or more organisms isolated in ascitic fluid (particularly anaerobes or fungi)
— At least two of the following findings in ascitic fluid:
  • Glucose <50 mg/dL
  • Protein >10 g/L
  • Lactic dehydrogenase >normal serum levels

in only a few cases, probably because SBP is usually diagnosed at very early stages of the infection, when the concentration of organisms in ascites is very low. In patients with hepatic hydrothorax in whom an infection is suspected and in whom SBP has been ruled out, a diagnostic thoracentesis should be performed given that spontaneous bacterial empyema may occur in the absence of ascites or SBP *(33)*.

Although the vast majority of cirrhotic patients with ascites and peritoneal infection have SBP, a small group of patients could have bacterial peritonitis secondary to perforation or acute inflammation of intraabdominal organs, abdominal wall infections, or previous abdominal surgical procedures. With the exception of the two latter conditions, the differential diagnosis between spontaneous and secondary peritonitis can occasionally be difficult, but it is very important because secondary peritonitis usually does not resolve unless patients are treated surgically. Secondary peritonitis should be suspected when there is one of the following conditions: lack of response to antibiotic treatment, more than one organism isolated from ascites (particularly when the growth of anaerobic bacteria or fungi is observed), and when in the ascitic fluid the glucose levels are below 50 mg/dL, the protein concentration is higher than 10 g/L and lactic dehydrogenase concentration is above normal serum levels *(34)* (Table 2). When secondary peritonitis is suspected, antibiotic treatment should include antimicrobial agents against anaerobic organisms and enterococci, and the presence of secondary peritonitis should be properly investigated.

MANAGEMENT OF SBP

The prognosis of SBP has varied to a great extent since its clinical description in 1971. In the 78 episodes of SBP analyzed in the study by Conn and Fessel, the hospital mortality rate was approx 95% *(35)*. Survival rates and resolution of infection rates improved dramatically in the 1980s to 37–77% and 50–85%, respectively. This trend has been confirmed in the reports of the last decade with corresponding figures of 74–83% and 83–92%, respectively *(36,37)* (Fig. 2). Early diagnosis and the initiation of prompt effective antibiotic therapy have played key roles in decreasing the mortality associated with SBP.

Because SBP is a serious infection that may precipitate numerous potentially lethal complications (septic shock, progressive circulatory and renal impairment, liver failure), empirical antibiotic therapy must be started as soon as the diagnosis of the infection is established, without prior knowledge of the causative organisms and their in vitro susceptibility. Because Gram-negative aerobic bacteria from the family of *Enterobacteriaceae* and nonenterococcal *Streptococcus* spp. are the most common causative organisms, the initial empirical antibiotic therapy of SBP should cover these organisms. Moreover, the

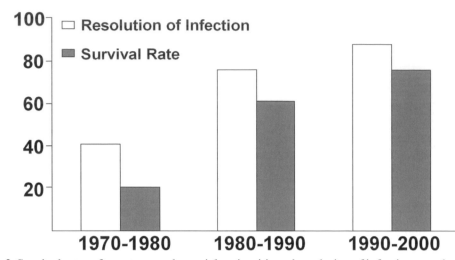

Fig. 2. Survival rates of spontaneous bacterial peritonitis and resolution of infection rates have been improved dramatically in the last decades. Early diagnosis and the initiation of prompt effective antibiotic therapy have played key roles in decreasing the mortality associated with spontaneous bacterial peritonitis.

pharmacokinetic properties of the antibiotics selected should be adequate to treat peritoneal infection, with an antibiotic concentration in ascitic fluid above MIC_{90} of causative microorganisms.

Cefotaxime and Other Cephalosporins

A landmark study comparing the combination ampicillin/tobramycin (a classic antibiotic regim) with cefotaxime demonstrated that cefotaxime was more effective and safer than the association of tobramycin-ampicillin and that the survival rate at the end of hospitalization was also greater in patients treated with cefotaxime *(38)*. This study set the stage for subsequent studies that established cefotaxime and other third-generation cephalosporins as the first choice antimicrobial agents in the treatment of SBP *(31)*. The cure rate with these antibiotics ranges between 80% and 94% *(31)*. The combination of amoxicillin and clavulanic acid (initially intravenous (iv) and then orally) has been shown to be as effective as cefotaxime in the treatment of SBP *(39)*.

Two randomized controlled trials assessing the optimal duration of therapy and dosage of cefotaxime in cirrhotic patients with SBP have been reported. One of these trials showed that 5-d therapy with cefotaxime (2 g iv every 8 h) was as effective as 10-d therapy in relation to the rate of resolution of infection (91.2% vs 93.1%), and hospital mortality rates (42.5% vs 32.6%) *(40)*. Another trial reported similar rates of SBP resolution and patient survival in cirrhotic patients with SBP receiving cefotaxime at a dose of either 2 g/6 h or 2 g/12 h *(41)*. The results of these two trials suggest that the high efficacy of cefotaxime in SBP can be maintained with short-course administration of this antimicrobial agent and with doses lower than those formerly used, with a significant reduction in the cost of the antibiotic. In Table 3 the results obtained with cefotaxime in the treatment of SBP are shown.

Table 3
Cefotaxime in the Treatment of Spontaneous Bacterial Peritonitis

	Spontaneous bacterial peritonitis resolution (%)	Hospital survival (%)
Felisart et al. *(38)* (2 g/4 h)	86	73
Runyon et al. *(40)*		
5 d treatment	93	67
10 d treatment	91	42
Rimola et al. *(41)*		
2 g/6 h	75	69
2 g/12 h	79	62

The rate of SBP resolution and patient survival has been found to be very high with the use of other cephalosporins, including ceftriaxone, cefonicid, ceftazidime, and ceftizoxime *(31)*, with no differences as compared to that reported with the use of cefotaxime.

Oral Antibiotics

In most instances, patients with SBP are in relatively good clinical condition and may be treated orally. Navasa et al. *(42)* reported the results of a randomized controlled trial in patients with nonseverely complicated SBP comparing oral ofloxacin (400 mg/12 h) to iv cefotaxime (2 g/6 h). The results of this study strongly suggest that oral ofloxacin is as effective as intravenous cefotaxime in the treatment of patients with uncomplicated SBP (no shock, ileus, gastrointestinal hamorrhage, profound hepatic encephalopathy, or serum creatinine >3 mg/dL). The investigators also suggest that a special small subgroup may be treated as outpatients. Although this idea carries great potential, clearly more such patients need to be studied before a general recommendation about outpatient can be made.

A study showed that iv ciprofloxacin was as useful as ciprofloxacin used intravenously during 2 d followed by oral ciprofoxacin *(43)*; however, resolution rates (76–78%) appeared to be lower than those reported in the earlier ofloxacin study (95%) or with the use of cefotaxime or with amoxicillin/clavulanate.

Aminoglycosides

As mentioned above, the usefulness of the association of ampicillin and tobramycin has been assessed in cirrhotic patients with severe infections *(38)*. Other combinations included cephalotin with either gentamicin or tobramycin, and mezlocillin with netilmicin *(44)*. The efficacy of these combinations is only moderate and, importantly, they are associated with a high incidence of nephrotoxicity. Cirrhotic patients are particularly prone to develop nephrotoxicity from aminoglycosides *(45)* and this is further supported by a recent retrospective case-control study that demonstrated that the presence of ascites and the use of aminoglycoside antibiotics were the only independent predictors of renal dysfunction in hospitalized cirrhotic patients *(46)*. Therefore, aminoglycosides should be avoided in cirrhotic patients and should only be considered as a last resort in the treatment of SBP and other infections in cirrhosis.

Table 4
Infections in Cirrhotic Patients in Relation to Norfloxacin Prophylaxis (50)

	No prophylaxis (n = 414)	Norfloxacin prophylaxis (n = 93)	P value
Gram-negative infections	46%	52%	N.S.
Quinolone-resistant	29%	65%	0.002
TMP-SMX*-resistant	44%	68%	0.02
Gram-positive infections	46%	42%	N.S.
Mixed infections	8%	6%	N.S.

*TMP-SMX: Trimethoprim-sulfamethoxazole.

Antibiotics in Patients on Chronic Quinolone Prophylaxis

At present, some patients developing SBP are receiving prophylaxis with quinolones. As expected, the use of norfloxacin prophylaxis has modified the microbial epidemiology of bacterial infections in cirrhosis. Duperyron et al. observed the presence of quinolone-resistant strains of Gram-negative bacteria in the stool of cirrhotic patients on norfloxacin (47), and this has recently been confirmed in a trial by Bauer et al. comparing daily norfloxacin to weekly rufloxacin in the prevention of SBP (48). In another study, Novella et al. showed that 90% of *E. coli* isolated (mostly from urinary infections) from patients on continuous long-term norfloxacin prophylaxis were resistant to quinolones (49). A large prospective study by Fernández et al. (50) showed that 65% of Gram-negative bacteria isolated from patients on long-term norfloxacin were quinolone-resistant compared to only 29% of Gram-negative bacteria from patients not on long-term norfloxacin. Importantly, trimethoprim/sulfamethoxazole resistance was also significantly more frequent in Gram-negative bacteria isolated from patients on long-term norfloxacin (68% vs 44%) (Table 4). An interesting point in the evolution of quinolone resistance in patients with cirrhosis receiving prophylaxis with norfloxacin has been the maintenance of a high efficacy despite the evidence that norfloxacin is unable to maintain a selective intestinal decontamination (48). Different explanations have been proposed for this phenomenon, including a reduction in the intestinal overgrowth, a diminution in the bacterial adhesion resulting in a decreased translocation capacity, and a favorable effect of quinolones upon nonspecific immune defenses. Additionally, the rate of methicillin-resistant *Staphylococcus aureus* (MRSA) infections has also been associated with prior antibiotic therapy and norfloxacin prophylaxis in cirrhotics (51,52).

Although there have been no prospective trials of SBP therapy in patients on prophylactic antibiotics, a large retrospective study compared clinical characteristics and response to therapy of patients with and without norfloxacin prophylaxis (53). Most (83%) patients in this study were treated with cefotaxime and there were no differences both in infection resolution between patients receiving or not receiving prophylaxis treatment (100 vs 91%) and in hospital mortality (20 vs 26%). In another report of 39 infections caused by *E. coli* resistant to norfloxacin, infections were shown to be equally severe than those caused by norfloxacin-sensitive *E. coli* and none were shown to be resistant to cefotaxime, whereas one was resistant to amoxicillin/clavulanate (54).

In a recent study that compared cefotaxime vs amoxicillin/clavulanate in the treatment of infections in cirrhosis, 22 patients were undergoing prophylaxis with norfloxacin (55).

Table 5
Hospital Mortality According to the Evolution of Kidney
Function in 231 SBP Episodes that Responded to Treatment *(56)*

SBP-RI status	Number	Deaths
Episodes without SBP-RI	166	12 (7%)
Episodes with SBP-RI	65	27 (42%)*
Transient SBP-RI	21	1 (5%)
Steady SBP-RI	26	8 (31%)*
Progressive SBP-RI	181	181 (100%)*

SBP-RI: Renal impairment induced by an episode of SBP; $*p = 0.001$ vs episodes without SBP-RI.

Infection resolution was achieved in all 10 patients in the amoxicillin/clavulanic acid group and in 10 of 12 patients in the cefotaxime group. This difference was not statistically significant but there was a trend for a higher resolution rate in the amoxicillin/clavulanate group, which will require confirmation in larger controlled trials.

Taking into account all of these results, for patients developing SBP while under quinolone prophylaxis, cefotaxime administration appears as the most adequate antibiotic regimen. However, given the higher rate of Gram-positive cocci infections, particularly MRSA, in patients on norfloxacin prophylaxis, the addition of vancomycin should be considered in patients who fail therapy and in whom ascites culture is negative.

Adjuncts to Antibiotic Therapy

In one-third of patients with SBP, renal impairment develops despite treatment of their infection with nonnephrotoxic antibiotics. This deterioration of renal function is the most sensitive predictor of in-hospital mortality *(56)* (Table 5). Renal impairment occurs in patients with the highest concentrations of cytokines in plasma and ascitic fluid and is associated with a marked activation of the renin-angiotensin system *(57)*. Therefore, it is considered that renal impairment in SBP occurs as a result of a further decrease in effective arterial blood volume, which in turn results from a cytokine-mediated aggravation of vasodilatation (Fig. 3).

Recently, a prospective randomized study comparing cefotaxime plus albumin with cefotaxime alone was performed in 126 patients with SBP with the objective of determining whether plasma volume expansion with albumin could prevent this impairment in renal function and improve survival in patients with SBP. The dose of albumin administered was 1.5 g/kg of body weight during the first 6 h after the diagnosis of SBP, followed by 1 g/kg on d 3. Although the rate of infection resolution was similar in both groups (94% in the cefotaxime group vs 98% in the cefotaxime + albumin group), patients who received albumin had significantly lower rates of renal dysfunction (10% vs 33%), in-hospital mortality (10% vs 29%), and 3-mo mortality (22% vs 41%) compared to patients who did not receive albumin *(58)*. Thus, in patients with cirrhosis and SBP, treatment with iv albumin in addition to an antibiotic reduces the incidence of renal impairment and death in comparison with an antibiotic alone. Patients treated with cefotaxime had higher levels of plasma renin activity than those treated with cefotaxime and albumin; patients with renal impairment had the highest values. Thus, the most likely explanation for the reduced

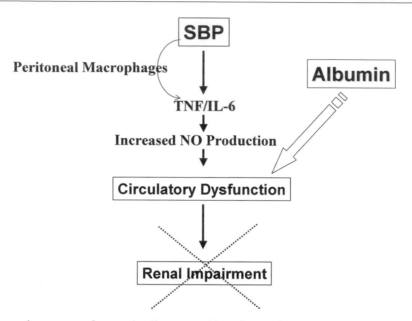

Fig. 3. Proposed sequence of events leading to renal impairment in patients with spontaneous bacterial peritonitis. Albumin administration prevents circulatory disfunction (i.e., maintaining the effective arterial blood volume) and the subsequent activation of vasoconstrictor systems.

rate of early mortality in patients who were treated with albumin is that such treatment prevents circulatory disfunction (i.e., maintaining the effective arterial blood volume) and the subsequent activation of vasoconstrictor systems. The in-patient mortality rate of 10% is the lowest described so far for SBP. The group of patients that appeared to be more likely to benefit from the addition of albumin was characterized by having a serum bilirubin level of >4 mg/dL and evidence of renal impairment at baseline (blood urea nitrogen >30 mg/dL and/or creatinine >1.0 mg/dL) (Fig. 4).

Intravenous albumin is expensive and has limited availability in some settings. Therefore, studies should be performed to determine whether treatment of SBP with lower doses of albumin or with artificial plasma expanders, which are less expensive, would have similar beneficial effects on renal function and survival. On the other hand, a prior study from the same investigators had identified a subgroup of patients with SBP that had an excellent prognosis (100% SBP resolution and 100% survival) with antibiotic therapy alone *(42)*. Probably, this subgroup would not require adjunctive therapy with albumin and is characterized by having a community-acquired SBP, no encephalopathy and a blood urea nitrogen <25 mg/dL (Table 6).

ROLE OF PROPHYLAXIS

As the gut appears to be the main source of bacteria that cause SBP, prophylaxis of SBP has been based on the oral administration of nonabsorbable or poorly absorbed antibiotics that will eliminate or reduce the concentration of Gram-negative gut bacteria without affecting Gram-positive organisms or anaerobes (selective intestinal decontamination). Long-term administration of orally administered norfloxacin, a poorly absorbed quinolone, has been shown to produce a marked reduction of GNB from the fecal flora of cirrhotic patients with no significant effects on GPC or anaerobic bacteria *(52)*.

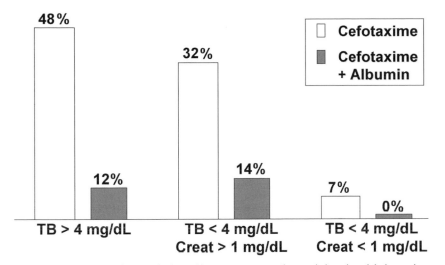

Fig. 4. Incidence of renal impairment induced by spontaneous bacterial peritonitis in patients treated with cefotaxime alone or associated with albumin administration grouped according different levels of total bilirubin and/or serum creatinine *(58)*.

Table 6
Predictors of Good Outcome
(100% of Infection Resolution and Survival)
of Spontaneous Bacterial Peritonitis *(42)*

— Uncomplicated Spontaneous Bacterial Peritonitis
  • No gastrointestinal hemorrhage
  • No severe hepatic encephalopathy
  • No septic shock
  • No ileus
  • Serum creatinine <3 mg/dL
— Community-acquired infection
— BUN <25 mg/dL
— No hepatic encephalopathy

Nevertheless, the high incidence of quinolone and trimethoprim/sulfamethoxazole resistant strains of *E. coli* isolated in decontaminated cirrhotic patients underlines the necessity of restricting the administration of prophylactic antibiotics only to those patients at the greatest risk of SBP. In addition, the increasing emergence of infections caused by quinolone and trimethoprim/sulfamethoxazole-resistant strains of Gram-negative bacilli also suggests that the effectiveness of selective intestinal decontamination will decrease with time owing to their widespread use. Thus, further studies are needed to evaluate alternative prophylactic measures such as other antibiotic regimes and nonantibiotic procedures in SBP prophylaxis.

Prevention of SBP Recurrence

Patients who have recovered from an episode of SBP are at a high risk of developing SBP recurrence. These patients have a 1-yr probability of SBP recurrence of 40–70% *(59,60)*.

In a double-blind placebo-controlled study, continuous oral norfloxacin was shown to significantly decrease the 1-yr probability of developing recurrent SBP from 68% (in the placebo group) to 20% (in the norfloxacin group). This was even more obvious for the probability of developing SBP caused by Gram-negative organisms, which was reduced from 60% to 3% *(60)*. Therefore, long-term selective intestinal decontamination dramatically decreases the rate of SBP recurrence in patients with SBP. Long-term prophylaxis with oral norfloxacin at a dose of 400 mg every day is indicated in patients who have recovered from an episode of SBP and should be initiated as soon as the course of antibiotics for the acute event is completed. Prophylaxis should be continuous until disappearance of ascites, death, or transplant *(31)*.

Prevention of Bacterial Infections in Cirrhotic Patients with Gastrointestinal Hemorrhage

All cirrhotic patients with upper gastrointestinal hemorrhage, independent of the presence or absence of ascites, are predisposed to develop severe bacterial infections, including SBP, within the first days of the hemorrhagic episode. Approximately 20% of these patients are already infected at admission to the hospital *(61)*, and between 30% and 40% of patients develop a nosocomial bacterial infection during hospitalization *(61, 62)*. This extremely high incidence of bacterial infections seems to be related to several dysfunctions that occur in bleeding patients as a consequence of the acute hemorrhage, such as depression of the activity of the reticuloendothelial system, alteration of intestinal permeability, and an increase in bacterial translocation. These alterations could be especially aggravated in patients with cirrhosis.

Because most microorganisms causing infection in cirrhotic patients are of enteric origin, the initial investigations addressed the effectiveness of prophylactic intestinal decontamination in these patients. Two randomized, controlled studies have demonstrated that selective intestinal decontamination with oral administration of antibiotics is effective in preventing bacterial infection in cirrhotic patients with gastrointestinal hemorrhage *(62,63)*. Three other studies show that iv antibiotics or fully absorbed oral antibiotics are also effective in preventing infections, including SBP, in cirrhotic patients with gastrointestinal bleeding *(64–66)* (Fig. 5).

A meta-analysis of these five randomized trials shows that short-term antibiotic prophylaxis significantly increased the mean percentage of patients free of infection (32% mean improvement rate, 95% confidence interval [CI]: 22–42; $p < 0.001$), bacteremia and/or SBP (19% mean improvement rate, 95% CI: 11–26; $p < 0.001$), and SBP (7% mean improvement rate, 95% CI: 2.1–12.6; $p = 0.006$). Antibiotic prophylaxis also significantly increased the mean survival rate (9.1% mean improvement rate, 95% CI: 2.9–15.3; $p = 0.004$), without significant heterogeneity *(67)*. Another more recent meta-analysis that also included two small randomized trials of antibiotic prophylaxis immediately prior to sclerotherapy also concluded that antibiotic prophylaxis for cirrhotic patients with gastrointestinal bleeding is efficacious in reducing the number of deaths and bacterial infections *(68)*.

Based on the above, short (7 d) prophylaxis is recommended in cirrhotic patients admitted with gastrointestinal hemorrhage, independent of the presence or absence of ascites, because this measure is effective in preventing bacterial infections and improving survival *(31)*. Although several antibiotic regimens are useful in these patients, oral administration of norfloxacin at a dose of 400 mg twice a day, appears to be the first-choice antibiotic

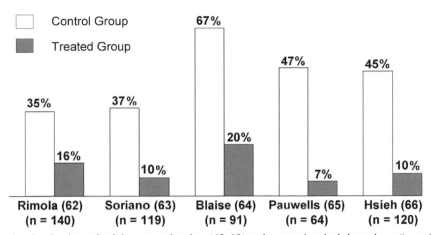

Fig. 5. Both selective intestinal decontamination *(62,63)* and systemic administration of prophylactic antibiotic agents *(64–66)* significantly decreased the mean percentage of patients free of infection in all five studies represented.

prophylaxis owing to its simpler administration and lower cost. In patients in whom it cannot be administered by mouth or through a nasogastric tube, systemic antibiotics can be administered.

Prophylaxis in Ascitic Cirrhotic Patients without Prior SBP or Gastrointestinal Hemorrhage

Ascites protein content has been shown to be a good predictor of SBP. Patients with a low (<1.0 g/dL) ascites protein (who receive short-term prophylaxis if and when they develop gastrointestinal hemorrhage) have a 1-yr probability of developing SBP of around 20% *(69)*, and of 40% (in patients who did not receive this prophylaxis) *(70)*. The risk of SBP in patients without a previous history of SBP and with an ascites protein content >1.0 g/dL is very low, with 1-yr and 3-yr probabilities of 0 and 3%, respectively *(69)*. Therefore, long-term prophylactic administration of antibiotics is not necessary because the risk of SBP in these patients is negligible provided adequate prophylaxis is administered if and when gastrointestinal hemorrhage develops in the course of the disease *(31)*.

Several studies have assessed the effect of prophylaxis of SBP in nonbleeding cirrhotic patients with ascites: two of them have used norfloxacin and other antibiotic regimens in the other two studies. The first study included 63 cirrhotic patients admitted to hospital for the treatment of an episode of ascites with an ascitic fluid total protein concentration lower than 15 g/L, some of whom had had a previous episode of SBP. In this inhomogeneous population, the administration of norfloxacin, 400 mg/d throughout the hospitalization period, decreased the in-hospital incidence of SBP from 22% in the control group to 0% in the treated group *(71)*. The second controlled double-blind trial of oral norfloxacin in the primary prophylaxis of SBP included cirrhotic patients with low ascites protein (<15 g/L) and no previous episodes of SBP. In this study, the 6-mo incidence of SBP was 0% in the group of patients prophylactically treated with norfloxacin, 400 mg/d, compared with 11% in patients treated with placebo. Nevertheless, the incidence of SBP caused by Gram-negative organisms (the only type that can be prevented by norfloxacin

Table 7
Indications and Duration of Selective Intestinal Decontamination
for the Prevention of Spontaneous Bacterial Peritonitis in Cirrhotic Patients (31)

Indications	Duration of prophylaxis
Cirrhotic Patients Recovering from a Previous Episode of SBP	Indefinitely or Until Disappearance of Ascites or Liver Transplantation
Cirrhotic Patients with Gastrointestinal Bleeding	7 d
Cirrhotic Patients with Ascites and Low Ascitic Fluid Protein Levels (<10 g/L)	No Consensus

prophylaxis) in the two groups was not statistically different: 0% in the norfloxacin group and 5% in the placebo group (72).

Other antibiotic regimes have been evaluated in the prevention of SBP in high-risk patients. A placebo-controlled study demonstrated that 6-mo prophylaxis with ciprofloxacin, 750 mg weekly, was effective in reducing the incidence of SBP in cirrhotic patients with low ascitic fluid protein concentration: 4% in the treated group and 22% in the placebo-control group (73). In this study, patients with and without a previous episode of SBP were included together and no attempt was made to evaluate the development of SBP in these two subgroups of patients separately. Finally, Singh et al. (74) have shown that trimethoprim/sulfamethoxazole is also effective in the prevention of SBP in 60 cirrhotic patients with ascites. The incidence of SBP during the study period (medium follow-up of only 90 d) was 3% in the treated group and 27% in the control group. Again, patients with different risk of SBP were analyzed together: patients with low and high ascitic fluid protein and patients with and without previous SBP episodes.

In patients with low protein content in ascitic fluid who have never had SBP the recommendation of antibiotic prophylaxis is difficult to establish, owing to the mentioned heterogeneity of the published studies, which included patients with low and high risk of SBP together. This is the main reason for the lack of consensus (30) because, despite the positive results of all the studies abovementioned, they have been unable to identify subsets of patients who clearly benefit from this therapy (Table 7).

In a recent study, Guarner et al. (75) have identified a subgroup of patients at high risk of developing a first episode of SBP, among 109 cirrhotic patients with ascites protein levels of <10 g/L. Patients with high serum bilirubin (>3.2 mg/dL) and/or low platelet count (<98,000/mm^3) present a 1-yr probability of developing a first episode of SBP of 55%, the highest reported so far, in comparison with 24% of patients with only low ascitic fluid protein levels. If these results are validated, this group of patients would be included in prophylactic (ideally placebo-controlled) trials.

Since survival expectancy is very much reduced after SBP (59), patients recovering from an episode of SBP should be considered as potential candidates for liver transplantation.

OTHER COMMON INFECTIONS IN CIRRHOSIS

Bacterial infection is one of the most important clinical problems in patients with decompensated cirrhosis. It is present at admission or develops during hospitalization in

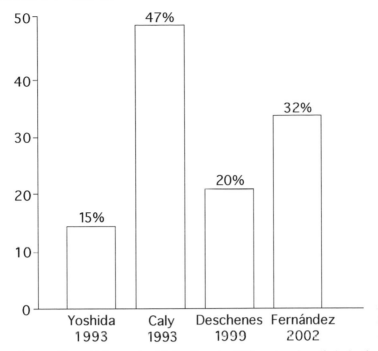

Fig. 6. Prevalence of hospital-acquired infections in different series of cirrhotic patients.

20% to 60% of the patients *(2,76–78)*. These figures contrast sharply with the hospital-acquired infections rate in a general hospital patient population (5–7%) (Fig. 6). On the other hand, between 7% and 25% of the deaths of cirrhotic patients are related to bacterial infections. Most studies assessing the etiology and clinical types of bacterial infections in cirrhosis were performed in the 1980s. At that time, the most frequent infections were urinary tract infections, pneumonia, and SBP; most infections were community acquired, and the great majority of the isolated microorganisms were Gram-negative bacilli.

During the last decade, practice in hepatology has considerably changed, and this may have influenced the epidemiology and frequency of bacterial infections in cirrhosis. In addition to the wide use of norfloxacin prophylaxis, treatment of cirrhotic patients with severe complications in intensive care units has been generalized, particularly with the extension of the liver transplantation programs, and new invasive treatments, such as variceal ligation, transjugular intrahepatic portosystemic shunt, and arterial embolization of hepatocellular carcinoma, have been developed and are widely used for specific complications of cirrhosis. The reported incidence of bacterial infections in recent, larger, prospective series performed in consecutively admitted cirrhotic patients, report bacterial infection rates of 32% *(50)* and 34% *(80)*. Patients with decompensated cirrhosis have been consistently shown to develop infections at a higher rate compared to compensated cirrhosis *(2)*. In another prospective study, admission for gastrointestinal bleeding and a low serum albumin were identified as the only two variables independently associated with the development of a bacterial infection *(79)*. Studies that have compared mortality in infected vs noninfected patients uniformly show that patients who develop an infection have a significant higher mortality *(2,80)*. Current evidence also suggests that infections predispose to recurrent variceal bleeding *(81–83)*. The largest prospective series of 572

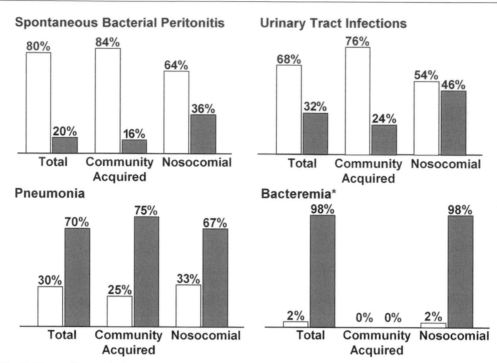

Fig. 7. Type of bacteria isolated in community-acquired and nosocomial infections in the study by Fernández et al. *(50)*. Infections caused by Gram-negative bacilli are represented in empty bars whereas those caused by Gram-positive cocci are represented in dashed bars. *Bacteremia associated with therapeutic invasive procedures and catheter sepsis.

consecutive infections in 405 cirrhotic patients hospitalized between 1998 and 2000 clearly indicates that the epidemiology of bacterial infections in cirrhosis has changed during the last decade *(50)*. Community-acquired infections are still more common (61%) but SBP was the most common infection, followed by urinary tract infection, pneumonia, and spontaneous bacteremia. Whereas Gram-negative bacilli were the main bacteria isolated in community-acquired infections, nosocomial infections were more frequently caused by Gram-positive cocci. In fact, Gram-positive cocci were the causative organisms in almost 50% of the infections, being the most frequently isolated bacteria in bacteremia, either associated to procedures (100%) or spontaneous (57%) and in nosocomial infections (60%). The increase in the number of infections caused by Gram-positive cocci can be explained by the higher degree of instrumentation of patients, and suggests that to reduce nosocomial infections in patients with cirrhosis, urinary and central venous catheters should be used only when necessary and removed as soon as possible. By contrast, Gram-negative bacteria continued to be the main organism responsible for SBP, independent of the site of infection acquisition, as well as in urinary tract infections (68%) and in community-acquired infections (60%) (Fig. 7). Another important finding of this study was that quinolone-resistant SBP constitutes an emergent problem in patients on long-term norfloxacin prophylaxis, with trimethoprim-sulfamethoxazole not being a valid alternative (Table 4). This observation should promote investigations aimed at identifying new prophylactic treatments in SBP.

Urinary Tract Infections

As in the noncirrhotic population, cirrhotics with indwelling catheters are highly predisposed to develop urinary tract infections. The incidence is markedly higher in female than in male cirrhotics *(84)*. The majority of these infections in cirrhotic patients are caused by Gram-negative bacilli *(50)*. Although urine culture are always recommended, cases requiring immediate therapy should be given a modern quinolone, or amoxicillin plus clavulanic acid or an oral cephalosporin *(85)*.

Pneumonia

Community-acquired pneumonia is a frequent complication in subjects with active alcoholism. Although *Streptococcus pneumoniae* is the most frequent causative organism, a significant number of cases of pneumonia are caused by other pathogens normally present in the oropharyngeal area, especially anaerobic bacteria or by Gram-negative bacilli. All of these organisms, together with the possibility of *Mycoplasma pneumoniae* or *Legionella* sp. should be considered when selecting empiric antibiotic therapy. Therefore, a suggested antibiotic regime could include erythromycin combined with one of the following antibiotics: cefotaxime, ceftriaxone, amoxicillin-clavulanic acid, or imipenem *(86)*. Because hospital-acquired pneumonia is predominantly caused by Gram-negative bacilli and staphylococci, the empiric administration of third-generation cephalosporins should be considered as the first choice of antibiotic. In the case of suspicion of aspiration, clindamycin should be added.

Other Infections

Soft tissue infections, particularly lymphangitis of the lower extremities and abdominal wall, are relatively frequent in cirrhotic patients with ankle edema or ascites. Although *Staphylococcus aureus* and *Streptococcus pyogenes* are the most frequent causative organisms, enterobacteriaceae and anaerobes may also be responsible for these infections. Cloxacillin has been considered the first choice antibiotic, but considering these causative organisms, amoxicillin-calvulanic acid may be a more adequate empiric antibiotic treatment.

Cirrhotic patients with hydrothorax can develop spontaneous bacterial empyema *(33)*. The pathogenesis is though to be the same as that of SBP, because the isolated bacteria are also the same. Therefore, patients with spontaneous bacterial empyema should be treated with the same antibiotic regimes.

REFERENCES

1. García-Tsao G. Spontaneous bacterial peritonitis. Gastroenterol Clin N Am 1992;21:257–275.
2. Caly WR, Strauss E. A prospective study of bacterial infections in patients with cirrhosis. J Hepatol 1993; 18:353–358.
3. Pinzello G, Simonetti R, Camma C, et al. Spontaneous bacterial peritonitis: an update. Gastroenterol Int 1993;6:54–60.
4. Berg RD, Garlington AW. Translocation of certain indigenous bacteria from the gastrointestinal tract to the mesenteric lymph nodes and other organs in a gnotobiotic mouse model. Infect Immun 1979;23: 403–411.
5. Steffen EK, Berg RD, Deitch EA. Comparison of translocation rates of various indigenous bacteria from the gastrointestinal tract to the mesenteric lymph nodes. J Infect Dis 1988;157:1032–1038.

6. Runyon BA, Squier SU, Borzio M. Translocation of gut bacteria in rats with cirrhosis to mesenteric lymph nodes partially explains the pathogenesis of spontaneous bacterial peritonitis. J Hepatol 1994;21: 792–796.

7. Llovet JM, Bartolí R, Planas R, et al. Bacterial translocation in cirrhotic rats: its role in the development of spontaneous bacterial peitonitis. Gut 1994;35:1648–1652.

8. Hamdani R, Chaparala R, Stauber RE, et al. PEG 600 absorption and urinary excretion identifies cirrhotics likely to die during hospitalization. Hepatology 1991;14:245A.

9. Lavo B, Colombel JF, Knutsson L, Hallgren R. Acute exposure of small intestine intestine to ethanol induces mucosal leakage and prostaglandin E2 synthesis. Gastroenterology 1992;102:468–473.

10. Payen JL, Cales P, Pienkowski P, et al. Weakness of mucosal barrier in portal hypertensive gastropathy of alcoholic cirrhosis. J Hepatol 1995;23:689–696.

11. Pantzar N, Bergqvist PBF, Bugge M, et al. Small intestinal absorption of polyethylene glycol 400 to 1000 in the portacaval shunted rat. Hepatology 1995;21:1167–1173.

12. Llovet JM, Bartolí R, Planas R, et al. Selective intestinal decontamination with norfloxacin reduces bacterial translocation in ascitic cirrhotic rats exposed to hemorrhagic shock. Hepatology 1996;23: 781–787.

13. Steffen EK, Berg RD. Relationship between cecal population levels of indigenous bacteria and translocation to the mesenteric lymph nodes. Infect Immun 1983;39:1252–1259.

14. Krause W, Matheis H, Wulf K. Fungemia and funguria after oral administration of Candida albicans. Lancet 1969;i:598–599.

15. Guarner C, Runyon BA, Young S, Heck M, Sheikh MY. Intestinal bacterial overgrowth and bacterial translocation in an experimental model of cirrhosis. J Hepatol 1997;26:1372–1378.

16. Chesta J, Defilippi C, Defilippi C. Abnormalities in proximal small bowel motility in patients with cirrhosis. Hepatology 1993;17:828–832.

17. Pérez-Páramo M, Muñoz J, Albillos A, et al. Effect of propranolol on the factors promoting bacterial translocation in cirrhotic rats with ascites. Hepatology 2000;31:43–48.

18. Pardo A, Bartoli R, Lorenzo-Zúûiga V, et al. Effect of cisapride on intestinal bacterial overgrowth and bacterial translocation in cirrhosis. Hepatology 2000;31:858–863.

19. Raedsch R, Stiehl A, Gundert-Remy U, et al. Hepatic secretion of bilirubin and biliary lipids in patients with alcoholic cirrhosis of the liver. Digestion 1983;26:80–88.

20. Lorenzo-Zúñiga V, Bartolí R, Planas R, et al. Oral bile acid administration reduces endotoxemia and bacterial translocation in ascitic cirrhotic rats. Hepatology 2003;37:551–557.

21. Rabinovitz M, Schade RR, Dindzans VJ, Belle SH, Van Thiel DH, Gavaler JS. Colonic disease in cirrhosis: an endoscopic evaluation in 412 patients. Gastroenterology 1990;99:195–199.

22. Wells CL, Maddaus MA, Simmons RL. Proposed mechanisms for the translocation of intestinal bacteria. Rev Infect Dis 1988;10:958–979.

23. Runyon BA, Morrissey R, Hoefs JC, Wyle F. Opsonic activity of human ascitic fluid: a potentially important protective mechanism againts spontaneous bacterial pritonitis. Hepatology 1985;5:634–637.

24. Agnello V. Complement deficiency states. Medicine 1978;57:1–23.

25. Laffi G, Carloni V, Baldi E, et al. Impaired superoxide anion, platelet-activating factor, and leukotriene B4 synthesis by neutrophils in cirrhosis. Gastroenterology 1993;106:170–177.

26. Rajkovic IA, Williams R. Abnormalities of neutrophil phagocytosis, intracellular killing, and metabolic activity in alcoholic cirrhosis and hepatitis. Hepatology 1986;6:252–262.

27. Rimola A, Soto R, Bory F, Arroyo V, Piera C, Rodés J. Reticuloendothelial system phagocytic activity in cirrhosis and its relation to bacterial infections and prognosis. Hepatology 1984;4:53–58.

28. Gómez P, Ruiz P, Schreiber AD. Impaired function of macrophage FC-gamma receptors and bacterial infection in alcoholic cirrhosis. N Engl J Med 1994;331:1122–1128.

29. Martini GA, Phear EA, Ruebner B, Sherlock S. The bacterial content of the small intestine in normal and cirrhotic subjects. Clin Sci 1957;16:35–51.

30. Morencos FC, de las Heras Costano G, Ramos LM, López-Arias MJ, Ledesma F, Romero FP. Small bowel bacterial overgrowth in patients with alcoholic cirrhosis. Dig Dis Sci 1995;40:1252–1256.

31. Rimola A, García-Tsao G, Navasa M, et al. Diagnosis, treatment and prophylaxis of spontaneous bacterial peritonitis: a consensus document. J Hepatol 2000;32:142–153.

32. Castellote J, López C, Gornals J, et al. Rapid diagnosis of spontaneous bacterial peritonitis by use of reagent strips. Hepatology 2003;37:893–896.

33. Xiol X, Castellvi JM, Guardiola J, et al. Spontaneous bacterial empyema in cirrhotic patients: a prospective study. Hepatology 1996;23:719–723.

34. Akriviadis EA, Runyon BA. Utility of an algorithm in differentiating spontaneous from secondary bacterial peritonitis. Gastroenterology 1990;98:127–133.

35. Conn HO, Fessel JM. Spontaneous bacterial peritonitis in cirrhosis: variations on a theme. Medicine 1971;50:161–197.

36. Curry N, McCallum RW, Guth PH. Spontaneous bacterial peritonitis in cirrhotic ascites: a decade of experience. Am J Dig Dis 1974;19:685–692.

37. García-Tsao G. Treatment of spontaneous bacterial peritonitis. In: Arroyo V, Bosch J, Bruix J, Ginès P, Navasa M, Rodés J, eds. Therapy in Hepatology. stm Editores, Barcelona, 2001, pp. 50–64.

38. Felisart J, Rimola A, Arroyo V, et al. Cefotaxime is more effective than is ampicillin-tobramycin in cirrhotics with severe infections. Hepatology 1985;5:457–462.

39. Ricart E, Soriano G, Novella M, et al. Amoxicillin-clavulanic acid versus cefotaxime in the therapy of bacterial infections in cirrhotic patients. J Hepatol 2000;32:596–602.

40. Runyon BA, Mc Hutchison JG, Antillon MR, Akriviadis EA, Montano AA. Short-course versus long-course antibiotic treatment of spontaneous bacterial peritonitis. A randomised controlled study of 100 patients. Gastroenterology 1991;100:1737–1742.

41. Rimola A, Salmerón JM, Clemente G, et al. Two different dossages of cefotaxime in the treatment of spontaneous bacterial peritonitis in cirrosis: results of a prospective, randomized, multicenter study. Hepatology 1995;21:674–679.

42. Navasa M, Follo A, Llovet JM, et al. Randomized, comparative study of oral ofloxacin versus intravenous cefotaxime in spontaneous bacterial peritonitis. Gastroenterology 1996;111:1011–1017.

43. Terg R, Cobas S, Fassio E, et al. Oral ciprofloxacin after a short course of intravenous ciprofloxacin in the treatment of spontaneous bacterial peritonitis: results of a multicenter, randomized study. J Hepatol 2000;33:564–569.

44. McCormick PA, Greenslade L, Kibbler CC, Chin JK, Burroughs AK, McIntyre N. A prospective randomized trial of ceftazidime versus nethylmicin plus mezlocillin in the empirical therapy of presumed sepsis in cirrhotic patients. Hepatology 1997;25:833–836.

45. García-Tsao G. Futher evidence against the use of aminoclycosides in cirrhotic patients. Gastroenterology 1998;114:612–613.

46. Hampel H, Bynum GD, Zamora E, et al. Risks factors for the development of renal dysfunction in hospitalized patients with cirrhosis. Am J Gastroenterol 2001;96:2206–2210.

47. Dupeyron C, Mangeney N, Sedrati L, et al. Rapid emergence of quinolone resistance in cirrhotic patients treated with norfloxacin to prevent spontaneous bacterial peritonitis. Antimicrob Agents Chemother 1994;38:340–344.

48. Bauer TM, Follo A, Navasa M, et al. Daily norfloxacin is more effective than weekly rufloxacin in prevention of spontaneous bacterial peritonitis recurrence. Dig Dis Sci 2002;47:1356–1361.

49. Novella M, Solà R, Soriano G, et al. Continuous versus inpatient prophylaxis of the first episode of spontaneous bacterial peritonitis with norfloxacin. Hepatology 1997;25:532–536.

50. Fernández J, Navasa M, Gómez J, et al. Bacterial infections in cirrosis: epidemiological changes with invasive procedures and norfloxacin prophylaxis. Hepatology 2002;35:140–148.

51. Campillo B, Dupeyron C, Richardet JP, et al. Epidemiology of severe hospital-acquired infections in patients with liver cirrhosis: effect of long-term administration of norfloxacin. Clin Infect Dis 1998;26:1066–1070.

52. Campillo B, Dupeyron C, Richardet JP. Epidemiology of hospital adquired infections in cirrhotic patients: effect of carriage of methicillin-resistant Staphylococcus aureus and influence of previous antibiotic therapy and norfloxacin prophylaxis. Epidemiol Infect 2001;127:443–450.

53. Llovet JM, Rodríguez-Iglesias P, Moitinho E, et al. Spontaneous bacterial peritonitis in patients with cirrhosis undergoing selective intestinal decontamination. A retrospective study of 229 spontaneous bacterial peritonitis episodes. J Hepatol 1997;26:88–95.

54. Ortiz J, Vila MC, Soriano G, et al. Infections caused by Esterichia coli resistant to norfloxacin in hospitalized cirrhotic patients. Hepatology 1999;29:1064–1069.

55. Campillo B, Richardet JP, Kheo T, et al. Nosocomial spontaneous bacterial peritonitis and bacteremia in cirrhotic patients: impacte of isolate type on prognosis and characteristics of infection. Clin Infect Dis 2002;35:1–10.

56. Follo A, Llovet JM, Navasa M, et al. Renal impairment after spontaneous bacterial peritonitis in cirrosis: incidence, clinical course, predictive factors and prognosis. Hepatology 1994;20:1495–1501.

57. Navasa M, Follo A, Filella X, et al. Tumor necrosis factor and interleukin-6 in spontaneous bacterial peritonitis in cirrosis: relationship with the development of renal impairment and mortality. Hepatology 1998;27:1227–1232.

58. Sort P, Navasa M, Arroyo V, et al. Effect of intravenous albumin on renal impairment and mortality in patients with cirrosis and spontaneous bacterial peritonitis. N Engl J Med 1999;341:403–409.

59. Tító L, Rimola A, Ginès P, Llach J, Arroyo V, Rodés J. Recurrence of spontaneous bacterial peritonitis in cirrhosis: frequency and predictive factors. Hepatology 1988;8:27–31.

60. Ginès P, Rimola A, Planas R, et al. Norfloxacin prevents spontaneous bacterial peritonitis recurrence in cirrhosis: results of a double-blind, placebo controlled trial. Hepatology 1990;12:716–724.

61. Bleichner G, Boulanger R, Squara P, Sollet JP, Parent A. Frequency of infections in cirrhotic patients presenting with acute gastrointestinal hemorrhage. Br J Surg 1986;73:724–726.

62. Rimola A, Bory F, Terès J, Pérez-Ayuso RM, Arroyo V, Rodés J. Oral, nonabsorbable antibiotics prevent infection in cirrhotics with gastrointestinal hemorrhage. Hepatology 1985;5:463–467.

63. Soriano G, Guarner C, Tomas A, et al. Norfloxacin prevents bacterial infection in cirrhotics with gastrointestinal hemorrhage. Gastroenterology 1992;103:1267–1272.

64. Blaise M, Pateron D, Trinchet JC, Levacher S, Beaugrand M, Pourriat JL. Systemic antibiotic therapy prevents bacterial infection in cirrhotic patients with gastrointestinal hemorrhage. Hepatology 1994;20:34–38.

65. Pauwels A, Mostefa-Kara N, Debenes B, Degoutte E, Levy VG. Systemic antibiotic prophylaxis after gastrointestinal hemorrhage in cirrhotic patients with a high risk of infection. Hepatology 1996;24:802–806.

66. Hsieh WJ, Lin HC, Hwang SJ, et al. The effect of ciprofloxacin in the prevention of bacterial infection in patients with cirrhosis after upper gastrointestinal bleeding. Am J Gastroenterol 1998;93:962–966.

67. Bernard B, Grange JD, Khac EN, et al. Antibiotic prophylaxis for the prevention of bacterial infections in cirrhotic patients with gastrointestinal bleeding: a metaanalysis. Hepatology 1999;29:1655–1661.

68. Soares-Weiser K, Brezis M, Tur-Kaspa R, et al. Antibiotic prophylaxis for cirrhotic patients with gastrointestinal bleeding (Cochrane Review). The Cochrane Library 2003, Issue 1.

69. Llach J, Rimola A, Navasa M, et al. Incidence and predictive factors of first episode of spontaneous bacterial peritonitis in cirrosis with ascites: relevance of ascitic fluid protein concentration. Hepatology 1992;16:724–727.

70. Andreu M, Sola R, Sitges-Serra A, et al. Risk factors for spontaneous bacterial peritonitis in cirrhotic patients with ascites. Gastroenterology 1993;104:1133–1138.

71. Soriano G, Guarner C, Teixidó M, et al. Selective intestinal decontamination prevents spontaneous bacterial peritonitis. Gastroenterology 1991;100:477–481.

72. Grange JD, Roulot D, Pelletier G, et al. Norfloxacin primary prophylaxis of bacterial infections in cirrhotic patients with ascites. A double-blind randomised trial. J Hepatol 1998;29:430–436.

73. Rolachon A, Cordier L, Bacq Y, et al. Ciprofloxacin and long-term prevention of spontaneous bacterial peritonitis: results of a prospective controlled trial. Hepatology 1995;22:1171–1174.

74. Singh N, Gayowski T, Yu VL, Wagener MM. Trimethoprim-sulfamethoxazole for the prevention of spontaneous bacterial peritonitis in cirrhosis: a randomized trial. Ann Intern Med 1995;122:595–598.

75. Guarner C, Solà R, Soriano G, et al. Risk of a first community-acquired spontaneous bacterial peritonitis in cirrhotics with low ascitic fluid protein levels. Gastroenterology 1999;117:414–419.

76. Rimola A, Bory F, Planas R, Xaubet A, Bruguera M, Rodés J. Infecciones bacterianas agudas en la cirrosis hepática. Gastroenterol Hepatol 1981;4:453–458.

77. Palazón JM, García A, Gómez A. Infecciones bacterianas en pacientes con cirrosis hepática. Gastroenterol Hepatol 1984;7:120–122.

78. Yoshida H, Hamada T, Inuzuka S, Ueno T, Sata M, Tanikawa K. Bacterial infection in cirrhosis, with and without hepatocellular carcinoma. Am J Gastroenterol 1993;88:2067–2071.

79. Deschenes M, Villeneuve JP. Risk factors for the development of bacterial infections in hospitalised patients with cirrhosis. Am J Gastroenterol 1999;94:2193–2197.

80. Borzio M, Salerno F, Piantoni L, et al. Bacterial infection in patients with advanced cirrhosis: a multicentre prospective study. Digest Liver Dis 2001;33:41–48.

81. Bernard B, Cadranel JF, Valla D, et al. Prognostic significance of bacterial infection in bleeding cirrhotic patients: a prospective study. Gastroenterology 1995;108:1828–1834.
82. Goulis J, Armonis A, Patch D, et al. Bacterial infection is independently associated with failure to control bleeding in cirrhotic patients with gastrointestinal hemorrhage. Hepatology 1998;27:1207–1212.
83. Vivas S, Rodríguez M, Palacio MA, et al. Presence of bacterial infection in bleeding cirrhotic patients is independently associated with early mortality and failure to control bleeding. Dig Dis Sci 2001;46: 2752–2757.
84. Burroughs AK, Rosenstein IJ, Epstein O, Hamilton-Miller JMT, Brumfit W, Sherlock S. Bacteriuria and primary biliary cirrhosis. Gut 1984;25:133–137.
85. Westphal J-F, Jehl F, Vetter D. Pharmacological, toxicological, and microbiological considerations in the choice of initial antibiotic therapy for serious infections in patients with cirrhosis of the liver. Clin Infect Dis 1994;18:324–335.
86. Levy M, Dromer F, Brion N, Leturdu F, Carbon C. Community-acquired pneumonia. Chest 1988;92: 43–48.

22

Diagnosis and Management of the Hepatorenal Syndrome

Kevin Moore

CONTENTS

INTRODUCTION
PATHOPHYSIOLOGY OF THE HEPATORENAL SYNDROME
MANAGEMENT OF THE HEPATORENAL SYNDROME
CONCLUSION
REFERENCES

INTRODUCTION

The hepatorenal syndrome (HRS) is defined as the development of renal failure in patients with severe liver disease in the absence of any other identifiable cause of renal pathology. Although classically associated with cirrhosis, it is now recognized that a similar syndrome occurs in patients with acute liver failure *(1)*. It is diagnosed following the exclusion of other causes of renal failure in patients with severe liver disease such as hypovolemia, drug nephrotoxicity, sepsis, or glomerulonephritis. The causes of renal failure in/and liver disease are listed in Table 1.

Diagnostic Criteria

The International Ascites Club group defined the diagnostic criteria for hepatorenal syndrome *(1)*, and these are listed in Table 2. Two patterns of the HRS are observed in clinical practice and these have been defined by the International Ascites club into type 1 and type 2 *(1)*. This classification is particularly useful in research as it enables direct comparison between studies.

Type 1 HRS is an acute form of HRS in which renal failure occurs in patients with severe liver disease and is rapidly progressive. It can occur spontaneously, e.g., as in acute alcoholic hepatitis or acute liver failure, or may be precipitated by a bacterial infection such as SBP *(3)*. Although, some investigators historically excluded such patients in whom there is a clear precipitating injury, many investigators in the field simply treat such patients with fluids and antibiotics, and if after 5 d renal failure develops or persists, they are labeled as having HRS. Personally I think this group of patients with a clear precipitating event should be separated (e.g., Type 1A and 1B) from those in whom HRS develops spontaneously

From: *Clinical Gastroenterology: Portal Hypertension*
Edited by: A. J. Sanyal and V. H. Shah © Humana Press Inc., Totowa, NJ

Table 1
Causes of Abnormal Liver and Renal Function

Sepsis in cirrhosis
Hypovolemia (overdiuresis, hemorrhage)
Hepatorenal syndrome
Glomerulonephritis (HCV, HBV)
IgA Nephropathy (alcohol)
Renal tubular acidosis (esp. PBC and Wilson's disease)
Chronic pyelonephritis (increased incidence)
Leptospirosis (Weil's disease)
Acetaminophen toxicity
Malaria
Sickle cell disease
Sepsis in normal subjects
Solvent abuse (carbon tetrachloride)

Table 2
Major Criteria

1. Chronic or acute liver disease with advanced hepatic failure and portal hypertension
2. Low GFR as indicated by serum creatinine >1.7 mg/dL or creatinine clearance <40 mL/min.
3. Absence of shock, on-going bacterial infection or recent treatment with nephrotoxic drugs. Absence of excessive fluid losses (including gastrointestinal bleeding).
4. No sustained improvement of renal function following expansion with 1.5 L of isotonic saline.
5. Proteinuria <0.5 g/d, and no ultrasonagraphic evidence of renal tract disease.

At the consensus conference, which decided the diagnostic criteria, there was widespread agreement about the above criteria. However, further additional criteria were defined (see below), but deemed to be unnecessary for the diagnosis. This may seem a curious anomaly in retrospect, but these "unnecessary criteria" were added primarily to satisfy various diehards and so that the meeting could finish! These are

1. Urine volume <500 mL/d
2. Urine sodium <10 mmoles/L
3. Urine osmolality > plasma osmolality
4. Urine RBC <50 per high per field
5. Serum Sodium <130 mmoles/L

Note: Low urinary sodium is not necessary for the diagnosis of HRS.

(usually during acute liver decompensation) to maintain homogeneity between groups so that research into disease mechanisms can be more easily interpreted.

Type 1 HRS is characterized by a marked reduction of renal function as defined by doubling of the initial serum creatinine to a level greater than 1.7 mg/dL, or a 50% reduction of the initial 24 h creatinine clearance to <20 mL/min within 2 wk. The development of type 1 HRS has a poor prognosis with 90% mortality at 4 wk *(2)* (Fig. 1). Renal function may recover spontaneously if there is a significant improvement of liver function. This is most frequently observed in acute liver failure or alcoholic hepatitis or following

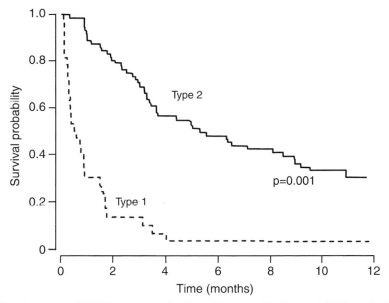

Fig. 1. The development of HRS is associated with a high mortality in type 1 HRS, and a 50% 6 month mortality in type 2 HRS. From Ref. 4.

acute decompensation on a background of cirrhosis, or recovery from bacterial infection. These patients are usually jaundiced with a significant coagulopathy. Death often results from a combination of hepatic and renal failure or variceal bleeding.

Type-2 HRS usually occurs in patients with diuretic resistant ascites. Renal failure has a slow course, in which it may deteriorate or improve over months. It is associated with a poor long-term (>1 yr) prognosis (4), with a mean mortality of 45% at 4 mo.

PATHOPHYSIOLOGY OF THE HEPATORENAL SYNDROME

The key to the logical therapy of HRS is to have a basic understanding of its pathophysiology. It is well recognized that the most important factor involved in the pathogenesis is severe reversible renal vasoconstriction and mild systemic hypotension (5). The kidneys are structurally normal, and at least in the early part of the syndrome, tubular function is intact, as reflected by avid sodium retention and oliguria. Moreover, kidneys from patients with HRS transplanted into a patient with end-stage renal failure and a healthy liver resumed normal function (6). Although many textbooks state that patients with HRS have low urinary sodium, it is well recognized that this is not always the case (7), and that electron microsopy (EM) studies of kidneys obtained from patients with HRS and sodium retention may have EM signs of acute tubular necrosis (8).

The cause of renal vasoconstriction is unknown but it seems to primarily involve a homeostatic response to systemic vasodilatation and mild hypotension with marked activation of the sympathetic nervous system, which sensitizes or shifts the renal autoregulatory curve so that renal blood flow is more critically dependent on blood pressure. Although this may be the predominant driving force in the majority of patients, in other patients, for example those with type 1 HRS, increased synthesis of vasoactive mediators, such as endothelin-1 or cysteinyl leukotrienes within the kidney, may decrease the glomerular filtration rate out of proportion to the reduction of renal blood flow, by causing contraction of mesangial cells and thereby decreasing the glomerular capillary ultrafiltration coefficient (K_f). This decreases the GFR out of proportion to the reduction of renal blood flow.

There are three factors predominantly involved in its pathogenesis (9).

1. Hemodynamic changes that decrease renal perfusion pressure.
2. Activation of the renal sympathetic nervous system (SNS).
3. Increased synthesis of humoral and renal vasoactive mediators.

The emphasis of each of the three pathogenic pathways probably varies from patient to patient, and between the acute (type 1) and the chronic form (type 2) of the hepatorenal syndrome. Each of these pathways are interrelated and, in practice, the pathophysiology of this process is more complicated. However, this outline provides a simple framework with which to understand the mechanisms involved.

Hemodynamic Changes

Systemic vasodilatation occurs in all patients with severe liver disease. Vasodilatation of the splanchnic circulation leads to a compensatory increase of plasma volume and cardiac output. However, cardiac compensation eventually fails, and some attribute this to the development of impaired cardiovascular responses to endogenous catecholamines. This failure of cardiac output to maintain blood pressure has been termed cirrhotic cardiomyopathy (10). This term is highly controversial, primarily because the heart does not exhibit histological changes such as fibrosis. Nevertheless, there is accumulating evidence that there is failure of the heart to adequately compensate for the systemic vasodilatation, and patients who develop HRS following SBP, have a reduction in cardiac output (11). Whatever the final pathway, there is a fall of mean arterial pressure (MAP) and reflex activation of the sympathetic nervous system. Several studies have consistently shown a progressive decrease in MAP with hepatic decompensation, with the lowest values (typically 60–65 mmHg) observed in patients with HRS (12), and prognostic studies in patients with cirrhosis have shown that arterial pressure is one of the best predictors of survival in patients with cirrhosis and ascites (13), with low arterial pressure being associated with a poor prognosis and increased risk of developing HRS.

It is a common misconception that modest reductions of blood pressure (BP) are insignificant in humans, and that renal autoregulation exists to prevent fluctuations in the renal blood flow (RBF) when BP decreases. Autoregulation of the renal circulation ensures a stable RBF during changes of renal perfusion pressure *above* ~75 mmHg (14). Below this pressure, RBF is directly proportional to perfusion pressure. Patients developing HRS have an activated sympathetic nervous system (SNS), and increased synthesis of several renal vasoconstrictors. Several studies have shown that activation of the SNS causes a rightward-shift in the autoregulatory curve (15), making RBF much more pressure dependent. These concepts are illustrated in Fig. 2. Thus, even modest decreases in mean BP may result in a marked fall of RBF. Understanding this important principle is essential in targeting pressor treatment because drugs that increase BP have a disproportionate effect on RBF and GFR in states associated with an activated SNS and lowered blood pressure. As a result, there is an interest in drugs which increase BP, and all have all been reported to increase urine output, sodium excretion, or GFR with variable success in patients with severe liver disease and HRS (16–23), and reviewed in ref. 19.

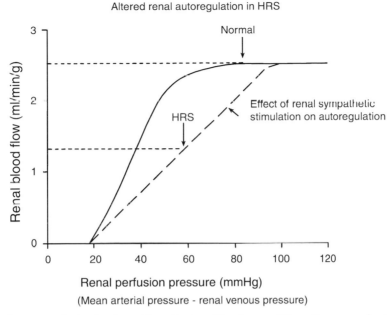

Fig. 2. Renal autoregulation is altered in patients with advanced liver disease and activation of the sympathetic nervous system, which renders renal blood flow much more dependent on renal perfusion pressure. Thus, a small increase in blood pressure can have a profound effect on renal blood flow, glomerular filtration and survival. From Ref. 9.

The presence of modest arterial hypotension raises the question about its cause. It is well established that severe liver disease is characterized by an increase in cardiac output and plasma volume, and decreased peripheral vascular resistance (5) owing to peripheral vasodilatation. Studies in animals and humans with cirrhosis indicate that the splanchnic circulation is the main vascular bed responsible for vasodilatation (24,25).

There is general acceptance that vascular reactivity is impaired in cirrhosis because isolated vessels have impaired responsiveness to vascular agonists. However, this may not apply to small vessels, and most studies have used aortic rings. Ultimately several mediators, either singly or in concert (NO, prostacyclin, glucagon, calcitonin gene-related peptide (CGRP) (26), or altered K^+ channel activation) may be responsible for the decreased vascular reactivity, or the opening of these anatomical shunts. Plasma levels of many endogenous vasodilatators, as well as vasoconstrictors are elevated in liver failure. Several potential mediators have been proposed and include the following:

1. *Nitric oxide*: NO is synthesized by several cell types including endothelial and vascular smooth muscle cells, and causes vasorelaxation (27). NO synthesis may be induced by shear stress, or in response to endotoxin-related cytokine expression (28–32). However, the concept that vasodilatation is secondary to induction of NOS by circulating endotoxins in humans has lost favor, with many now advocating an increase in activity of eNOS, perhaps owing to increased levels of tetrahydrobiopterin as a result of activation of GTP cyclohydrolase. Studies in patients with decompensated cirrhosis show increased plasma nitrite/nitrate indicative of increased NO production (33). Pharmacological studies using isolated vascular rings or the mesenteric vasculature have shown decreased vascular reactivity

tacyclin is increased in HRS, but that the urinary excretion of its metabolite is decreased by the presence of renal failure *(42)*. These compensatory mechanisms are important because inhibition or antagonism of their actions frequently causes further deterioration of renal function.

Pressure Effects of Tense Ascites: Gross or tense ascites increases the IVC pressure and thus the renal venous pressure. Studies have shown that the renal venous pressure may increase to >25 mmHg *(75)*. In this situation, increased venous pressure may further compromise renal blood flow, and thus renal function.

SNS

The SNS is highly activated in patients with the hepatorenal syndrome and causes renal vasoconstriction and increases sodium retention *(76–78)*. Several studies have shown that there is increased secretion of catecholamines in the renal and splanchnic vascular beds *(79–81)*.

An important concept to emerge in the early 1990s was that of a hepatorenal neural reflex arc. In fact, this concept really first arose in 1980s, when Kostreva et al. *(82)* observed that an increase in intrahepatic pressure resulted in a greater efferent renal sympatho-adrenergic activity. Vasoconstriction of the afferent arterioles of the kidney led to a reduction in renal plasma flow and glomerular filtration rate and to an increased reabsorbtion of tubular sodium and water. Hepatic denervation was effective in delaying, but not preventing, the increased tubular reabsorption of sodium in portal hypertension, and Levy et al. *(83)* discovered that the onset of ascites formation was delayed in dogs with bile duct ligation following hepatic denervation. This concept was expanded and developed by Hausinger's group *(84)*, who observed that infusion of glutamine into the internal jugular vein had no effect on renal function, whereas it caused a significant decrease of both GFR and RBF when infused into the portal vein, unless there was renal denervation, when such responses were not observed. They postulated that infusion of glutamine into the portal vein caused swelling of hepatcytes and activation of the hepatorenal sympathetic neural reflex arc. In support of this concept in humans, studies by Jalan and colleagues have shown that acute occlusion of the TIPS shunt is associated with an acute reduction of renal blood flow in patients with cirrhosis *(85)*. In another study, temporary lumbar sympathectomy with local anesthesia increased GFR in five of eight cirrhotic patients with HRS *(86)* suggesting that increased renal sympathetic nervous activity decreased GFR in some patients. Such data may explain why patients who undergo liver transplantation for HRS frequently show a dramatic recovery of renal function.

Humoral and Renal Vasoactive Mediators

It is unlikely that the development of HRS is purely a consequence of renal vasoconstriction. If one examines the relationship between RBF, and the presence of HRS or hepatic decompensation ± ascites, there is considerable overlap of RBF between these groups *(87)* (Fig. 3). Thus, some patients with preserved renal function may have a lower RBF than those with HRS, indicating that other factors are involved.

The observation that two patients may have a comparable decrease of RBF, and yet have either HRS or "near-normal renal function" suggests that other factors must be involved which decrease the filtration fraction. The renal glomeruli are dynamic structures, invaginated with mesangial cells which, in a similar way to hepatic stellate cells, may contract in response to several agonists such as endoethin-1, and, thus, reduce the surface area avail-

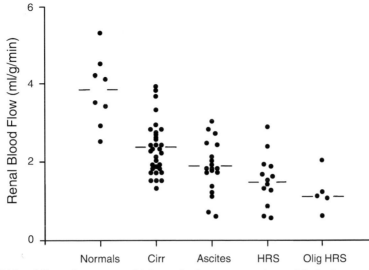

Fig. 3. Renal blood flow decreases with hepatic decompensation, with the lowest RBF observed in patients with HRS. However, there is a considerable overlap between RBF observed in patients with Ascites, but "normal" renal function and HRS, suggesting that other factors must be involved, such as contraction of mesangial cells (see Fig. 5). From Ref. *87*.

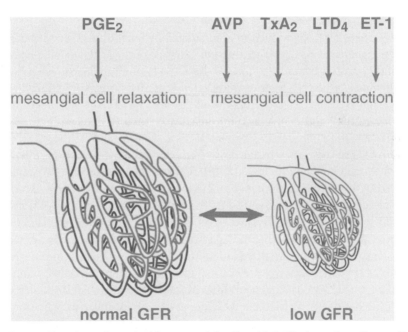

Fig. 4. The glomeruli are invaginated with mesangial cells which, like hepatic stellate cells, express actin,. And can contract in response to physiological or pathological stimuli such as endothelin-1 (ET-1) or the cysteinyl-leukotriene LTD4.

able for glomerular filtration (Fig. 4). Many studies have now shown that there is increased synthesis of several vasoactive mediators, which have the important added effect of causing mesangial cell contraction, hence lowering the glomerular capillary ultrafiltration coefficient (K_f), and thus the filtration fraction. Such factors involved may include:

1. *Endothelin*: This 21-amino-acid peptide is a potent renal vasoconstrictor, and a potent agonist of mesangial cell contraction. Endothelin-1 (ET-1) concentrations are increased in the hepatorenal syndrome, and correlate with creatinine clearance in decompensated liver disease *(88,89)*. The cause of increased plasma ET-1 concentrations is unknown. One possibility is altered redox state because oxidative stress is known to occur in HRS *(90)*, and products of lipid peroxidation such as oxidized LDL and F2-isoprostanes have been shown to induce ET-1 synthesis in vitro *(92)*, but whether this causes increased plasma ET-1 concentrations is unknown. Recent studies in which ET-1 has been infused into the forearm of patients with advanced (Child–Pugh C) cirrhosis have suggested that ET-1 may paradoxically cause vasodilatation *(93)*. This unexpected observation may have a profound impact on the viability of clinical studies using ET-1 antagonists in patients with HRS.

2. *Cysteinyl leukotrienes*: Leukotrienes C_4 and D_4 are produced by inflammatory cells of the myeloid series, and can be synthesized by the isolated kidney *(94)*. They are potent renal vasoconstrictors, and cause contraction of mesangial cells in vitro. Endotoxemia, activation of complement, or various cytokines may stimulate their synthesis. There is good evidence that systemic, and probably renal synthesis of cysteinyl leukotrienes is increased in the hepatorenal syndrome. Urinary leukotriene E_4 is markedly elevated, as well as N-acetyl LTE_4 in HRS *(95–97)*. Plasma concentrations are too low to have a direct effect on the renal circulation, but renal leukotriene synthesis may be an important modulator of renal function in HRS, and isolated pig kidneys have been shown to synthesize cysteinyl leukotrienes in vitro *(94)*.

3. *Thromboxane A_2*: TXA_2 production is stimulated by renal ischemia and causes both vasoconstriction and mesangial cell contraction. It has been suggested that the balance between vasodilatory prostaglandins and thromboxane A_2 might critically favor vasoconstriction *(98)*. However, when TXB2 excretion is corrected for renal function, urinary TXB2 excretion has been shown to correlate with the severity of liver disease, rather than HRS *(42)*. Further, inhibition of TXA_2 synthesis with dazoxiben does not improve renal function *(99)*.

4. *F_2-isoprostanes*: The F_2-isoprostanes are formed by lipid peroxidation. Their role in liver disease has recently been reviewed *(100)*. One of the major F_2-isoprostanes formed in vivo namely 8-iso-PGF_2 is a potent renal vasoconstrictor. In the first study measuring the plasma concentrations of F_2-isoprostanes in any human disease, we observed a marked increased synthesis of the F_2-isoprostanes in patients with HRS indicative of increased lipid peroxidation *(90)*. Whether the F_2-isoprostanes themselves are important mediators of renal vasoconstriction in HRS is unknown, but it is difficult to prove. However, the synthesis of several vasoactive mediators, which have been implicated in the pathogenesis of HRS, are regulated through products of lipid peroxidation or through redox changes of signaling pathways. Thus, the development of oxidant stress may be important as the final pathway leading to increased synthesis of many of the mediators discussed above.

MANAGEMENT OF THE HEPATORENAL SYNDROME

Measures to Prevent the Development of Renal Failure in Cirrhosis

Prophylaxis against bacterial infections: Bacterial infections occur in approx 40% of patients with variceal hemorrhage and antibiotic prophylaxis improves survival by approx 10% *(101)*. Patients who have had a previous episode of SBP have a 68% chance of recurrent infection at 1 yr, and this carries an 30% chance of developing renal failure *(3)*.

Because bacterial infections are an important cause of renal dysfunction in cirrhotic patients, prophylaxis with antibiotics is recommended in two clinical settings, namely variceal bleeding and a history of previous SBP.

Volume expansion postparacentesis or during SBP: To prevent the development of renal failure in patients who develop SBP, recent studies have suggested that these patients should be given plasma volume expansion with 20% albumin (1–1.5 g/kg over 1–3 d) at diagnosis to prevent circulatory dysfunction, renal impairment, and mortality *(102)*. However, the control groups were not given volume support with either crystalloid or colloid, and, therefore, further studies are needed before the unequivocal use of albumin is recommended. The use of salt poor albumin or other colloids in patients undergoing large volume paracentesis (>5 L) is essential to prevent paracentesis induced circulatory dysfunction and renal impairment *(103,104)*.

Avoid overdiuresis: Identifying the lowest effective diuretic for any individual patient is important because diuretic-induced renal impairment occurs in approx 20% of patients with ascites. It develops when the rate of diuresis exceeds the rate of ascites reabsorption, leading to intravascular volume depletion. Diuretic-induced renal impairment is usually moderate and is normally rapidly reversible following diuretic withdrawal.

Avoid the use of nephrotoxic drugs: Patients with cirrhosis and ascites are predisposed to develop acute tubular necrosis during use of aminoglycosides, with renal failure occurring is approx 33% of patients as compared with 3–5% in the general population *(105)*. Another important cause of renal failure is the use of NSAIDs. These drugs inhibit formation of intrarenal PGE_2 or PGI_2 causing a marked decline of renal function and salt and water excretion in cirrhotic patients with ascites. Therefore, when confronted with a patient with liver disease and renal failure, always look at the drug chart to ensure that your patient is not being poisoned by a well-meaning doctor who has prescribed an NSAID for back pain caused by gross ascites.

Treatment of Patients with Hepatorenal Syndrome

Renal function rarely recovers in patients with HRS (as opposed to volume depletion) in the absence of recovery of liver function. The key goal in the management of these patients is to exclude reversible or treatable lesions (mainly hypovolemia or sepsis), and to support the patient until liver recovery (e.g., from alcoholic hepatitis), hepatic regeneration (acute liver disease), or until liver transplantation. Even terminally ill patients can have reversal of HRS, albeit temporarily (e.g., 1–3 wk), which may enable them to set their affairs in order. The treatment of HRS is directed at reversing the hemodynamic changes induced by modest lowering of blood pressure, stimulation of the sympathetic nervous system, and increased synthesis of humoral and renal vasoconstrictor factors.

Initial Management

- Optimize fluid management: All patients should be given a fluid challenge with colloid or crystalloid (usually 1–1.5 L). It is important to recognize that saline-based fluids contain high amounts of chloride, and may cause hyperchloremic acidosis, which can cause further renal vasoconstriction, if given in large amounts (>3 L over a few hours), in which case a balance salt solution such as Hartman's or Ringer's lactate may be preferable *(106)*. The volume used depends on clinical circumstances and response, but most patients with advanced liver disease act like fluid sumps, with increased venous compliance *(107)*. In practical terms, this means that if one infuses 1 L of crystalloid or colloid rapidly, there is a transient increase in central venous pressure, and then the venous system expands to absorb the volume, and CVP decreases. Fluid replacement should be based on clinical response, urine output, blood pressure, and CVP or PCWP. Generally speaking, one should avoid giving fluids to achieve a CVP goal, because this can result in fluid overload because of abnormal venous compliance (i.e., CVP does not have a sustained increase despite adequate fluid load).

- Exclude precipitating or iatrogenic causes of renal failure: Stop diuretic therapy (diuretics do not work in patients with HRS, and will only exacerbate renal failure). Check the drug chart for other drugs that may have been prescribed overnight or without your knowledge such as NSAIDs, gentamicin, or vancomycin.
- Investigate and treat potential sepsis: Evidence of sepsis should be sought by culture of blood, ascites, cannulae, and urine, and fungal cultures requested. Because undiagnosed sepsis is an important cause of renal failure in cirrhosis, all patients should be started on nonnephrotoxic broad-spectrum antibiotics, regardless of overt or other evidence of sepsis, e.g., iv cefotaxime, or oral ciprofloxacin plus amoxycillin.

Optimization of Blood Pressure and Renal Haemodynamics

Terlipressin: Following volume expansion, the mean arterial pressure should be increased to >85 mmHg by infusing vasopressor drugs. There have been no studies to evaluate which mean arterial pressure should be attained during vasopressor therapy, but based on renal autoregulatory curves and personal experience, it should generally be above 85 mmHg, or any level at which diuresis starts and is maintained. Most studies have used terlipressin, but this is not available in Canada or the US.

The first study, carried out at the Royal Free Hospital, London, in 1972 by Sheila Shelock's group showed that octapressin could improve renal blood flow *(16)*. Subsequently, Lentz et al. showed that infusion of vasopressin transiently increases GFR in patients with HRS during a short term infusion *(17)*, and various agents have since been used with some success *(16–23)*. Terlipressin (glypressin), which is injected as an iv bolus, has an effect lasting from 2–4 h. There are uncontrolled data to suggest that terlipressin is less effective unless given with albumin support *(108)*. Further studies are needed, however, before such treatment is recommended. However, all patients should be fluid replete, having been given a volume challenge, before commencing terlipressin. Most experts start terlipressin at 0.5 mg iv every 6 h, increasing in frequency and dose to a maximum dose of 2 mg hourly. At such high doses, digital ischemia and coronary artery spasm become more common. There have now been several open studies using terlipressin, and its action is twofold. First, it increases arterial blood pressure, and places the patient back into a position where RBF increases in response to increases in blood pressure, second, it suppresses activation of the sympathetic nervous system *(23)* (Fig. 5). Thus, for every minor increment of arterial pressure, there is a corresponding increase in renal blood flow. This is illustrated in Fig. 2. However, several studies have now shown improved survival with terlipressin, with a comprehensive study from Moreau et al. in which survival with terlipressin therapy was reported as 55% *(109)*. In one of the very few randomized studies in HRS, it has recently been shown that terlipressin increases survival from 0 to 42% *(110)*.

NOREPINEPHRINE INFUSION

As long ago as 1963, Laragh et al. had shown that infusion of norepinephrine into patients with HRS could improve renal function in some patients *(61)*. Most recently, Duvoux

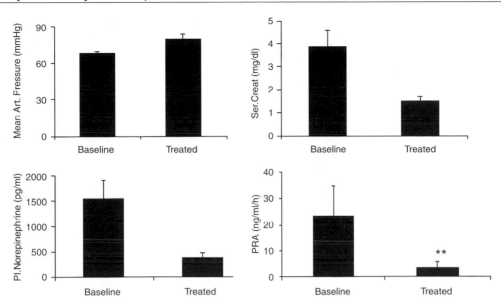

Fig. 5. Administration of terlipressin with albumin support improves mean arterial pressure, suppresses activation of the sympathetic nervous system, and improves renal function. From Ref. *23.*

et al. have shown that infusion of norepinephrine and furosemide into patients with HRS improves renal function *(111)*. The rationale for the inclusion of furosemide in the regime was never clear, and unless there is a need to try and enhance the diuresis, e.g., owing to fluid overload, it is probably best to keep the regimen simple by infusion of norepinephrine alone at a dose sufficient to increase BP. There are no head-to-head studies with terlipressin.

MIDODRINE AND OCTREOTIDE

Terlipressin is not licensed in the US at present, and, therefore, alternative therapies have been used. These include infusion of norepinephrine or oral administration of midodrine ± iv octroetide *(21)*. Midodrine is an orally active α-adrenergic agent, and octreotide is a long-acting analog of somatostatin, which has a variable effect on splanchnic haemodynamics. The data on its use in HRS are limited, to a recent publication by Angeli et al. *(21)* in patients with type 1 HRS, although more data from Florence Wong's group will be published soon. Angeli demonstrated that combined long-term administration of midodrine and octreotide, together with albumin, support to increase mean arterial pressure by 15 mmHg, resulted in a significant improvement of renal function. No significant side effects were observed.

What To Do If There Is Fluid Overload in a Patient with HRS

Occasionally, one is faced with a patient with fluid overload and oliguric HRS. In the first instance, if they have tense ascites, this should be drained acutely without albumin or colloid support. This will cause an immediate decrease in right atrial pressure *(112)*. Second, many clinicians have serious concerns about the use of loop diuretics. However, in a patient who is overloaded, a bolus of frusemide (100 mg iv) may convert a patient with oliguria, and difficult fluid management, into a patient who is passing urine, and easier to manage in terms of fluid balance. Loop diuretics increase renal PGE2 synthesis. Finally, begin terlipressin or other vasopressor therapy to increase mean arterial pressure to >85 mmHg, or to a lower pressure if urine output increases adequately.

N-Acetylcysteine

There has been one series of 12 patients (9 of whom had alcoholic cirrhosis) with HRS where N-acetylcysteine was given iv for 5 d *(113)*. This treatment was well tolerated, with no side effects. At baseline, following aggressive fluid replacement, the mean creatinine clearance was 24 ± 3 mL/min, rising to 43 ± 4 mL/min following the 5 d of therapy. This was associated with an increase in urine output, and a significant increase in sodium excretion from 1.2 ± 0.5 to 1.8 ± 0.6 mmol/h ($p < 0/05$). High survival figures of 67% (8/12) at 1 mo and 58% (7/12) at 3 mo were observed. This included two patients who underwent successful orthotopic liver transplantation after improvement in their renal function *(113)*. The mechanism of action is unknown, but may involve an improvement of cardiac function, as this has been observed in rats with impaired cardiac function (unpublished). Recent studies have shown that NAC therapy also prevents radio-contrast nephropathy *(114)*.

Renal Support and MARS

Renal support should only be given when there is a clear goal of management and potential positive outcome, and when the above therapeutic maneuvers have failed. Thus, renal support should only be offered where there is a realistic possibility of hepatic regeneration, hepatic recovery, or liver transplantation. Renal support otherwise merely prolongs the dying process. Renal support is generally given as continuous hemofiltration because intermittent hemodialysis causes hemodynamic instability. The survival of patients with severe alcoholic hepatitis given renal support is approx 15% (unpublished). The Molecular Adsorbent Recirculating System (MARS) is a modified dialysis method, using albumin-containing dialysate that is recirculated and perfused online through charcoal and anion exchanger columns. MARS enables the elective removal of albumin-bound substances. Mitzner et al. *(115)* in a randomized controlled trial compared standard therapy consisting of volume expansion, dopamine, and hemofiltration vs the same plus MARS dialysis. They found a significant improvement in standard liver and kidney test function in the MARS group. Mortality rates where 100% in the control group and 62.5% in the MARS group at d 7. Further studies are needed, as the possibility of a type 2 error in this study is high.

Surgical Maneuvers, Transjugular Portosystemic Shunts (TIPS), and Liver Transplantation

There are few case reports of TIPS in patients with HRS and the results are mixed. Some patients with type 2 HRS have a delayed response (after 4 wk), with improvement of renal function. However, the largest series show improvement in renal function in most, and the German series had 6 of 16 patients with type 1 syndrome. Three-month survival rate was 75%. Recently, the long-term follow-up of this group with a larger cohort (median follow up 2 yr) has been published *(116,117)*. Thirty-one patients with HRS received TIPS (14 patients HRS type I, 17 HRS type II). Following TIPS total survival rates at 3 and 12 mo were 63% and 39%, respectively. These results are encouraging, but controlled trials are required to confirm improvement in prognosis. TIPS may serve as a bridge to liver transplant allowing kidney function to recover and clinical status.

The only effective and permanent treatment for the HRS is orthotopic liver transplantation (OLT). Gonwa et al. compared survival following OLT of 56 patients with HRS with 513 patients controls (non-HRS), They observed a 1- and 4-yr survival of 71 and 60% for HRS patients, and 83 and 70%, respectively, for non-HRS patients *(118)*. The same retrospective study also considered the long-term evolution of renal function following OLT for both groups of patients. Both cyclosporin and FK506 (used following OLT) also impair renal function. As a consequence, in 407 non-HRS patients, GFR decreased from 94 to 60 mL/min at 1 yr following transplantation. In 34 patients with HRS, GFR increased from 14 to 44 mL/min at 1 yr following transplantation. The preoperative and postoperative morbidity in HRS patients was higher. Dialysis was required in 32% of HRS patients prior to OLT, and 10% remained on dialysis following transplantation. Overall mean posttransplant hospital stay is 42 d for patients with HRS compared to 27 d for those without HRS *(119)*. Hence, it seems currently clear that eligible patients with HRS can safely benefit from liver replacement at the price of increased time spent in the hospital and modest impact on long-term survival *(118)*.

CONCLUSION

The hepatorenal syndrome is a syndrome of renal failure owing to advance acute or chronic liver disease. It is caused by impaired renal perfusion pressure, stimulation of the renal sympathetic nervous system, and increased synthesis of several vasoactive mediators, causing mesangial contraction and reduced filtration fraction. Patients with the HRS should be treated by supportive measures (blood pressure support and antibiotics), and hemofiltration or renal support only given if recovery of liver function is likely, either spontaneously or following liver transplantation.

REFERENCES

1. Arroyo V, Gines P, Gerbes AL, et al. Definition and diagnostic criteria of refractory ascites and hepatorenal syndrome in cirrhosis. Hepatology 1996;23:164–176.
2. Gines A, Escorsell A, Gines P, et al. Incidence, predictive factors, and prognosis of the hepatorenal syndrome in cirrhosis with ascites. Gastroenterology 1993;105:229–236.
3. Follo A, Llovet JM, Navasa M, et al. Renal impairment after sponatneous bacterial peritonitis in cirrhosis: predictive factors of infection resolution and survival in patients with cefotaxime. Hepatology 1993;251–257.
4. Guevara PM, Arroyo V, Rodes J. Hepatorenal syndrome. Lancet 2003;362:1819–1827.
5. Schrier RW, Arroyo V, Bernardi M, Epstein M, Henriksen JH, Rodes J. Peripheral arterial vasodilation hypothesis: a proposal for the initiation of renal sodium and water retention in cirrhosis. Hepatology 1988;8:1151–1157.
6. Koppel MH, Coburn JM, Mims MM, et al. Transplantation of cadaveric kidneys from patients with hepatorenal syndrome. Evidence for the functional nature of renal failure in advanced liver disease. N Engl J Med 1969;280:1367–1371.
7. Dudley FJ, Kanel GC, Wood LJ, Reynolds TB. Hepatorenal syndrome without avid sodium retention. Hepatology 1986;6:248–251.
8. Mandal AK, Lansing M, Fahmy A. Acute tubular necrosis in hepatorenal syndrome: an electron microscopy study. Am J Kidney Dis 1982;2:363–374.
9. Moore K. The hepatorenal syndrome. Clin Sci 1997;92:433–443.
10. Ma Z, Lee SS. Cirrhotic cardiomyopathy: getting to the heart of the matter. Hepatology 1996;24:451–459.
11. Ruiz-del-Arbol L, Urman J, Fernandez J, et al. Systemic, renal, and hepatic hemodynamic derangement in cirrhotic patients with spontaneous bacterial peritonitis. Hepatology 2003;38:1210–1218.

12. Fernanadez-Seara J, Prieto J, Quiroga J, et al. Systemic and regional haemodynamics in patients with liver cirrhosis and ascites with and without functional renal failure. Gastroenterology 1989;97:1304–1312.

13. Llach J, Gines J, Arroyo V, et al. Prognostic value of arterial pressure, endogenous vasoactive systems, and renal function in cirrhotic patients admitted to the hospital for the treatment of ascites. Gastroenterology 1988;94:482–487.

14. Navar LG. Renal autoregulation: perspectives from whole kidney and single nephron studies. [Review]. Am J Physiol 1978;234:357–370.

15. Person PB, Ehmeke H, Naf B, Kircheeim HR. Sympathetic modulation of renal autoregulation by carotid occlusion in conscious dogs. Am J Physiol 1990;258:F364–F370.

16. Kew MC, Varma RR, Sampson DJ, Sherlock S. The effect of octapressin on renal and intrarenal blood flow in cirrhosis of the liver. Gut 1972;13:293–296.

17. Evrard P, Ruedin P, Installe E, Suter PM. Low-dose ornipressin improves renal function in the hepatorenal syndrome. Critical Care Med 1994;22:363–366.

18. Ganne-Carri N, Hadengue A, Mathurin P, et al. Hepatorenal syndrome: long-term treatment with terlipressin as a bridge to liver transplantation. Digest Dis Sci 1996;41:1054–1056.

19. Guevara M, Gines P, Fernandez-Esparrach G, et al. Reversibility of hepatorenal syndrome by prolonged administration of ornipressin and plasma volume expansion. Hepatology 1998;27:35–41.

20. Dagher L, Patch D, Marley R, Moore K, Burroughs AK. Pharmacological treatment of the hepatorenal syndrome in cirrhotic patients. Alimentary Pharmacology & Therapeutics 2000;14:515–521.

21. Angeli P, Volpin R, Piovan D, et al. Acute effects of the oral administration of midodrine, an alpha-adrenergic agonist, on renal hemodynamics and renal function in cirrhotic patients with ascites. Hepatology 1998;28:937–943.

22. Lenz K, Hortnagl H, Druml W, et al. Ornipressin in the treatment of functional renal failure in decompensated liver cirrhosis. Gastroenterology 1991;101:1060–1067.

23. Uriz J, Cardenas A, Sort P, et al. Telipressin plus albumin infusion: an effective and safe therapy of hepatorenal syndrome. J Hepatol 2000;33:43–48.

24. Maroto A, Gines P, Arroyo V, et al. Brachial and femoral artery blood flow in cirrhosis: relationship to kidney dysfunction. Hepatology 1993;17:788–793.

25. Sato S, Ohnishi K, Sugita S, Okuda K. Splenic artery and superior mesenteric artery blood flow: nonsurgical Doppler US measurement in healthy subjects and patients with chronic liver disease. Radiology 1987;164:347–352.

26. Bendtsen F, Schifter S, Henriksen JH. Increased circulating calcitonin gene-related peptide (CGRP) in cirrhosis. J Hepatol 1991;12:118–123.

27. Vallance P, Moncada S. Hyperdynamic circulation in cirrhosis: a role for nitric oxide? Lancet 1991; 337:776–778.

28. Hecker M, Mülsch A, Bassenge E, Busse R. Vasoconstriction and increased flow: two principle mechhanisms of shear stress-dependent endothelial autacoid release. Am J Physiol 1993;265:H828–H833.

29. Stark ME, Szurszewski JH. Role of nitric oxide in gastrointestinal and hepatic function and disease. Gastroenterology 1992;103:1928–1949.

30. Bomzon A, Blendis LM. The nitric oxide hypothesis and the hyperdynamic circulation in cirrhosis. Hepatology 1994;20:1343–1350.

31. Groszmann RJ. Hyperdynamic circulation of liver disease 40 years later: pathophysiology and clinical consequences. Hepatology 1994;20:1359–1363.

32. Pierre-Yves M, Gines P, Schrier R. Nitric Oxide as a mediator of haemodynamic abnormalities and sodium and water retention in cirrhosis. N Engl J Med 1998;339:533–541.

33. Guarner C, Soriano G, Tomas A, et al. Increased serum nitrite and nitrate levels in patients with cirrhosis: relationship to endotoxemia. Hepatology 1993;18:1139–1143.

34. Claria J, Jimenez W, Ros J, et al. Increased nitric oxide-dependent vasorelaxation in aortic rings of cirrhotic rats with ascites. Hepatology 1994;20:1615–1621.

35. Mathie RT, Ralevic V, Moore KP, Burnstock G. Mesenteric vasodilator responses in cirrhotic rats: a role for nitric oxide? Hepatology 1996;23:130–136.

36. Pizcueta MP, Pique JM, Fernandez M, et al. Modulation of the hyperdynamic circulation of cirrhotic rats by nitric oxide inhibition. Gastroenterology 1992;103:1909–1915.

37. Forrest EH, Jones AL, Dillon JF, Walker J, Hayes PC. The effect of nitric oxide synthase inhibition on portal pressure and azygous blood flow in patients with cirrhosis. J Hepatol 1995;23:254–258.

38. Atucha NM, Shah V, Garcia-Cardena G, Sessa WE, Groszmann RJ. Role of endothelium in the abnormal response of mesenteric vessels in rats with portal hypertension and liver cirrhosis. Gastroenterology 1996;111:1627–1632.

39. Ottesen LH, Harry D, Frost M, et al. Increased formation of S-nitrothiols and nitrotyrosine in cirrhotic rats during endotoxemia. Free Radic Biol Med 2001;31:790–798.

40. Marley R, Feelisch M, Holt S, Moore K. A chemiluminescense-based assay for S-nitrosoalbumin and other plasma S-nitrosothiols. Free Radic Res 2000;32:1–9.

41. Guarner F, Guarner C, Prieto J, et al. Increased synthesis of systemic prostacyclin in cirrhotic patients. Gastroenterology 1996;90:687–694.

42. Moore K, Ward P, Taylor G, Williams R. Systemic and renal production of thromboxane A2 and prostacyclin in decompensated liver disease and hepatorenal syndrome. Gastroenterology 1991;100: 1069–1077.

43. Bruix J, Bosch J, Kravetz D, Mastai R, Rodés J. Effects of prostaglandin inhibition on systemic and hepatic hemodynamics in patients with cirrhosis of the liver. Gastroenterology 1985;88:430–435.

44. Moreau R, Komeichi H, Kirstetter P, Ohsuga M, Cailmail S, Lebrec D. Altered control of vascular tone by adenosine triphosphate sensitive potassium channels in rats with cirrhosis. Gastroenterology 1994;106:1016–1023.

45. Moreau R, Komeichi H, Cailmail S, Lebrec D. Blockade of ATP-sensitive K+ channels by glibenclamide reduces portal pressure and hyperkinetic circulation in portal hypertensive rats. J Hepatol 1992;16:215–218.

46. Moreau R, Lebrec D. Endogenous factors involved in the control of arterial tone in cirrhosis. J Hepatol 1995;22:370–376.

47. Wilkinson SP, Moodie H, Stamatakis JD, Kakkar VV, Williams R. Endotoxaemia and renal failure in cirrhosis and obstructive jaundice. Br Med J 1976;2:141–158.

48. Bourgoignie JJ, Valle GA. Endotoxin and renal dysfunction in liver disease. In: Epstein M, ed. The Kidney in Liver Diseases. Williams and Wilkins, Baltimore, MD, 1988, pp. 486–507.

49. Lumsden AB, Henderson JM, Kutner MH. Endotoxin levels measured by a chromogenic assay in portal hepatic and peripheral venous blood in patients with cirrhosis. Hepatology 1988;8:232–236.

50. Sheron N, Bird G, Koskinas J, et al. Circulating and tissue levels of the neutrophil chemotaxin interleukin 8 are elevated in severe acute alcoholic hepatitis, and tissue levels correlate with neutrophil infiltration. Hepatology 1993;18:41–46.

51. Sheron N, Bird G, Goka J, Alexander G, Williams R. Elevated plasma interleukin6 and increased severity and mortality in alcoholic hepatitis. Clin Experi Immunol 1991;84:449–453.

52. LopezTalavera JC, Merrill WW, Groszmann RJ. Tumor necrosis factor alpha: a major contributor to the hyperdynamic circulation in prehepatic portalhypertensive rats. Gastroenterology 1995;108: 761–767.

53. Fernando B, Marley R, Holt S, et al. Acetylcysteine prevents development of the hyperdynamic circulation in the portal hypertensive rat. Hepatology 1998;28:689–694.

54. Lopez-Talavera JC, Levitzki A, Martinez M, Gazit A, Esteban R, Guardia E. Tyrosine kinase inhibition ameliorates the hyperdynamic state and decreases nitric oxide production in cirrhotic rats with portal hypertension and ascites. J Clin Invest 1997;100:664–670.

55. Batkai S, Jarai Z, Wagner JA, et al. Endocannabinoids acting at vascular CB1 receptors mediate the vasodilated state in advanced liver cirrhosis. Nat Med 2001;7:827–832.

56. Ros J, Claria J, To-Figueras J, et al. Endogenous cannabinoids: a new system involved in the homeostasis of arterial pressure in experimental cirrhosis in the rat. Gastroenterology 2002:122:85–93.

57. Orliac ML, Peroni R, Celuch SM, Adler-Graschinsky E. Potentiation of anandamide effects in mesenteric beds isolated from endotoxemic rats. J Pharmacol Exp Ther 2003;304:179–184.

58. Varga K, Lake KD, Huangfu D, Guyenet PG, Kunos G. Mechanism of the hypotensive action of anandamide in anesthetized rats. Hypertension 1996;28(4):682–686.

59. Wilkinson SP, Williams R. Renin-angiotensin-aldosterone system in cirrhosis. Gut 1980;21:545–554.

60. Schroeder ET, Eich RH, Smulyan H, et al. Plasma renin level in hepatic cirrhosis: relation to functional renal failure. Am J Med 1970;49:189–191.

61. Laragh JH, Cannon PJ, Bentzel CJ, Sicinski AM, Meltzer J. Angiotensin II, norepinephrine and renal transport of electrolytes and water in normal man and in cirrhosis with ascites. J Clin Invest 1963;42: 1179–1192.

62. Cobden I, Shore A, Wilkinson R, Record CO. Captopril in the hepatorenal syndrome. J Clin Gastroenterol 1985;7:354–360.

63. Gentilini P, Romanelli RG, La Villa G, et al. Effects of low dose captopril on renal haemodynamics and function in patients with cirrhosis of the liver. Gastroenterology 1993;104:588–594.

64. Pariente EA, Bataille C, Bercoff E, Lebrec D. Acute effects of captopril on systemic and renal haemodynamics and renal function in cirrhotic patients with ascites. Gastroenterology 1985;88:1255–1259.

65. Wood LJ, Goergen S, Stockigt JR, et al. Adverse effects of captopril in treatment of resistant ascites, a state of functional bilateral renal artery stenosis. (Letter) Lancet 1985;2:1008–1009.

66. Schroeder ET, Anderson GH. Effect of blockade of angiotensin II on blood pressure, renin and aldosterone in cirrhosis. Kid Int 1976;9:511–519.

67. Schneider AW, Kalk FJ, Klein CP. Effect of Losartan, an Angiotensin II receptor antagonist on portal pressure in cirrhosis. Hepatology 1999;29:334–339.

68. Garcia-Tsao G. Angiotensin II receptor antagonist in the pharmacological therapy: a caution. Gastroenterology 1999;117:740–742.

69. Epstein M. Renal prostaglandins and the control of renal function in liver disease. Am J Med 1986; 80:46–61.

70. Guarner C, Colina I, Guarner F, Corzo J, Prieto J, Vilardi F. Renal prostaglandins in cirrhosis of the liver. Clin Sci 1986;70:477–484.

71. Laffi G, La Villa G, Pinzani M, et al. Altered renal and platelet arachidonic acid metabolism in cirrhosis. Gastroenterology 1986;90:274–282.

72. Rimola A, Gines P, Arroyo V, et al. Urinary excretion of 6-keto-prostaglandin F1alpha, thromboxane B2 and prostaglandin E2 in cirrhosis with ascites: relationship to functional renal failure (hepatorenal syndrome). J Hepatol 1986;3:111–117.

73. Zipser R, Hoefs J, Speckart P, Zia P, Horton R. Prostoglandins: modulators of renal function and pressor resistance in chronic liver disease. J Clin Endocrinol Metab 1979;48:895–900.

74. Boyer T, Zia P, Reynold T. Effect of indomethacin and prostaglandin A, on renal function and plasma renin activity in alcoholic liver disease. Gastroenterology 1979;77:215–222.

75. Mullane JF, Gliedman ML. Elevation of the pressure in the abdominal inferior vena cava as a cause of a hepatorenal syndrome in cirrhosis. Surgery 1966;59:1135–1146.

76. Henriksen JH. Hepatorenal disorders: role of the sympathetic nervous system. Sem Liver Dis 1994; 14:35–43.

77. Zambraski EJ, DiBona GF. Sympathetic nervous system in hepatic cirrhosis. The kidney in the liver disease. Williams and Wilkins, Baltimore, 1988, pp. 469–485.

78. Bichet DG, Van Putten VJ, Schrier RW. Potential role of increased sympathetic activity in impaired sodium and water excretion in cirrhosis. N Engl J Med 1982;307:1552–1557.

79. Gaudin C, Braillon A, Poo JL, Moreau R, Hadengue A, Lebrec D. Regional sympathetic activity, severity of liver disease and hemodynamics in patients with cirrhosis. J Hepatol 1991;13:161–168.

80. Henriksen JH, Ring-Larsen H, Christensen NJ. Kidney, lower limb, and whole-body uptake and release of catecholamines in alcoholic liver disease. Clin Physiol 1988;8:203–210.

81. Henriksen JH, Christensen NJ, Ring-Larsen H. Noradrenaline and adrenaline concentrations in various vascular beds in patients with cirrhosis. Relation to haemodynamics. Clin Physiol 1981;1:293–304.

82. Kostreva D, Castaner A, Kampine J. Reflex effects of hepatic baroreceptors on renal and cardiac sympathetic nerve activity. Am J Physiol 1980;238:R390–R394.

83. Levy M, Wexler MJ. Hepatic denervation alters first-phase urinary sodium excretion in dogs with cirrhosis. Am J Physiol 1987;253:F664–F671.

84. Lang F, Tschernko E, Schulze E, et al. Hepatorenal reflex regulating kidney function. Hepatology 1991;14:590–594.

85. Jalan R, Forrest EH, Redhead DN, Hayes PC. Reduction in renal blood flow with acute increase of portal pressure gradient. Evidence for the hepatorenal reflex? Hepatology 1994;20.

86. Solis-Herruzo JA, Duran A, Favelza V, et al. Effects of lumbar sympathetic block on kidney function in cirrhotic patients with hepatorenal syndrome. J Hepatol 1987;5:167–173.

87. Ring-Larsen H. Renal blood flow in cirrhosis: relation to systemic and portal haemodynamics and liver function. Scand J Clin Lab Invest 1977;37:635–642.

88. Uchihara M, Izumi N, Sato C, Marumo F. Clinical significance of elevated plasma endothelin concentration in patients with cirrhosis. Hepatology 1992;16:95–99.

89. Moore K, Wendon J, Frazer M, Karani J, Williams R, Badr K. Plasma endothelin immunoreactivity in liver disease and the hepatorenal syndrome. N Engl J Med 1992;327:1774–1778.

90. Morrow JD, Moore KP, Awad JA, et al. Marked overproduction of non-cyvclooxygenase derives prostanoids (F2-isoprostanes) in the hepatorenal syndrome. J Lipid Mediators 1993;6:417–420.

91. Boulanger CM, Tanner FC, Bea ML, Hahn AW, Werner A, Luscher TF. Oxidized low density lipoproteins induce mRNA expression and release of endothelin from human and porcine endothelium. Circ Res 1992;70:1191–1197.

92. Yura T, Fukunaga M, Khan R, Nassar GN, Badr KF, Montero A. Free-radical-generated F2-isoprostane stimulates cell proliferation and endothelin-1 expression on endothelial cells. Kidney Int 1999;56:471–478.

93. Vaughan RB, Angus PW, Chin-Dusting JP. Evidence for altered vascular responses to exogenous endothelin-1 in patients with advanced cirrhosis with restoration of the normal vasoconstrictor response following successful liver transplantation. Gut 2003;52:1505–1510.

94. Moore KP, Taylor GW, Gove C, et al. Synthesis and metabolism of cysteinyl leukotrienes by the isolated pig kidney. Kid Int 1992;41:1543–1548.

95. Moore KP, Taylor GW, Maltby NH, et al. Increased production of cysteinyl leukotrienes in hepatorenal syndrome. J Hepatol 1990;11:263–271.

96. Uemura M, Buchholz U, Kojima H, et al. Cysteinyl leukotrienes in the urine of patients with liver diseases. Hepatology 1994;20:804–812.

97. Huber M, Kastner S, Scholmerich J, Gerok W, Keppler D. Analysis of cysteinyl leukotrienes in human urine: enhanced excretion in patients with liver cirrhosis and hepatorenal syndrome. Europ J Clin Invest 1989;19:53–60.

98. Zipser RD, Radvan GH, Kronborg IJ, Duke R, Little TE. Urinary thromboxane B2 and prostaglandin E2 in the hepatorenal syndrome: evidence for increased vasoconstrictor and decreased vasodilator factors. Gastroenterology 1983;84:697–703.

99. Zipser RD, Kronborg I, Rector W, Reynolds T, Daskalopoulos G. Therapeutic trial of thromboxane synthesis inhibition in the hepatorenal syndrome. Gastroenterology 1984;87:1228–1232.

100. Guha IN, Moore K. F2-isoprostanes and the liver. Prostaglandins and other Lipid Mediators 2003; 72:73–84.

101. Goulis J, Patch D, Burroughs AK. Bacterial infection in the pathogenesis of variceal bleeding. Lancet 1999;353:139–142.

102. Sort P, Navasa M, Arroyo V, et al. Effect of intravenous albumin on renal impairment and mortality in patients with cirrhosis and spontaneous bacterial peritonitis. N Engl J Med 1999;341:403–409.

103. Gines P, Tito L, Arroyo V, et al. Randomized comparative study of therapeutic paracentesis with and without intravenous albumin in cirrhosis. Gastroenterology 1988;84:1493–1502.

104. Gines P, Fernandez-Esparrach G, Monescillo A, et al. Randomized trial comparing albumin, dextran 70, and polygeline in cirrhotic patients with ascites treated by paracentesis. Gastroenterology 1996;111:1002–1010.

105. Cabrera J, Arroyo V, Ballesta AM, et al. Aminoglycoside toxicity in cirrhosis. Value of urinary beta-2 microglobulin to discriminate functional renal failure from acute tubular damage. Gastroenterology 1982;82:97–105.

106. Martin G, Bennett-Guerrero E, Wakeling H, et al. A prospective, randomized comparison of thromboelastographic coagulation profile in patients receiving lactated Ringer's solution, 6% hetastarch in a balanced-saline vehicle, or 6% hetastarch in saline during major surgery. J Cardiothorac Vasc Anesth 2002;16:441–446.

107. Hadengue A, Moreau R, Gaudin C, Bacq Y, Champigneulle B, Lebrec D. Total effective vascular compliance in patients with cirrhosis: a study of the response to acute blood volume expansion. Hepatology 1992;15:809–815.

108. Ortega R, Gines P, Uriz J, et al. Terlipressin therapy with and without albumin for patients with hepatorenal syndrome: results of a prospective, nonrandomized study. Hepatology 2002;36:941–948.

109. Moreau R, Durand F, Poynard T, et al. Terlipressin in patients with cirrhosis and type 1 hepatorenal syndrome: a retrospective multicenter study. Gastroenterology 2002;122:923–930.

110. Solanki P, Chawla A, Garg R, Gupta R, Jain M, Sarin SK. Beneficial effects of terlipressin in hepatorenal syndrome: a prospective, randomized placebo-controlled clinical trial. J Gastroenterol Hepatol 2003;18:152–156.

111. Duvoux C, Zanditenas D, Hezode C, et al. Effects of noradrenalin and albumin in patients with type I hepatorenal syndrome: a pilot study. Hepatology 2002;36:374–380.
112. Panos MZ, Moore K, Vlavianos P, et al. Single, total paracentesis for tense ascites: sequential hemodynamic changes and right atrial size. Hepatology 1990;11:662–667.
113. Holt S, Marley R, Fernando B, Harry D, Moore K. Improvement of renal function in hepatorenal syndrome with N-acetyl cysteine. Lancet 1999;353:294.
114. Tepel M, van der Giet M, Schwarzfeld C, Laufer U, Liermann D, Zidek W. Prevention of radiographic-contrast-agent-induced reductions in renal function by acetylcysteine. N Engl J Med 2000; 343:180–184.
115. Mitzner S, Stange J, Klammt S, et al. Improvement of hepatorenal syndrome with extracorporeal albumin dialysis MARS: results of a prospective, randomized, controlled trial. Liver Transplantation 2000;6:277–286.
116. Ochs A, Rossle M, Haag K, et al. The transjugular intrahepatic portosystemic stent-shunt procedure for refractory ascites. N Engl J Med 1995;332:1192–1197.
117. Brensing KA, Textor J, Perz J, et al. Long term outcome after transjugular intrahepatic portosystemic stent-shunt in non-transplant cirrhotics with hepatorenal syndrome: a phase II study. Gut 2000;47: 288–295.
118. Gonwa TA, Morris CA, Goldstein RM, Husberg BS, Klinthalm GB. Long-term survival and renal function following liver transplantation in patients with and without hepatorenal syndrome-experience in 300 patients. Transplantation 1991;51:428–430.
119. Le Moine O. Hepatorenal syndrome outcome after liver transplantation. Nephrology, Dialysis Transplant 1998;13:20–22.

VI EVALUATION AND TREATMENT IN SPECIAL CIRCUMSTANCES OF PORTAL HYPERTENSION

23 Pregnancy and Portal Hypertension

Bimaljit Sandhu, MD and Arun J. Sanyal, MD

CONTENTS

INTRODUCTION
HEMODYNAMICS IN NORMAL PREGNANCY
PATHOPHYSIOLOGY OF PORTAL HYPERTENSION
PORTAL VENOUS FLOW CHANGES IN PREGNANCY
COMPLICATIONS AS A RESULT OF PORTAL HYPERTENSION
   IN PREGNANCY
FETAL WASTAGE
PERINATAL FETAL LOSS
IMPACT OF PREGNANT STATE ON PREEXISTING LIVER DISEASE
   AND PORTAL HYPERTENSION
MATERNAL COMPLICATIONS
NATURAL HISTORY OF PORTAL HYPERTENSION DURING PREGNANCY
OTHER COMPLICATIONS
MANAGEMENT OF PREGNANCY COEXISTING WITH PORTAL
   HYPERTENSION
PRECONCEPTION COUNSELING AND MANAGEMENT
ROLE OF SURVEILLANCE ENDOSCOPY IN PREGNANT PATIENTS
   WITH PORTAL HYPERTENSION
PRIMARY PROPHYLAXIS
SECONDARY PROPHYLAXIS
ANTENATAL MANAGEMENT
MANAGEMENT OF ACTIVE VARICEAL HEMORRHAGE
PERINATAL MANAGEMENT
SPLENIC ARTERY ANEURYSM (SAA) IN PREGNANCY
   WITH PORTAL HYPERTENSION
SUMMARY
REFERENCES

INTRODUCTION

Pregnancy is a normal physiological state characterized by numerous hemodynamic changes. These hemodynamic changes, although necessary for a normal pregnancy, pose a special problem in the presence of portal hypertension. In North America, cirrhosis of the liver is the most common cause of portal hypertension. Although rare, the occurrence

From: *Clinical Gastroenterology: Portal Hypertension*
Edited by: A. J. Sanyal and V. H. Shah © Humana Press Inc., Totowa, NJ

Table 1
Physiological Changes During Pregnancy

Increased Blood Volume
    Sodium and Water Retention
    Increased Red Blood Cell Volume
Changes in Venous Return
    Increased owing to Increased Blood Volume
    Decrease as a result of Vena Cava Compression by Gravid Uterus
Increased Cardiac Output
    Increased Heart Rate
    Increased Stroke Volume
Decreased Blood Pressure
    Systemic Vasodilation
    Placental Circulation

of pregnancy is not altogether unknown in this population. This is caused by reduced fertility as a consequence of anovulatory cycles, altered endocrine metabolism, and a relatively older age of these patients *(1–6)*. Most women with well-compensated early chronic liver disease and those with the liver disease in remission, can expect to have normal fertility *(3,7)*. Subjects with liver diseases that progress slowly, such as primary biliary cirrhosis, are particularly likely to have preserved fertility until the disease becomes quite advanced *(8–12)*. Also, in patients with noncirrhotic portal hypertension (NCPH) the hepatic synthetic functions are relatively well preserved and so is the fertility *(13,14)*. Pregnancy in a patient with portal hypertension is a unique problem that needs specialized care to prevent potentially life-threatening complications such as gastrointestinal hemorrhage. It is therefore important to understand the effect of pregnancy on portal hypertension and vice versa so that untoward incidents like fetal morbidity and mortality and gastrointestinal hemorrhage can be avoided.

HEMODYNAMICS IN NORMAL PREGNANCY

Many systemic hemodynamic alterations occur during pregnancy as indicated in Table 1. These changes not only maintain tissue perfusion but also provide the growing fetus with nutrients and oxygen. These changes are evident as early as the beginning of the first trimester and peak in the second trimester *(15)*. These changes also serve as a reserve to protect the mother from hypovolemia related to blood loss during delivery and the puerperium. The physiologic changes, however, take on special significance in patients with underlying portal hypertension because they set the mother up for variceal hemorrhage, which constitutes a major threat to her well being, as well as the baby's *(14)*.

One of the earliest changes is an increase in plasma volume which increases by 40–50% starting by the 6th week of gestation and peaking around the 32nd wk *(16)*. This increase in blood volume is contributed to by retention of approx 1000 mEq of Na, which occurs despite an increase in the glomerular filtration rate *(17)*. Plasma renin activity (PRA) increases by up to tenfold and the plasma aldosterone levels increase by two to three times. These substances along with increased estrogen, deoxycortisone, and placental lactogen increase tubular Na reabsorption *(18,19)*. There is also an approx 20–30% increment in red cell mass, but hemoglobin levels drop owing to the net dilution effects from the relatively greater increase in plasma volume *(20,21)*.

Maternal cardiac output increases by 30–50% due to the increase in stroke volume and the heart rate. The stroke volume increases by up to 75 mL per stroke and the heart rate by 15–20 beats per minute (bpm) *(9,22,23)*. The systemic vascular resistance declines progressively because of both systemic vasodilation produced by progesterone and other hormones and the development of the placenta which adds another active, highly perfused vascular bed to the circulation. Consequently, the diastolic blood pressure declines during the first 24 wk. A hyperdynamic circulatory state (HCS) with increased pulse pressure results from a decreased systemic vascular resistance and increased cardiac output *(24)*.

PATHOPHYSIOLOGY OF PORTAL HYPERTENSION

Portal hypertension is said to exist when the portal pressure exceeds 5 mmHg as measured from the hepatic venous pressure gradient (HVPG). HVPG is the difference between the free hepatic venous pressure (FHVP) and the wedged hepatic venous pressure (WHVP). WHVP indicates the sinusoidal pressure (portal pressure) in the absence of obstruction and the FHVP corrects for the intraabdominal pressure. The pathogenesis of portal hypertension takes into account the relationship between the portal venous blood flow and the resistance offered to the blood flow within the portal system. It is the pressure difference or the gradient along the length of the portal system that drives the blood within the portal system. The pressure gradient involving any vascular system, as expressed by the Ohm's law, is the product of portal blood flow (Q) and resistance (R) offered by the vascular system to blood flow *(25)*.

$$\Delta P = Q \times R$$

The splanchnic and the splenic venous blood flow accounts for the entire inflow to the portal vein. The delivery of blood from the splanchnic circulation to the portal system, in turn, has a direct correlation to the resistance offered in the splanchnic arterioles. Furthermore, the resistance in the splanchnic bed is dependent on the presence of effective circulating blood volume and a normal cardiac output. An increased resistance in the portal venous system is responsible for causing portal hypertension and its sequelae. The increased resistance in the portal system could be at the presinusoidal, sinusoidal, or postsinusoidal level, depending on the cause of portal hypertension. Despite the state of portal hypertension due to increased resistance to the flow of blood in the portal system, there is also paradoxically increased portal venous inflow due to mesenteric arteriolar dilatation *(26)*.

Portal hypertension has myriad clinical consequences that are directly or indirectly related to the formation of collaterals mainly in the form of esophageal and gastric varices. The varices are known to occur above a threshold of 11–12 mmHg of HVPG (portal pressure). Although the threshold of 11–12 mmHg is required for the varices to develop, many patients with HVPG in excess of 12 mmHg do not have varices *(27)*. Because varices are not seen in patients with an HVPG less than 11–12 mmHg, variceal bleeding is seldom, if ever, encountered at HVPG values below this threshold. At the same time, it is important to add that there are many patients who have HVPG greatly in excess of this threshold and still never bleed *(28)*. The risk of bleeding from the varices depends on the wall tension as depicted by Laplace's law, which is calculated as

$$\text{Wall tension} = (P1 - P2) \times r/w$$

where $P1 - P2$ is the gradient between the intravariceal luminal pressure and the esophageal luminal pressure, r is the radius of the varix, and w is the variceal wall thickness. The pressure gradient, for all practical purposes, is taken as the portal pressure, which obeys Ohm's law. Variceal wall tension can thus be redefined as

$$\text{Wall tension} = (\text{Variceal flow} \times \text{collateral resistance}) \times r/w$$

The likelihood of a varix to rupture, therefore, would be higher when the varix has a larger diameter, thin wall, and a higher pressure. Local conditions in the esophagus, like esophagitis, may increase the likelihood to bleed although this remains controversial (28).

PORTAL VENOUS FLOW CHANGES IN PREGNANCY

Transient portal hypertension, even leading to the development of esophageal varices, has been described in two-thirds of healthy pregnant women (29). This has been ascribed mainly to splanchnic blood flow which results from the hyperdynamic circulatory state in pregnancy. In addition, the increased intraabdominal pressure during the second and third trimesters increases postsinusoidal resistance and impedes blood flow in the inferior vena cava in supine position. This causes diversion of blood flow via the azygous system toward the gastroesophageal collateral channels. This scenario, although transient, is somewhat similar to the postsinusoidal portal hypertension (1). In those with preexisting portal hypertension, the normal transient rise in portal pressures during pregnancy causes an additional burden on the collateral circulation. This worsens portal hypertension and can precipitate variceal hemorrhage. The incidence of variceal bleeding in pregnant patients with portal hypertension has been reported to range from 6 to 44%; this increases to 62–78% in those who have portal hypertension with demonstrable varices before conception occurs (1–3,30).

The overall risk of variceal bleeding in pregnant women with portal hypertension is almost 400 times greater than in pregnant women without portal hypertension (1). In a patient with preexisting portal hypertension, the tendency for variceal hemorrhage during pregnancy is increased due to the increased intraabdominal pressure caused by the growing fetus, and also due to Valsalva's maneuver during labor. The second trimester of pregnancy is the period during which the systemic and portal circulatory changes peak. Consequently, the risk of variceal hemorrhage is greatest during this period. During labor, postsinusoidal resistance increases as a result of increased thoracic pressures owing to Valsalva's maneuver. This may also contribute to the risk of variceal rupture (29). Rare instances of precipitation of variceal hemorrhage have been attributed to violent retching in the first trimester because of morning sickness (1).

COMPLICATIONS AS A RESULT
OF PORTAL HYPERTENSION IN PREGNANCY

Owing to a paucity of data, the true incidence of various types of complications caused by cirrhosis and portal hypertension in the pregnant females is not known (Table 2). There is a general belief that the patients with chronic liver disease are incapable of conception (1–6). The incidence of pregnancy in cirrhosis is very low and has been reported to be approx 1 in 5950 pregnancies from an Indian series (31).

Table 2
Causes of Fetal Complications

Early Termination of Pregnancy ($\leq$20 wk)
　　Spontaneous Abortion (10–18%)
　　Therapeutic Abortion
　　Hysterotomy
Premature Termination of Pregnancy (21–37 wk)
　　Maternal Death
　　Variceal Hemorrhage
　　Therapeutic Abortion
Perinatal Deaths
　　Still Birth
　　Prematurity
　　Intrauterine Growth Retardation
　　Complicated Labor

FETAL WASTAGE

The outcome of pregnancy in patients with portal hypertension due to noncirrhotic causes is similar to the general population except for an increased incidence of abortion *(13)*. In an Indian series, the pregnant women with NCPH have an outcome similar to the normal population, except for a higher rate of abortion (20%) *(32)*. Similar outcomes as in patients with EHPVO are expected in patients of cirrhosis with relatively preserved liver synthetic functions, provided the risk of variceal hemorrhage is obviated by either endoscopic therapy or portal decompression prior to conception *(3,33–37)*. The incidence of spontaneous abortion in this population has been reported to vary from 3% to 6% suggesting that this subset of patients have a lower risk of this complication *(4,13,14,32)*.

There is a high incidence of fetal wastage in the patients with cirrhosis, ranging from 9.6% to 66% *(2,4,38,39)*. Most of the cases of early termination of pregnancy are caused by spontaneous abortions *(2)*. The rate of spontaneous abortion in patients with cirrhosis is in the range of 15–20% *(3,39)*. As seen in normal women, spontaneous abortions occur most often in the first trimester, in subjects with cirrhosis. In contrast, it has been reported that 60% of spontaneous abortions in pregnant women with NCPH occur in the second trimester *(13,40)*. There are scant data on rates of loss of pregnancy in the third trimester, in both those with cirrhosis and noncirrhotic portal hypertension. The early interruption of pregnancy because of therapeutic abortion, hysterotomy, and hysterectomy, although reported, is relatively rare. Early termination of pregnancy due to maternal death is also rare. Premature termination of pregnancy (21–37 wk) is comparable among the patients with cirrhotic and noncirrhotic portal hypertension (20.51 vs 18.75%) *(2)*.

PERINATAL FETAL LOSS

Perinatal mortality is higher (11–33.3%) in patients with portal hypertension owing to both cirrhotic and noncirrhotic causes, as compared to normal pregnant women *(3,32, 39)*. This is mainly a result of a high incidence of stillbirths in patients with portal hypertension (17.85% in cirrhotic and 11.53% in noncirrhotic portal hypertension). The likelihood of perinatal loss is closely related to the severity of the underlying liver disease and not to its cause or the degree of portasystemic shunting. The specific complications contributing to perinatal mortality include variceal hemorrhage, progressive liver failure, toxemia, high blood pressure, severe anemia, and worsening renal function (2,30). The fetal wastage in the patients with NCPH, on the other hand, has been reported to range from 7.9% to 20% in different series (13,32,40).

Perinatal mortality caused by variceal hemorrhage can be effectively reduced in patients who are diagnosed to have portal hypertension before pregnancy by adoption of effective means for variceal eradication. Good fetal outcome and a comparatively low perinatal mortality has been reported by the use of endoscopic variceal eradication during pregnancy by sclerotherapy, glue injection, and band ligation (13,33,35–37,41–45). A better outcome has also been shown in the subgroup of patients with relatively preserved liver functions who underwent a preconception decompressive shunt operation (13,38,46–48). However, emergency portosystemic anastomotic shunts have been performed during pregnancy, followed by arrest of variceal hemorrhage and uneventful delivery (49–53). Successful TIPS has been performed for recurrent variceal bleeding due to liver cirrhosis in a pregnant woman at 20-wk gestation (34).

There is no controlled trial to compare the efficacy of one procedure over another for preventing variceal hemorrhage. However, the endoscopic variceal band ligation is widely available and quite effective with relatively minor morbidity and mortality (33,35). This modality is therefore often used for this purpose. However, the choice of the procedure for a given patient at a given center has to be individualized according to the patient's circumstances and the expertise available.

IMPACT OF PREGNANT STATE ON PREEXISTING LIVER DISEASE AND PORTAL HYPERTENSION

There are limited data on the effect of pregnancy on chronic liver disease. It is generally agreed that pregnancy does not appear to unduly stress the cirrhotic liver and does not constitute a risk for worsening of chronic liver disease uncomplicated by portal hypertension (54). However, slight worsening of jaundice, impairment in liver functions, and/or hepatic decompensation have been reported during pregnancy, although these changes do not occur consistently (55).

Whereas liver functions are well preserved during pregnancy in those with NCPH, the data for cirrhotic subjects are more mixed. It has been reported that 54.02% pregnancies in cirrhotic patients had no deterioration, 41.37% had slight worsening, and 4.59% had an improvement in the liver functions (2). Importantly, there are no consistent pattern of changes from one pregnancy to the next for the same person. Clinical improvement in the liver functions of patients with Wilson's disease has been reported in the later stages of pregnancy, probably because of the diminution in tissue copper levels from mobilization to meet the requirements of the growing fetus (2,56,57). A patient who has deterioration of liver functions during one pregnancy may never encounter these changes in subsequent pregnancies (2).

MATERNAL COMPLICATIONS

Maternal complications occur in 30–50% of patients with preexisting portal hypertension. These are more common in patients with cirrhosis as compared to patients with NCPH (4,58). Many complications are encountered in such patients including variceal hemorrhage, hepatic failure, postpartum hemorrhage, rupture of splenic artery aneurysm, rupture of splenorenal shunts, spontaneous bacterial peritonitis, and maternal death. When acute hepatic failure develops on a background of cirrhosis and pregnancy, it is associated with a high mortality with nearly one-third of subjects dying within 48 h of the onset of acute liver failure *(3,13,14,38,40)*. Hypersplenism may cause anemia and its related complications. It also poses an added risk of bleeding due to thrombocytopenia during pregnancy in such patients *(13)*. The presence of underlying liver disease does not affect the risk of toxemia of pregnancy which occurs with similar frequency in cirrhotic (7.69%) vs noncirrhotic (9.37%) patients *(2)*.

NATURAL HISTORY OF PORTAL HYPERTENSION DURING PREGNANCY

General consensus exists about the increased risk of bleeding from esophageal varices during pregnancy. Variceal hemorrhage occurs in around 19–45% of patients with portal hypertension who become pregnant *(3,46)*. Importantly, almost 78% of the patients who have detectable varices during pregnancy are likely to bleed during the index gestation *(3,32,46)*. In an individual patient, bleeding occurs unpredictably in terms of both its timing and severity. However, in general, it is more frequent in the second and third trimester and also during labor. This has been attributed to both the increase in intraabdominal pressures due to the enlarged gravid uterus and the hemodynamic changes associated with pregnancy which peak in the second trimester. During labor, the expulsive efforts associated with the 2nd stage causes a further rise in intraabdominal pressure which compresses the inferior vena cava and causes increased blood flow through gastroesophageal collaterals and azygous system *(1,29)*. Reflux esophagitis that commonly occurs in pregnancy in conjunction with retching because of morning sickness has been reported to precipitate variceal hemorrhage in the first trimester *(13)*.

It is difficult to predict which women with preexisting varices will bleed during pregnancy. It is, however, more likely that those with large varices are more likely to bleed than those with small varices. Whereas this was refuted in one study *(30)*, it is generally held that variceal size and the presence of endoscopic red signs are markers for increased risk of bleeding. Although, a positive history of preconception variceal bleeding also has been shown to have little predictive value in terms of bleeding during pregnancy in one study *(1)*, other reports suggest that a prior variceal bleed is an important risk factor for rebleeding during pregnancy *(3)*. Bleeding is approx seven times more likely to occur in those who have not had a portal decompressive procedure compared to those who have had such a procedure *(55)*. Although some reports have failed to find a difference in the incidence of variceal hemorrhage between cirrhotic and noncirrhotic portal hypertensive pregnant patients *(1)*, others have reported a higher rate of bleeding in those with extrahepatic portal hypertension (43.7%) compared to cirrhotic subjects (19.6%) *(2)*. Interestingly, whereas the mortality in the latter group was around 61.5%, it was negligible in the latter *(2)*.

Individual bleeding patterns in both cirrhotic and noncirrhotic portal hypertensive patients are not predictive of bleeding during the gestation, suggesting that the patients who have bled during pregnancy might, or might not bleed during subsequent pregnancies *(1)*. Maternal mortality associated with variceal hemorrhage in the perinatal period in the pregnant patients with cirrhotic portal hypertension ranges from 18% to 61.5%, whereas the maternal mortality in pregnant women with NCPH is in the range of 2–7.1% *(13,59)*.

Given the differences in these studies and existing literature on the natural history of variceal hemorrhage, it is difficult to clearly demonstrate a higher risk of mortality from variceal hemorrhage in pregnant vs nonpregnant subjects *(59)*.

OTHER COMPLICATIONS

Pregnant cirrhotic patients have a high likelihood of postpartum hemorrhage, ranging from 7% to 26%, as a result of coagulopathy and thrombocytopenia due to hypersplenism *(2,39)*. The coagulopathy is due mainly caused by a deficiency of factors V and VII, with ocassional true prothrombin deficiency *(2)*. Increased postpartum hemorrhage is also seen in the pregnant cirrhotics after porto-caval shunt surgery owing to an increased tendency to fibrinolysis after the anastomosis *(39)*. Worsening of the already compromised hepatic function because of variceal hemorrhage contributes to a great extent in the morbidity and mortality of pregnant women. Acute variceal hemorrhage can cause acute worsening of liver function in those with preexisting chronic liver disease. This may manifest as worsening jaundice, hepatic encephalopathy, ascites, spontaneous bacterial peritonitis, or renal failure. Hypotension and compromised liver blood supply are important factors that further contribute to worsening liver failure *(25,28)*.

Rupture of a splenic artery aneurysm is another potentially life-threatening condition during pregnancy in a patient with portal hypertension and carries a considerably high fetal, as well as maternal, mortality. This complication is addressed to in greater detail in the later part of this chapter.

MANAGEMENT OF PREGNANCY COEXISTING WITH PORTAL HYPERTENSION

Pregnancy in a patient with preexisting portal hypertension is a unique problem that requires a hepatologist, neonatologist, and obstetrician to team up and work in a closely coordinated manner. The management of such patients should ideally be done at the centers equipped with facilities and expertise for gastrointestinal endoscopy and portal vascular surgery, high-risk obstetric care, and intensive perinatal care. The optimal management starts with preconception advice about the potential complications that are likely to occur and the associated risks to both the mother and the fetus because of these complications. The management of such patients continues through the gestation in to the perinatal period.

PRECONCEPTION COUNSELING AND MANAGEMENT

The most important aspect of preconception counseling is to get a sense for the patients' desire to have children even after understanding the potential risks related to it. After making an unbiased assessment about the desire to have children, the patients' psychologic and social situation should also be assessed to determine whether the patients' stated desire to have children is motivated by undue social pressures. It is generally advisable to talk to both prospective parents together and separately. The potential risks to both the mother and the fetus should be explained to both prospective parents *(4)*.

A complete medical history, physical examination, and laboratory investigations to assess the liver, renal, hematologic, and coagulation functions should be undertaken in addition to the routine investigations done in normal women planning a pregnancy. A preconception endoscopy should be performed in all the patients with portal hypertension or chronic liver disease with substantial fibrosis who plan to conceive. The cause of the portal hypertension must also be taken in to consideration because of the specific problems encountered in different types of portal hypertension and appropriate laboratory studies to determine the cause of liver disease should be performed if they are already available. Genetic counseling should be provided when necessary. In the case of infectious diseases such as hepatitis B and C, the risks of transmission to the offspring should be explained. Patients with chronic hepatitis B or C, while on Interferon and Ribavarin therapy should be advised against conception because of the toxicity and teratogenic effects of these drugs *(4)*. Autoimmune liver diseases usually do not flare up during pregnancy because of the immunosuppressive effects of pregnancy.

Pruritis of chronic cholestatic liver disease often worsens during pregnancy. Anticipation by the physician and preparedness of the mother is vital for the optimal care of this potentially disabling symptom. More importantly, pregnancy should be planned when the liver disease is stable and reliable contraception should be encouraged until conception is desired and recommended. Pregnancy should be avoided in the patients with prospects for liver transplantation in near future, until the transplant has been done. However, this is rarely a clinical issue owing to the poor fertility of such individuals.

ROLE OF SURVEILLANCE ENDOSCOPY IN PREGNANT PATIENTS WITH PORTAL HYPERTENSION

A major objective is to find out the subgroup of patients who are at high risk for bleeding. Surveillance endoscopy in the preconceptional period should be performed in all portal hypertensive patients planning conception *(3,60)*. The general management of portal hypertension is not substantively different in pregnant subjects compared to nonpregnant subjects (Fig. 1). According to the protocol followed for the nonpregnant portal hypertensive patients, the bigger size of varices at endoscopy and the presence of a previous variceal bleeding increases the likelihood of variceal hemorrhage *(14,61,62)*.

PRIMARY PROPHYLAXIS

Until more conclusive data are available, the primary prophylaxis of the variceal bleeding (varices that have never bled) by a nonselective β-receptor antagonist drug remains the therapy of choice. The role of endoscopic variceal ligation (EVL) for primary prophylaxis of variceal hemorrhage in the setting of pregnancy requires further evaluation as there are only anecdotal data in support of these endoscopic treatment *(25,37,62,63)*. Beta-adrenergic receptor antagonist drugs are relatively safe but need fetal monitoring for bradycardia and growth retardation *(4)*. Those who are intolerant of β blockers may be treated with endoscopic variceal band ligation, particularly if their varices are large. There is currently no role or justification for the use of prophylactic shunt surgery in those who have never bled *(55)*.

SECONDARY PROPHYLAXIS

The patients with a previous variceal bleeding and borderline liver functions are more likely to develop another episode of variceal hemorrhage during pregnancy with its attendant risks of going into hepatic failure. Appropriate contraception should be advised in

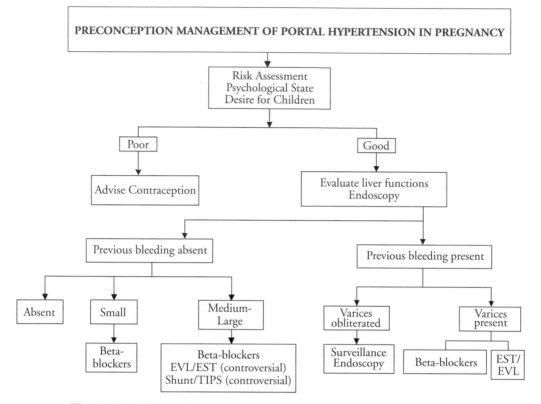

Fig. 1. Algorithm to the management of portal hypertension in pregnancy.

these patients until the liver functions have stabilized and the variceal obliteration achieved using EVL. EVL has replaced endoscopic sclerotherapy for this purpose *(64)*.

ANTENATAL MANAGEMENT

When a pregnancy occurs in a female with portal hypertension, the expectant mother should be evaluated both by the hepatologist and the obstetrician and proper risk assessment be done. In case of an unplanned conception, the risks should be explained again to the expectant parents and the desire for a child must be balanced against the risks of pregnancy. The decision to terminate pregnancy is a complicated one and should involve careful consideration of the medical risks to the mother, fetus, as well as the religious and ethical issues surrounding such a decision *(4)*. The duration of gestation is also a key factor in making this decision. The further along the pregnancy is, the more difficult such a decision becomes. In general, most physicians support the pregnancy if it is more than 10–12 wk along unless the mother's life is in immediate jeopardy.

The routine antenatal care given during any pregnancy should be given in addition to the special considerations related to management of portal hypertension. Fetal development should be closely monitored at regular intervals to detect intrauterine growth retardation and fetal distress at the earliest, so that an effective management plan can be implemented to improve both the maternal and fetal outcomes. Immunosuppressive drugs in post-liver transplant patients should be carefully titrated to lowest effective dose so as to prevent the intrauterine growth retardation and neonatal immunosuppression *(65,66)*.

The adaptation of the mother to the hemodynamic and other changes during the pregnancy have effects on preexisting cirrhosis and/or portal hypertension. Renal Na and water retention can contribute to several complications such as pulmonary edema, and generalized convulsive seizures. Such hemodynamic changes have been described in both the cirrhotic and noncirrhotic pregnant patients *(3)*. In subjects with either a history of ascites, Na restriction is advised *(3)*.

The assessment of the variceal size and liver functions must be done once the conception is confirmed in the patients in whom it has been missed in the preconception period so that an appropriate management plan may be outlined. An ultrasound and Doppler examination should be performed to look for the porto-splenic vessels. Special effort must be made to look for a splenic artery aneurysm due to the potential for their rupture and life-threatening hemorrhage during the course of pregnancy *(4)*. Early detection of the varices during gestation may help in deciding the future course of management in these patients *(3)*. The management of varices should follow the guidelines described above (Fig. 1). Nonselective β-adrenergic receptor antagonists are the first line of therapy for primary prophylaxis of the high risk varices. Intolerance to these drugs is an indication for EVL. In those who experience bleeding, the management of the active bleed should follow standard guidelines with pharmacologic treatment with Octreotide and endoscopic sclerotherapy or band ligation. Once bleeding is controlled, variceal eradication should be achieved using weekly or two weekly endoscopic sessions *(67)*.

MANAGEMENT OF ACTIVE VARICEAL HEMORRHAGE

The development of active variceal hemorrhage is a medical emergency. This warrants the emergency control of variceal bleeding by the EVL or EST, along with use of Octreotide. Both EST and EVL have been shown to be safe and effective means to control bleeding during pregnancy *(33,35–37,41,44,15)*. Vasopressin and its analogs should be avoided owing to the risks of inducing labor. Pharmacologic therapy with somatostatin or its analogs are a valuable adjunct to the endoscopic therapy with minimal side effects. The pharmacologic therapy is of particular value to control the variceal bleeding alone when the patient is too unstable for the endoscopic procedure. These drugs have been safely used for 5–7 d with an effective control of variceal bleeding *(25)*. Balloon tamponade is often used to stabilize patients who fail to respond to the endoscopic and the pharmacologic therapy and are hemodynamically unstable. This is just a temporary measure to bridge the gap of time until more definitive therapy as shunt surgery or TIPS is undertaken *(25)*. Emergency portosystemic anastomotic shunts have been performed during pregnancy, followed by arrest of variceal hemorrhage and uneventful delivery *(49–53)*. Successful TIPS has also been performed for recurrent variceal bleeding caused by liver cirrhosis in a pregnant woman at 20 weeks gestation. TIPS procedure is not absolutely contraindicated during pregnancy. The risks of TIPS placement must be considered on a case-by-case basis taking the severity of the underlying maternal disease and risks of radiation exposure to the fetus *(34)*.

The management of the cause of portal hypertension must continue. Pruritis associated with liver disease often worsens during pregnancy. Management with ursodeoxycholoic acid (UDCA), mild antihistamines, ultraviolet radiation, and phenobarbital are considered as to be safe options in pregnancy *(4)*. Although interferon therapy for hepatitis B and C is not advisable because of the risks associated with these drugs during pregnancy,

Lamivudine, a nucleoside analog is a safe and effective antiviral drug that can be used in hepatitis B virus infections with a positive hepatitis B e antigen or a high DNA load. Lamivudine, given in the perinatal period, effectively prevents the vertical transmission of virus in addition to the benefit of viral eradication in the mother *(68)*. Expectant management with regular monitoring may be undertaken in diseases like Wilson's disease where clinical improvement in the liver functions has been reported in the later stages of pregnancy *(2,56,57)*.

PERINATAL MANAGEMENT

The perinatal management of a pregnant portal hypertensive mother has to be individualized according to the status of the liver disease and the size of the esophageal varices. Elective abdominal delivery by cesarean section in an attempt to minimize the stress on the circulatory system is reserved only for the usual obstetric indications *(2)*. Vaginal delivery is generally attempted unless there is an obstetric indication for cesarean section *(2,38)*. The patient should be carefully sedated and should avoid straining, especially when full cervical dilatation has not been attained. Oversedation should be avoided. Fetal monitoring is required if maternal sedation is provided. Shortening of the second stage of labor by forceps or other obstetric techniques is advisable and strongly recommended. Adequate amount of blood and a tube for balloon tamponade should be kept by the bedside in case of a variceal hemorrhage during or after delivery *(2,4)*. Volume overloading by overzealous fluid administration can be catastrophic and should be avoided. Coagulopathy due to the liver disease should be corrected.

In case abdominal delivery by cesarean section becomes mandatory, a vascular surgeon with expertise should be available to take care of the uncontrolled variceal bleeding or ectopic varices in the operative field *(4)*. Postpartum hemorrhage should be anticipated and adequately managed.

SPLENIC ARTERY ANEURYSM (SAA) IN PREGNANCY WITH PORTAL HYPERTENSION

Pregnancy-related rupture of arterial aneurysm is an unusual complication that is associated with a considerably high maternal and fetal morbidity and mortality. Rupture of aortic, cerebral artery, splenic artery, renal artery, hepatic artery, coronary artery, and ovarian artery aneurysms have all been reported during pregnancy *(69,70)*. SAAs are specifically more common during pregnancy in a portal hypertensive mother. The exact etiopathogenesis of this phenomenon is not very clear.

The actual incidence of SAA is unknown. It has been reported to range from 0.16% in a series of unselected autopsies to 10.4% in patients who died above 60 yr of age *(71,72)*. SAA are the third most common intraabdominal artery aneurysm after aortic and iliac artery aneurysms *(71,73)*. This condition is more prevalent in females with a male-to-female ratio of 1 to 4–5 *(70,74)*.

Pregnancy is not the sole cause of SAA. Certain congenital abnormalities (like Marfan's syndrome, Ehler–Danlos syndrome), inherited vascular disorders, inflammatory processes, arterial degeneration, and trauma can also cause arterial aneurysms. Factors as portal hypertension, pancreatitis, grand multiparity, and trauma have been associated with the formation and rupture of SAA in the nonpregnant population. Portal hypertension has been especially linked with the SAA and is present in 19–33% of the cases of ruptured

SAA (75–77). On the other hand, the incidence of SAA rupture in all cases of pregnancy is only 2.6% (2). It has been postulated that SAAs result from the hyperkinetic circulation associated with pregnancy. Pregnancy is also associated with hyperplasia of the arterial intima with fragmentation and fibrodysplasia of the media. These degenerative changes may lead to mural outpouchings especially in the setting of a hyperdynamic circulation as seen in pregnancy. Relaxin, a hormone secreted during the third trimester for relaxation of pubic symphysis, has also been implicated in this process (69,78).

SAA rupture is most common in pregnancy and commonly occurs in the age group ranging from 15 to 41 yr. The incidence of rupture increases during pregnancy from approx 12% in the first two trimesters to 69% in the third trimester (79). The risk declines to 13% during labor and 6% in the puerperium.

The SAA are most commonly (71%) solitary lesions located most commonly (79%) in the distal third of the artery, usually at the bifurcation. These are usually saccular and calcified in around 72% cases (80). Nearly 95% of the SAA are clinically silent. The patients may have intermittent epigastric or left upper quadrant pain radiating to back or left shoulder as a prodrome to rupture. Pain may occur days to weeks in either shoulder prior to aneurysm rupture caused by the enlarging aneurysm. Some patients develop right upper quadrant pain that is mistaken as cholecystitis. The rupture of SAA may have variable presentations mimicking common conditions as amniotic fluid embolism, placental abruption, uterine rupture, pulmonary thromboembolism, peptic ulcer perforation, renal colic, cholecystitis, and rarely, appendicitis (74,81,82). Nonspecific symptoms like nausea and vomiting may also be encountered. The physical signs suggestive of a SAA are splenonegaly (44%), a left upper quadrant bruit (<10%), or very rarely, a palpable aneurysmal mass. The SAA are occasionally incidentally detected as curvilinear or signet ring opacity in the left upper quadrant on abdominal roentgenogram obtained for unrelated reasons (80,82–84).

SAA usually (75%) rupture freely into the peritoneal cavity. Rarely the rupture is in the form of a "Double-Rupture" syndrome where the rupture initially occurs in the lesser omental sac accompanied by syncope, hypotension, and flank pain. Partial tamponade occurs once the lesser sac is full of blood clot, thereby allowing partial recovery of the patient's blood pressure. After a period ranging from minutes to weeks, the second rupture occurs when the clot escapes from the lesser sac into the peritoneum via the foramen of Winslow permitting free peritoneal bleeding. There is rapid worsening of pain and hemodynamic collapse occurs (76,80). SAA have also been reported to rupture into the gastrointestinal tract causing gastrointestinal bleeding and into the common bile duct causing acute pancreatitis and hemobilia (78,83).

There has to be a high index of suspicion to diagnose a SAA rupture. Ultrasonography with pulsed Doppler and computed tomography are less invasive modes of diagnosis, and, hence, are more commonly used in the diagnosis of SAA, but are less reliable. Arteriography and magnetic resonance imaging (MRI) have facilitated in the incidental clinical identification of the SAA. Once a pregnant patient has presented with acute abdomen, and the presumptive diagnosis of intraabdominal bleeding is made, exploratory laparotomy becomes mandatory. Splenectomy and ligation of the splenic artery is performed for ruptured SAA. Ruptured SAAs are associated with a very high maternal and fetal mortality (nearly 75 and 95%, respectively). However, there are few case reports where good fetal and maternal outcome have been reported (78,85–87).

Varying opinions exist with respect to the management of the asymptomatic SAA. Some experts advise elective surgical repair when the aneurysm is >2 cm or when pregnancy is anticipated *(74)*. Others stress that even a small SAA warrants preemptive obliteration by surgery, embolization, or laparoscopic ligation to avoid the very high maternal and fetal loss *(88)*.

SUMMARY

As emphasized earlier, pregnancy in a patient with portal hypertension is a unique problem because of the effects of the hemodynamic chages that occur to maintain a normal perfusion and nutrition of the growing fetus. This situation needs specialized care to prevent potentially life-threatening complications such as gastrointestinal hemorrhage. The risk of bleeding from the esophageal varices in a patient with portal hypertension is almost 400 times greater than a nonportal hypertensive mother, with the greatest risk being during the second trimester. Almost 78% of the patients who have detectable varices during pregnancy would bleed during the index gestation. It is not possible to predict which women with preexisting varices would bleed during the present pregnancy and also there is no correlation of size of varices to the risk of variceal hemorrhage and its severity. Coordination by a hepatologist, an obstetrican, and a neonatologist is required for the adequate management of this condition and starts with a preconception advice about the potential complications and associated risks to both the mother and the fetus. The management of such patients continues through the gestation, the antenatal period, up to the perinatal period. Surveillance endoscopy in the preconceptional period is an absolute must. At present, primary prophylaxis of the variceal bleeding by a nonselective β-receptor antagonist drug is safe and remains the therapy of choice. The role of EST and EVL as modalities for primary prophylaxis of variceal hemorrhage requires further evaluation. As a modality for secondary prophylaxis EVL has gained an edge over EST. The concept of a prophylactic shunt leading to improved survival has been disapproved.

Other complications encountered in such patients beside the variceal hemorrhage are hepatic failure, postpartum hemorrhage, rupture of splenic artery aneurysm, rupture of splenorenal shunts, spontaneous bacterial peritonitis, and maternal death. It is, therefore, important to understand the effect of pregnancy on portal hypertension and vice versa so that untoward incidents like fetal morbidity and mortality and gastrointestinal hemorrhage can be avoided. SAAs are more common during pregnancy and is one of the commonest visceral artery aneurysm during pregnancy. A high index of suspicion is required for making an early diagnosis and management of such cases. SAA is associated with a considerably high maternal and fetal morbidity and mortality.

REFERENCES

1. Britton RC. Pregnancy and esophageal varices. Am J Surg 1982;143(4):421–425.
2. Cheng YS. Pregnancy in liver cirrhosis and/or portal hypertension. Am J Obstet Gynecol 1977;128(7): 812–822.
3. Varma RR, Michelsohn NH, Borkowf HI, Lewis JD. Pregnancy in cirrhotic and noncirrhotic portal hypertension. Obstet Gynecol 1977;50(2):217–222.
4. Sandhu BS, Sanyal AJ. Pregnancy and liver disease. Gastroenterol Clin North Am 2003;32(1):407–436.
5. Pajor A, Lehoczky D. Pregnancy in liver cirrhosis. Assessment of maternal and fetal risks in eleven patients and review of literature. Gynecol Obstet Invest 1994;38:45–50.
6. Lloyd CW, Williams RH. Endocrine changes associated with laennec's cirrhosis of the liver. Am J Med 1948;4:315–330.
7. Lee WM. Pregnancy in patients with chronic liver disease. Gastroenterol Clin North Am 1992;21(4): 889–903.

8. Goh SK, Gull SE, Alexander GJ. Pregnancy in primary biliary cirrhosis complicated by portal hypertension: report of a case and review of the literature. BJOG 2001;108(7):760–762.

9. Restaino A, Campobasso C, D'Aloya A, Abbruzzese AD, Valerio A, Pansini F. Cirrhosis and pregnancy. A case report and review of the literature. Clin Exp Obstet Gynecol 1996;23(4):240–247.

10. McMichens TT, Robichaux AG3, Smith JW. Successful pregnancy outcome in a patient with congenital biliary atresia. Obstet Gynecol 1992;80(3 Pt 2).

11. Wong KK, Goh KL. Pregnancy in primary biliary cirrhosis. Europ J Obstet Gynecol Reprod Biol 1992; 45(2):149–151.

12. Misra S, Sanyal AJ. Pregnancy in a patient with portal hypertension. Clin Liver Dis 1999;3:147–162.

13. Pajor A, Lehoczky D. Pregnancy and extrahepatic portal hypertension. Review and report on the management. Gynecol Obstet Invest 1990;30(4):193–197.

14. Thompson E, Williams R, Sherlock S. Liver function in extra-hepatic portal obstruction. Lancet 1964; ii:1352–1356.

15. Evans IM, Hoyuen B, Anderson FH. Bleeding esophageal varices in pregnancy. Obstet Gynecol 1972; 40(3):377–380.

16. Cruickshank D, Wigton T, Hays P. Maternal physiology in pregnancy. In: Gabb S, NJSJ, ed. Obstetrics: Normal and Problem Pregnancies. Churchill Livingstone, New York, 1996, pp. 91–119.

17. Pritchard JA. Changes in blood volume during pregnancy and delivery. Anaesthesiology 1965;26:393.

18. Wilson M, Morganti AA, Zervoudakis I, et al. Blood pressure, the renin-aldosterone system and sex steroids throughout normal pregnancy. Am J Med 1980;68:97–104.

19. Davison JM, Dunlop W. Renal function in pregnancy. Contrib Nephrol 1981;25:4–9.

20. Royek A, Parisi V. Maternal biological adaptations to pregnancy. In: Reece EA HJ, ed. Medicine of the Fetus and Mother. Lippincott-Raven, Philadelphia, 1999, pp. 903–920.

21. Clark CL, Cotton DB, Pivarnik JM, et al. Position change and central hemodynamic profile during normal third-trimester pregnancy and post partum. Am J Obstet Gynecol 1991;164:883–887.

22. Capeless EL, Clapp JF. Cardiovascular changes in early phase of pregnancy. Am J Obstet Gynecol 1989;161:1449–1453.

23. Vorobioff J, Bredfeldt JE, Groszmann RJ. Hyperdynamic circulation in portal hypertensive rat model: a primary factor for maintenance of chronic portal hypertension. Am J Physiol 1983;244:G52–G57.

24. Hytten F, Lind T. Indices of renal function. Diagnostic indices in pregnancy. Basel (Switzerland): Documenta Geigy 1973:18.

25. Bass NM, Yao FY. Portal Hypertension and variceal bleeding. In: Feldman M FLSM, ed. Gastrointestinal and Liver Disease. Saunders (Elsevier Science), Philadelphia, 2002, pp. 1487–1516.

26. Palmer E. Effect of valsalva maneuver on portal pressure. Am J Med 1961;242:223–225.

27. Garcia-Tsao G, Groszmann R, Fisher R, et al. Portal pressure, presence of gastroesophageal varices and variceal bleeding. Hepatology 1985;5:419.

28. Groszmann RJ, Franchis R. Portal hypertension. In: Schiff ER SMMW, ed. Schiff's Diseases of the Liver. Lippincott-Raven, Philadelphia, 1999, pp. 387–442.

29. Scott D, Kerr M. Inferior vena cava pressure in late pregnancy. BJOG 1963;24:305–308.

30. Homburg R, Bayer I, Lurie B. Bleeding esophageal varices in pregnancy. A report of two cases. J Reprod Med 1988;33(9):784–786.

31. Aggarwal N, Sawnhey H, Suril V, Vasishta K, Jha M, Dhiman RK. Pregnancy and cirrhosis of the liver. Aust N Z J Obstet Gynaecol 1999;39(4):503–506.

32. Aggarwal N, Sawhney H, Vasishta K, Dhiman RK, Chawla Y. Non-cirrhotic portal hypertension in pregnancy. Int J Gynaecol Obstet 2001;72(1):1–7.

33. Dhiman RK, Biswas R, Aggarwal N, Sawhney H, Chawla Y. Management of variceal bleeding in pregnancy with endoscopic variceal ligation and N-butyl-2-cyanoacrylate: report of three cases. Gastrointest Endosc 2000;51(1):91–93.

34. Wildberger JE, Vorwerk D, Winograd R, Stargardt A, Busch N, Gunther RW. New TIPS placement in pregnancy in recurrent esophageal varices hemorrhage—assessment of fetal radiation exposure. Rofo Fortschr Geb Rontgenstr Neuen Bildgeb Verfahr 1998;169(4):429–431.

35. Starkel P, Horsmans Y, Geubel A. Endoscopic band ligation: a safe technique to control bleeding esophageal varices in pregnancy. Gastrointest Endosc 1998;48(2):212–214.

36. Iwase H, Morise K, Kawase T, Horiuchi Y. Endoscopic injection sclerotherapy for esophageal varices during pregnancy. J Clin Gastroenterol 1994;18(1):80–83.

37. Kochhar R, Goenka MK, Mehta SK. Endoscopic sclerotherapy during pregnancy. Am J Gastroenterol 1990;85(9):1132–1135.

38. Whelton MJ, Sherlock S. Pregnancy in patients with hepatic cirrhosis. management and outcome. Lancet 1968;2(7576):995–999.

39. Whelton MJ, Sherlock S. Pregnancy in patients with cirrhosis of the liver. Obstet Gynecol 1970;36: 315–324.

40. Kochhar R, Kumar S, Goel RC, Sriram PV, Goenka MK, Singh K. Pregnancy and its outcome in patients with noncirrhotic portal hypertension. Dig Dis Sci 1999;44(7):1356–1361.

41. Zeeman GG, Moise KJ Jr. Prophylactic banding of severe esophageal varices associated with liver cirrhosis in pregnancy. Obstet Gynecol 1999;94(5(Pt 2)):842.

42. Shertsinger AG, Kitsenko EA, Shipkova TI, Minasian SL. Management strategy for pregnant women with portal hypertension syndrome. Akush Ginekol (Mosk) 1994;1:16–18.

43. Pauzner D, Wolman I, Niv D, Ber A, David MP. Endoscopic sclerotherapy in extrahepatic portal hypertension in pregnancy. Am J Obstet Gynecol 1991;164(1 Pt 1):152–153.

44. Augustine P, Joseph PC. Sclerotherapy for esophageal varices and pregnancy. Gastrointest Endosc 1989;35(5):467–468.

45. Salena BJ, Sivak MV Jr. Pregnancy and esophageal varices. Gastrointest Endosc 1988;34(6):492–493.

46. Russell MA, Craigo SD. Cirrhosis and portal hypertension in pregnancy. Semin Perinatol 1998;22(2): 156–165.

47. Marpeau L, Peraudeau-Daoud P, Castiel J, et al. Normal pregnancy after a Budd-Chiari syndrome treated by shunting: apropos of a case, review of the literature. J Gynecol Obstet Biol Reprod (Paris) 1987;16(8):1045–1052.

48. Hanker JP, Beckmann M. Pregnancy after portocaval shunt operation. A case of report and review of the literature (author's transl) [Article in German]. Geburtshilfe Frauenheilkd 1979;39(1):78–79.

49. Chattopadhyay TK, Kapoor VK, Iyer KS, Sarathy VV. Successful splenorenal shunt performed during pregnancy. Jpn J Surg 1984;14(5):405–406.

50. Salam AA, Warren WD. Distal splenorenal shunt for the treatment of variceal bleeding during pregnancy. Arch Surg 1972;105(4):643–634.

51. Brown AA. Emergency portacaval anastomosis in pregnancy. Proc R Soc Med 1971;64(8):809.

52. Reisman TM, O'Leary JA. Portacaval shunt performed during pregnancy. A case report. Obstet Gynecol 1971;37(2):253–254.

53. Jochimsen PR, Castaneda AR. Emergency mesocaval shunt performed during pregnancy, followed by arrest of variceal hemorrhage and uneventful delivery. Surgery 1968;63(4):601–603.

54. Paternoster DM, Floreani AR, Paggioro A, Laureti E. Portal hypertension in a pregnant woman. Minerva Ginecol 1996;48(6):243–245.

55. Schreyer P, Caspi E, El-Hindi JM, Eshchar J. Cirrhosis—pregnancy and delivery: a review. Obstet Gynecol Surv 1982;37(5):304–312.

56. Bihl JH. The effect of pregnancy on hepatolenticular degeneration (Wilson's disease). Am J Obstet Gynecol 1959;78:1182.

57. Dreifuss FE, Mckinney WM. Wilson's disease (hepatolenticular degeneration) and pregnancy. JAMA 1966;195:960.

58. Oyarzun E, Gonzalez R, Vesperinas G, Macaya R, Gomez R, Llanos O. Pregnancy and portal hypertension. Rev Med Chil 1993;121(5):548–552.

59. Britton RC. Management of complications of portal hypertension. Modern Treatment 1969;6:175–190.

60. O'Grady J, Day E, Toole A. Splenic artery aneurysm in pregnancy. Obstet Gynecol 1977;57:255–257.

61. deFranchis R. Prediction of first variceal hemorrhage in patients with cirrhosis of liver and esophageal varices. N Engl J Med 1988;319:983–989.

62. Colombo M, deFranchis R, Tommasini M, Sangiovanni A, Dioguardi N. Beta-blockade prevents recurrent gastrointestinal bleeding in well compensated patients with alcoholic cirrhosis: a multicenter randomized controlled trial. Hepatology 1989;9:433–438.

63. Sanyal AJ, Shiffman M. The pharmacologic treatment of portal hypertension. Curr Clin Topn Gastrointestl Pharmacoly 1997;1:242–275.

64. Laine L, Cook D. Endoscopic ligation compared with sclerotherapy for treatment of esophageal variceal bleeding. A meta-analysis. Ann Intern Med 1995;123:280–287.

65. Crawford J, Johnson K, Jones K. Pregnancy outcome after transplantation in women maintained on cyclosporin immunosuppression. Repro Toxicol 1993;7:156.
66. Haagsma EB, Visser GH, Klompmaker IJ, Verwer R, Slooff MJ. Successful pregnancy after orthotopic liver transplantation. Obstet Gynecol 1989;74:442–443.
67. Grace ND. Diagnosis and treatment of gastrointestinal bleeding secondary to portal hypertension. American College of Gastroenterology Practice Parameters Committee. Am J Gastroenterol 1997;92: 1081–1091.
68. vanNunen AB, deMan RA, Heijtink RA, Niesters HG, Schalm SW. Lamivudine in the last 4 weeks of pregnancy to prevent perinatal transmission in highly viremic chronic hepatitis B patients. J Hepatol 2000;32:1040–1041.
69. Barrett JM, Van Hooydonk JE, Boehm FH. Pregnancy-related rupture of arterial aneurysms. Obstet Gynecol Surv 1982;37(9):557–566.
70. Messina LM, Shanley CJ. Visceral artery aneurysms. Surg Clin North Am 1997;77:425–442.
71. Hunsaker DM, Turner S, Hunsaker JC3. Sudden and unexpected death resulting from splenic artery aneurysm rupture: two case reports of pregnancy-related fatal rupture of splenic artery aneurysm. Am J Forensic Med Pathol 2002;23(4):338–341.
72. Sheps SG, Spittel JA, Fairbairn JF, Edwards JE. Aneurysms of splenic artery with special reference to bland aneurysms. Proc Staff Meet Mayo Clin 1958;33:381–389.
73. Wagner WH, Allins AD, Treiman RL, et al. Ruptured visceral artery aneurysms. Ann Vasc Surg 1997; 11:342–347.
74. Williams JJ. Splenic artery aneurysm rupture: An uncommon obstetrical catastrophe. J Fam Pract 1998; 25:73–75.
75. Martinez E, Menendez AR, Ablanedo P. Splenic artery aneurysms. Int Surg 1986;71(2).95–99.
76. Owens J, Coffey R. Aneurysm of splenic artery, including a report of 6 additional cases. Int Abst Surg 1953;97:313.
77. Boijsen E, Efsing O. Aneurysm of splenic artery. Acta Radiol (Diagn) 1969;8:29.
78. Angelakis EJ, Bair WE, Barone JE, Lincer RM. Splenic artery aneurysm rupture during pregnancy. Obstet Gynecol Surv 1993;48(3):145–148.
79. Mavfarlane J, Thorbjarnarson B. Rupture of splenic artery aneurysm during pregnancy. Am J Obstet Gynecol 1966;95:1025.
80. Trastek V, Pairolero P, Joyce J, et al. Splenic artery aneurysms. Surgery 1982;91:694.
81. Barrett JM, Caldwell BH. Association of portal hypertension and ruptured splenic artery aneurysm in pregnancy. Obstet Gynecol 1981;57(2):255–257.
82. Lowry SM, O'Dea T, Gallagher D, et al. Splenic artery aneurysm rupture: The seventh instance of maternal and fetal survival. Obstet Gynecol 1986;67:291.
83. Lambert CJ, Williamson JW. Splenic artery aneuyrsm: a rare cause of upper gastrointestinal bleeding. Am Surg 1990;56:543.
84. MacFarlane JR, Thorbjarnarson B. Rupture of splenic artery aneurysm during pregnancy. Am J Obstet Gynecol 1966;95:1025.
85. Dunlop W, Iwanicki S, Akierman A, PJ, Higgin JR. Spontaneous rupture of splenic artery aneurysm: maternal and fetal survival. Can J Surg 1990;33(5):407–408.
86. Caillouette JC, Merchant EB. Ruptured splenic artery aneurysm in pregnancy. Twelfth reported case with maternal and fetal survival. Am J Obstet Gynecol 1993;168(6 Pt 1):1810–1811.
87. Herbeck M, Horbach T, Putzenlechner C, Klein P, Lang W. Ruptured splenic artery aneurysm during pregnancy: a rare case with both maternal and fetal survival. Am J Obstet Gynecol 1999;181(3): 782–783.
88. Hallet JW Jr. Splenic artery aneurysms. Semin Vasc Surg 1995;8:321–326.

24 Causes and Management of Portal Hypertension in the Pediatric Population

Frederick C. Ryckman, MD,
Maria H. Alonso, MD, and Greg Tiao, MD

INTRODUCTION

The survival of children with portal hypertension has improved over the past decade owing to significant improvements in both medical and surgical therapy. These improvements have included progress in the pharmacologic control of acute portal hypertensive hemorrhage and improved efficacy and safety of endoscopic methods to treat acute esophageal variceal hemorrhage. However, despite these changes, there remains a significant role for advanced surgical therapy using portocaval shunts in children with gastrointestinal

This chapter is reprinted from *Clinics in Liver Disease*, V5(3): 789–818, Ryckman et al.,
©2001, Elsevier Inc., with permission from Elsevier.

From: *Clinical Gastroenterology: Portal Hypertension*
Edited by: A. J. Sanyal and V. H. Shah © Humana Press Inc., Totowa, NJ

hemorrhage were significant sequela of portal hypertension. In addition, patience with both irreversible liver disease and portal hypertension have benefited from the improved success with pediatric liver transplantation as a definitive treatment for children with end-stage liver disease. This review will primarily examine the role of surgical therapy for children with progressive portal hypertension.

DEFINITION, ETIOLOGY

Portal hypertension is defined as an elevation of the portal pressure above 10–12 mmHg. In healthy children, portal pressure rarely exceeds 7 mmHg. Elevation of the portal pressure is commonly classified by the anatomic location of the obstructed portal venous flow, subdivided as presinusoidal, sinusoidal, or postsinusoidal block, although increased splanchnic blood flow may contribute in some cases. The response to increased portal venous pressure is similar to adults, with the development of collateral circulatory pathways connecting the high-pressure portal vasculature to the low-pressure systemic venous system. The most common communications occur within the esophageal wall, connecting the coronary and short gastric veins to the esophageal venous plexus, which communicate with the intercostal, azygous, and hemiazygous veins. As portal pressure increases, esophageal varices developing within this plexus become the site with the highest risk for massive hemorrhage. Less-threatening collateral communications can develop between the recanalized umbilical vein and abdominal wall systemic veins (caput medusa), the inferior -rectal veins as hemorrhoids, and around the retroperitoneal pancreas and duodenum. In addition, any surgical union between the portal and systemic venous circulation, such as occurs with intestinal stomas or previous incision sites, can become problematic collateral sites. Favorable collaterals developing within the tissues surrounding the pancreas, duodenum, and left kidney form "spontaneous" spleno-renal shunts. The possibility that these collaterals play a significant role in ultimately decreasing portal venous pressure and preventing variceal hemorrhage has been suggested, but remains unproven. In our opinion, their radiographic and physical appearance exceeds their hemodynamic importance and benefit.

The progressive development of collaterals connecting the portal and systemic circulation has the theoretical beneficial effect of decreasing portal pressure. However, this effect is ameliorated by the concurrent development of a hyperdynamic circulatory state (1). Portal hypertension has been associated with the presence of autonomic nervous system dysfunction, and an excess of circulating cytokines leading to tachycardia, decreased systemic, and splanchnic vascular resistance secondary to vasodilatation, plasma volume expansion, increased cardiac output, and subsequently, increased portal inflow.

The combination of increasing portal inflow, venous outflow obstruction, and the remarkable collateral circulation that develops account for many of the complications associated with portal hypertension. Superficial submucosal varices, especially those in the esophagus and stomach, and, to a lesser extent, those in the duodenum, colon, or rectum, are prone to rupture and bleeding. In addition, prominent submucosal arteriovenous communications between the muscularis mucosa and dilated precapillaries and veins within the stomach result in vascular ectasia, or congestive hypertensive gastropathy, significantly contributing to the risk of hemorrhage from the stomach.

Each of the causes of elevated portal pressure shares the common mechanism of increased resistance to blood flow from the visceral/splanchnic portal circulation to the right atrium.

In children, the location of this increased resistance can be: (1) *prehepatic (or presinusoidal)*—usually within the portal vein and its primary feeding branches; (2) *intrahepatic* —due to presinusoidal obstructions (congenital hepatic fibrosis, congenital or acquired arterial-portal fistula, or schistosomiasis), postsinusoidal cirrhosis, or venoocclusive disease; or (3) *posthepatic*—secondary to hepatic vein obstruction. Although this anatomic description is helpful to structurally organize a differential diagnosis, the primary factor influencing the prognosis and treatment algorithm is the intrinsic status of the liver. Presinusoidal obstruction does not result in impairment of hepatic synthetic function, coagulopathy is usually absent or only mildly affected. Treatment should be directed toward the prevention of hemorrhage through palliative interventional procedures while spontaneous collateral venous channels develop. In contrast, postsinusoidal obstruction is characterized by hepatic synthetic compromise, coagulopathy, and progressive hepatic failure. Although intervention to prevent or treat potentially fatal complications may be necessary, definitive correction with liver transplantation is often required. Table 1 reviews the diseases associated with portal hypertension in children *(2)*.

PRESINUSOIDAL OBSTRUCTION

The most common type of presinusoidal obstruction is extrahepatic portal vein obstruction (EPVO) at any level of the portal vein. Umbilical vein infection in infancy, with or without umbilical vein cannulation, has been associated with the development of occult thrombosis of the portal vein. Infection can spread from the umbilical vein to the left branch of the portal vein, and eventually the main portal venous channels, leading to phlebitis and subsequent thrombosis. Similar infections in older children, such as perforated appendicitis, primary peritonitis, and inflammatory bowel disease have also been identified as predisposing factors, as have primary biliary tract infections or cholangitis. Inherited abnormalities predisposing to hypercoagulability play a significant role in "spontaneous thrombosis" in childhood. A complete evaluation of the thrombotic system should be undertaken in each case, with attention directed toward factor V Leiden mutation, protein C, protein S, and antithrombin III deficiencies. In addition, hyperviscosity/polycythemia in infancy can lead to secondary thrombosis, especially when accompanied by neonatal dehydration or systemic infection and phlebitis *(2,3)*. Ando et al. suggested that embryological malformations resulting in tortuous, poorly developed portal veins could be a primary cause for EPVO or predispose to an increased risk of thrombosis *(4)*. Rare congenital anatomic abnormalities can also include webs or diaphragms within the portal vein leading to obstruction. The potential role of congenital abnormalities in EPVO is supported by the concurrent presence of other congenital anomalies in 40% of children with no postnatal etiology for EPVO compared to an incidence of only 12% of children with a defined etiology such as umbilical vein catheterization *(2,5)*. Presinusoidal obstruction can also result from congenital hepatic fibrosis, schistosomiasis, hepato-portal sclerosis, and rare cases where increased portal blood flow is attributed to congenital or acquired arteriovenous fistula within the portal system *(6)*. Despite thorough evaluation, over one-half of reported EPVO cases have no identifiable cause.

POSTSINUSOIDAL OBSTRUCTION

Postsinusoidal obstruction to the portal venous system is caused by intrinsic liver disease, secondary to cirrhosis, or obstruction to the hepatic vein outflow from the liver.

Table 1
Pediatric Diseases Associated with Portal Hypertension (2)

Presinusoidal
Venous Obstructions
  Portal vein thrombosis/cavernous transformation
  Splenic vein thrombosis
  Portal vein malformation (Congenital)
Congenital hepatic fibrosis
Arteriovenous fistula
Schistosomiasis
Hepatoportal sclerosis
Sinusoidal
Hepatocellular Disease
  Autoimmune hepatitis
  Hepatitis B, C
  Wilson's disease
  α_1–antitrypsin deficiency
  Glycogen storage disease–Type IV
  Toxins and drugs
  Histiocytosis X
  Gaucher's disease
  Peliosis
Biliary Tract Disease
  Biliary atresia
  Cystic fibrosis
  Choledochal cyst
  Intrahepatic cholestasis syndromes
  Sclerosing cholangitis
Sinusoidal venoocclusive disease
Postsinusoidal
Budd–Chiari Syndrome
Inferior vena cava obstructions
Chronic congestive heart failure
Venoocclusive disease (s/p bone marrow transplantation)
Prothrombotic disease

Cirrhosis resulting from primary liver diseases is the most common etiology of post-sinusoidal portal hypertension in children, with venous obstruction arising secondary to intrahepatic scarring. The numerous causes of cirrhosis include recognized disorders such as extrahepatic biliary atresia, metabolic liver disease such as α-1 antitrypsin deficiency, Wilson's disease, glycogen storage disease type IV, hereditary fructose intolerance, and cystic fibrosis. As many of these conditions are associated with progressive liver failure, the primary treatment in most cases is liver transplantation. Successful transplantation corrects the portal hypertension and its complications such as hypersplenism, ascites, and synthetic liver failure. In the clinical situation where hepatic synthetic failure is not present or only slowly progressive, direct treatment of portal hypertension or its complications is indicated.

Hepatic vein obstruction (Budd–Chiari syndrome) can occur secondary to obstruction to the hepatic veins at any point from the sinusoids to the entry of the hepatic veins into the right atrium/inferior vena cava. Although a specific etiology is often not found, thrombosis can complicate neoplasms, collagen vascular disease, infection, trauma, or hypercoagulability states. Veno-occlusive disease has emerged as one of the most frequent causes of hepatic vein obstruction in children. In this disorder, occlusion of the centrilobular venules or sublobular hepatic veins occurs. Most cases occur after total body irradiation with or without cytotoxic drug therapy associated with bone marrow transplantation (7). This condition has also occurred after the ingestion of herbal remedies containing the pyrrolizidine alkaloids, which are sometimes taken as medicinal teas (8).

DIAGNOSIS AND EVALUATION

Clinical history and examination should concentrate on identifying factors that predispose to the development of cirrhosis, including a family history of inherited metabolic disease, and possible exposure to viral or toxic pathogens. Clinical examination findings suggesting underlying liver disease (ascites, liver size/contour, nutritional status), hypersplenism (spleen size, bruising), or hepatopulmonary syndrome (spider angiomas, clubbing, cyanosis) contribute to diagnostic evaluation and therapeutic planning. Historical events preceding portal vein thrombosis should be sought. Hypercoagulability and its complications should be evaluated in both the patient and family members due to the inherited basis for these protein abnormalities.

Imaging tests are essential to confirm the presence of portal hypertension, define the portal venous anatomy, and formulate options for future therapy. Initial screening with ultrasound can suggest the presence of chronic liver disease and should determine portal venous patency. Doppler examination can depict both the direction of portal flow and the degree of hepatopetal flow, which correlates with the risk of variceal hemorrhage. The branches of the portal venous system are examined to exclude splenic vein thrombosis, or widespread portal system thrombosis. Magnetic resonance angiography (MRA) or contrast-enhanced computed tomography have replaced mesenteric angiography when further definition of portal anatomy is necessary, such as when liver transplantation or portal–systemic shunt procedures are planned (9).

Upper gastrointestinal endoscopy is the most accurate and reliable method for detecting esophageal varices and for detecting the source of acute gastrointestinal hemorrhage. This is especially valuable in the presence of acute hemorrhage, where up to one-third of patients with known varices may have bleeding from other sources such as portal hypertensive gastropathy or gastric/duodenal ulcerations. In addition, endoscopy can identify features associated with an increased risk for future hemorrhage, such as large varices, "red spots" apparent over varices representing fragile telangiectasis within the shallow submucosa, and portal hypertensive gastropathy. Endoscopy is also used to initiate treatment when acute bleeding varices are identified (10).

Liver biopsy may be helpful in determining the etiology of intrinsic liver disease and in defining further therapy or need for transplantation.

TREATMENT OF PORTAL HYPERTENSIVE COMPLICATIONS

The decision to undertake pharmacological, endoscopic, or surgical treatment for portal hypertension must be based on the natural history of the disease and the possibility of life-threatening complications. The prognosis is related to the primary etiology of the portal hypertension. It has generally been accepted in patients with portal hypertension due to EPVO that the risk of acute variceal bleeding decreases with age, concurrent with the development of spontaneous portosystemic collaterals. This postulated natural history has been the primary argument supporting conservative management of hemorrhage in these patients, using endoscopic therapy to obliterate esophageal varices while awaiting the development of favorable retroperitoneal and peripancreatic collaterals. However, when the natural history of patients with EPVO was studied by Lykavieris et al., they found little to support this theory *(11)*. Their review of 44 patients, followed for a mean of 8 yr after their twelfth birthday, showed that the actuarial risk of hemorrhage increased with age from 49% at 16 yr to 76% at 24 yr. Children who had experienced bleeding complications prior to age 12 had a significantly greater chance of bleeding again by age 23, compared to those who had not bled by 12 yr of age (93% vs 56%; $p = 0.007$). In those with grade II or III varices, the actuarial risk of hemorrhage was 60% at age 18, and 85% at age 23, compared to patients with no esophageal varices or grade I varices at 12 years of age who experienced no episodes of hemorrhage. This high rate of bleeding in adolescence and early adulthood challenges the assumption that these complications inevitably decrease with time, and suggests that a high-risk population for rebleeding can be identified and selected for preemptive effective treatment. A similar conclusion was reached by Orloff et al. who noted in their 40-yr experience that 42 out of 94 adult patients who underwent portosystemic shunt procedures for portal vein thrombosis had the onset of their bleeding episodes in childhood *(12)*. In this series, an average of 5.4 bleeding episodes occurred prior to portosystemic shunting. Data to conclusively supported the concept that extrahepatic portal hypertension and its complications will be "outgrown" are presently lacking although the concept persists.

In patients with intrinsic liver disease, therapeutic choices are influenced by the probability of progression of their disease and their potential need for liver transplantation in the future. A significant number of these patients will require temporizing endoscopic treatment or surgical portosystemic shunt therapy to treat complications or maintain stability prior to needing liver replacement.

The most common portal hypertensive complication is gastrointestinal bleeding. Regardless of the site and mechanism, initial therapy for portal hypertensive bleeding is directed toward fluid resuscitation and, when necessary, blood replacement. A nasogastric tube should be placed to confirm the upper GI tract as the source of bleeding, and for evacuation of blood from the stomach. An H2 receptor blocker or proton-pump inhibitor should be administered to decrease the risk of further bleeding from gastric erosions. In patients with hepatic synthetic dysfunction and coagulopathy, administration of vitamin K, fresh frozen plasma, or cryoprecipitate, and platelets when thrombocytopenia is present may also be necessary. Adequate volume resuscitation is essential; however, volume overload from excessive transfusion or crystaloid administration is counterproductive, as this leads to a further increase in portal pressure and continued hemorrhage.

PHARMACOLOGIC TREATMENT

Pharmacologic intervention to decrease portal pressure may be considered in pediatric patients with continued bleeding. A variety of options are now available when intervention is required are similar to those used in adult patients.

Vasopressin

Vasopressin increases splanchnic vascular tone, decreasing splanchnic arterial inflow, thus decreasing portal venous pressure. It is administered as an initial bolus of 0.3 µg/kg over 20 min followed by a continuous infusion of 0.002–0.005 µg/kg/min. Intraarterial infusion into the superior mesenteric artery has no advantage over intravenous routes. Several randomized controlled trials in adults have verified the significant beneficial effect of vasopressin in controlling variceal hemorrhage *(13)*. Although vasopressin infusion has been associated with control of variceal hemorrhage in 53–85% of cases in children, its use has been limited by the associated systemic vasoconstriction to the heart, bowel, and kidneys, impairing cardiac function, and exacerbating fluid retention *(10)*. Nitroglycerin has been used to augment the decrease in portal pressure and ameliorate the untoward systemic effects, but is inappropriate when systemic blood pressure is unstable. Because of these limitations, vasopressin is uncommonly used in the pediatric setting.

Somatostatin and Octreotide

Somatostatin, a 14-amino-acid peptide, also reduces splanchnic blood flow by selective mesenteric vascular smooth muscle constriction, and therefore does not precipitate the systemic vasoconstriction seen with vasopressin infusions. Its short half-life complicated treatment, leading to the development of octreotide, an 8-amino-acid synthetic somatostatin analog. Octreotide can be administered subcutaneously, but is best used as a continuous intravenous (iv) drip (25–50 µg/m^2/h, or 1.0 µg/kg/h). In adult studies, both somatostatin and octreotide have achieved excellent results in controlling acute variceal hemorrhage compared to vasopressin or mechanical tamponade *(13)*. Studies in children to confirm this success have not been undertaken, and its use and efficacy in children can only be inferred.

MECHANICAL TAMPONADE

Mechanical tamponade using balloon catheter tubes (Sengstaken–Blakemore or Minnesota tubes) provide mechanical compression of esophageal and gastric fundal varices. These must be carefully placed by an individual skilled in their use, often with fluoroscopic assistance. Monitoring is necessary to keep the esophageal balloon pressure below mean arterial blood pressure to avoid mucosal ischemia during long-term placement. Suction of secretions from the upper esophagus and pharynx is necessary to prevent aspiration. Endotracheal intubation is inevitably required in children. Although balloon tamponade is usually successful in stopping refractory hemorrhage, the effect is often transient and recurrence following removal is common. This high rate of complications has limited their use to emergency control until other measures or surgical intervention can be instituted.

ENDOSCOPIC INTERVENTION FOR ESOPHAGEAL VARICES

In most cases, variceal hemorrhage can be controlled in children with fluid resuscitation, correction of coagulation, and pharmacologic support. However, the risk of recurrent hemorrhage and the need for accurate diagnosis of the site of hemorrhage often mandate endoscopy during the early posthemorrhage period. When variceal hemorrhage is confirmed or strongly suspected, variceal sclerotherapy or variceal band ligation can be used to eradicate the present or future sites of bleeding.

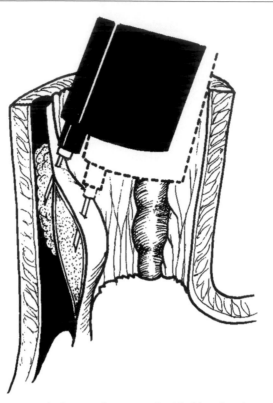

Fig. 1. Injection sclerotherapy techniques—intravascular (dark) and perivascular (dotted) techniques. Reprinted with permission *(60)*.

ENDOSCOPIC SCLEROTHERAPY–ENDOSCOPIC BAND LIGATION

The use of endoscopic methods to control acute variceal hemorrhage is well established. Endoscopic sclerotherapy (EST) has been widely used as the primary treatment for refractory variceal bleeding due to its high success rate (>90%) and the ability to institute initial treatment at the time of diagnostic endoscopy. The procedure is successful using both intravariceal and perivariceal injection techniques (Fig. 1). In children, 5% ethanolamine, 1–1.5% tetradecyl sulfate, or 5% sodium morrhuate have been used with equal success. Most patients require 3–6 sessions at intervals of 2–4 wk to eradicate esophageal varicies. Minor early complications, which occur in almost all patients, include retrosternal pain, fever, and transient dysphagia. Esophageal ulceration at the site of injection, a direct consequence of the procedure, is seen in 70–80% of patients and can be the source of recurrent bleeding. Serious complications such as esophageal strictures, esophageal perforation, or mediastinitis occur in 10–20% of patients. Despite these risks, emergency sclerotherapy has been successful in terminating acute variceal hemorrhage. The long-term outcome following EST is related to the primary liver disease. In children with EPVO, recurrent variceal bleeding developed in 31% of patients followed for a mean period of 8.7 yr; however, in children with intrahepatic disease, the rate was 75% *(14,15)* (Table 2).

In an attempt to overcome these complications but preserve the treatment success of EST, esophageal band ligation (EBL) of varices has been developed, using techniques

Table 2
Pediatric Experience with Endoscopic Sclerotherapy

Author	N	Obliterated %	Rebleed %	Recurrence %	Esophageal ulceration	Esophageal stricture	Mean # treatments	% gastric varicies (G.V.)
Dilawari (64)	38	92	23	16	23	10	—	—
Yachha (65)	50	88	26	10	20	6	8	70% G.V.
Horigome (66)	7	100	14	29	0	0	2.3	—
Maksoud (67)	62	45	53	—	—	—	—	—
	45	96	18	—	—	3	—	18% G.V.
(prophylactic)	49		6	—	—	—	—	—
Howard (68)								
(prophylactic)	108	92 EPVO 75 Intrahep	39	12	29	16	6–6	—
(prophylactic)	17		65	—	—	—	3.8	
Stringer (15)	36	80	31	28	—	3	—	13% G.V.
Thapa (69)	30	90	10	13	20	20	5	13% G.V.
Gonclaves (18)	50	94	24	—	—	—	—	12% G.V. 16% C.H.G.
Hill (70)	33	100	36	33	13	12	4–5	—

391

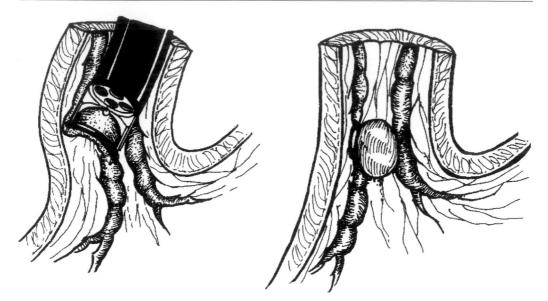

Fig. 2. Endoscopic band ligation technique—(**A**) Varix is drawn into the band ligator using suction to facilitate band placement; (**B**) Band applied to varix to occlude proximal and distal flow. Reprinted with permission *(60)*.

similar to those for banding internal hemorrhoids (Fig. 2). Band ligation has the advantage of ligating only the submucosal venous varices, without harming the submucosal lining. This should minimize the technical complications associated with injection of the submucosa and esophageal wall during sclerotherapy. Several bands are placed during each procedure, requiring multiple passes of the endoscope as it may bear only a single band at a time.

Experience with EBL in children is less extensive but reports similar success to the 90–96% control rate for acute variceal hemorrhage seen in adults *(14,16,17)* (Table 3). Variceal obliteration was achieved in 73–100% of cases, rebleeding prior to completion of obliteration was less common then with EST; however, recurrence was seen in 75% of patients with intrahepatic disease. In addition, the small size of the child's esophagus limits the number of O-rings that can be placed at one treatment session, requiring multiple treatments. The thinner esophageal wall of small (<1 yr old) children makes full-thickness ligation a risk, precluding EBL below this age *(14)*.

Both EST and EBL have been used for the primary prophylaxis of variceal hemorrhage. Prophylactic EST decreased the incidence of bleeding in children from 42% to 6% in the controlled randomized trial by Goncalves et al., using EST every 21 d until initial obliteration was complete *(18)*. However, following successful EST, 16% developed congestive hypertensive gastropathy and 38% bled from this lesion. This was in contrast to the control group where only 6% had congestive hypertensive gastropathy, with no gastropathy associated bleeding episodes. Prophylactic EST did not alter patient survival compared to the control group. When this trial was expanded as a controlled prospective randomized trial of prophylactic sclerotherapy, identical conclusions were reached *(18)*. EBL has also had used for primary prophylaxis in a limited number of children. When undertaken for intrahepatic disease, 72% of varices were eradicated or

Table 3
Pediatric Experience with Variceal Band Ligation

Author	N	Etiology	Obliterated %	Rebleed %	Recurrence %	Follow-up mean	Band failure	Mean # treatments	% gastric varicies
Price (17)	22	36% EPVO 64% Hepatic	66	33	9	5.3 yr	0	4	—
Nijhawan (16)	15	100% EPVO	93	7	—	9 mo	0	1.8	—
Sasaki (19)	11	100% Biliary Atresia	18 54 improved	—	—	—	1	—	—
Fox (14)	7	100% Intrahepatic	100	33	75	13.8 mo	0	4	33% G.V.

improved, but two-thirds required combined EST in addition to EBL to achieve control. Varices were not controlled or recurred in 27%, and the emergence of congestive hypertensive gastropathy was noted as well *(19)*. Long-term control with EST seems to exceed that with EBL, and a combination of both may be more effective than EBL alone. The risk of accelerated formation of gastric varices may overshadow any prophylactic benefit for either EST or EBL; however, sufficient experience is not available to assess this risk at the present time.

PORTOSYSTEMIC SHUNTS

Numerous surgical procedures have been devised to divert portal blood into the low-pressure systemic venous circulation, thereby decreasing the portal venous pressure. Enthusiasm for the use of portosystemic shunting in children was limited due to several concerns whose validity can now be questioned. Early reports suggested that children less than 8 yr of age, and those with vessels for the shunt anastomosis less than 8–10 mm, would be unsuitable candidates because of the high risk of shunt thrombosis *(12,20)*. Recent experience in centers skilled in pediatric vascular reconstruction has established that a high rate of success can be achieved with minimal complications even in small pediatric patients. To achieve these goals, we have found that the following principles should be followed: (1) anastomosis should be constructed using fine (6.0–7.0) monofilament sutures with provision for growth; (2) sufficient mobilization of vessels is necessary to prevent kinking or twisting of the shunt after the viscera are returned to their normal location; (3) postreconstructive venography should be performed to ensure division of all collaterals and adequate shunt flow; (4) selective postoperative anticoagulation should be performed and antiplatelet drugs administered; and (5) the surgical team should be skilled at pediatric portal vascular reconstruction. We believe present success supports the recommendation that successful portosystemic shunt therapy can be undertaken whenever clinical indications are met.

A second concern regarded the possibility of encephalopathy developing following portosystemic shunting in children. The primary reports from Voorhees et al. suggested a high incidence of neuropsychiatric disturbances following nonselective shunts in children *(21,22)*. These conclusions were derived from studies performed on a single day in eight highly selected patients chosen from a pool of 100 patients who had undergone portosystemic shunts or through a retrospective chart review have not been substantiated in most clinical series. Alagille et al. conducted a detailed evaluation of portosystemic shunts in 42 children with EHPO 18 and 24 mo following surgery *(23)*. No evidence of encephalopathy or loss of intellectual capacity was detected. A similar absence of encephalopathy was found in Orloff's extensive follow-up series, even though all 200 of their patients had central nonselective shunts *(12)*.

In general, portosystemic shunts can be classified into two groups—*nonselective* and *selective* shunts.

Nonselective shunts are constructed to communicate with the entire portal venous system, and, therefore, have the potential to divert blood from the normal antegrade perfusion to the liver. Historically, the most commonly used shunt in children was the mesocaval shunt (Clatworthy shunt), where the distal inferior vena cava (IVC) was ligated and divided, and its proximal portion was then anastomosed to the side of the superior mesenteric vein (SMV). This was often complicated by the development of transient lower extremity edema, but had the advantage of using a larger sized vein for the shunt anastomosis. A

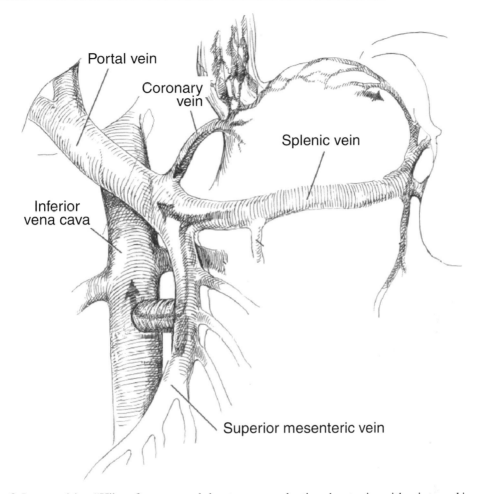

Portal vein

Coronary vein

Splenic vein

Inferior vena cava

Superior mesenteric vein

Fig. 3. Interposition "H" graft mesocaval shunt—a nonselective shunt using either internal jugular vein harvested from the patient, or PTFE vascular graft material. This shunt allows the superior mesenteric vein to communicate with the infrarenal inferior vena cava. Reprinted with permission (modified from) *(61)*.

similar nonselective shunt, the H-graft mesocaval shunt, uses a short segment of internal jugular vein to connect the SMV or splenic vein and the IVC. This has now replaced the mesocaval shunt, retaining the advantage of a larger vessel for the anastomosis, and avoiding ligation of the IVC *(24)* (Fig. 3). Excellent patency (93%) and no episodes of encephalopathy support its use in pediatric patients *(24)*. The limited intraabdominal dissection needed to complete the H-Graft mesocaval shunt contributes to its technical ease, and if liver transplantation is needed, the shunt can be easily occluded at that time. Other nonselective shunts have significant disadvantages in children because of the need for splenectomy (proximal splenorenal), or dissection of the main portal vein which compromises liver transplantation (end-to-side, side-to-side portocaval shunts).

Selective shunts are constructed to divert the "gastrosplenic" portion of the portal venous flow into a systemic vein, most frequently the left renal vein or the immediately adjacent IVC. Communication between the "central" mesenteric portal circulation which

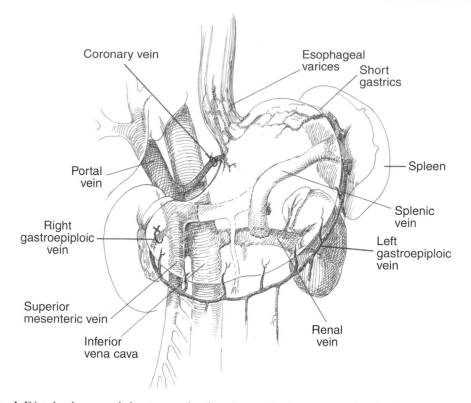

Fig. 4. Distal splenorenal shunt—a selective shunt allowing communication between the splenic vein and the left renal vein. The esophagogastric venous complex communicates via the short gastric veins, decompressing esophageal varicies without decreasing perfusion through the mesenteric portal system to the liver. Reprinted with permission *(61)*.

perfuses the liver, and the gastrosplenic portal circulation, is severed by dividing the gastroepiploic veins, the coronary vein termination at the portal vein, and the retroperitoneal pancreatic collaterals. The most common selective shunt, the distal splenorenal shunt (DSRS) (Warren shunt), preserves antegrade perfusion to the liver within the mesenteric portion of the portal circulation, while decompressing the esophageal venous plexus through the short gastric veins and splenic vein (Fig. 4). This theoretical "selective" advantage can unfortunately be lost over time as the high-pressure mesenteric component progressively decompresses into the lower pressure gastrosplenic compartment. Complete isolation of the pancreas from the splenic vein will decrease the frequency and rapidity of this change *(20,25)*. Despite this potential for progressive loss of selectivity, we use this shunt as a primary option in children. When the adrenal vein is appropriately located and dilated, it serves as an alternative anastomotic site to access the left renal vein *(26,27)*.

When performed in centers experienced in complex vascular reconstruction of the portal system, as is necessary in pediatric liver transplantation, shunt patency has ranged from 83% to 100% *(12,28–30)* (Table 4). When shunt patency is maintained, recurrence of variceal bleeding is uncommon, although decompressed varices may still be identifiable on endoscopy. Encephalopathy is uncommon in children following successful porto-

Table 4
Pediatric Experience with Portosystemic Shunt Procedures

Author	N	Type of shunt	% Patency	Encephalopathy	Survival
Maksoud (67)	42	DSRS	Case 1–7 = 71% Case 8–42 = 92%	—	100% peri-op survival
Bernard (71)	92 EPVO 17 CHF 37 Cirrhosis 12 B-C Syndrome	M.C.-I.J.V.	93 94 84 83	0 0 29 0	100 100 81 75
Orloff (28)	162 EPVO	SS–SR–75 PSR–34 MC–53	100 88 100	0 0 0	99%—5 yr 96%—10 yr
Orloff (12)	200 EPVO 148 symptomatic prior to 18 yr of age	SS–SR–94 PSR–40 MC–56	100 88 100	0 0 0	99%—5 yr 97%—10 yr 95%—15 yr
Gauthier (24)	84 (59 EPVO, 23 Intrahepatic disease. 4 B-C Syndrome)	SR–20 MC–55 PC–4 Makeshift – 7	93	0	100% peri-op survival
Kato (30)	12	DSRS – 10 PC – 1 MC – 1	100 (2 revisions) 100 100	1 ? case overall in autistic child	100% @ 2–4 yr
Evans (72)	9	DSRS – 8 MCS – 1	75% 100%	1–after MCS	2 Deaths 3 OLTx
Hasegawa (20)	5	DSRS	100%	0	100% 4–12 yr
Sigalet (73)	Biliary atresia 20 (21 shunts)	H-Graft Int. Jugular Vn.	95% One revised	2 transient	95%
Mazariegos (26) Cincinnati CH	12 40	DS-Adrenal	83%	8%	100%, 1 OLTx
Authors Series	(20 EPVO, 18 Intrahepatic disease, 2B-C Syndrome)	DSRS–25 CSRS–6 MC–9	95% 100% 89%	0 0 11%	100% peri-op, 92% 83% 100% peri-op, 89%

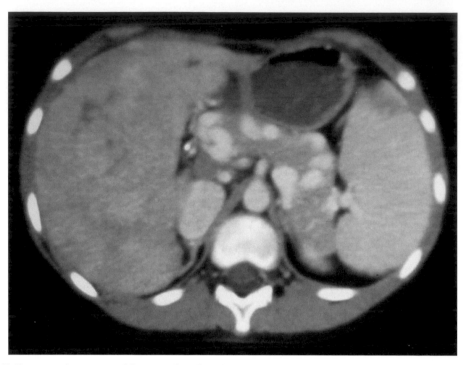

Fig. 5. Computed tomographic scan showing the development of peripancreatic collateral venous channels connecting the mesenteric portal venous system to the decompressed esophagogastric system in a patient with primary extrahepatic portal venous obstruction 8 yr post-op following a distal splenorenal shunt without pancreatic isolation.

systemic shunting, even in patients with intrinsic liver disease. In these children, this is controlled with lactulose and dietary protein restriction *(31)*.

Methods to directly reconstruct the portal circulation in patients with EPVO into the left branch of the portal vein have been described and represent ideal solutions *(32–34)*. This mesentericoportal shunt (Rex shunt) reestablishes normal portal inflow into the intrahepatic portal vein, using either an interposition jugular venous graft or the dilated coronary vein (Fig. 5). Candidates for this procedure must fulfill three conditions: the liver parenchyma must be normal, they must not have a hypercoagulable state, and the umbilical portion of the left portal vein must be accessible and patent. Attempts to identify the intrahepatic portal vein and prove patency have been frustrating and often unsuccessful. Because of the small diameter and low flow within these residual veins, both Doppler and MR scanning may not clearly visualize these branches. The best assessment of patency is through direct visualization of the left portal vein branch and the Rex recess at the time of exploration. Rapid enlargement of these branches occurs with reestablishment of normal portal blood flow into the left portal vein, with mean portal vein diameters increasing 33% over the first year *(32)*. The procedure is unique in that it restores hepatopetal portal perfusion and the inflow of hepatatrophic substances to the liver. Patients with diffuse portal vein thrombosis are not candidates for this reconstruction. Doppler ultrasound and direct portography would suggest, however, that approximately two-thirds of children with EPVO have sufficient left portal vein patency to undergo this procedure. In the reported experience (Table 5), all shunts have maintained initial patency, although

Table 5
Experience with Portal System Reconstruction (Mesenterico-Left Portal Bypass) (REX Shunt) in Pediatric Patients

Author	N	Shunt material	Patency	Follow-up	Complications
de Ville de Goyet (74)	7	5 – L. internal jugular vein	100%	7 mo to 3 yr	None
		1 – R. gastroepoploic vein (direct)	100%	(1.5 yr median)	None
		1 – L. int. jug + venous allograft	allograft sclerosis (4 mo)		Gortex redo
de Ville de Goyet (34) Brussels, Belgium Series	11	9 – L. int. jugular vein + above (allograft, excess tension)	100% – 2 sclerosis	1–32 mo	Revise 2 grafts (6,9 mo)
Gehrke (75)	13	13 L. internal jugular vein	100%	6–24 mo (1 yr median)	
Bambini (32)	5	4 – L. internal jugular vein	100% @ 6 mo	7–21 mo	2 late failures
		1 – Cadaveric iliac vein graft	40% late occlusions		1 revised
Mack (35) Chicago Series	11	As above	100% @ 1 yr	1 yr	1 stenosis
Fuchs (76) Hannover, Germany	7	7 – L. internal jugular vein	100%	3–28 mo (15 mo mean)	

399

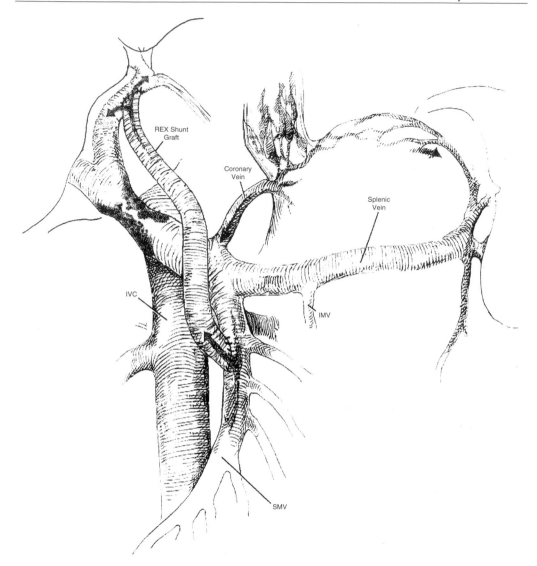

Fig. 6. Mesentericoportal shunt to restore portal blood flow to the left branch of the intrahepatic portal vein. This shunt returns portal blood flow directly to the hepatic portal circulation, and is useful only in patients with EPVO and a patent intrahepatic portal venous system. An interposition jugular venous graft is preferred.

several have required revision secondary to stenosis. Hypertensive gastropathy resolved, and variceal bleeding did not recur. In these selected patients, this option should be considered despite the more complex technical challenge it presents.

An interesting observation from the Chicago group suggests that the coagulation abnormalities routinely seen in their series prior to Rex shunting in patients with portal vein thrombosis are reversible; these abnormalities are primarily represented by abnormal prothrombin time, factor V, factor VIII, protein C, and protein S deficiency results following restoration of normal portal blood flow. This suggests that portal blood flow

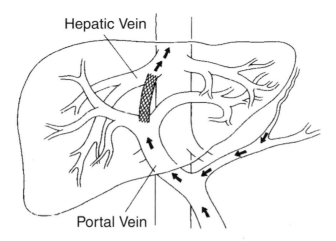

Hepatic Vein

Portal Vein

Fig. 7. Transjugular intrahepatic portosystemic shunt (TIPS) procedure. Reprinted with permission *(62)*.

assists with normalization of clotting indices, and they postulate that gut derived factors in portal blood are responsible for this improvement *(35)*.

The indications for portosystemic shunting have been altered by the growing success of endoscopic methods to control variceal bleeding, and the improvements in pediatric liver transplantation. We now consider the following children to be candidates for portosystemic shunting: (1) children with documented variceal hemorrhage who have progressive or continued esophageal variceal bleeding despite endoscopic intervention, and who have preserved hepatic synthetic function; (2) children who fail endoscopic treatment and have intrinsic liver disease, but have adequate liver synthetic function to predict that liver transplantation will not be needed for several years (selective shunt only); (3) severe portal hypertension in patients with cystic fibrosis and variceal hemorrhage whose microbiologic flora compromise liver transplant survival *(36)*; (4) children with severe portal hypertension who reside a great distance from emergency medical care endangering their survival should significant hemorrhage occur; and (5) children with EPVO and uncontrolled hypersplenism.

TRANSJUGULAR INTRAHEPATIC PORTOSYSTEMIC SHUNT (TIPS)

The introduction of TIPS has added another therapeutic option for the physician confronted with complex portal hypertension. This procedure uses interventional radiographic techniques to place an intrahepatic expandable metallic shunt between a portal vein branch and the hepatic vein, forming a central nonselective portocaval shunt. The procedure is undertaken using access via the right internal jugular vein. The hepatic veins are identified and a fluoroscopic/ultrasonographic-guided puncture from the hepatic vein into an intrahepatic portion of the portal vein is undertaken. This tract is then dilated and an expandable coaxial mesh stent is placed, forming a communication between the intrahepatic portal vein and the hepatic vein branch (Fig. 7). Technical difficulties in establishing a safe but large enough tract for sufficient shunt flow limit the usefulness of this procedure in infants. In children with biliary atresia, the close proximity of the biliary Roux-en-Y conduit to the portal vein and the often diminutive size of the portal vein increase the risk of stent perforation, malposition, or perforation *(37)*. This procedure has great benefit in the control of refractory portal hypertensive bleeding unresponsive to the pharmacologic methods, and in patients needing temporary portal decompression prior to liver transplantation *(38–40)*. The ability to embolize bleeding varices from the coronary vein at the time of TIPS placement assists in achieving primary control of bleeding sites.

The two principal long-term complications of TIPS are encephalopathy and shunt occlusion. Being a central nonselective shunt, this procedure can precipitate hepatic encephalopathy, especially when used in patients with severe intrinsic liver disease. The overall risk of encephalopathy ranges from 5% to 35% in adult patients, a rate similar to that seen with side-to-side surgical shunts. Most episodes of encephalopathy can be controlled with dietary protein restriction and lactulose administration. Selection of a shunt size to allow sufficient portal decompression without shunting excessive amounts of blood from the liver is also a theoretical solution. Stenosis of the shunt or shunt thrombosis remains a major complication following TIPS. Shunt stenosis occurs in 25–75% of cases, with shunt patency decreasing with the length of time that the shunt is in place. Intimal hyperplasia or incorrect shunt placement most commonly causes the stenosis. Stent transgression of the bile duct radicle at the time of shunt placement can also contribute to recurrent shunt thrombosis. Regular monitoring for shunt patency and periodic shunt dilation or restenting is necessary *(39)*.

Pediatric experience with TIPS is still limited, primarily due to a lack of appropriate candidates for the procedure. The majority of children with biliary atresia and ineffective portoenterostomy procedure develop end-stage cirrhosis within their first 2 yr of life. These patients are poor candidates by virtue of both their size and the frequency of portal vein abnormalities within this population. The majority of experience is in children over 5 yr of age (Table 6). Success rates appear to approximate the adult experience, with 75–90% initial success in TIPS placement. The smaller size of the liver and its venous structures requires special skill and equipment. Shorter stent lengths and smaller diameter stents have been constructed for pediatric applications; however, the risks of hepatic perforation and stent malposition are greater in small patients. Postprocedural encephalopathy seems to be less common in children, although limited clinical experience and the difficulties in diagnosing subtle encephalopathy in children makes this observation tentative. The complications of shunt stenosis are equally problematic, and patient growth over time may cause the initial shunt to be too short, requiring revision or restenting to maintain access to both the portal and hepatic venous circulation. These limitations and risks make TIPS a reasonable and suitable treatment for acute unresponsive variceal hemorrhage in children with established intrinsic liver disease, often while awaiting liver transplantation. It is particularly helpful when used as a bridge to achieve stability by controlling refractory hemorrhage in patients awaiting liver transplantation *(40)*. Long-term decompression is better achieved through surgical shunts at the present time, and TIPS is not indicated in patients with extrahepatic portal vein occlusion.

TIPS has recently been used for adult patients with progressive or fulminant Budd–Chiari syndrome. Access via the hepatic vein stump is possible, or direct puncture from the IVC into the right portal vein serves as an alternative route for stent placement. Although plagued as expected by thrombotic complications, successful decompression of portal hypertension and prolonged survival was achieved. Similar experience in children has not been reported *(41)*.

Table 6
Pediatric Experience with TIPS

Author	Age	Diagnosis	Follow-up	Complications
Kerns (77)	13 yr	cystic fibrosis	6 mo	Encephalopathy
Wang (37)	21 mo	biliary atresia		OLTx
	4 yr	—		
	2.5 yr	—		
Cao (78)	10 mo	biliary atresia	—	
Schweizer (79)	7 patients 3–13 yr	biliary atresia	4–24 mo	1 liver capsule puncture
Astfalk (80)	4.5 yr	biliary atresia	5 mo	Shunt occlusion (angioplasty)
Lagier (81)	7 yr	pseudoobstruction	4 mo	
Berger (82)	14 yr	cystic fibrosis	11 mo	
	10, 11 yr	biliary atresia	4, 9 mo	1 occluded
Johnson (40)	6 yr	cholestasis		
	7 yr	congenital hepatic fibrosis		
	11 yr	biliary atresia		
Weinberg (83)	2.5, 4 yr	short gut syndrome	1,10 mo	1 Small Bowel Transplant @ 1 mo
Azoulay (7)	10 patients	bone marrow transplant	6 mo	1 Survivor
Fleet (38)	14 yr	cystic fibrosis	30 mo	Shunt stenosis–revised
	10 yr	cystic fibrosis	2 yr	Died–Pulmonary disease
Steventon (84)	9 yr	autoimmune hepatitis		
Sergent (85)	15 mo	cystic fibrosis	22 d	Died–Sepsis
Heyman (86)	4 patients 5,5,7,12 yr	biliary atresia	5,6,66,0 d	OLTx 3, 12 y/o occluded–DSRS
	5 patients 7,9,10,15,15 yr	cirrhosis	0,24,40,35,800 d	3 occluded, 2 revised, and 1 DSRS, 1 bleed, 1 OLTx
Hackworth (87)	4 patients 2,3,7,9 yr	biliary atresia	9–127 d to OLTx	10 OLTx, 1 replaced
	8 patients 5,7,9,9,10,15,16 yr	cirrhosis (7), ascites (1)	301,357 d Non OLTx	
Ong (88)	10 yr	cystic fibrosis	35 d	Hepatic encephalopathy, death
Kimura (89)	2 yr	biliary atresia	7 mo	Occluded 2x, 2 d, and 6 mo, revised
Pozler (90)	5 patients	cystic fibrosis	15–81 mo	6 recurrent hemorrhages
	8–18 yr			15 asymptomatic stenosis dilated
				Oltx–1 15 mo, deaths 4.5, 6.7 yr

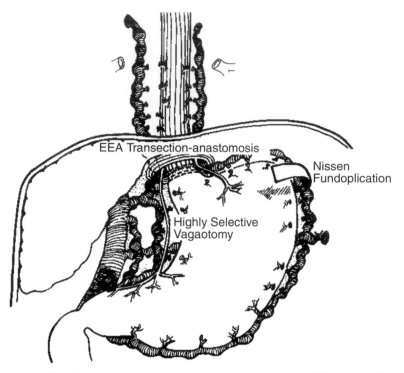

Fig. 8. Sugiura procedure for gastroesophageal devascularization, modified for pediatric patients to include division of the short gastric veins without splenectomy. Reprinted with permission *(63)*.

NONSHUNT PROCEDURES FOR PORTAL HYPERTENSION

The use of nonshunt surgical procedures for the management of portal hypertension does not offer the same success as is enjoyed by shunt therapy. These operations have included both direct variceal ligation through a transthoracic or abdominal approach, gastroesophageal devascularization procedures (Sugiura procedure), or, rarely, translocation of the spleen into the thorax *(42–44)*. In general, these procedures have been abandoned except in cases where widespread thrombosis of the mesenteric venous vasculature makes shunt therapy or transplantation poor alternatives.

The Sugiura procedure has been used with the most success in children (Fig. 8). This procedure includes devascularization of the upper two-thirds of the greater and lesser curvatures of the stomach, and ligation of the left gastroepiploic, short gastric, and left gastric vessels. Ligation of all retrogastric collaterals, transhiatal devascularization of the lower esophagus, esophageal transection with fundoplication, and pyloroplasty if the vagus nerves are damaged *(43)*. Splenectomy was advocated in the original descriptions of this procedure as well. However, splenectomy has been associated with a greater risk of intraoperative bleeding, need for intraoperative blood transfusions, and postoperative portal vein thrombosis. Because of these risks and the known increased potential for postoperative infectious complications of splenectomy, we do not routinely perform splenectomy in children. Specific indications for splenectomy during nonshunt operations are severe hypersplenism, massive splenomegaly, and splenic vein thrombosis *(45)*. Following extensive devascularization to achieve portal–azygos disconnection, rebleeding rates of 5–10% can be achieved during long-term follow-up *(42)*. Five-year survival following these operations has been reported to be 88% and 80% at 10 yr *(43)*. This is a safe alternative for variceal control in patients with anatomy unsuitable for shunting, or when the expertise for emergency portocaval shunt or liver transplantation is not available.

Portopulmonary shunting, induced by splenopneumopexy, is intended to produce collateral circulation between the portal system and the pulmonary veins. This communication is created by amputating the superior pole of the spleen, transposing it through an opening in the left hemidiaphragm, and exposing the raw splenic surface to the left lower lung. Splenic artery occlusion by angiographic or direct ligation is also undertaken *(46)*. A parenchymatous anastomosis is induced between the splenic pulp veins and the pulmonary venous structures. This uncommon procedure has been successfully used in children with EPVO, hepatic fibrosis, intrinsic cirrhosis, and Budd–Chiari syndrome. A decrease in splenic pulp pressure of 25% has been reported in most cases where this was recorded. Indications for this procedure are limited to the treatment of children with widespread occlusion of the portal vein and its radicals *(44,46,47)*.

LIVER TRANSPLANTATION

The progressive improvement in both the operative techniques and the immunosuppression management of children who have undergone liver transplant have led to 1-yr survival rates approaching 90% in many centers, with 5-yr survival rates of 85% *(48–53)*. Regardless of the primary etiology of portal hypertension, liver transplantation successfully reverses the portal flow obstruction and allows the resolution of hypersplenism and hypertensive portal gastropathy. The introduction of innovative surgical procedures to allow transplantation of liver segments and reduced-size grafts has improved and increased donor availability and donor access for children of all ages *(53,54)*. However, the use of primary transplantation as a treatment modality for portal hypertension is limited by the availability of suitable donor organs and the long-term risks of immunosuppression, opportunistic infections, and lymphoproliferative disease. When children have progressive intrinsic hepatic disease, the course of their progression and the amount of hepatic functional reserve should determine the use of primary transplantation compared to temporizing treatments such as sclerotherapy or surgical shunts. At present, primary transplantation is recommended for children who have significant portal hypertensive complications such as bleeding, hypersplenism, or hepatopulmonary syndrome, and those who have progressive hepatic synthetic failure. Children with intrinsic liver disease but preserved hepatic synthetic function, who may not require transplantation for several years, will achieve excellent palliation with selective DSRS. TIPS is reserved for patients who have unresponsive variceal bleeding as a therapeutic bridge to transplantation, allowing them to achieve suitable stability while awaiting transplant donor organ availability.

PULMONARY SYNDROMES ASSOCIATED WITH PORTAL HYPERTENSION

Hepatopulmonary syndrome (HPS), a syndrome associated with hepatic dysfunction, hypoxemia, and pulmonary vascular dilatations, characteristically occurs in children with long-standing liver disease and portal hypertension. This constellation of symptoms is thought to be secondary to the effects of vasoactive substances, normally inactivated in the liver, on the pulmonary vasculature. Although this syndrome is usually seen in patients with portal hypertension and spontaneous portosystemic communications, it has been reported following surgical portosystemic shunting as well *(55,56)*. Progressive hypoxemia, which is exacerbated by the horizontal position (orthodeoxia and platypnea), is commonly seen on evaluation. Hypoxemia does not correct with 100% oxygen ventilation, confirming the presence of intrapulmonary shunts contributing to the alveolar perfusion abnormalities. Abnormal extrapulmonary (brain) uptake of $(^{99m})$Tc macroaggregated albumin (MAA) after lung perfusion scanning, or the presence of early microbubble perfusion on echocardiography are diagnostic and predictive of morbidity with general anesthesia or liver transplant *(57)*. Present experience suggests that these abnormalities are reversible following successful liver transplantation *(55,57)*.

Pulmonary hypertension has been associated with severe liver disease and portal hypertension in 1–2% of patients. In the presence of spontaneous or surgically created portosystemic communication, pulmonary vasoconstrictive substances can pass directly into the systemic circulation, bypassing hepatic metabolism. Possible agents include histamine, serotonin, purine, pyrimidine, neuropeptide Y, and thromboxanes *(58)*. Symptoms of dyspnea, exercise intolerance, and palpitation occur; however, many patients remain asymptomatic until late in the course of their disease. Initial treatment with oxygen and vasodilators is occasionally helpful. The pathologic lesion, plexogenic pulmonary arteriopathy, results in increased smooth muscle, increased thickness of the media, concentric luminal fibrosis, and eventually fibrinoid necrosis. Case reports suggest that liver transplantation may assist in reversal, provided diagnosis, and transplantation are undertaken at the early stages of pathologic evolution *(58,59)*. In later stages, resolution can not be anticipated.

SUMMARY

Therapeutic options for children with portal hypertension now include a broad range of pharmacologic, endoscopic, and surgical procedures. Thoughtful application of all of these options can improve quality of life by decreasing the complications of portal hypertension, and decrease mortality by preventing the consequences of variceal hemorrhage. The development of portal hypertensive gastropathy following palliative procedures such as endoscopic sclerotherapy and band ligation may limit their long-term success in children. The excellent results now obtained with selective portosystemic shunts and liver transplantation assure that definitive surgical treatments will continue to be a critical component in the treatment of children with portal hypertensive complications or progressive liver disease. Evolving procedures, such as TIPS, represent excellent short-term life preserving techniques to stabilize critical patients while awaiting liver transplantation. Their role in the future long-term management of children is yet to be defined.

REFERENCES

1. Karrer FM, Price MR, Bensard DD, et al. Long-term results with the Kasai operation for biliary atresia. Arch Surg 1996;131(5):493–496.
2. Ryckman FC, Alonso MH. Causes and management of portal hypertension in the pediatric population. In: Sanyal AJ, ed. Clinics in Liver Disease, vol. 5. W.B. Sanders, Philadelphia, 2001, pp. 789–818.
3. Dubuisson C, Boyer-Neumann C, Wolf M, et al. Protein C, protein S and antithrombin III in children with portal vein obstruction. J Hepatol 1997;27(1):132–135.
4. Ando H, Kaneko K, Ito F, et al. Anatomy and etiology of extrahepatic portal vein obstruction in children leading to bleeding esophageal varices. J Am Coll Surg 1996;183(6):543–547.

5. Odievre M, Pige G, Alagille D. Congenital abnormalities associated with extrahepatic portal hypertension. Arch Dis Child 1977;52(5):383–385.

6. Carson JA, Tunell WP, Barnes P, Altshuler G. Hepatoportal sclerosis in childhood: a mimic of extrahepatic portal vein obstruction. J Pediatr Surg 1981;16(3):291–296.

7. Azoulay D, Castaing D, Lemoine A, et al. Transjugular intrahepatic portosystemic shunt (TIPS) for severe veno-occlusive disease of the liver following bone marrow transplantation. Bone Marrow Transpl 2000;25(9):987–992.

8. Sperl W, Stuppner H, Gassner I, et al. Reversible hepatic veno-occlusive disease in an infant after consumption of pyrrolizidine-containing herbal tea. Eur J Pediatr 1995;154(2):112–116.

9. Kreft B, Strunk H, Flacke S, et al. Detection of thrombosis in the portal venous system: comparison of contrast-enhanced MR angiography with intraarterial digital subtraction angiography. Radiology 2000;216(1):86–92.

10. Karrer FM, Narkewicz MR. Esophageal varices: current management in children. Semin Pediatr Surg 1999;8(4):193–201.

11. Lykavieris P, Gauthier F, Hadchouel P, et al. Risk of gastrointestinal bleeding during adolescence and early adulthood in children with portal vein obstruction. J Pediatr 2000;136(6):805–808.

12. Orloff MJ, Orloff MS, Girard B, Orloff SL. Bleeding esophagogastric varices from extrahepatic portal hypertension: 40 years' experience with portal-systemic shunt. J Am Coll Surg 2002;194(6):717–728; discussion 728–730.

13. D'Amico G, Pagliaro L, Bosch J. The treatment of portal hypertension: a meta-analytic review. Hepatology 1995;22(1):332–354.

14. Fox VL, Carr-Locke DL, Connors PJ, Leichtner AM. Endoscopic ligation of esophageal varices in children. J Pediatr Gastroenterol Nutr 1995;20(2):202–208.

15. Stringer MD, Howard ER. Longterm outcome after injection sclerotherapy for oesophageal varices in children with extrahepatic portal hypertension. Gut 1994;35(2):257–259.

16. Nijhawan S, Patni T, Sharma U, et al. Endoscopic variceal ligation in children. J Pediatr Surg 1995; 30(10):1455–1456.

17. Price MR, Sartorelli KH, Karrer FM, et al. Management of esophageal varices in children by endoscopic variceal ligation. J Pediatr Surg 1996;31(8):1056–1059.

18. Goncalves ME, Cardoso SR, Maksoud JG. Prophylactic sclerotherapy in children with esophageal varices: long-term results of a controlled prospective randomized trial. J Pediatr Surg 2000;35(3): 401–405.

19. Sasaki T, Hasegawa T, Nakajima K, et al. Endoscopic variceal ligation in the management of gastroesophageal varices in postoperative biliary atresia. J Pediatr Surg 1998;33(11):1628–1632.

20. Hasegawa T, Tamada H, Fukui Y, et al. Distal splenorenal shunt with splenopancreatic disconnection for portal hypertension in biliary atresia. Pediatr Surg Int 1999;15(2):92–96.

21. Voorhees AB Jr, Chaitman E, Schneider S, et al. Portal-systemic encephalopathy in the noncirrhotic patient. Effect of portal-systemic shunting. Arch Surg 1973;107(5):659–663.

22. Voorhees AB Jr, Price JB Jr. Extrahepatic portal hypertension. A retrospective analysis of 127 cases and associated clinical implications. Arch Surg 1974;108(3):338–341.

23. Alagille D, Carlier JC, Chiva M, et al. Long-term neuropsychological outcome in children undergoing portal-systemic shunts for portal vein obstruction without liver disease. J Pediatr Gastroenterol Nutr 1986;5(6):861–866.

24. Gauthier F, De Dreuzy O, Valayer J, Montupet P. H-type shunt with an autologous venous graft for treatment of portal hypertension in children. J Pediatr Surg 1989;24(10):1041–1043.

25. Miura H, Kondo S, Shimada T, et al. Long-term effects of distal splenorenal shunt with splenopancreatic and gastric disconnection on hypersplenism due to liver cirrhosis. Hepatogastroenterology 1999; 46(29):2995–2998.

26. Mazariegos GV, Reyes J. A technique for distal splenoadrenal shunting in pediatric portal hypertension. J Am Coll Surg 1998;187(6):634–636.

27. Kulkarni VM, Nagral SS, Mathur SK. Use of adrenal vein conduit for splenorenal shunts: a case report. Hepatogastroenterology 1999;46(27):2033–2034.

28. Orloff MJ, Orloff MS, Rambotti M. Treatment of bleeding esophagogastric varices due to extrahepatic portal hypertension: results of portal-systemic shunts during 35 years. J Pediatr Surg 1994;29(2):142–151; discussion 151–154.

29. Reyes J, Mazariegos GV, Bueno J, et al. The role of portosystemic shunting in children in the transplant era. J Pediatr Surg 1999;34(1):117–122; discussion 122,123.
30. Kato T, Romero R, Koutouby R, et al. Portosystemic shunting in children during the era of endoscopic therapy: improved postoperative growth parameters. J Pediatr Gastroenterol Nutr 2000;30(4): 419–425.
31. Shun A, Delaney DP, Martin HC, et al. Portosystemic shunting for paediatric portal hypertension. J Pediatr Surg 1997;32(3):489–493.
32. Bambini DA, Superina R, Almond PS, et al. Experience with the Rex shunt (mesenterico-left portal bypass) in children with extrahepatic portal hypertension. J Pediatr Surg 2000;35(1):13–18; discussion 18,19.
33. de Ville de Goyet J, Clapuyt P, Otte JB. Extrahilar mesenterico-left portal shunt to relieve extrahepatic portal hypertension after partial liver transplant. Transplantation 1992;53(1):231,232.
34. de Ville de Goyet J, Alberti D, Falchetti D, et al. Treatment of extrahepatic portal hypertension in children by mesenteric-to-left portal vein bypass: a new physiological procedure. Eur J Surg 1999;165(8): 777–781.
35. Mack CL, Superina RA, Whitington PF. Surgical restoration of portal flow corrects procoagulant and anticoagulant deficiencies associated with extrahepatic portal vein thrombosis. J Pediatr 2003;142(2): 197–199.
36. Debray D, Lykavieris P, Gauthier F, et al. Outcome of cystic fibrosis-associated liver cirrhosis: management of portal hypertension. J Hepatol 1999;31(1):77–83.
37. Wang J, Cox KL, Dake M, et al. Transjugular intrahepatic portosystemic shunt placement in a child complicated by perforated Roux-en-Y portoenterostomy. J Pediatr Gastroenterol Nutr 1997;25(4): 421–425.
38. Fleet M, Stanley AJ, Forrest EH, et al. Transjugular intrahepatic portosystemic stent shunt placement in a patient with cystic fibrosis complicated by portal hypertension. Clin Radiol 2000;55(3):236,237.
39. Heyman MB, LaBerge JM. Role of transjugular intrahepatic portosystemic shunt in the treatment of portal hypertension in pediatric patients. J Pediatr Gastroenterol Nutr 1999;29(3):240–249.
40. Johnson SP, Leyendecker JR, Joseph FB, et al. Transjugular portosystemic shunts in pediatric patients awaiting liver transplantation. Transplantation 1996;62(8):1178–1181.
41. Perello A, Garcia-Pagan JC, Gilabert R, et al. TIPS is a useful long-term derivative therapy for patients with Budd-Chiari syndrome uncontrolled by medical therapy. Hepatology 2002;35(1):132–139.
42. Mathur SK, Shah SR, Nagral SS, Soonawala ZF. Transabdominal extensive esophagogastric devascularization with gastroesophageal stapling for management of noncirrhotic portal hypertension: long-term results. World J Surg 1999;23(11):1168–1174; discussion 1174,1175.
43. Ohashi K, Kojima K, Fukazawa M, et al. Long-term prognosis of non-shunt operation for idiopathic portal hypertension. J Gastroenterol 1998;33(2):241–246.
44. Reese JC, Fairchild RB, Brems JJ, Kaminski DL. Splenopneumopexy to treat portal hypertension produced by venous occlusive disease. Arch Surg 1992;127(9):1129–1132.
45. Orozco H, Mercado MA, Martinez R, et al. Is splenectomy necessary in devascularization procedures for treatment of bleeding portal hypertension? Arch Surg 1998;133(1):36–38.
46. Sakoda K, Ono J, Kawada T, et al. Portopulmonary shunt by splenopneumopexy for portal hypertension in children. J Pediatr Surg 1988;23(4):323–327.
47. Akita H, Sakoda K. Portopulmonary shunt by splenopneumopexy as a surgical treatment of Budd-Chiari syndrome. Surgery 1980;87(1):85–94.
48. Alonso MH, Ryckman FC. Current concepts in pediatric liver transplant. Semin Liver Dis 1998;18(3): 295–307.
49. Balistreri WF, Grand R, Hoofnagle JH, et al. Biliary atresia: current concepts and research directions. Summary of a symposium. Hepatology 1996;23(6):1682–1692.
50. Balistreri WF. Transplantation for childhood liver disease: an overview. Liver Transpl Surg 1998;4 (5 Suppl 1):S18–S23.
51. Goss JA, Shackleton CR, McDiarmid SV, et al. Long-term results of pediatric liver transplantation: an analysis of 569 transplants. Ann Surg 1998;228(3):411–420.
52. Busuttil RW, Goss JA. Split liver transplantation. Ann Surg 1999;229(3):313–321.
53. Otte JB. The availability of all technical modalities for pediatric liver transplant programs. Pediatr Transplant 2001;5(1):1–4.

54. Ryckman FC, Flake AW, Fisher RA, et al. Segmental orthotopic hepatic transplantation as a means to improve patient survival and diminish waiting-list mortality. J Pediatr Surg 1991;26(4):422–427; discussion 427,428.

55. Hannam PD, Sandokji AK, Machan LS, et al. Post-surgical shunt hepatopulmonary syndrome in a case of non-cirrhotic portal hypertension: lack of efficacy of shunt reversal. Eur J Gastroenterol Hepatol 1999;11(12):1425–1427.

56. Krowka MJ, Wiseman GA, Burnett OL, et al. Hepatopulmonary syndrome: a prospective study of relationships between severity of liver disease, PaO(2) response to 100% oxygen, and brain uptake after (99m)Tc MAA lung scanning. Chest 2000;118(3):615–624.

57. Krowka MJ. Hepatopulmonary syndrome: recent literature (1997 to 1999) and implications for liver transplantation. Liver Transpl 2000;6(4 Suppl 1):S31–S35.

58. Soh H, Hasegawa T, Sasaki T, et al. Pulmonary hypertension associated with postoperative biliary atresia: report of two cases. J Pediatr Surg 1999;34(12):1779–1781.

59. Losay J, Piot D, Bougaran J, et al. Early liver transplantation is crucial in children with liver disease and pulmonary artery hypertension. J Hepatol 1998;28(2):337–342.

60. Terblanche J, Kringe J. Endoscopic therapy in the management of esophageal varicies: injection sclerotherapy and variceal ligation. In: Nyhus LM BR, Fischer JE, eds. Mastery of Surgery, vol. 2. Boston, Little, Brown and Company, Boston, 1997, pp. 1329–1349.

61. Zollinger R, Zollinger R. Atlas of Surgical Operations. Macmillan, New York, 1975.

62. Shneider BL, Groszmann R. Portal hypertension. In: Suchy FJ, ed. Liver Disease in Children. Mosby, St. Louis, 1994, pp. 249–266.

63. Superina RA, Weber JL, Shandling B. A modified Sugiura operation for bleeding varices in children. J Pediatr Surg 1983;18(6):794–799.

64. Dilawari JB, Chawla YK, Ramesh GN, et al. Endoscopic sclerotherapy in children. J Gastroenterol Hepatol 1989;4(2):155–160.

65. Yachha SK, Sharma BC, Kumar M, Khanduri A. Endoscopic sclerotherapy for esophageal varices in children with extrahepatic portal venous obstruction: a follow-up study. J Pediatr Gastroenterol Nutr 1997;24(1):49–52.

66. Horigome H, Nomura T, Saso K, et al. Endoscopic injection sclerotherapy for esophagogastric variceal bleeding in children with biliary atresia. Hepatogastroenterology 1999;46(30):3060–3062.

67. Maksoud JG, Goncalves ME. Treatment of portal hypertension in children. World J Surg 1994;18(2):251–258.

68. Howard ER, Stringer MD, Mowat AP. Assessment of injection sclerotherapy in the management of 152 children with oesophageal varices. Br J Surg 1988;75(5):404–408.

69. Thapa BR, Mehta S. Endoscopic sclerotherapy of esophageal varices in infants and children. J Pediatr Gastroenterol Nutr 1990;10(4):430–434.

70. Hill ID, Bowie MD. Endoscopic sclerotherapy for control of bleeding varices in children. Am J Gastroenterol 1991;86(4):472–476.

71. Bernard O, Alvarez F, Brunelle F, et al. Portal hypertension in children. Clin Gastroenterol 1985;14(1):33–55.

72. Evans S, Stovroff M, Heiss K, Ricketts R. Selective distal splenorenal shunts for intractable variceal bleeding in pediatric portal hypertension. J Pediatr Surg 1995;30(8):1115–1118.

73. Sigalet DL, Mayer S, Blanchard H. Portal venous decompression with H-type mesocaval shunt using autologous vein graft: a North American experience. J Pediatr Surg 2001;36(1):91–96.

74. de Ville de Goyet J, Alberti D, Clapuyt P, et al. Direct bypassing of extrahepatic portal venous obstruction in children: a new technique for combined hepatic portal revascularization and treatment of extrahepatic portal hypertension. J Pediatr Surg 1998;33(4):597–601.

75. Gehrke I, John P, Blundell J, et al. Meso-portal bypass in children with portal vein thrombosis: rapid increase of the intrahepatic portal venous flow after direct portal hepatic reperfusion. J Pediatr Surg 2003;38(8):1137–1140.

76. Fuchs J, Warmann S, Kardorff R, et al. Mesenterico-left portal vein bypass in children with congenital extrahepatic portal vein thrombosis: a unique curative approach. J Pediatr Gastroenterol Nutr 2003;36(2):213–216.

77. Kerns SR, Hawkins IF Jr. Transjugular intrahepatic portosystemic shunt in a child with cystic fibrosis. Am J Roentgenol 1992;159(6):1277,1278.

78. Cao S, Monge H, Semba C, et al. Emergency transjugular intrahepatic portosystemic shunt (TIPS) in an infant: a case report. J Pediatr Surg 1997;32(1):125–127.
79. Schweizer P, Brambs HJ, Schweizer M, Astfalk W. TIPS: a new therapy for esophageal variceal bleeding caused by EHBA. Eur J Pediatr Surg 1995;5(4):211–215.
80. Astfalk W, Huppert PE, Schweizer P, Plinta-Zgrabczynski A. Recurrent intestinal bleeding from jejunojejunostomy caused by portal hypertension following hepatoportojejunostomy in extra hepatic biliary atresia (EHBA)—successful treatment by transjugular intrahepatic portosystemic shunt (TIPS). Eur J Pediatr Surg 1997;7(3):147,148.
81. Lagier E, Rousseau H, Maquin P, et al. Treatment of bleeding stomal varices using transjugular intrahepatic portosystemic shunt. J Pediatr Gastroenterol Nutr 1994;18(4):501–503.
82. Berger KJ, Schreiber RA, Tchervenkov J, et al. Decompression of portal hypertension in a child with cystic fibrosis after transjugular intrahepatic portosystemic shunt placement. J Pediatr Gastroenterol Nutr 1994;19(3):322–325.
83. Weinberg GD, Matalon TA, Brunner MC, et al. Bleeding stomal varices: treatment with a transjugular intrahepatic portosystemic shunt in two pediatric patients. J Vasc Interv Radiol 1995;6(2):233–236.
84. Steventon DM, Kelly DA, McKiernan P, et al. Emergency transjugular intrahepatic portosystemic shunt prior to liver transplantation. Pediatr Radiol 1997;27(1):84–86.
85. Sergent G, Gottrand F, Delemazure O, et al. Transjugular intrahepatic portosystemic shunt in an infant. Pediatr Radiol 1997;27(7):588–590.
86. Heyman MB, LaBerge JM, Somberg KA, et al. Transjugular intrahepatic portosystemic shunts (TIPS) in children. J Pediatr 1997;131(6):914–919.
87. Hackworth CA, Leef JA, Rosenblum JD, et al. Transjugular intrahepatic portosystemic shunt creation in children: initial clinical experience. Radiology 1998;206(1):109–114.
88. Ong TJ, Murray FE, Redhead DN, et al. Colonic stricture in cystic fibrosis unmasked by successful transjugular intrahepatic portosystemic stent shunt (TIPSS). Scott Med J 1996;41(4):113,114.
89. Kimura T, Hasegawa T, Oue T, et al. Transjugular intrahepatic portosystemic shunt performed in a 2-year-old infant with uncontrolled intestinal bleeding. J Pediatr Surg 2000;35(11):1597–1599.
90. Pozler O, Krajina A, Vanicek H, et al. Transjugular intrahepatic portosystemic shunt in five children with cystic fibrosis: long-term results. Hepatogastroenterology 2003;50(52):1111–1114.

25 Noncirrhotic Portal Hypertension and Portal Vein Thrombosis

Shiv K. Sarin, MD, DM
and Manav Wadhawan, MD

CONTENTS

INTRODUCTION
NONCIRRHOTIC PORTAL FIBROSIS (NCPF)
EXTRAHEPATIC PORTAL VEIN OBSTRUCTION (EHPVO)
NODULAR REGENERATIVE HYPERPLASIA (NRH)
 AND PARTIAL NODULAR TRANSFORMATION
CONGENITAL HEPATIC FIBROSIS (CHF)
REFERENCES

INTRODUCTION

Noncirrhotic portal hypertension (NCPH) encompasses a group of diseases of varied etiology. The characteristic features of this group are increase in portal pressure caused by prehepatic or intrahepatic causes, with absence of liver cirrhosis, as well as of hepatic venous outflow obstruction. The wedged hepatic venous pressure is normal or only mildly elevated. Table 1 lists the common causes of NCPH. The most commonly encountered diseases in this group are noncirrhotic portal fibrosis (NCPF) [alternatively called idiopathic portal hypertension (IPH)] and extrahepatic portal vein obstruction (EHPVO). Together, these two entities constitute 20–30% of total cases of portal hypertension (PHT) in developing countries like India *(1–3)*. In the following discussion, we will describe these two conditions in detail. Other prominent causes of NCPH like schisosamiasis, Nodular regenerative hyperplasia, and Partial nodular transformation will be described briefly.

The underlying lesion in both NCPF and EHPVO is considered to be vascular in origin. Although the precise etiopathogenesis of the two conditions is not clear, a common pathway with different outcomes has been previously proposed (Fig. 1) *(1)*. In a genetically predisposed individual, an infection or a prothrombotic event could precipitate thrombosis in portal vein or its radicals. If it is a major thrombotic event occurring early in life, the main portal vein is occluded leading to EHPVO. If there are repeated microthrombotic events, the small or medium sized venous channels are affected leading to development of NCPF.

From: *Clinical Gastroenterology: Portal Hypertension*
Edited by: A. J. Sanyal and V. H. Shah © Humana Press Inc., Totowa, NJ

Table 1

Common Causes of Noncirrhotic Portal Hypertension

Extra hepatic portal venous obstruction (EHPVO)
Noncirrhotic portal fibrosis (NCPF) or idiopathic portal hypertension (IPH)
Nodular regenerative hyperplasia
Partial nodular transformation
Congenital hepatic fibrosis
Schistosomiasis
Peliosis hepatitis

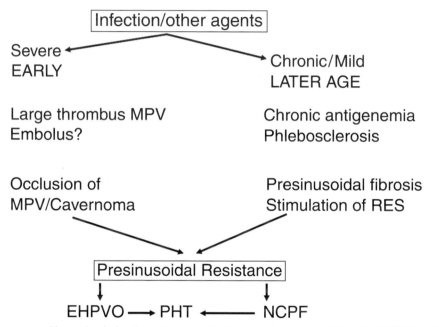

Fig. 1. A proposed hypothesis for the pathogenesis of noncirrhotic portal fibrosis (NCPF) and extra-hepatic portal vein obstruction (EHPVO).

NONCIRRHOTIC PORTAL FIBROSIS (NCFP)

Nomenclature

The first reports of a condition which may now be thought to represent NCPF were published in late 19th century by Banti *(4)*. He described a condition characterized by anemia, congestive splenomegaly with or without gastrointestinal bleed. This clinico-pathologic entity as a cause of portal hypertension was initially recognized in India in the mid-20th century *(5)*. In 1965, Mikkelsen et al. described 36 patients with PHT with-out cirrhosis, who had phlebosclerosis of intra- and extrahepatic portal veins and termed this condition hepatoportal sclerosis *(6)*. Boyer et al. initially used the term idiopathic portal hypertension (IPH) for this condition *(7)*. In 1969, a workshop organized by the Indian Council of Medical Research reviewed all available information on this condition and renamed this distinct entity as noncirrhotic portal fibrosis (NCPF) *(8)*. In other parts of the world, including Japan, a somewhat similar entity is termed as IPH *(9,10)*. It is not very clear whether NCPF and IPH are the same disorders described in different populations.

Etiopathogenesis

The pathogenesis of NCPF is not clearly understood. Several hypotheses have been proposed, which may be contributory in variable degree to the genesis of the disease.

INFECTIVE HYPOTHESIS

NCPF is more commonly seen in patients from low socioeconomic strata. Subjects in this stratum receive poor antenatal and perinatal care and have a high incidence of umbilical sepsis, bacterial infections, and diarrheal episodes in infancy and early childhood. Such repetitive insults result in portal pyemia and may lead to small vessel pylephlebitis, resulting in thrombosis, sclerosis, and obstruction of these venous channels. Repeated intraportal injection of killed *Escherichia coli* produce histological lesions similar to those seen in NCPF/IPH in rabbits and dogs *(11–13)*.

EXPOSURE TO TRACE METALS AND CHEMICALS

Chronic ingestion of arsenic has been incriminated in the causation of NCPF *(14)*. Liver biopsy in these patients reveals periportal fibrosis, incomplete septal cirrhosis with or without development of neovascularization within the expanded portal zones, findings similar to those in NCPF. Administration of Fowler's solution, which is rich in arsenic, was reported in 8 of 47 patients admitted with NCPH in one of the studies *(15)*.

The histological picture similar to NCPF has been observed following chronic exposure to vinyl chloride monomers, copper sulfate (vineyard sprayers), protected treatment with methotrexate, hypervitaminosis A, and in renal allograft recipients receiving treatment with 6-mercaptopurine, azathioprine, and corticorteroids *(1,16,17)*.

IMMUNOLOGIC HYPOTHESIS

Immunologic activity directed against small venous radicals has also been investigated. In a study from Japan, endothelial cells of the smaller venous radicals more frequently expressed HLA-DR antigen in IPH than in chronic active hepatitis, cirrhosis, and normal liver *(18)*. In another study from our center, the high frequency of HLA-DR3 was found in subjects with NCPF *(19)*. These data raise the possibility that the smaller venous radicles in the small- and medium-sized portal tracts are targets of immunologic attack in idiopathic portal hypertension.

Other evidence supporting an immunologic hypothesis is (a) reduction in the suppressor/cytotoxic T lymphocytes in NCPF patients; (b) reduced T4:T8 ratio *(20)*; (c) poor autologous mixed lymphocyte reaction (MLR) *(21)*; (d) frequent association of IPH (Japan) with autoimmune disorders *(22,23)*.

Pathology

In NCPF, liver size may be normal to enlarged. The surface is smooth but it may be nodular in 10–15% of the cases *(26)*. This variant assumes special significance as these patients have deranged liver function tests (LFTs) in contrast with most of the patients with NCPF *(26)*. The portal vein and its branches are prominent and have sclerosed walls. Autopsy series show thrombosis in the medium and small (diameter < 300 mcm) portal vein branches *(21,22)*.

Table 2
Liver Histology in IPH

Parameter	Frequency
Dense portal fibrosis and portal venous obliteration	
Mild	48
Moderate to severe	52
Portal Inflammation	47
Irregular intimal thickening of portal veins	75–100*
Organizing thrombhic and/or recanalization of portal veins	20–100*
Nodular hyperplasia of parenchyma	40
Abnormal blood vessels in lobules	75
Intra lobular fibrous septa	95
Subcapsular atrophy	70
Periductal fibrosis of interlobular bile ducts	50

Modified from Nakanuma et al. *(25)* based on study of 66 patients with IPH.
*100% abnormalities were in autopsy specimens.

Histology of NCPF has been aptly described as obliterative portovenopathy of liver *(24)*. There is marked but patchy and segmental subendothelial thickening of the large- and medium-sized branches of the portal vein. Table 2 describes the histologic findings described in NCPF/IPH *(25)*. The intimal thickening of intrahepatic portal venous channels, associated with obliteration of small portal venules and emergence of new aberrant vessels is characteristic feature of NCPF. Subgroup of patients with nodular transformation have extensive subhepatic and portal fibrosis *(26)*. Rarely, progression of NCPF/IPH to incomplete septal cirrhosis (ISC) has been reported. ISC, characterized by slender incomplete fibrous septae from inconspicuous nodules, may represent a late manifestation of NCPF *(27–29)*.

Hemodynamics

The intrasplenic and portal vein pressures are markedly elevated in patients with NCPF. The wedged hepatic venous pressure (WHVP) may be normal or slightly elevated in about half the patients. Two sites of obstruction (Fig. 2) have been identified; a pressure gradient between the spleen (intrasplenic pressure, ISP) and the liver (intrahepatic pressure, IHP), and between the liver and WHVP (IHP–WHVP) (Fig. 3) *(30,31)*. Intravariceal pressure in NCPF has been found to be comparable to that in cirrhotic PHT *(30–32)*.

Clinical Features

NCPF is a disease of young patients affecting them in the third and fourth decade of life. It is more commonly seen people of lower socioeconomic background. Most of the studies from India show a slight male preponderance *(30,33,34)*. However, one center from north India has consistently reported a female preponderance *(35,36)*, as is seen in IPH reported from Japan. Patients present with one or more episodes of gastrointestinal hemorrhage, mass in the left upper quadrant (splenomegaly) and consequences of hypersplenism (Table 3) *(37)*. Of all the causes of PHT, massive splenomegaly is most com-

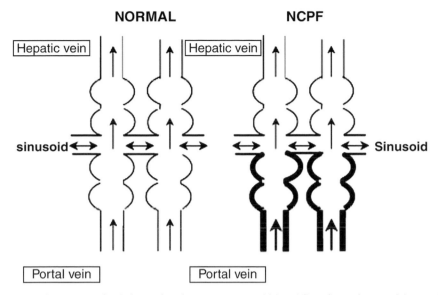

Fig. 2. The patho-anatomical sites of resistance to portal blood flow in patients with noncirrhotic portal fibrosis (NCPF), the presinusoidal and perisinusoidal, caused by thickening and obstruction to the medium and small branches of portal veins and the collagenization of the Space of Disse, respectively.

monly seen in NCPF. Like cirrhosis, NCPF may have atypical presentation like glomerulonephritis *(38)* or hypoxemia *(39).*

NCPF patients generally have preserved liver function tests, including semiquantitative tests of liver function such as monoethylglycinexylidide (MEGX) extraction *(40).* However, the nodular variant of NCPF, which constitutes nearly 10% of these patients, may present with jaundice, mild ascites, and low albumin *(26).* Anemia is a common finding in a majority of these patients, usually microcytic, hypochronic (due to gastrointestinal blood loss). Patients may have evidence of hypersplenism in the form of normocytic, normochromic anemia, leukopenia (<4,000/mm^3) and thrombocytopenia (<50,000/mm^3). Asymptomatic hypersplenism is quite common in NCPF, in contrast, symptomatic disease is very rare *(41).* Coagulation and platelet function abnormailites have been observed in NCPF patients (Table 4) *(42,43).* Autonomic dysfunction has been increasingly observed in cirrhosis. We have recently observed these anomalies in NCPF patients as well *(44).*

Diagnosis

The diagnostic criteria for NCPF are (1) splenomegaly; (2) normal or near normal liver function tests; (3) varices on UGI endoscopy (seen in 85–95% cases); (4) patent portal and hepatic veins; (5) normal or mildly elevated WHVP; and (6) no evidence of cirrhosis on liver biopsy. A doppler ultrasound abdomen would show typically dilated portal vein (Fig. 4) with massively increased spleen size and presence of splenorenal and other shunts (Fig. 5), as well as a dilated paraumbilical vein. Raised portal venous pressure can only be measured direct catheterization of portal vein, which can only be achieved by percutaneous transhepatic route. The other way is to measure indirectly by splenic

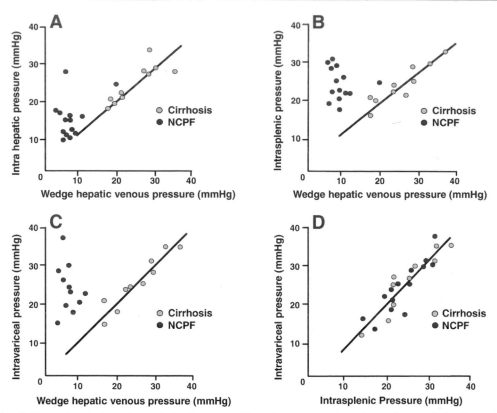

Fig. 3. Hemodynamics of noncirrhotic portal fibrosis, a comparison to cirrhosis of the liver. (a) Correlation of wedged hepatic venous pressure (WHVP) with intrahepatic pressure; (b) Correlation of WHVP with intrasplenic pressure; (c) Correlation of WHVP with intravariceal pressure; (d) Intrasplenic pressure and intravariceal pressure. The latter correlates well with the intrasplenic pressure and is, therefore, recommended as the single hemodynamic measurement for patients with NCPF.

Table 3
Profile of NCPF and EHPVO Patients: G.B. Pant Hospital Experience

Parameter	NCPF ($n = 207$)	EHPVO ($n = 236$)
Mean age, years	30.7	13.9
Male:Female	117:90	168:68
Hemetemesis/melena (%)	84.5	94.5
Mass in LUQ (%)	13.5	3.5
Ascites (transient) (%)	10	12.7
Jaundice (%)	—	12.7
Liver functions tests	Near normal	Near normal
Esophageal varices (%)	92	94
Gastric varices (%)	22.3	40.7
Portal gastropathy		
Presclerotherapy (%)	1.6	0.5
Postsclerotherapy (%)	17	15
Portal biliopathy (%)	40	90
Portal colopathy (%)	40	44

Table 4
Coagulation and Platelet function in Noncirrhotic Portal Hypertension

Parameter (Normal Range)	NCPF (n = 18)	EHPVO (n = 18)
International Normalized Ratio (INR)	1.8 ± 0.68	1.7 ± 0.4*
Partial thromboplastin time (28–31 s)	29 ± 4.2	30 ± 4.2*
Fibrinogen (250–350 mg%)	196 ± 57**	199 ± 61**
Fibrinogen degradation products (<8 µg/mL)	<8	>8**
Platelet aggregation (40–60%)	33 ± 16.5	22 ± 11.3**
Platelet malondialdehyde (MDA) (6–12 nmol/mL)	9.0 ± 3.6	9.6 ± 3.8

*$p < 0.05$ w.r.t. controls.
**$p < 0.001$ w.r.t. controls.

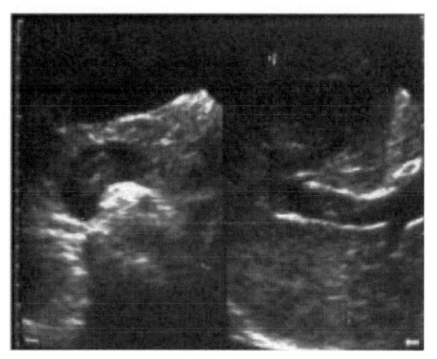

Fig. 4. Ultrasound showing thrombus in the left branch of portal vein in a patient with noncirrhotic portal fibrosis.

puncture for splenic pulp pressure or hepatic puncture for hepatic pressure. A liver biopsy reveals absence of cirrhosis with other findings detailed previously.

Treatment and Prognosis

As the liver function is relatively well preserved, the major cause of death is variceal bleeding. Accordingly, the management of NCPF revolves around control of bleeding. For acutely bleeding patients, endoscopic variceal ligation (EVL) and endoscopic sclerotherapy (EST) are equally efficacious (95% success in control of acute bleed) *(45)*.

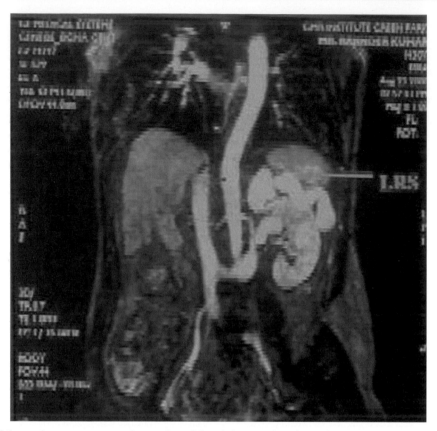

Fig. 5. Magnetic resonance angiography of the abdomen showing a large spontaneous shunt in a patient with noncirrhotic portal fibrosis.

Emergency shunt surgery is required in less than 5% of cases. The modes of prevention of rebleed in these patients are β-blockers and variceal obliteration by EVL. There are anecdotal case reports of response to propranolol in NCPH patients. The only controlled trial of β-blockers in NCPH patients is in patients of schistosomiasis *(46)*. In a recently concluded trial from our center (*Digestive Disease and Sciences,* accepted), the rate of rebleed in NCPH patients was significantly lower on EVL as compared to propranolol and ISMN combination. Primary prophylaxis variceal bleeding in NCPH patients is desirable, as >95% of them have variceal hemorrhage sometime in the course of their disease. Again, the options are β-blockers and variceal obliteration. In our recently reported experience of primary prophylaxis using β blocker or EVL, both the modalities were found to be comparable and efficacious even in noncirrhotic patients *(47)*. Some surgeons, especially from Japan, prefer a prophylactic decompressive surgery for portal decompression in these patients. The risk of operative mortality is very low as liver function is well preserved. However, there are no controlled trials comparing between repeated EVL and prophylactic surgery as the primary management of these patients.

The other complication that needs intervention in NCPH patients is hypersplenism. The usual treatment offered to these patients is splenectomy with possibly a proximal splenorenal shunt. The other options like partial splenic artery embolization have not been systematically studied in these patients.

The prognosis of these patients is excellent. The mortality from acute bleed in NCPH is significantly lower than that observed in cirrhotic patients. After successful eradication of esohagogastric varices, a 2- and 5-yr survival of 100% has been observed in these patients.

EXTRAHEPATIC PORTAL VEIN OBSTRUCTION (EHPVO)

Definition

EHPVO, a common cause of major upper gastrointestinal bleeding in children, is defined as obstruction in the portal vein, usually caused by a thrombus. The entire length of the portal vein is usually occluded with extension into the splenic vein and sometimes into the upper portion of the superior mesenteric vein. In a small proportion, only the terminus of the portal vein at the hepatic hilum is occluded *(48)*. The most common site of a block is at the portal vein formation (90%), and total block of the splenoportal axis is seen in only 10% *(49)*. Isolated thrombosis of splenic vein without portal vein involvement is not included in this disease. Portal vein thrombosis (PVT) commonly occurs as a complication in cirrhotics, but is usually asymptomatic and is not included in the definition of EHPVO.

Etiology and Pathogenesis

The etiopathogenesis of occlusion of the portal vein is obscure in approx 50% of patients *(50–53)*. The known causes of portal vein obstruction can be divided into three main categories: Patients with underlying cirrhosis or hepatocellular carcinoma deserve special mention.

CONDITIONS THAT LEAD TO PORTAL VEIN INJURY

These conditions directly lead to portal vein injury and subsequent obstruction. These include omphalitis, umbilical vein catheterization, neonatal peritonitis, abdominal trauma, iatrogenic operative trauma to the portal vein, and cysts and tumors encroaching upon the portal vein within the porta hepatis. The most common neonatal and childhood causes of EHPVO are omphalitis and intraabdominal sepsis *(50–52,54)*. Although, several investigators believe that umbilical vein cannulation and umbilical sepsis are responsible for PVT *(50,55)*, others disagree *(56,57)*.

DEVELOPMENTAL ANOMALIES

Rare anomalies such as portal vein stenosis, portal vein atresia, or agenesis constitute this category. Obstruction can occur anywhere along the line of left and right vitelline veins from which the portal vein develops. The hypothesis of the congenital origin of EHPVO is supported by the presence of other congenital defects, usually of the cardiovascular system *(50,58,59)*.

FACTORS INDIRECTLY ASSOCIATED WITH PORTAL VEIN THROMBOSIS

This subgroup includes conditions such as neonatal systemic sepsis from nonintraabdominal sources, dehydration, multiple exchange transfusions, and hypercoagulable states. The latter includes myeloproliferative disorders such as polycythemia vera, inherited deficiencies of natural anticoagulants such as antithrombin III, protein C and protein S, activated protein C resistance (APCR), and prothrombin gene (G20210A) mutation. Underlying prothrombotic states have been conclusively shown to predispose to EHPVO

Table 5
Frequency of Hypercoagulable States in Patients with Extrahepatic Portal Vein Obstruction

Characteristics	Valla et al. (1988)	Denninger et al. (1997)	Sexias et al. (1997)	Mahmoud et al. (1997)	Chaomouard et al. (2000)	Egesel et al. (2000)	Jansen et al. (2000)
Number of patients	33	46	20	32	10	23	92
Factor V leiden mutation	NE	9	0	3	10	30	8
Prothrombin gene mutation	NE	NA	NE	NE	40	NE	3
Protein C deficiency	NE	NA	NE	NE	NE	26	7
Protein S deficiency	NE	NA	NE	NE	NE	43	2
Antithrombin III deficiency	NE	NA	NE	NE	NE	26	1
Myeloproliferative disorders	12	24	NE	NE	NE	NE	17

(Table 5) *(60–67)*. The prothrombotic mutations create an inherited predisposition for PVT, and overt thrombosis develops once a thrombotic stimulus such as infection, use of oral contraceptives, pregnancy, abdominal surgery, or myeloproliferative disease is superimposed.

CIRRHOSIS AND OTHER CAUSES

In adults, cirrhosis has long been considered a major cause of PVT. Cirrhosis has been present in 24–32% of patients with PVT *(73)*. The reported incidence of PVT in cirrhotic patients varies widely from 0.6% to 17%. The pathogenesis of PVT in patients with cirrhosis is uncertain, although it has been suggested that decreased portal blood flow and the presence of periportal lymphangitis and fibrosis in these patients promotes the formation of thrombus. The other principal cause of PVT in adults is neoplastic disease. Pancreatic cancer and hepatocellular carcinoma constitute majority of these cases. PVT may occur as a consequence of direct invasion of the portal vein by tumor, extrinsic compression, or periportal fibrosis following surgery or radiotherapy. A hypercoagulable state secondary to malignancy may further predispose these patients to develop PVT. Infection is also an important cause of PVT in adults, although much less common than in children. In adults, the reported etiologies include intraabdominal sepsis, biliary tract disease, pylephlebitis, subacute bacterial endocarditis, postoperative infection and abdominal wound infections *(68)*. Intraabdominal inflammatory diseases also may precipitate PVT in the absence of infection. Pancreatitis is the most common inflammatory disease, others include cholecystitis, alcoholic hepatitis, and appendicitis.

Pathology

Liver pathology is not very characteristic. Macroscopic appearance varies from normal to finely granular surface. The architectural pattern is preserved, concentric condensation of reticulin fibers around portal tracts is seen, which could form septae extending into the parenchyma *(69)*. Such periportal fibrosis could arise from an extension of the extrahepatic thrombophlebitic process into the intrahepatic radicals of the portal vein or chemical irritation as a result of hepatocellular breakdown products or bile imbibition.

The characteristic abnormality in patients with EHPVO is cavernomatous transformation of the portal vein. The portal vein is made up of a cluster of different-sized vessels arranged haphazardly within a connective tissue support, and the original portal vein is not identifiable. Phlebothrombosis of intrahepatic portal vein branches, although much less common than in NCPF, is a common pathogenic denominator in NCPF and EHPVO *(70)*.

Hemodynamics

The level of block in EHPVO patients is presinusoidal and most likely prehepatic. Wedged hepatic venous pressure is normal and intrasplenic pressure is significantly elevated *(71)*. Intravariceal pressure closely represents the portal and intrasplenic pressure. The hepatic blood flow is normal or decreased *(69,71)*. Portoportal collateral vessels bypassing the obstructed area and hepatic artery buffer response contribute to the hepatic blood flow in these patients. Systemic vascular resistance is significantly lower, and cardiac output is significantly higher in patients with EHPVO, indicating a hyperkinetic circulatory state *(71)*. It is suggested that extensive portal–systemic venous collateral circulation may be responsible for this state. Cardiovascular autonomic reflexes have been shown to be impaired in EHPVO patients *(44,72)*. The role of autonomic nervous dysfunction in the pathogenesis of characteristic hemodynamic disturbances of portal hypertension is controversial.

Clinical Features

Patients with EHPVO may present from 6 wk to adulthood, with varied manifestations. The precipitating condition influences the clinical presentation of PVT. The most common presentation is of a child with well-tolerated variceal bleeding and splenomegaly. Cirrhotic patients with PVT also tend to experience variceal hemorrhage, but tolerate the bleed poorly with deterioration of liver function, intractable ascites, encephalopathy, and even death. On the other hand, patients with underlying malignant disease are less likely to survive long enough to develop the complication of variceal bleed as a result of PVT. Finally, in a subset of patients, clinical features of acute PVT develop such as progressive ascites, abdominal pain, and intestinal ischemia.

The common presentations in infancy are variceal bleeding, ascites, and growth failure. Later in childhood and early adult life, variceal bleeding, growth retardation, and hypersplenism are the main presenting clinical problems. Persistent anemia, abdominal pain, and thrombocytopenia caused by splenomegaly are common. Sometimes, incidentally detected splenomegaly may be the only manifestation. Rare problems seen in adults with PVT include venous infarction of the intestines, massive hemobilia, and pulmonary emboli. Ascites, which is high gradient, is usually transient, following hemorrhage or surgery. Ten to fifteen percent of EHPVO patients develop ascites sometime during the course of the disease *(50,74)*. EHPVO patients very often develop significant growth retardation. It has been attributed to reduced portal blood supply to the liver and deprivation of hepatotrophic hormones regulating liver growth and function *(75)*. Resistance to the action of growth hormone is also suggested as a possible cause *(76)*.

Jaundice may rarely be a presenting feature of portal vein occlusion and is most often caused by portal biliopathy. Portal biliopathy, which refers to abnormalities of the extrahepatic and intrahepatic bile ducts and gallbladder wall in patients with portal hypertension,

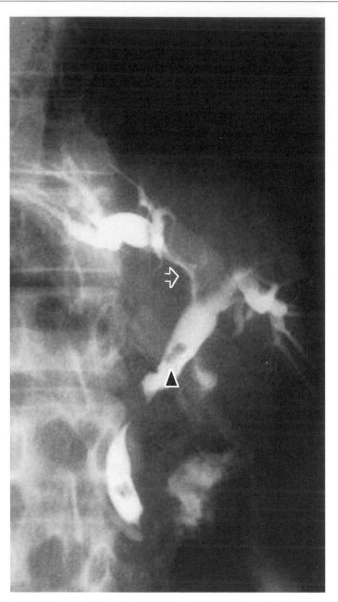

Fig. 6. ERCP showing portal biliopathic changes with common bile duct stones (*arrowhead*) and left hepatic duct stricture (*open arrow*).

is seen in 80–100% of patients with EHPVO (Fig. 6) *(77–81)*. The biliary abnormalities may be explained either by compression of bile ducts by prominent paracholedochal and epicholedochal collateral vessels (indentations and wall irregularities) or ischemic injury of the bile ducts as a result of thrombosis of veins draining the bile duct (stricture formation). Although biliary abnormalities have been reported in 80–100% of cases, only a few patients present with jaundice or pain. Symptomatic patients are usually adults, indicating that portal biliopathy develops in patients with long-standing disease. The presence of increased alkaline phosphatase (usually two to five times the upper limit of normal

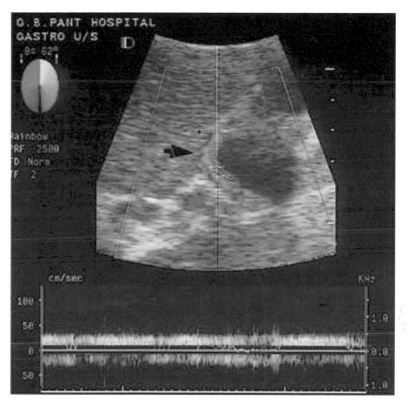

Fig. 7. Ultrasonogram showing gallbladder varices (*arrow*).

for age) could help in the selection of patients for workup for portal biliopathy. Gallbladder varices (Fig. 7) were observed in 34% of patients, and they appear as tortuous, dilated vessels in or around the wall of the gallbladder or in the bed of the gallbladder fossa. These varices do not alter gallbladder contractility *(82)*.

Abnormalities in prothrombin time, partial thromboplastin time, and platelet function have been reported in a few studies *(83–85)*. It may result from mild compensated disseminated intravascular coagulation secondary to portosystemic shunting. Splenomegaly is the second most common initial manifestation of EHPVO and eventually develops in almost all patients. Mild hypersplenism as manifested by thrombocytopenia and leukopenia, is seen in 40–80% of patients and raises the issue of splenectomy, even prior to variceal bleeding. Humoral immunity is normal in patients with EHPVO whereas it is grossly abnormal in cirrhotics. Cell-mediated immunity shows qualitatively similar defects in patients with EHPVO and chronic liver disease *(86–88)*. The defects in cell-mediated immunity result in part from sequestration of T cells by the spleen and partly from the presence in serum of factors that influence the kinetics of lymphocyte response.

Esophageal varices are seen in 90–95% and gastric varices in about 35–40% of patients with EHPVO. The frequency of isolated gastric varices is about 6%. The frequency of portal hypertensive gastropathy (PHG) is low in EHPVO patients as compared to cirrhotics. Bleeding is rarely seen as a result of PHG. Anorectal varices are significantly more frequent in patients with EHPVO than in patients with cirrhosis and NCPF. They are

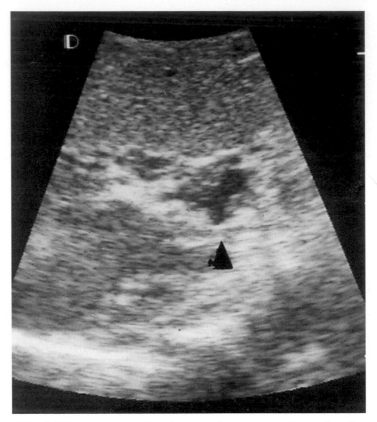

Fig. 8. Ultrasonogram showing portal cavernoma (*arrowhead*).

observed in 80–90% of cases. They rarely bleed (incidence 0.5–10%), but when bleeding does occur, it usually is massive and life threatening.

Diagnosis

As described previously, liver function tests are generally normal in young patients with EHPVO. However, in patients with long-standing disease, synthetic dysfunction in the form of deranged prothrombin time and reduction in serum albumin level has been observed. The gold standard for diagnosis of EHPVO is Doppler ultrasound examination of the upper abdomen. A fresh thrombus within the portal vein can be identified as an echogenic material within the lumen. Cavernous transformation of the portal vein (Fig. 8) produces a distinctive tangle of tortuous vessels in the porta hepatis.

Splenoportography (Fig. 9) or arterial portography provides good images of the portal venous system to permit identification of the site of obstruction, extent of obstruction, location and extent of collateral circulation, but are rarely performed these days. Doppler ultrasonography has largely replaced these investigations. The other techniques include computed tomographic (CT) arterial portography, CT percutaneous transsplenic portography, iv CT portography, magnetic resonance (MR) studies, and MR angiography of the upper abdomen. These investigations (MR angiography, CT portogram, or angiography) are performed only if Doppler is of suboptimal quality.

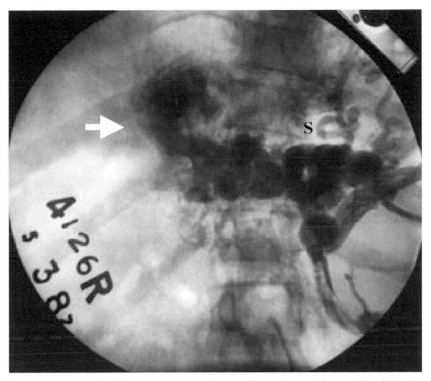

Fig. 9. Splenoportogram showing cavernomatous transformation of the portal vein (*white arrow*). *S,* splenic vein; *I,* inferior mesenteric vein.

Treatment

The management of variceal bleeding and hypersplenism is similar to that detailed in NCPF. A few issues especially important in the management of EHPVO patients are portal biliopathy and growth retardation. Another aspect, which has recently gained importance, is anticoagulation for recent portal vein thrombosis.

Endoscopic therapy is the first line of treatment for variceal bleeding, failing which surgical shunt is required. EST and EVL are effective in the control of acute esophageal variceal bleeding in 90–95% of patients. Most of the acute bleeds can be controlled by endoscopic means alone. Secondary prophylaxis is possible with either β-blockers or EVL/EST. Endoscopic methods also achieve variceal obliteration in 80–90% of patients *(89–93).* The beneficial effect of β-blockers on gastrointestinal bleeding in EHPVO patients has not been tested conclusively in clinical trials. The question of primary prophylaxis of variceal bleeding in EHPVO patients is yet unanswered, but is logically desirable, as 90–95% of these patients have variceal hemorrhage in their lifetime. In addition to endoscopic variceal obliteration, β-blockers are also an option for that. We have recently reported that both the modalities are equally efficacious in EHPVO patients, although the number of patients was small *(47).* However, endoscopic therapy, especially EST, carries a risk of extension of the thrombus into the splenic or mesenteric vein because of flow of the sclerosant into the collateral vessels. Furthermore, variceal obliteration alone without alleviation of portal hypertension cannot ameliorate anorectal varices and ectopic varices, promote normal growth, or prevent the development of portal biliopathy.

Surgery is primarily indicated in patients with variceal bleeding who fail to respond to endoscopic management. Also, patients with ectopic variceal and/or portal hypertensive gastropathy bleeding or portal biliopathy may require surgery. Emergency surgery for control of acute bleeding is usually a devascularisation procedure. Elective surgical procedure is a portosystemic shunt, which may be selective or total. The main problems with a shunt are a high rebleeding rate after surgery, mortality, and a risk of hepatic encephalopathy. Recent surgical series have shown a rebleeding rate of 2–11%, with mortality rates of 0–2% (95–97). Shunts (except mesocaval) cannot be performed in patients who have extensive thrombosis of the whole splenoportal axis. Moreover, a theoretical risk of ongoing thrombosis is there, especially in patients with prothrombotic states. Hypersplenism is rarely severe enough to require specific treatment. Only patients with spontaneous ecchymosis or bleeding/severe anemia requiring blood transfusions merit treatment for hypersplenism. Selective, as well as total, shunts result in a reduction in the spleen volume and an increase in the platelet count postoperatively. Other therapies like partial splenic embolization and teletherapy (splenic irradiation with cobalt 60) has not been evaluated in EHPVO patients with hypersplenism.

Symptomatic portal biliopathy is a definite indication for intervention as if obstruction remains unrelieved, there is a risk of secondary biliary cirrhosis. Portosystemic shunting with/without hepaticojejunostomy is required as a definitive procedure (98). The role of surgery in overcoming growth retardation remains to be confirmed, but a few studies have shown increase in growth velocity in EHPVO patients after a portosystemic shunt.

ANTICOAGULATION IN PVT

Once the role of prothrombotic disorders was recognized in the pathogenesis of PVT, it led to the suggestion that long-term anticoagulation might prevent both extension of thrombosis in the splanchnic veins and thrombosis in other deep veins. The most convincing evidence in favor of anticoagulation in cases of PVT in noncirrhotic population arises from a study by Condat et al. (99). They showed that anticoagulant therapy in these patients did not increase the risk or the severity of bleeding, whereas underlying prothrombotic state and absence of anticoagulant therapy were independent predictors for thrombosis. Although the results are preliminary and unconfirmed by further studies, they raise a possibility of anticoagulation in these patients. The same group also has reported recanalization of recent PVT (101). There are a few anecdotal reports of anticoagulation in cirrhotics with PVT (100), but already deranged liver functions and high risk of subsequent bleed preclude its routine use in cirrhotic patients. Acute PVT can be treated by thrombolysis (102), by removal of the thrombus through the transjugular route (103). Patients with signs of intestinal infarction require laparotomy with excision of any necrotic bowel.

NODULAR REGENERATIVE HYPERPLASIA (NRH) AND PARTIAL NODULAR TRANSFORMATION

Both nodular regenerative hyperplasia (NRH) and partial nodular transformation are rare disorders of poorly understood etiologies. Among series with noncirrhotic portal hypertension, NRH was responsible for 27% of the patients in Europe (104) and 14% in Japan (25). Although NRH has been found in 0.7–2.6% of all autopsies (105,110), only a minority of the patients have evidence of portal hypertension. The most frequent presentation is with variceal bleeding and/or symptoms of hypersplenism. Few patients may have ascites. In NRH, 1–2 mm nodules of regenerating hepatocytes are seen diffusely scttered in the liver, compressing the intervening parenchyma and, hence, causing portal hypertension. These nodules do not have surrounding fibrous septae. Reticulin staining shows micronodularity with maintained acinar structure and shows atrophy in the center of the liver with crowding caused by regenerative activity at the periphery *(104)*. NRH seems to be vascular in origin, the characteristic feature being the presence of obliterative lesions in small portal veins *(105,106)*. Patients with partial nodular transformation have large regenerative nodules near the hepatic hilum. A new classification of nodular transformation is proposed that encompasses the spectrum of lesions described previously as focal nodular hyperplasia and partial nodular transformation. The major conclusion is that NRH is a secondary and nonspecific tissue adaptation to heterogeneous distribution of blood flow and does not represent a specific entity *(107)*.

Treatment is mainly directed at portal hypertension and the usual measures including endoscopic treatment, β-blockers, surgical shunt, and TIPS provide satisfactory results. Portocaval shunting can be done but this can lead to severe encephalopathy requiring shunt closure and even hepatic failure necessitating liver transplantation *(108)*. The prognosis of these patients is generally good if variceal obliteration can be achieved. However, progressive course with hepatic decompensation leading to OLT has been described *(109)*

CONGENITAL HEPATIC FIBROSIS (CHF)

CHF, an autosomal reccesive disease, presents in late childhood with hepatomegaly, portal hypertension in the form of variceal bleeding, and normal liver function tests. The liver is enlarged and firm, with a fine reticular pattern of portal fibrosis. It is characterized by diffuse periportal fibrosis of varied thickness. There are numerous ectatic bile ducts in an interrupted circular arrangement (ductal plate malformation). Portal hypertension is caused by presinusoidal obstruction. As LFTs are normal, variceal bleds are well tolerated. Congenital hepatic fibrosis may be associated with Caroli's disease, adult polycystic kidney disease, and choledochal cysts.

In summary, patients suffering from NCPH, be it caused by NCPF or IPH or EHPVO have significant portal hypertension with near normal hepatic parenchymal function. Whereas in NCPF patients, variceal obliteration suffices in EHPVO patients, subsequent development of gastric or ecotopic varices, portal biliopathy, growth retardation, and slow hepatic dysfunction do reduce the overall survival. There is a need to identify the precise etiopathogensis and natural history of these diseases to reduce their incidence and improve the management.

REFERENCES

1. Sarin SK, Kapoor D. Non-cirrhotic portal fibrosis: current concepts and management. J Gastroenterol Hepatol 2002;17:526–534.
2. Sama SK, Bhargawa S, Gopi Nath N, et al. Non-cirrhotic portal fibrosis. Am J Med 1971;51:160–169.
3. Sarin SK, Sachdev Group, Nanda R. Follow-up of patients after variceal eradication. A comparison of patients with cirrhosis, non-cirrhotic portal fibrosis and extrahepatic obstruction. Ann Surg 1986; 202:78–82.
4. Banti G. Splenomegalic mit Leberzirrhose. Beitrage sur pathologischen. Anat allgemeinen Pathol 1889;24:21–33.
5. Mikkelsen WP, Edmondson HA, Peters RL, Redekar AG, Reynolds TB. Extra and intrahepatic portal hypertension without cirrhosis (hepatoportal sclerosis). Ann Surg 1965;162:602–620.

6. Ramalingaswamy B, Wig KL, Sama SK. Cirrhosis of liver in northern India. A clinicopathologic study. Arch Intern Med 1962;110:350–358.

7. Boyer JL, Sengupta KP, Biswas SK, et al. Idiopathic portal hypertension: comparison with portal hypertension of cirrhosis and extrahepatic portal vein obstruction. Ann Intern Med 1967;66:41–68.

8. Proceeding of the workshop on non-cirrhotic portal fibrosis. Indian Council of Medical Research, New Delhi, India, 1969.

9. Kobayashi Y, Inokuchi K, Saku M. Epidemiology of idiopathic portal hypertension based on a nationwide survey. In: Suguira M, ed. Report of the Ministry of Health and Welfare Research Committee on Idiopathic Portal Hypertension. Japan Ministry of Health and Welfare, Tokyo, Japan, 1976, pp. 10–15.

10. Okuda K, Kono K, Onishi K, Kimura K, Omata M, Koen H. Clinical study of eighty-six cases of idiopathic portal hypertension and comparison with cirrhosis with splenomegaly. Gastroenterology 1984;86:600–608.

11. Sugita S, Ohnishi K, Saito M, Okuda K. Splanchnic hemodynamics in portal hypertensive dogs with portal fibrosis. Am J Physiol Gastrointest Liver Physiol 1987;252:G748–G754.

12. Kohno K, Ohnishi K, Omata M, et al. Experimental portal fibrosis produced by intraportal injection of killed nonpathogenic Escherichia coli in rabbits. Gastroenterology 1988;94:787–796.

13. Kathayat R, Pandey GK, Malhotra V, Omanwar S, Sharma BK, Sarin SK. Rabbit model of non-cirrhotic portal fibrosis with repeated immunosensitization by rabbit splenic extract. J Gastroenterol Hepatol 2002;17:1312–1316.

14. Guha Mazumdar DN, Gupta JD Das. Arsenic and non-cirrhotic portal hypertension. J Hepatol 1991; 13:376.

15. Nevens F, Fevery J, Steenbergen Van W, et al. Arsenic and non-cirrhotic portal hypertension. A report of eight cases. J Hepatol 1990;11:80–85.

16. Pimentel JC, Menezes AP. Liver disease in vineyard sprayers. Gastroenterology 1977;72:275–283.

17. Thomas LB, Popper H, Berk PD, Selikoff I, Falk H. Vinyl-chloride-induced liver disease. From idiopathic portal hypertension (Banti's syndrome) to Angiosarcomas. N Engl J Med 1975;292:17–22.

18. Terada T, Nakanuma Y, Hoso M, Obata H. Expression of HLA-DR antigen on hepatic vascular endothelial cells in idiopathic portal hypertension. Clin Exp Immunol 1991;84:303–307.

19. Sarin SK, Mehra NK, Agarwal A, Malhotra V, Anand BS, Taneja V. Familial aggregation in non-cirrhotic portal fibrosis: a report of four families. Am J Gastroenterol 1987;82:1130–1133.

20. Nayyar AK, Sharma BK, Sarin SK, et al. Characterization of peripheral blood lymphocytes in patients with non-cirrhotic portal fibrosis: a comparison with cirrhotics and healthy controls. J Gastroenterol Hepatol 1990;5:554–559.

21. Okuda K, Obata H. Idiopathic portal hypertension (hepatoportal sclerosis). In: Okuda K, Benhamou JP, eds. Portal Hypertension. Clinical and Physiological Aspects. Springer, Tokyo, 1992, pp. 271–287.

22. Nakanuma Y, Nonomura A, Hayashi M, et al. Pathology of the liver in "idiopathic portal hypertension" associated with autoimmune disease. Acta Pathol Jpn 1989;39:586–592.

23. Saito K, Nakanuma Y, Takegoshi K, et al. Non-specific immunological abnormalities and association of autoimmune diseases in idiopathic portal hypertension. A study by questionnaire. Hepatogastroenterology 1993;40:163–166.

24. Nayak NC, Ramalingaswamy V. Obliterative portal venopathy of liver. Arch Pathol 1979;87:359–369.

25. Nakanuma Y, Hoso M, Sasaki M, et al. Histopathology of the liver in non-cirrhotic portal hypertension of unknown aetiology. Histopathology 1996;28:195–204.

26. Tandon BN, Nundy Study, Nayak NC. Non-cirrhotic portal hypertension in northern India. Clinical features and liver function tests. In: Okuda K, Omata M, eds. Idiopathic Portal Hypertension. University of Tokyo Press, Tokyo, 1983, pp. 377–386.

27. Bernard PH, Le Bail B, Cransac M, et al. Progression from idiopathic portal hypertension to incomplete septal cirrhosis with liver failure requiring liver transplantation. J Hepatol 1995;22:495–499.

28. Ludwig J, Hashimoto E, Obata H, Baldus WP. Idiopathic portal hypertension: a histopathological study of 26 Japanese cases. Histopathology 1993;22:227–234.

29. Sciot R, Staessen D, Van Damme B, et al. Incomplete septal cirrhosis: histopathological aspects. Histopathology 1988;13:593–603.

30. Sarin SK, Sethi KK, Nanda R. Measurement and correlation of wedged hepatic, intrahepatic, intrasplenic and intravariceal pressure in patients with cirrhosis of liver and non-cirrhotic portal fibrosis. Gut 1987;28:260–266.

31. Ohnishi K, Saito M, Sato S, et al. Portal hemodynamics in idiopathic portal hypertension (Banti's syndrome). Comparison with chronic persistent hepatitis and normal subjects. Gastroenterology 1987; 92:751–758.

32. El Atti EA, Nevens F, Bogaerts K, Verbeke G, Fevery J. Variceal pressure is a strong predictor of variceal haemorrhage in patients with cirrhosis as well as in patients with non-cirrhotic portal hypertension. Gut 1999;45:618–621.

33. Sama SK, Bhargawa S, Gopi Nath N, et al. Non-cirrhotic portal fibrosis. Am J Med 1971;51:160–169.

34. Habibullah CM, Rao GN, Murthy DK, et al. Non-cirrhotic portal fibrosis in Andhra Pradesh. J Assoc Phys Ind 1978;26:379–382.

35. Dhiman RK, Chawla Y, Vasishta RK, et al. Non-cirrhotic portal fibrosis (idiopathic portal hypertension): experience with 151 patients and a review of the literature. J Gastroenterol Hepatol 2002;17: 6–16.

36. Koshy A. Relationship between NCPF and EHO. In: Okuda K, Omata M, eds. Idiopathic Portal Hypertension. University of Tokyo Press, Tokyo, 1982, pp. 13–18.

37. Sarin SK, Agarwal SR. Idiopathic portal hypertension. Digestion 1998;59:420–423.

38. Kumar A, Bhuyan UN, Nundy S. Glomerulonephritis complicating non-cirrhotic portal fibrosis. J Gastroenterol Hepatol 1998;13(Suppl 1):271–275.

39. Babbs C, Warnes TW, Haboubi NY. Non-cirrhotic portal hypertension with hypoxaemia. Gut 1998; 29:129–131.

40. Misra A, Guptan RC, Sarin SK. Monoethylglycinexylidide (MEGX): a sensitive noninvasive method to differentiate NCPF and Child's study A Chronic liver disease. Indian J Gastroenterol 1997;16(Suppl 2):A101.

41. Mehta S, Gondal R, Saxena S, Sarin SK. Profile of hypersplenism in cirrhosis and non-cirrhotic portal hypertension. Hepatology 1994;20:A217.

42. Bajaj JS, Bhattacharjee J, Sarin SK. Coagulation profile and platelet functions in patients with extraheptic portal vein obstruction and non-cirrhotic portal fibrosis and influence of hypersplenism. J Gastroenterol Hepatol 2001;16:641–646.

43. Sheth SG, Deo AM, Bichile SK, Amarapurkar DN, Chopra KB, Mehta PJ. Coagulation abnormalities in non-cirrhotic portal fibrosis and extra hepatic portal vein obstruction. J Assoc Physicians India 1996;44:790,791.

44. Rangari M, Sinha S, Kapoor D, Mohan JC, Sarin SK. Prevalence of autonomic dysfunction in cirrhotic and noncirrhotic portal hypertension. Am J Gastroenterol 2002;97:707–713.

45. Sarin SK, Govil A, Jain AK, et al. Prospective randomized trial of endoscopic sclerotherapy versus variceal band ligation for esophageal varices: influence on gastropathy, gastric varices and variceal recurrence. J Hepatol 1997;26:826–832.

46. Kiire CF. Controlled trial of propranolol to prevent recurrent variceal bleeding in patients with non-cirrhotic portal fibrosis. Br Med J 1989;298:1363–1366.

47. Sarin SK, Lamba GS, Kumar M, Misra A, Murthy NS. Comparison of endoscopic ligation and propranolol for the primary prevention of variceal bleeding. N Engl J Med 1999;340:988–993.

48. Rosch J, Dotter CT. Extrahepatic portal obstruction in childhood and its angiographic diagnosis. Am J Radiol 1981;112:143–149.

49. Mitra SK, Kumar V, Dutta DV. Extrahepatic portal hypertension: a review of 70 cases. J Pediatr Surg 1978;13:51–54.

50. Webb LJ, Sherlock S. The aetiology, presentation and natural history of extra-hepatic portal venous obstruction. Q J Med 1979;192:627–639.

51. Househam KC, Bowie MD. Extrahepatic portal venous obstruction. S Afr Med J 1983;64:234–236.

52. Cardin F, Graffeo M, McCormick PA. Adult "idiopathic" extrahepatic venous thrombosis: importance of putative "latent" myeloproliferative disorders and comparison with cases with known etiology. Dig Dis Sci 1992;37:335–339.

53. Stringer MD, Heaton ND, Karani J. Patterns of portal vein occlusion and their aetiological significance. Br J Surg 1994;81:1328–1331.

54. Maddrey WC, Basu Mallik HC, Iber FL. Extrahepatic portal obstruction of the portal venous system. Surg Gynaecol Obstet 1968;127:989–998.

55. Gibson JB, Johnson GW, Rodgers HW. Extrahepatic portal venous obstruction. Br J Surg 1965;152: 129–139.

56. Guimaraes H, Castelo L, Guimaraes J. Does umbilical vein catheterization to exchange transfusion lead to portal vein thrombosis? Eur J Pediatr 1998;157:461–463.

57. Yadav S, Dutta AK, Sarin SK. Do umbilical vein catheterization and sepsis lead to portal vein thrombosis?—A prospective, clinical and sonographic evaluation. J Pediatr Gastroenterol Nutr 1993;17: 392–396.

58. Alvarez F, Bernard O, Brunelle F. Portal obstruction in children. I. Clinical investigations and hemorrhage risk. J Pediatr 1983;103:696–702.

59. Odievre M, Pige G, Alagille D. Congenital abnormalities associated with extrahepatic portal hypertension. Arch Dis Child 1977;52:383–385.

60. Valla D, Casadevall N, Huisse MG. Myeloproliferative disorders in portal vein thrombosis in adults. Gastroenterology 1988;94:1063–1069.

61. Denninger MH, Helley D, Valla D. Prospective evaluation of the prevalence of factor V Leiden mutation in portal or hepatic vein thrombosis. Thromb Haemost 1997;78:1297–1298.

62. Mahmoud AEA, Elias E, Beauchamp N. Prevalence of the factor V Leiden mutation in hepatic and portal vein thrombosis. Gut 1997;40:798–800.

63. Seixas CA, Hessel G, Ribeiro CC. Factor V Leiden is not common in children with portal vein thrombosis. Thromb Haemost 1997;77:258–226.

64. Chamouard P, Pencreach E, Maloisel F. Frequent factor II G20210A mutation in idiopathic portal vein thrombosis. Gastroenterology 1999;116:144–148.

65. Jansen HLA, Meinardi JR, Vleggaar FP. Factor V Leiden mutation, prothrombin gene mutation, and deficiencies in coagulation inhibitors associated with Budd-Chiari syndrome and portal vein thrombosis: results of a case-control study. Blood 2000;96:2364–2368.

66. Egesel T, Buyukasik Y, Dundar SV. The role of natural anticoagulant deficiencies and factor V Leiden in the development of idiopathic portal vein thrombosis. J Clin Gastroenterol 2000;30:66–71.

67. Mohanty D, Shetty S, Ghosh K, Pawar A, Abraham P. Hereditary thrombophilia as a cause of Budd-Chiari syndrome: a study from Western India. Hepatology 2001;34:666–670.

68. Valla DC, Condat B. Portal vein thrombosis in adults: pathophysiology, pathogenesis and management. J Hepatol 2000;32:865–871.

69. Sengupta KP, Basu Mallik KC, Maddrey WC. Liver changes in extrahepatic portal venous obstruction. Ind J Med Res 1968;56:1643–1650.

70. Mikkelsen WP, Edmondson HA, Peters RL. Extra and intrahepatic portal hypertension without cirrhosis (hepatopetal sclerosis). Ann Surg 1965;162:602–620.

71. Lebrec D, Bataille C, Bercoff E. Hemodynamic changes in patients with portal venous obstruction. Hepatology 1983;3:550–553.

72. Voigt MD, Trey G, Levitt NS. Autonomic neuropathy in extra-hepatic portal vein thrombosis: evidence for impaired autonomic reflex arc. J Hepatol 1997;26:634–641.

73. Okuda K, Ohnishi K, Kimura K. Incidence of portal vein thrombosis in liver cirrhosis. An angiographic study in 708 patients. Gastroenterology 1985;89:279–286.

74. Sarin SK, Agarwal SR. Idiopathic portal hypertension. Digestion 1998;59:420–423.

75. Sarin SK, Bansal A, Sasan S. Portal-vein obstruction in children leads to growth retardation. Hepatology 1992;15:229–233.

76. Mehrotra RN, Bhatia V, Dabadghao P. Extrahepatic portal vein obstruction in children: anthropometry, growth hormone, and insulin-like growth factor 1. J Paediatr Gastroenterol Nutr 1997;25: 520–523.

77. Sarin SK, Bhatia V, Makwane U. "Portal biliopathy" in extrahepatic portal vein obstruction. Ind J Gastroenterol 1992;11:82.

78. Dilawari JB, Chawla YK. Pseudosclerosing cholangitis in extrahepatic portal venous obstruction. Gut 1992;33:272–276.

79. Khuroo MS, Yattoo GN, Zargar SA. Biliary abnormalities associated with extrahepatic portal venous obstruction. Hepatology 1993;17:807–813.

80. Malkan GH, Bhatia SJ, Bashir K. Cholangiopathy associated with portal hypertension: diagnostic evaluation and clinical implications. Gastrointest Endosc 1999;49:344–348.

81. Nagi B, Kochhar R, Bhasin D. Cholangiopathy in extrahepatic portal venous obstruction. Acta Radiol 2000;41:612–615.

82. Chawla A, Dewan R, Sarin SK. The frequency and influence of gallbladder varices on gallbladder functions in patients with portal hypertension. Am J Gastroenterol 1995;90:2010–2014.

83. Sheth SG, Deo AM, Bichile SK. Coagulation abnormalities in non-cirrhotic portal fibrosis and extra hepatic portal vein obstruction. J Assoc Phys Ind 1996;44:790–791.

84. Robson SC, Kahn D, Kruskal J. Disordered hemostasis in extrahepatic portal hypertension. Hepatology 1993;18:853–857.

85. Bajaj JS, Bhattacharjee J, Sarin SK. Coagulation profile and platelet function in patients with extrahepatic portal vein obstruction and non-cirrhotic portal fibrosis. J Gastroenterol Hepatol 2001;16:641–646.

86. Webb LJ, Ross M, Markham RL. Immune function in patients with extrahepatic portal venous obstruction and the effect of splenectomy. Gastroenterology 1980;79:99–103.

87. Robson SC, Saunders RH, Kruskal JB. Immune dysfunction in extrahepatic portal hypertension-identification of immunosuppressive factors. Hepatology 1988;8:1428.

88. Seth A, Yadav S, Sasan S. Systemic and gut mucosal immunity in children with extrahepatic portal vein obstruction. Ind J Gastroenterol 1992;11:81.

89. Kahn D, Terblanche J, Kitane S. Injection sclerotherapy in adults with extrahepatic portal venous obstruction. Br J Surg 1987;74:600–602.

90. Howard ER, Stringer MD, Mowat AP. Assessment of injection sclerotherapy in management of 152 children with esophageal varices. Br J Surg 1988;75:404–408.

91. Dilawari JB, Chawla YK, Ramesh GN. Endoscopic sclerotherapy in children. J Gastroenterol Hepatol 1989;4:155–160.

92. Chawla YK, Dilawari JB, Ramesh GN. Sclerotherapy in extrahepatic portal venous obstruction. Gut 1990;31:213–216.

93. Bhargava DK, Dasarathy S, Sundaram KR. Efficacy of endoscopic sclerotherapy on long-term management of oesophageal varices: a comparative study of results in patients with cirrhosis of the liver, non-cirrhotic portal fibrosis (NCPF) and extrahepatic portal venous obstruction (EHO). J Gastroenterol Hepatol 1991;6:471–475.

94. Yachha SK, Sharma BC, Kumar M. Endoscopic sclerotherapy for esophageal varices in children with extrahepatic portal venous obstruction: a follow-up study. J Pediatr Gastroenterol Nutr 1997;24:49–52.

95. Orloff MJ, Orloff MS, Rambotti M. Treatment of bleeding esophagogastric varices due to extrahepatic portal hypertension: results of portal systemic shunts during 35 years. J Paediatr Surg 1994;29:142–154.

96. Mitra SK, Rao KLN, Narasimhan KL. Side-to-side lienorenal shunt without splenectomy in non-cirrhotic portal hypertension in children. J Pediatr Surg 1993;28:398–402.

97. Prasad SA, Gupta S, Kohli V. Proximal splenorenal shunts for extrahepatic portal venous obstruction in children. Ann Surg 1994;219:193–196.

98. Chaudhary A, Dhar P, Sarin SK. Bile duct obstruction due to portal biliopathy in extrahepatic portal hypertension: surgical management. Br J Surg 1988;85:326–329.

99. Condat B, Pessione F, Hillaire S, et al. Current outcome of portal vein thrombosis in adults: risk and benefit of anticoagulant therapy. Gastroenterology 2001;120:490–497.

100. Romero-Gomez M, Gutierrez-Tous R, Delgado-Mije D. Anticoagulation therapy for recent portal vein thrombosis in a patient with liver cirrhosis suffering from variceal rebleeding. Gastroenterology 2001;120:490–497.

101. Condat B, Pessione F, Helene DM, Hillaire S, Valla D. Recent portal or mesenteric venous thrombosis: increased recognition and frequent recanalization on anticoagulant therapy. Hepatology 2000;32:466–470.

102. Tateishi A, Mitsui H, Oki T, et al. Extensive mesenteric vein and portal vein thrombosis successfully treated by thrombolysis and anticoagulation. J Gastroenterol Hepatol 2001;16:1429–1433.

103. Uflacker R. Applications of percutaneous mechanical thrombectomy in transjugular intrahepatic portosystemic shunt and portal vein thrombosis. Tech Vasc Interv Radiol 2003;6:59–69.

104. Naber AHJ, VanHaelst U, Yap SH. Nodular regenerative hyperplasia of the liver: an important cause of portal hypertension in non-cirrhotic patients. J Hepatol 1990;12:94–99.

105. Wanless IR. Micronodular transformation (nodular regenerative hyperplasia) of the liver: a report of 64 cases among 2.500 autopsies and a new classification of benign hepatocellular nodules. Hepatology 1990;11:787–797.

106. Shimamatsu K, Wanless IR. Role of ischemia in causing apoptosis, atrophy, and nodular hyperplasia in human liver. Hepatology 1997;26:343–350.
107. International Working Party: terminology of nodular hepatocellular lesions. Hepatology 1995;22:983.
108. Blanc JF, Bernard PH, Le Bail B, et al. Vascular pathology of the portal vein distal branches: a rare cause of liver transplantation and a protean clinical presentation. Gastroenterol Clin Biol 2000;24:667–670.
109. Dumortier J, Bizollon T, Scoazec JY, et al. Orthotopic liver transplantation for idiopathic portal hypertension: indications and outcome. Scand J Gastroenterol 2001;36:417–422.
110. Nakanuma Y. Nodular regenerative hyperplasia of the liver: retrospective survey in autopsy series. J Clin Gastroenterol 1990;12:460–465.

26

Hepatic Venous Outflow Obstruction

Budd–Chiari Syndrome and Veno-Occlusive Disease (Sinusoidal Obstruction Syndrome)

Hugo E. Vargas, MD and Thomas D. Boyer, MD

CONTENTS

INTRODUCTION
BUDD–CHIARI SYNDROME (BCS)
SINUSOIDAL OBSTRUCTIVE SYNDROME (SOS)
   (HEPATIC VENO-OCCLUSIVE DISEASE)
REFERENCES

INTRODUCTION

The liver is very susceptible to increases in venous pressure because of its unique architecture. In contrast to most organs, the liver has large endothelial pores and lacks a basement membrane. Thus, any increase in venous pressure leads to the rapid movement of large volumes of fluid from the vascular space into the interstitial space. The ability of the hepatic lymphatics to remove this excess fluid is limited and, therefore, the excess fluid enters the peritoneal cavity. Thus, obstruction to the venous outflow of the liver [Budd–Chiari syndrome (BCS)] presents clinically with signs of congestion of the liver including ascites, hepatomegaly, and right upper quadrant abdominal pain. It is perhaps this typical presentation that has led clinicians over the years to lump together all vascular obstruction into one general classification regardless of the vessels involved. In this chapter, we will make use of recent classifications of hepatic venous obstruction that allow for a better understanding of how each disease causing the BCS is different in its presentation and management. The term BCS will include hepatic vein occlusion, including combined occlusion of the hepatic veins and the vena cava. Hepatic veno-occlusive disease (VOD) also termed sinusoidal occlusion syndrome (SOS) will be considered separately. Cardiac causes of hepatic outflow obstruction will not be considered.

BUDD–CHIARI SYNDROME (BCS)

History of BCS

The first description of large hepatic vein obstruction dates back to George Budd's classic textbook of liver disease, wherein he described four cases of hepatic vein endophlebitis

From: *Clinical Gastroenterology: Portal Hypertension*
Edited by: A. J. Sanyal and V. H. Shah © Humana Press Inc., Totowa, NJ

Table 1
Differences Between HVT and MOVC in BCS

Variable	HVT	MOVC
Epidemiology	More common in West	Developing countries
Etiology	Prothrombotic disorder	Unknown or prothrombotic disorder
Presentation	Acute to chronic with hepatomegaly and ascites	More insidious with hepatomegaly and subcutaneous collaterals
Hepatoma	No increased risk	Common
Histology	Congestion with loss hepatocytes	Congestion with fibrosis or cirrhosis

Adapted from ref. 8.
HVT-hepatic vein thrombosis.
MOVC-membranous obstruction of vena cava.

and thrombosis *(1,2)*. Hans Chiari, an illustrious pathologist then working in Prague, described the pathological changes, linked them to the clinical findings described by Budd before him, and earned his eponymous place in medicine *(3)*. The entity of hepatic venous occlusion was firmly established for modern medicine by a landmark article by Parker *(2,4)*. At that time and as late as the mid-1970s, the prognosis for these cases was uniformly poor *(5)*. This was in part due to the lack of understanding of the etiology of BCS, the inability to make early diagnoses, and the limited experience with surgical techniques to decompress the liver *(2,5)*.

Until recently, the etiology of BCS was unclear. In the early and mid-20th century, as few as 30% of patients diagnosed with BCS had a recognizable etiological factor *(4,5)*. An increasing understanding of myeloproliferative and prothrombotic disorders has led to a better understanding of the etiological factors that lead to BCS. Currently, the cause of BCS can be identified in as many as 75% of patients and two factors may coexist in up to 25% of patients *(6)*.

Definition of BCS

The heterogeneous nature of BCS has resisted efforts by many investigators to rename the entity *(7,8)*. A recent European expert panel proposed that the name BCS be retained because it has been widely used and because it is more succinct than the other proposed names that define the location of the obstructive process. BCS is defined as hepatic venous outflow obstruction at any level from the small hepatic veins to the junction of the inferior vena cava (IVC) and the right atrium, regardless of the cause of obstruction *(6)*. Outflow obstruction caused by SOS or cardiac disease is explicitly excluded *(6)*. Another classification was developed by Okuda et al. *(8)* and Table 1 contains that classification. The advantage of this classification is that the presentation, complications, and therapies differ for the two causes of BCS, i.e., hepatic vein thrombosis (HVT) and membranous obstruction of the vena cava (MOVC).

ETIOLOGY OF BCS

BCS arising from endoluminal blockage of the hepatic veins that originates in the vein is considered *primary* BCS or HVT. HVT is more common in Western countries and is associated with a prothrombotic disorder in most cases. MOVC is more common in the Far East, is associated with the development of hepatocellular carcinoma and has a more

Table 2
Thrombophilias in Patients with BCS

Hematologic disorder	Western countries	India
Myeloproliferative	49.4%	NA
Antiphospholipid	12.5%	11.3%
PNH	1.5%	NA
Factor V Leiden mutation	28.9%	26.4%
Factor II mutation	5.5%	0%
Protein C deficiency	17.4%	13.2%
Protein S deficiency	6.3%	5.7%
Antithrombin deficiency	4.4%	3.8%
Pregnancy	6.4%	11.7%
Oral contraceptives	52.2%	5.9%

Data taken from ref. *20*.
PNH-paroxysmal nocturnal hemoglobinuria.

subacute or chronic presentation as compared to HVT *(8,9)*. *Secondary* BCS refers to hepatic vein occlusion where the obstruction occurs as a result of a process that does not originate in the venous system, such as infiltrating tumor, compression of the vessels by extrinsic mass, parasitic infestation or following liver transplantation *(6,8,9)*.

SEVERITY BCS

The duration of disease or the rate of symptom progression has been used widely, but without consistency to classify BCS. The terms "acute," "subacute," and "chronic" are abundant, yet no consensus exists on the exact timing required for their use. Further confusion is added when the terms "fulminant" and "subfulminant" are used. This terminology needs to be defined carefully, and its application will be dependent on its utility with respect to prognosis and treatment *(6)*. However, despite this lack of clarity, BCS can present with acute hepatic failure or as an indolent disease suggestive of cirrhosis and an awareness of these different presentations is required so that a correct diagnosis can be made quickly.

Etiological Causes of BCS

Beginning with the first descriptions of the BCS in modern medical literature, hematological disorders have frequently been linked with BCS. Notably, polycythemia rubra vera and paroxysmal nocturnal hemoglobinuria have been diagnosed consistently in many patients with HVT *(4,5,10)*. In recent years, the recognition of familial traits that predispose to prothrombotic disorders have been increasingly recognized as an causative factor in HVT *(11–13)*. The association between HVT and the use of prothrombotic therapies, such as oral contraceptives, has been well documented *(13)*. The development of the web lesion in the IVC that causes MOVC is thought to follow thrombosis. The propensity for this lesion to develop near the diaphragm is thought to be related to diaphragmatic movement *(8,20)*. Whereas Indian series report high incidence of thrombophilias, the Japanese and Chinese series have a striking number of idiopathic cases of MOVC *(8,14–19)*. Table 2 outlines the most common single factors that predispose to HVT. Note that because of low prothrombotic potential, often times these factors coexist or are encountered in patients with local factors that lead to BCS *(20)*.

Table 3
Initial Evaluation for the Diagnosis of BCS

Complete medical history	Focus on current medications and presence of a systemic disease
Complete blood count	Bone marrow biopsy, flow cytometry, and determination of total red cell mass if PRV considered
Factor V and prothrombin gene defect analysis	
Antiphospholipid antibodies	
Lupus anticoagulant	
Protein C and protein S levels	May need to take into consideration the presence of hepatic insufficiency
Homocysteine level	There may be a role for MTHFR polymorphism analysis

PRV-polycythemia rubra vera.

Diagnosis of BCS

The numerous ways that BCS can present, along with its relative infrequency require that clinicians consider the disease in a variety of clinical settings so that the diagnosis can be made relatively quickly. Patients presenting with ascites, hepatomegaly, and right upper quadrant abdominal pain, patients with any of the known prothrombotic disorders and new onset ascites, patients with acute hepatic failure and ascites, or patients with what appears to be cryptogenic cirrhosis should be thoroughly evaluated for BCS *(6,21)*. Table 3 outlines the elements requisite in the initial evaluation.

IMAGING OF BCS

Imaging modalities are paramount for the diagnosis of BCS *(22,23)*. Sonography in combination with Doppler analysis may confirm BCS with a sensitivity of 87.5% *(24)*. The ready availability and relatively low cost make ultrasound with Doppler a logical first step in the assessment of vascular anatomy in this patient group *(25)*. Color Doppler evaluation of the liver can reveal the following: (a) enlargement of the hepatic veins without evidence of flow; (b) large intrahepatic collaterals; (c) spider web-like vascular pattern in the vicinity of the ostia of the hepatic veins; (d) hyperechoic cord replacing the lumen of the vein; and (e) loss of hepatic vein wave signal. Magnetic resonance imaging (MRI) and computed tomography (CT) also provide very accurate means to evaluate the vascular anatomy of the liver *(26)* (see Fig. 1A). Both modalities may enhance the evaluation because they add information about the status of the liver and may point to local factors that contribute to the development of BCS *(6,26)*. Furthermore, visualization of an enlarged caudate lobe may help to further raise the degree of suspicion for BCS. The use of venography may be necessary in the minority of cases where the diagnosis remains in question or there is uncertainty as to the patency of the IVC. Venous pressure gradient measurement and histological sampling to ascertain hepatic damage should be performed at the time of venography *(6)* (see Fig. 1B).

HISTOLOGY OF BCS

The necessity of liver biopsy in the management of BCS is the subject of considerable debate *(27,28)*. The pathological features of BCS have been very nicely outlined using

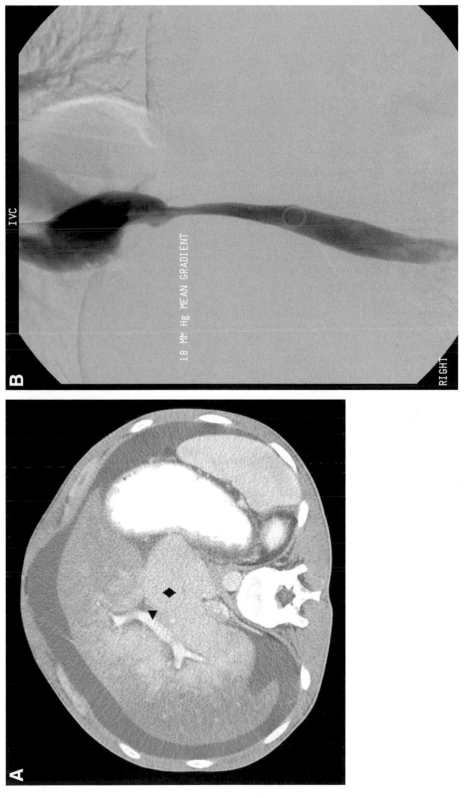

Fig. 1. This 25 yr-old healthy man presented with new onset ascites and right quadrant pain. At presentation patient had intractable ascites, coagulopathy and renal insufficiency. (**A**) CT scan (arterial phase) revealed shrunken liver, with notable exception of caudate lobe (◆), which is notably hypertrophied. Note portal system is open (arrow) and there is poor enhancement of parenchyma except in the caudate lobe. (**B**) Venographic image in same patient. Note the effective caval narrowing with subsequent increased flow gradient.

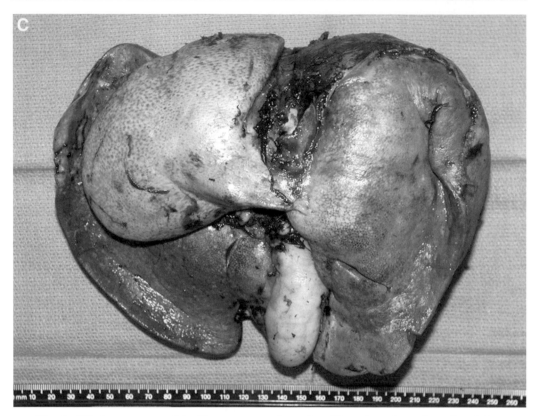

Fig. 1. (**C**) Appearance of the liver on transplantation. Note the enlarged caudate lobe.

available explants from liver transplantation *(9,27–29)*. On gross examination, the livers are noted to be enlarged, with Segment I (caudate lobe) hypertrophy (see Fig. 1C). The classic microscopic description of the injury includes sinusoidal ectasia with centrilobular necrosis *(9,27–29)* (see Figs. 1Di and 1Dii). Fibrosis classically follows leading to so-called reverse cirrhosis or venocentric cirrhosis *(29)*, terms used to describe fibrous bands connecting central veins without bridging to portal tracts. Affected livers can be also divided into two groups: those that exhibit large regenerative nodules with features of focal nodular hyperplasia and those without any nodules. The latter is seen more commonly in patients with short duration of symptoms and fresh clots. The development of focal nodular hyperplasia is thought to be caused by decreases in portal perfusion in association with arterial hyperemia *(9,29)*.

In practical terms, the patient with suspected BCS should undergo a liver biopsy, particularly when the decompensation has been rapid and the optimal therapeutic intervention is in question *(27)*. This approach is particularly important in patients who have underlying cirrhosis, where the diagnosis is uncertain *(20)*. Some groups recommend that bilobar samples be obtained, as the parenchymal involvement may be uneven as not all hepatic veins may be occluded *(30)*.

Therapy of BCS

The management of BCS hinges on two basic premises: first, treatment of the etiological cause if possible, and second, decompression of the liver. It had been believed

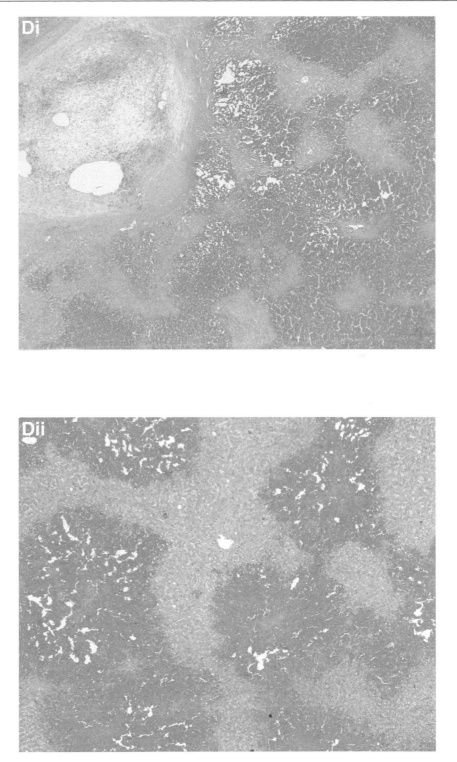

Fig. 1. (D) Microscopic appearance in the same patient. i. Low power view. Note the confluent necrosis centered around the central veins, sparing the portal tracts. ii. Note the very prominent congestion and necrosis around the central veins. Work-up revealed Factor V Leiden defect (heterozygous). Patient has normal Factor V levels 2 yr after LT.

previously that decompression of the liver was the critical component in the management of patients with BCS. The realization that most of the patients seen in Western countries had an underlying prothrombotic disorder has lead to a reconsideration of how these patients should be managed. Life-long anticoagulation is necessary in the majority of cases reported in Western countries, because approx 75% of cases will have disorders of coagulation *(20)*. This decision is more difficult in the setting of liver failure but certainly needs to be considered after definitive therapy has been selected. Treatment of the underlying medical disorder alone has been successful in well-selected patients *(20)*. Reports from large centers in Europe and the United States confirm that 33–60% of patients can be managed primarily by treating their underlying hematological condition without resorting to decompressive procedures *(31,32)*. If the thrombosis can be documented to be recent, some investigators have reported limited success with thrombolysis accompanied by long-term anticoagulation *(33–36)*. International consensus favors the stepwise approach to the patient, particularly if clinical stability can be achieved with initial anticoagulation, with subsequent use of more invasive decompressive maneuvers *(6,20)*. There are no precise criteria, however, for defining when a patient has failed anticoagulant therapy and is in need of hepatic compression.

Decompressive modalities all have a common goal of creating a new conduit for venous drainage. The extent of the thrombosis, i.e., whether or not some hepatic veins are partially open, and the patency of the IVC will influence the choice of therapies. Multispecialty expertise is needed to afford the BCS patient who fails medical therapy or who presents with rapidly progressive hepatic decompensation the procedure most likely to achieve ultimate long-term therapeutic success. The approaches that are well accepted are outlined below under the individual disciplines.

INTERVENTIONAL RADIOLOGY

Interventional radiology teams have a prominent role in the management of BCS. Distinguishing between HVT and MOVC will influence which approach is taken by the interventional radiologists. There are several reports of balloon dilation and stent placement followed by anticoagulation that are very promising especially in those with MOVC *(36–38)*. In the typical Western patient, transjugular intrahepatic portosystemic shunts (TIPS) can serve as an effective decompressive procedure or in patients with more advanced disease as a bridge to liver transplantation. BCS presents unique technical problems if the hepatic veins do not allow for the formation of the connection to the vena cava or if the hypertrophy of the caudate lobe causes compression of the intrahepatic vena cava *(32,39)*. The technique needs to be modified to allow the clinician to form direct portocaval connections through the hepatic parenchyma that successfully decompress the hepatic sinusoids *(40)*. TIPS may even be performed in patients with acute hepatic failure caused by BCS, however, mortality in this group of patients is quite high and liver transplantation, if possible, is the preferred approach *(41,42)*. In instances where the caudate lobe has been congested and causes compression of the vena cava, TIPS can be used to decompress the liver sinusoids into the suprahepatic cava. The experience in a large European center suggests that TIPS may even rescue surgical shunts that fail to decompress the liver fully *(32)*.

SURGERY

There is a considerable body of literature in support of surgical decompression for BCS *(30,37,43–48)*. A side-to-side shunt is required to decompress the liver. The approaches

Table 4
Long-Term Outcome of Liver Transplantation for BCS

Institution	Year	No. of patients	Actuarial survival (%)		
			1 yr	3 yr	5 yr
Pittsburgh (52)	1990	23	69	45	45
Hanover (54)	1994	43	69	69	69
Cambridge (53)	1991	26	69	69	50
Los Angeles/Dallas (46)	1992	14	86	76	NA
London (Kings) (56)	1999	19	95	95	95
London (Ontario) (57)	1994	11	NA	64	64

commonly used today include side-to-side portocaval and mesocaval shunts. In cases of BCS that present with infrahepatic IVC obstruction, mesoatrial or cavoatrial shunts are used (44). Another more radical procedure, dorsocranial hepatic resection with anastomosis of the liver capsule and the right atrium (Senning's procedure) has been described but is rarely used (49). The ultimate choice of decompressive surgery rests with the expertise of the surgical team and a careful assessment of the patients clinical condition.

LIVER TRANSPLANTATION

The introduction of liver transplantation for BCS in 1976 has opened a new modality that allows salvage of the worst cases if all other treatment modalities fail (50). It became apparent early on that this treatment was not a panacea, as many patients had recurrence of their thrombosis (51–53). Most centers have implemented postoperative anticoagulation protocols that are safe and have led to very reasonable success rates in later series (54,55). The survival for this indication is 60–95% at five years (43,46,53,54,56,57) (see Table 4). A small number of patients with BCS have undergone living donor transplantation as well (58).

Prognosis and Management Recommendations

BCS requires very early and aggressive diagnostic work-up. The availability of effective medical therapy makes a solid diagnosis imperative. Patients in Western countries require a thorough evaluation by a Hematology team and early management of thrombophilias and myeloproliferative disorders. Ideally, venographic analysis can be performed, at which time pressures across stenoses can be checked and liver samples obtained. Histology may not predict the outcome reliably, but the presence of extensive necrosis will help the clinician expedite care and proceed with decompression. TIPS and surgical shunts can be considered and, depending on the extent of the thrombosis and the experience of the surgical team, an optimal choice can be made. Liver transplantation should be reserved for those patients with very rapid decompensation or those who fail medical and decompressive therapy. TIPS serves a useful role in stabilizing the sickest patient until such a time as a liver graft becomes available.

Despite the documented effectiveness of surgical management on the outcome of BCS, Zeitoun et al. demonstrated in a retrospective multivariate analysis of 120 consecutive patients seen over 22 yr, that only age, response of ascites to diuretics, Child–Pugh score,

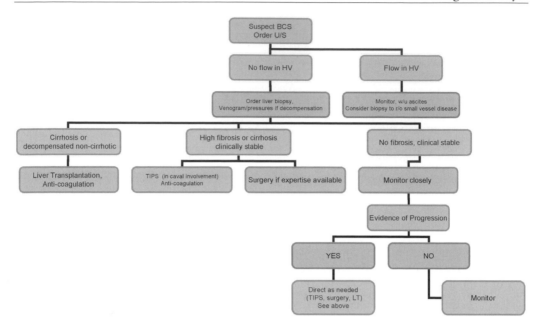

Fig. 2. A management algorithm.

and renal function were independent predictors of survival. Using these variables, a model was developed that accurately predicted survival on a subset of new patients referred to this center. Surprisingly, medical or surgical interventions were not found to be an important predictive factors in patient outcomes *(47)*. This model has been further modified to include clinical features suggesting an acute vs a chronic presentation. Patients with both acute and chronic features had the worse prognosis and the addition of this variable to the prognostic index improved its predictive power *(59)*. Patients with a good prognostic index can be managed medically, whereas those with a poor index should be considered for a TIPS or perhaps liver transplantation. An individualized approach to patients is paramount to successful management of the BCS patient. Rapid diagnosis and close follow-up are pivotal in the separating those patients who will have rapid progression of disease from those who will respond to medical therapy. Figure 2 illustrates a management algorithm that takes into account all the measures described above.

SINUSOIDAL OBSTRUCTIVE SYNDROME (HEPATIC VENO-OCCLUSIVE DISEASE)

Introduction

The similarities in clinical presentation between BCS and SOS make it tempting to group these two entities; however, they are clearly quite different both as to cause and response to therapy. The most commonly used term to describe this syndrome is VOD but the term SOS has recently been suggested to be more descriptive of this condition. This change in terminology reflects the realization that the primary pathophysiologic event is an alteration in the liver microcirculation which may occur in the absence of vascular occlusion *(60)*. SOS will be the term utilized in this chapter.

SOS was initially described by physicians treating epidemic liver injury in patients who had ingested tea or flour contaminated by pyrrolizine alkaloids *(61–64)*. Today, SOS is seen in Western countries in patients receiving antineoplastic regimens, including, but not limited to, hematopoietic stem cell transplantation (HSCT) conditioning regimens *(65–67)*. Many links to antimetabolites [azathioprine *(68)*, 6-mercaptopurine *(69)*, 6-thioguanine *(70)*, and cytosine arabinoside], alkylating agents [dacarbazine *(71)*, cyclophosphamide, carmustine, and busulfan *(72)*], and antilymphocyte antibodies *(73,74)* used outside of stem cell transplantation have been established. There are also reports of SOS in the management of Wilm's tumor in children, which requires combination radiation and chemotherapy *(75–77)* and in liver transplantation *(78,79)*.

Pathophysiology of SOS

Understanding the type of injury to the hepatic vasculature is pivotal to understanding SOS pathophysiology. The description of histological patterns of injury evolved from seminal autopsy studies arising from the early HSCT experience from the Seattle group *(67,80)*. The authors correlated their pathological findings with the clinical severity and symptoms observed in their patient cohort. The earliest histologic findings in livers of SOS patients include marked centrilobular hemorrhagic necrosis, with subsequent narrowing of the terminal hepatic venules *(67)*. This damage leads to extravasation of red cells and cellular debris into the space of Disse, with evident hepatocyte necrosis and macrophage recruitment *(67)*. Outflow impairment facilitates retrograde flow of cellular debris into portal radicals and perhaps embolization of damaged central veins. Liver biopsies obtained 2 wk after the onset of clinical symptoms demonstrate more significant deposition of cellular matrix materials in sinusoidal and subendothelial spaces *(60, 81)*. There is also stellate cell activation and increased fibrogenic activity soon after the initial injury *(82)*. Single lesions can be seen in asymptomatic individuals, however, there is a relationship between the number of lesions and the severity of SOS *(68,80)*.

Until recently, much debate has surrounded the causal mechanism for SOS. Given the clinical scenarios where SOS is seen, direct toxic effects to the hepatocytes and endothelial cells of the drugs administered to these patients were always suspect. Indirect evidence also implicated disorders of coagulation favoring a procoagulant balance *(83)*. It was not until the recent development of a rat model of SOS that damage to the sinusoidal cell has emerged as the key step in the development of this syndrome *(84)*. The animals were fed a pyrrolizidine alkaloid, monocrotaline, that induced findings parallel to human SOS, with hepatomegaly, ascites formation, and hyperbilirubinemia *(84)*. Electron microscopy of livers from this model revealed that the initial change is sinusoidal cell distortion, leading to disruption of the fenestrae, red cell movement into the space of Disse, and tearing of the sinusoidal lining. The resulting cellular debris then sloughs off and disrupts the microcirculation leading to sinusoidal obstruction *(60,84)*. Three complimentary events may explain many of the changes. The first is activation of matrix metalloproteinases that allow for the disruption of the sinusoidal epithelium, the first change in SOS *(60)*. Second, depletion of glutathione appears to play a role in the disruption of the sinusoidal cells as prevention of depletion of glutathione reduces the injury *(85)*. Last, inhibition of nitric oxide synthesis in the sinusoid, possibly as a result of decreased flow through the sinusoid and perhaps linked to metalloproteinase activation, may accentuate the obstruction to flow and, thus, worsen the injury *(86,87)*.

The possibility of a distinct contribution from a preexisting or acquired impairment of coagulation in SOS has been raised and continues to be considered an important factor. Levels of factor VIII, vonWillebrand factor (vWF), and fibrinogen increase in the period following HSCT *(83)*. Tissue necrosis factor α (TNFα) levels have also been noted to be increased after conditioning regimens, leading to an intriguing theoretical mechanism of injury. Salat et al. *(88)* proposed that the initial injury exposes hepatic venular surface, which leads to the production of endothelial factors such as factor VIII and vWF. The neutropenia that follows allows for bacterial translocation in the gut, resulting in endotoxemia, release of TNFα, and other prothrombotic agents from the endothelium, which cause further vascular perturbations *(88)*. Future therapeutic efforts are likely to benefit from these new insights and will include cytoprotective therapies that have the potential to prevent SOS.

Clinical Picture of SOS

As many as 50% of patients receiving HSCT develop SOS of clinical significance *(89, 90)*. The clinical triad of weight gain, painful hepatomegaly, and jaundice (generally in that sequence) appearing within 20 d of inductive therapy defines the syndrome clinically *(89–94)*. However, SOS has been described later in the course of HSCT as well *(95)*. SOS usually resolves spontaneously in the majority of patients but it can progress to multiorgan system failure, usually congestive heart failure, renal insufficiency/failure, gastrointestinal bleeding, and encephalopathy *(90,96)*. The renal insufficiency generally represents hepatorenal syndrome, but its appearance may follow use of known nephrotoxic agents such as amphotericin-B and calcineurin inhibitors *(90)*. Mortality is usually the result of one of the ensuing complications *(90,94)*. The onset of multiorgan failure requiring mechanical ventilation and pressors or hemodialysis portends a very grim prognosis *(60,97)*.

Risk Factor Assessment in SOS

Several large series have identified characteristics that increase of the risk of developing SOS following HSCT *(89,90,98)*. Table 5 lists the most significant recipient and transplantation-related risk factors for the development of SOS. Factors that are solidly established include the use of allogeneic stem cells, the degree of histocompatibility, the use of total body irradiation and its dose, and the use of busulfan in the conditioning regimen. Less solidly established risk factors include the presence of underlying liver disease or presence of liver metastases *(91)*.

Laboratory Findings in SOS

SOS patients generally will develop jaundice of variable proportions, normally owing to direct hyperbilirubinemia *(89,90,94)*. Serum alkaline phosphatase and serum transaminase levels can also be elevated *(90)*. Thrombocytopenia appears early in the course of the syndrome and may be related to the increase in portal hypertension but can also be secondary to a failure of engraftment of the transplant *(98)*. Creatinine generally increases in the most severe cases and can signal impending renal failure.

Several groups have investigated the use of coagulation factor levels as indicators of SOS *(83,90,94)*. It is well recognized that vWF and thrombomodulin levels are elevated in these patients, as well as factor VIII and plasminogen *(90,99)*. Anticoagulants such as protein C and antithrombin III are decreased in SOS patients *(83,90,94)*. However, none

Table 5
Risk Factors for Development of VOD

Risk Factor	Factors that increase risk of SOS
Transplant Type	Allogeneic
Donor	Non-related donor
Grade of HLS compatibility	Poor match
Diagnosis	Transplant performed for malignancy
Conditioning regimen	Nonfractionated high dose TBI, conditioning regimens that contain busulfan and cyclophosphamide
Age	Older recipients
Sex	Male
Liver factors	Abnormal liver injury tests, tumor laden liver, and prior irradiation
Cytomegalovirus	Present

Adapted from ref. 90.
TBI-total body irradiation.

of these factors is a reliable diagnostic marker of SOS (83). The level of plasminogen activator-I has been described as a good early discriminator of patients with SOS, particularly in the pediatric population (100–102). A recent report suggests that the use of serum levels of hyaluronic acid can help in the diagnosis of SOS in patients undergoing HSCT (103).

Histological Studies in SOS

Although histology remains the gold standard to accurately diagnose early SOS (as described above), the presence of SOS in patients without any discernible venular occlusion coupled with potential bleeding complications, make liver biopsy an option that is not routinely considered in patients suspected of having SOS (90,94). If a liver biopsy is needed, then the transjugular approach is the safest.

Hemodynamic Studies

In cases where the typical time-course is not followed and in cases where underlying hepatic disease may be present, transjugular liver biopsy and measurement of hepatic venous pressure gradient (HVPG) may be helpful to establish the diagnosis (104,105). There are several reports of correlation between high HVPG and increased mortality. The presence of high HVPG (>10 mmHg) and the absence of preexisting liver disease can diagnose SOS with reasonable certainty (106).

Imaging in SOS

Whereas ultrasonography may confirm the presence of ascites, hepatomegaly, and anomalies in hepatic outflow, it does not offer many specific findings that help in the diagnosis (107–109). Ultrasonography can certainly eliminate entities that may mimic SOS and has the added advantage of being portable and easily used in a sterile environment (109). MRI has been used although some of the limitations of ultrasonography apply to this modality as well. Many of the findings in SOS that can be seen by MRI develop late in the course of the disease and are of limited use (110,111).

Table 6
Diagnostic Criteria for SOS

Seattle Criteria *(65)*	Development of 2/3 features below before 30 d from transplantation
	Jaundice
	Hepatomegaly with right upper quadrant pain
	Ascites and/or unexplained weight gain
Modified Seattle	Development of 2/3 features below before 20 d from transplantation
Criteria *(81)*	Hyperbilirubinemia with serum bilirubin >2 mg/dL
	Hepatomegaly with right upper quadrant pain
	Weight gain >2% from baseline due to fluid retention
Baltimore	Development of serum bilirubin >2 mg/dL within 21 d from
Criteria *(112)*	transplantation and at least 2 of the findings below
	Hepatomegaly
	Weight gain >5% from baseline
	Ascites

Diagnosis of SOS

For many of the reasons outlined above, the use of clinical criteria to make the diagnosis has been adopted. Two sets of criteria have been widely used, the so-called Seattle criteria *(65)* and the Baltimore criteria *(112)*. A modification of the Seattle criteria has been recently proposed that decreases the time to onset of symptoms and better defines the weight gain and jaundice *(81)* (see Table 6). The reliability of the different criteria using histological confirmation of SOS was determined and both were found to have identical predictive value. Both methods lacked sensitivity, which is not too surprising, as the process must become quite extensive before clinical symptoms appear *(113)*. Strong clinical suspicion and the consideration of a wide differential diagnosis are very important factors in the diagnosis of SOS. Table 7 lists the differential diagnosis for SOS.

Prevention of SOS

The identification of SOS risk factors has led to changes in the performance of HSCT in individuals with high-risk profiles. Prophylactic regimens have been extensively investigated in an effort to help those HSCT patients in whom there are identified risk factors for SOS. Attempts to prevent depletion of glutathione, and the tissue injury resulting from microthrombi/emboli and fibrin deposition are all steps which have been targeted in therapeutic trials with varied success *(114)*. Heparins (both low-molecular-weight and unfractionated) have been used in a number of trials. A randomized trial revealed that prophylactic heparin reduced the incidence of SOS, but did not prevent the development of severe SOS *(115)*. A nonrandomized study of patients at high risk showed that heparin was ineffective *(116)*. Low-molecular-weight heparin may have fewer side effects, but its benefit is unclear *(117,118)*. The use of L-glutamine and N-acetylcysteine as sources of glutathione have not yet been explored fully, although they hold promise on the basis of experimental evidence *(85,119–121)*. Ursodeoxycholic acid has also been used and has failed to demonstrate a significant survival effect, despite apparent effectiveness in decreasing the rate of SOS *(122,123)*. Pentoxifylline, a TNFα antagonist, has been used alone and as adjuvant and has shown no effectiveness in the prevention of SOS *(124,125)*.

Table 7
Differential Diagnosis of SOS

Sepsis-related jaundice
Drug hepatotoxicity
Hepatic graft-vs-host disease
Viral hepatitis
Fungal hepatitis
Total parental nutrition related jaundice
Tumor infiltration of the liver
Right heart failure
Hemolysis

Treatment of Established SOS

In making the decision to treat patients with suspected or confirmed SOS, it has to be remembered that a large percentage of patients have a mild course and the disease resolves spontaneously (94). Despite efforts by large centers to derive a model that will help to stratify patients likely to benefit most from treatment that goal has not been reached (126). Several approaches have been taken to treat the more seriously ill patients. The use of tissue plasminogen activator was aggressively studied with the hope of addressing what was then felt to be the primary pathological event (127). Although some patients benefited, the very high risk of hemorrhage has made the therapy unacceptable. Defibrotide has recently emerged as a promising agent. This agent is a polydeoxyribonucleotide with adenosine receptor agonist activity (128,129). Initial trials were encouraging and have led to a large multicenter trial (128,129). Defibrotide administration increases endothelial prostaglandins, thrombomodulin, and endogenous tissue plasminogen activator levels, with concomitant decrease in levels of plasminogen activator inhibitor-1; all of this occurs without anticoagulant activity or significant toxicity (130). Thirty-six percent of treated patients resolved their severe SOS, with survival beyond 100 d of 35% (130). Given the severity of the SOS in these patients these results are encouraging. New, yet unproven, therapies for SOS include administration of N-acetylcysteine (131), antithrombin III (132,133), charcoal hemofiltration (134), and lately, TIPS (135–137). Although TIPS was effect in decompressing the liver, there was no benefit on survival and this approach has been abandoned by most centers. Liver transplantation has been occasionally used in the rescue of patients with SOS (138–140). This approach depends on the availability of very scarce resources, and given the high recurrence rates of the hematological malignancies which led to HSCT in the first place, few patients would be considered appropriate transplant candidates.

REFERENCES

1. Budd G. On diseases of the liver. John Churchill, London, UK, 1845.
2. Reuben A. Illustrious, industrious, and perhaps notorious. Hepatology 2003;38:1065–1069.
3. Chiari H. Phlebitis obliterans der Haupstamme der Venae hepaticae als Todersursache. Beitrage zur pathologischen Anatomie und zur allgemeinen. Pathologie 1899;26:1–17.
4. Parker R. Occlusion of the hepatic veins in man. Medicine 1959;38:369–402.
5. Tavill AS, Wood EJ, Kreel L, Jones EA, Gregory M, Sherlock S. The Budd-Chiari syndrome: correlation between hepatic scintigraphy and the clinical, radiological, and pathological findings in nineteen cases of hepatic venous outflow obstruction. Gastroenterology 1975;68:509–518.

6. Janssen HL, Garcia-Pagan JC, Elias E, Mentha G, Hadengue A, Valla DC. Budd-Chiari syndrome: a review by an expert panel. J Hepatol 2003;38:364–371.

7. Ludwig J, Hashimoto E, McGill DB, van Heerden JA. Classification of hepatic venous outflow obstruction: ambiguous terminology of the Budd-Chiari syndrome. Mayo Clinic Proc 1990;65:51–55.

8. Okuda K, Kage M, Shrestha SM. Proposal of a new nomenclature for Budd-Chiari syndrome: hepatic vein thrombosis versus thrombosis of the inferior vena cava at its hepatic portion. Hepatology 1998; 28:1191–1198.

9. Cazals-Hatem D, Vilgrain V, Genin P, et al. Arterial and portal circulation and parenchymal changes in Budd-Chiari syndrome: a study in 17 explanted livers. Hepatology 2003;37:510–519.

10. Valla D, Dhumeaux D, Babany G, et al. Hepatic vein thrombosis in paroxysmal nocturnal hemoglobinuria. A spectrum from asymptomatic occlusion of hepatic venules to fatal Budd-Chiari syndrome. Gastroenterology 1987;93:569–575.

11. Valla D, Casadevall N, Lacombe C, et al. Primary myeloproliferative disorder and hepatic vein thrombosis. A prospective study of erythroid colony formation in vitro in 20 patients with Budd-Chiari syndrome. Ann Intern Med 1985;103:329–334.

12. Janssen HL, Meinardi JR, Vleggaar FP, et al. Factor V Leiden mutation, prothrombin gene mutation, and deficiencies in coagulation inhibitors associated with Budd-Chiari syndrome and portal vein thrombosis: results of a case-control study [comment]. Blood 2000;96:2364–2368.

13. Denninger MH, Helley D, Valla D, Guillin MC. Prospective evaluation of the prevalence of factor V Leiden mutation in portal or hepatic vein thrombosis.[comment]. Thromb Haemost 1997;78:1297, 1298.

14. Mohanty D, Shetty S, Narayanan TS, Abraham P. Factor V leiden mutation and Budd-Chiari syndrome. Blood 1998;92:1838,1839.

15. Dayal S, Pati HP, Pande GK, Sharma MP, Saraya AK. Multilineage hemopoietic stem cell defects in Budd Chiari syndrome. J Hepatol 1997;26:293–297.

16. Dayal S, Pati HP, Sharma MP. Tissue plasminogen activator and plasminogen activator inhibitor status in Budd-Chiari syndrome. Haemostasis 1996;26:284–287.

17. Okuda H, Yamagata H, Obata H, et al. Epidemiological and clinical features of Budd-Chiari syndrome in Japan. J Hepatol 1995;22:1–9.

18. Okuda K. Obstructive disease of the inferior vena cava—an idiopathic type of Budd-Chiari syndrome. Trop Gastroenterol 1997;18:91,92.

19. Chan P, Lee CP, Yang CY, Hung JS. Complete membranous obstruction of the inferior vena cava: clinical characteristics of Chinese patients. J Int Med 1993;234:501–505.

20. Valla DC. The diagnosis and management of the Budd-Chiari syndrome: consensus and controversies. Hepatology 2003;38:793–803.

21. Ganguli SC, Ramzan NN, McKusick MA, Andrews JC, Phyliky RL, Kamath PS. Budd-Chiari syndrome in patients with hematological disease: a therapeutic challenge. Hepatology 1998;27:1157–1161.

22. Spritzer CE. Vascular diseases and MR angiography of the liver. Mag Reson Imag Clin N Am 1997;5: 377–396.

23. Murphy FB, Steinberg HV, Shires GT, 3rd, Martin LG, Bernardino ME. The Budd-Chiari syndrome: a review. (AJR) Am J Roentgenol 1986;147:9–15.

24. Bolondi L, Gaiani S, Li Bassi S, et al. Diagnosis of Budd-Chiari syndrome by pulsed Doppler ultrasound. Gastroenterology 1991;100:1324–1331.

25. Millener P, Grant EG, Rose S, et al. Color Doppler imaging findings in patients with Budd-Chiari syndrome: correlation with venographic findings. (AJR) Am J Roentgenol 1993;161:307–312.

26. Miller WJ, Federle MP, Straub WH, Davis PL. Budd-Chiari syndrome: imaging with pathologic correlation. Abdom Imag 1993;18:329–335.

27. Henderson JM, Warren WD, Millikan WJ Jr, et al. Surgical options, hematologic evaluation, and pathologic changes in Budd-Chiari syndrome. Am J Surg 1990;159:41–48; discussion 48–50.

28. Tang TJ, Batts KP, de Groen PC, et al. The prognostic value of histology in the assessment of patients with Budd-Chiari syndrome. J Hepatol 2001;35:338–343.

29. Tanaka M, Wanless IR. Pathology of the liver in Budd-Chiari syndrome: portal vein thrombosis and the histogenesis of veno-centric cirrhosis, veno-portal cirrhosis, and large regenerative nodules. Hepatology 1998;27:488–496.

30. Klein AS, Molmenti EP. Surgical treatment of Budd-Chiari syndrome. Liver Transpl 2003;9:891–896.
31. Min AD, Atillasoy EO, Schwartz ME, Thiim M, Miller CM, Bodenheimer HC Jr. Reassessing the role of medical therapy in the management of hepatic vein thrombosis.[comment]. Liver Transplant Surg 1997;3:423–429.
32. Perello A, Garcia-Pagan JC, Gilabert R, et al. TIPS is a useful long-term derivative therapy for patients with Budd-Chiari syndrome uncontrolled by medical therapy.[comment]. Hepatology 2002;35:132–139.
33. Valla DC. Hepatic vein thrombosis (Budd-Chiari syndrome). Semin Liver Dis 2002;22:5–14.
34. Ilan Y, Oren R, Shouval D. Postpartum Budd-Chiari syndrome with prolonged hypercoagulability state. Am J Obstet Gynecol 1990;162:1164,1165.
35. Suzuoki M, Kondo S, Ambo Y, et al. Treatment of Budd-Chiari syndrome with percutaneous transluminal angioplasty: report of a case. Surg Today 2002;32:559–562.
36. Frank JW, Kamath PS, Stanson AW. Budd-Chiari syndrome: early intervention with angioplasty and thrombolytic therapy. Mayo Clinic Proc 1994;69:877–881.
37. Fisher NC, McCafferty I, Dolapci M, et al. Managing Budd-Chiari syndrome: a retrospective review of percutaneous hepatic vein angioplasty and surgical shunting. Gut 1999;44:568–574.
38. Kohli V, Pande GK, Dev V, Reddy KS, Kaul U, Nundy S. Management of hepatic venous outflow obstruction. Lancet 1993;342:718–722.
39. Blum U, Rossle M, Haag K, et al. Budd-Chiari syndrome: technical, hemodynamic, and clinical results of treatment with transjugular intrahepatic portosystemic shunt. Radiology 1995;197:805–811.
40. Ochs A, Sellinger M, Haag K, et al. Transjugular intrahepatic portosystemic stent-shunt (TIPS) in the treatment of Budd-Chiari syndrome.[comment]. J Hepatol 1993;18:217–225.
41. Shrestha R, Durham JD, Wachs M, et al. Use of transjugular intrahepatic portosystemic shunt as a bridge to transplantation in fulminant hepatic failure due to Budd-Chiari syndrome. Am J Gastroenterol 1997;92:2304–2306.
42. Mancuso A, Fung K, Mela M, et al. TIPS for acute and chronic Budd-Chiari syndrome: a single-center experience. J Hepatol 2003;38:751–754.
43. Orloff MJ, Daily PO, Orloff SL, Girard B, Orloff MS. A 27-year experience with surgical treatment of Budd-Chiari syndrome. Ann Surg 2000;232:340–352.
44. Millikan WJ Jr, Henderson JM, Sewell CW, et al. Approach to the spectrum of Budd-Chiari syndrome: which patients require portal decompression? Am J Surg 1985;149:167–176.
45. Bismuth H, Sherlock DJ. Portasystemic shunting versus liver transplantation for the Budd-Chiari syndrome. Ann Surg 1991;214:581–589.
46. Shaked A, Goldstein RM, Klintmalm GB, Drazan K, Husberg B, Busuttil RW. Portosystemic shunt versus orthotopic liver transplantation for the Budd-Chiari syndrome. Surg Gynecol Obstet 1992;174:453–459.
47. Zeitoun G, Escolano S, Hadengue A, et al. Outcome of Budd-Chiari syndrome: a multivariate analysis of factors related to survival including surgical portosystemic shunting. Hepatol 1999;30:84–89.
48. Singh V, Sinha SK, Nain CK, et al. Budd-Chiari syndrome: our experience of 71 patients. J Gastroenterol Hepatol 2000;15:550–554.
49. Sauvanet A, Panis Y, Valla D, Vilgrain V, Belghiti J. Budd-Chiari syndrome with extensive portal thrombosis: treatment with Senning's procedure. Hepato-Gastroenterol 1994;41:174–176.
50. Putnam CW, Porter KA, Weil R 3rd, Reid HA, Starzl TE. Liver transplantation of Budd-Chiari syndrome. JAMA 1976;236:1142–1143.
51. Seltman HJ, Dekker A, Van Thiel DH, Boggs DR, Starzl TE. Budd-Chiari syndrome recurring in a transplanted liver. Gastroenterology 1983;84:640–643.
52. Halff G, Todo S, Tzakis AG, Gordon RD, Starzl TE. Liver transplantation for the Budd-Chiari syndrome. Ann Surg 1990;211:43–49.
53. Jamieson NV, Williams R, Calne RY. Liver transplantation for Budd-Chiari syndrome, 1976–1990. Annal Chirurg 1991;45:362–365.
54. Ringe B, Lang H, Oldhafer KJ, et al. Which is the best surgery for Budd-Chiari syndrome: venous decompression or liver transplantation? A single-center experience with 50 patients. Hepatology 1995;21:1337–1344.
55. Gordon RD. Liver transplantation and venous disorders of the liver. Liver Transplant Surg 1997;3:S41–S51.

56. Srinivasan P, Rela M, Prachalias A, et al. Liver transplantation for Budd-Chiari syndrome. Transplantation 2002;73:973–977.

57. Sakai Y, Wall WJ. Liver transplantation for Budd-Chiari syndrome: a retrospective study. Surg Today 1994;24:49–53.

58. Yasutomi M, Egawa H, Kobayashi Y, Oike F, Tanaka K. Living donor liver transplantation for Budd-Chiari syndrome with inferior vena cava obstruction and associated antiphospholipid antibody syndrome. J Pediatric Surg 2001;36:659–662.

59. Langlet P, Escolano S, Valla D, et al. Clinicopathological forms and prognostic index in Budd-Chiari syndrome. J Hepatol 2003;39:496–501.

60. DeLeve LD, Shulman HM, McDonald GB. Toxic injury to hepatic sinusoids: sinusoidal obstruction syndrome (veno-occlusive disease). Semin Liver Dis 2002;22:27–42.

61. Tandon BN, Tandon HD, Tandon RK, Narndranathan M, Joshi YK. An epidemic of veno-occlusive disease of liver in central India. Lancet 1976;2:271,272.

62. Mohabbat O, Younos MS, Merzad AA, et al. An outbreak of hepatic veno-occlusive disease in northwestern Afghanistan. Lancet 1976;2:269–271.

63. Ridker PM, McDermott WV. Comfrey herb tea and hepatic veno-occlusive disease. Lancet 1989;1:657,658.

64. Steenkamp V, Stewart MJ, Zuckerman M. Clinical and analytical aspects of pyrrolizidine poisoning caused by South African traditional medicines. Therapeut Drug Monitor 2000;22:302–306.

65. McDonald GB, Sharma P, Matthews DE, Shulman HM, Thomas ED. Venocclusive disease of the liver after bone marrow transplantation: diagnosis, incidence, and predisposing factors. Hepatology 1984;4:116–122.

66. Berk PD, Popper H, Krueger GR, Decter J, Herzig G, Graw RG Jr. Veno-occlusive disease of the liver after allogeneic bone marrow transplantation: possible association with graft-versus-host disease. Ann Intern Med 1979;90:158–164.

67. Shulman HM, McDonald GB, Matthews D, et al. An analysis of hepatic venocclusive disease and centrilobular hepatic degeneration following bone marrow transplantation. Gastroenterology 1980;79:1178–1191.

68. Read AE, Wiesner RH, LaBrecque DR, et al. Hepatic veno-occlusive disease associated with renal transplantation and azathioprine therapy. Ann Intern Med 1986;104:651–655.

69. Merino JM, Casanova F, Saez-Royuela F, Velasco A, Gonzalez JB. Veno-occlusive disease of the liver associated with thiopurines in a child with acute lymphoblastic leukemia. Pediat Hematol Oncol 2000;17:429–431.

70. Kao NL, Rosenblate HJ. 6-Thioguanine therapy for psoriasis causing toxic hepatic venoocclusive disease. J Am Acad Dermatol 1993;28:1017,1018.

71. Paschke R, Heine M. Pathophysiological aspects of dacarbazine-induced human liver damage. Hepatogastroenterology 1985;32:273–275.

72. Hanel M, Kroger N, Sonnenberg S, et al. Busulfan, cyclophosphamide, and etoposide as high-dose conditioning regimen in patients with malignant lymphoma. Ann Hematol 2002;81:96–102.

73. Giles FJ, Kantarjian HM, Kornblau SM, et al. Mylotarg (gemtuzumab ozogamicin) therapy is associated with hepatic venoocclusive disease in patients who have not received stem cell transplantation. Cancer 2001;92:406–413.

74. Giles F, Garcia-Manero G, O'Brien S, Estey E, Kantarjian H. Fatal hepatic veno-occlusive disease in a phase I study of mylotarg and troxatyl in patients with refractory acute myeloid leukemia or myelodysplastic syndrome. Acta Haematolog 2002;108:164–167.

75. Bisogno G, de Kraker J, Weirich A, et al. Veno-occlusive disease of the liver in children treated for Wilms tumor. Med Pediat Oncol 1997;29:245–251.

76. Czauderna P, Katski K, Kowalczyk J, et al. Venoocclusive liver disease (VOD) as a complication of Wilms' tumour management in the series of consecutive 206 patients. Europ J Pediat Surg 2000;10:300–303.

77. Hazar V, Kutluk T, Akyuz C, Varan A, Yaris N, Buyukpamukcu M. Veno-occlusive disease-like hepatotoxicity in two children receiving chemotherapy for Wilms' tumor and clear cell sarcoma of kidney. Pediat Hematol Oncol 1998;15:85–89.

78. Nakazawa Y, Chisuwa H, Mita A, et al. Life-threatening veno-occlusive disease after living-related liver transplantation. Transplantation 2003;75:727–730.

79. Sebagh M, Debette M, Samuel D, et al. "Silent" presentation of veno-occlusive disease after liver transplantation as part of the process of cellular rejection with endothelial predilection. Hepatology 1999;30:1144–1150.

80. Shulman HM, Fisher LB, Schoch HG, Henne KW, McDonald GB. Veno-occlusive disease of the liver after marrow transplantation: histological correlates of clinical signs and symptoms. Hepatology 1994;19:1171–1181.

81. Shulman HM, Hinterberger W. Hepatic veno-occlusive disease—liver toxicity syndrome after bone marrow transplantation. Bone Marrow Transplant 1992;10:197–214.

82. Sato Y, Asada Y, Hara S, et al. Hepatic stellate cells (Ito cells) in veno-occlusive disease of the liver after allogeneic bone marrow transplantation. Histopathology 1999;34:66–70.

83. Korte W. Veno-occlusive disease of the liver after bone marrow transplantation: is hypercoagulability really part of the problem? Blood Coagulat Fibrinolysis 1997;8:367–381.

84. DeLeve LD, McCuskey RS, Wang X, et al. Characterization of a reproducible rat model of hepatic veno-occlusive disease. Hepatology 1999;29:1779–1791.

85. Wang X, Kanel GC, DeLeve LD. Support of sinusoidal endothelial cell glutathione prevents hepatic veno-occlusive disease in the rat. Hepatology 2000;31:428–434.

86. DeLeve LD, Wang X, Kanel GC, et al. Decreased hepatic nitric oxide production contributes to the development of rat sinusoidal obstruction syndrome. Hepatology 2003;38:900–908.

87. Eberhardt W, Beeg T, Beck KF, et al. Nitric oxide modulates expression of matrix metalloproteinase-9 in rat mesangial cells. Kidney Int 2000;57:59–69.

88. Salat C, Holler E, Kolb HJ, et al. Plasminogen activator inhibitor-1 confirms the diagnosis of hepatic veno-occlusive disease in patients with hyperbilirubinemia after bone marrow transplantation. Blood 1997;89:2184–2188.

89. Bearman SI. The syndrome of hepatic veno-occlusive disease after marrow transplantation. Blood 1995;85:3005–3020.

90. Carreras E. Veno-occlusive disease of the liver after hemopoietic cell transplantation. Europ J Haematol 2000;64:281–291.

91. McDonald GB, Shulman HM, Sullivan KM, Spencer GD. Intestinal and hepatic complications of human bone marrow transplantation. Part I. Gastroenterology 1986;90:460–477.

92. McDonald GB, Shulman HM, Sullivan KM, Spencer GD. Intestinal and hepatic complications of human bone marrow transplantation. Part II. Gastroenterology 1986;90:770–784.

93. McDonald GB, Shulman HM, Wolford JL, Spencer GD. Liver disease after human marrow transplantation. Semin Liver Dis 1987;7:210–229.

94. Kumar S, DeLeve LD, Kamath PS, Tefferi A. Hepatic veno-occlusive disease (sinusoidal obstruction syndrome) after hematopoietic stem cell transplantation. Mayo Clinic Proc 2003;78:589–598.

95. Lee JL, Gooley T, Bensinger W, Schiffman K, McDonald GB. Veno-occlusive disease of the liver after busulfan, melphalan, and thiotepa conditioning therapy: incidence, risk factors, and outcome. Biol Blood Marrow Transplant 1999;5:306–315.

96. Bearman SI. Veno-occlusive disease of the liver. Curr Opin Oncol 2000;12:103–109.

97. Rubenfeld GD, Crawford SW. Withdrawing life support from mechanically ventilated recipients of bone marrow transplants: a case for evidence-based guidelines. Ann Intern Med 1996;125:625–633.

98. McDonald GB, Hinds MS, Fisher LD, et al. Veno-occlusive disease of the liver and multiorgan failure after bone marrow transplantation: a cohort study of 355 patients. Ann Int Med 1993;118:255–267.

99. Lee JH, Lee KH, Kim S, et al. Relevance of proteins C and S, antithrombin III, von Willebrand factor, and factor VIII for the development of hepatic veno-occlusive disease in patients undergoing allogeneic bone marrow transplantation: a prospective study. Bone Marrow Transplant 1998;22:883–888.

100. Salat C, Holler E, Kolb HJ, et al. The relevance of plasminogen activator inhibitor 1 (PAI-1) as a marker for the diagnosis of hepatic veno-occlusive disease in patients after bone marrow transplantation. Leuk Lymph 1999;33:25–32.

101. Kaleelrahman M, Eaton JD, Leeming D, et al. Role of plasminogen activator inhibitor-1 (PAI-1) levels in the diagnosis of BMT-associated hepatic veno-occlusive disease and monitoring of subsequent therapy with defibrotide (DF). Hematology 2003;8:91–95.

102. Lee JH, Lee KH, Kim S, et al. Plasminogen activator inhibitor-1 is an independent diagnostic marker as well as severity predictor of hepatic veno-occlusive disease after allogeneic bone marrow transplantation in adults conditioned with busulphan and cyclophosphamide. Br J Haematol 2002;118:1087–1094.

103. Fried MW, Duncan A, Soroka S, et al. Serum hyaluronic acid in patients with veno-occlusive disease following bone marrow transplantation. Bone Marrow Transplant 2001;27:635–639.

104. Shulman HM, Gooley T, Dudley MD, et al. Utility of transvenous liver biopsies and wedged hepatic venous pressure measurements in sixty marrow transplant recipients. Transplantation 1995;59:1015–1022.

105. Carreras E, Granena A, Navasa M, et al. Transjugular liver biopsy in BMT. Bone Marrow Transplant 1993;11:21–26.

106. Carreras E, Garcia-Pagan JC, Bosch J, Rozman C. Transvenous liver biopsies in marrow transplant recipients. Transplantation 1995;60:1375.

107. Hommeyer SC, Teefey SA, Jacobson AF, et al. Venocclusive disease of the liver: prospective study of US evaluation. Radiology 1992;184:683–686.

108. Lassau N, Leclere J, Auperin A, et al. Hepatic veno-occlusive disease after myeloablative treatment and bone marrow transplantation: value of gray-scale and Doppler US in 100 patients. Radiology 1997;204:545–552.

109. Lassau N, Auperin A, Leclere J, Bennaceur A, Valteau-Couanet D, Hartmann O. Prognostic value of doppler-ultrasonography in hepatic veno-occlusive disease. Transplantation 2002;74:60–66.

110. van den Bosch MA, van Hoe L. MR imaging findings in two patients with hepatic veno-occlusive disease following bone marrow transplantation. Europ Radiol 2000;10:1290–1293.

111. Mortele KJ, Van Vlierberghe H, Wiesner W, Ros PR. Hepatic veno-occlusive disease: MRI findings. Abdom Imag 2002;27:523–526.

112. Jones RJ, Lee KS, Beschorner WE, et al. Venoocclusive disease of the liver following bone marrow transplantation. Transplantation 1987;44:778–783.

113. Carreras E, Granena A, Navasa M, et al. On the reliability of clinical criteria for the diagnosis of hepatic veno-occlusive disease. Ann Hematol 1993;66:77–80.

114. Bearman SI. Avoiding hepatic veno-occlusive disease: what do we know and where are we going? Bone Marrow Transplantation 2001;27:1113–1120.

115. Attal M, Huguet F, Rubie H, et al. Prevention of hepatic veno-occlusive disease after bone marrow transplantation by continuous infusion of low-dose heparin: a prospective, randomized trial. Blood 1992;79:2834–2840.

116. Bearman SI, Hinds MS, Wolford JL, et al. A pilot study of continuous infusion heparin for the prevention of hepatic veno-occlusive disease after bone marrow transplantation. Bone Marrow Transplant 1990;5:407–411.

117. Simon M, Hahn T, Ford LA, et al. Retrospective multivariate analysis of hepatic veno-occlusive disease after blood or marrow transplantation: possible beneficial use of low molecular weight heparin. Bone Marrow Transplant 2001;27:627–633.

118. Or R, Nagler A, Shpilberg O, et al. Low molecular weight heparin for the prevention of veno-occlusive disease of the liver in bone marrow transplantation patients. Transplantation 1996;61:1067–1071.

119. DeLeve LD, Ito Y, Bethea NW, McCuskey MK, Wang X, McCuskey RS. Embolization by sinusoidal lining cells obstructs the microcirculation in rat sinusoidal obstruction syndrome. Am J Physiol Gastrointest Liver Physiol 2003;284:G1045–G1052.

120. Goringe AP, Brown S, O'Callaghan U, et al. Glutamine and vitamin E in the treatment of hepatic veno-occlusive disease following high-dose chemotherapy. Bone Marrow Transplant 1998;21:829–832.

121. Shulman HM, Luk K, Deeg HJ, Shuman WB, Storb R. Induction of hepatic veno-occlusive disease in dogs. Am J Pathol 1987;126:114–125.

122. Essell JH, Schroeder MT, Harman GS, et al. Ursodiol prophylaxis against hepatic complications of allogeneic bone marrow transplantation. A randomized, double-blind, placebo-controlled trial. Ann Int Med 1998;128:975–981.

123. Ohashi K, Tanabe J, Watanabe R, et al. The Japanese multicenter open randomized trial of ursodeoxycholic acid prophylaxis for hepatic veno-occlusive disease after stem cell transplantation. Am J Hematol 2000;64:32–38.

124. Clift RA, Bianco JA, Appelbaum FR, et al. A randomized controlled trial of pentoxifylline for the prevention of regimen-related toxicities in patients undergoing allogeneic marrow transplantation. Blood 1993;82:2025–2030.

125. Ferra C, de Sanjose S, Lastra CF, et al. Pentoxifylline, ciprofloxacin and prednisone failed to prevent transplant-related toxicities in bone marrow transplant recipients and were associated with an increased incidence of infectious complications. Bone Marrow Transplant 1997;20:1075–1080.

126. Bearman SI, Anderson GL, Mori M, Hinds MS, Shulman HM, McDonald GB. Venoocclusive disease of the liver: development of a model for predicting fatal outcome after marrow transplantation. J Clin Oncol 1993;11:1729–1736.

127. Bearman SI, Lee JL, Baron AE, McDonald GB. Treatment of hepatic venocclusive disease with recombinant human tissue plasminogen activator and heparin in 42 marrow transplant patients. Blood 1997; 89:1501–1506.

128. Richardson PG, Elias AD, Krishnan A, et al. Treatment of severe veno-occlusive disease with defibrotide: compassionate use results in response without significant toxicity in a high-risk population. Blood 1998;92:737–744.

129. Chopra R, Eaton JD, Grassi A, et al. Defibrotide for the treatment of hepatic veno-occlusive disease: results of the European compassionate-use study. Br J Haematol 2000;111:1122–1129.

130. Richardson PG, Murakami C, Jin Z, et al. Multi-institutional use of defibrotide in 88 patients after stem cell transplantation with severe veno-occlusive disease and multisystem organ failure: response without significant toxicity in a high-risk population and factors predictive of outcome. Blood 2002; 100:4337–4343.

131. Ringden O, Remberger M, Lehmann S, et al. N-acetylcysteine for hepatic veno-occlusive disease after allogeneic stem cell transplantation. Bone Marrow Transplant 2000;25:993–996.

132. Morris JD, Harris RE, Hashmi R, et al. Antithrombin-III for the treatment of chemotherapy-induced organ dysfunction following bone marrow transplantation. Bone Marrow Transplant 1997;20:871–878.

133. Mertens R, Brost H, Granzen B, Nowak-Gottl U. Antithrombin treatment of severe hepatic veno-occlusive disease in children with cancer. Europ J Pediat 1999;158:S154–S158.

134. Tefferi A, Kumar S, Wolf RC, et al. Charcoal hemofiltration for hepatic veno-occlusive disease after hematopoietic stem cell transplantation. Bone Marrow Transplant 2001;28:997–999.

135. Azoulay D, Castaing D, Lemoine A, Hargreaves GM, Bismuth H. Transjugular intrahepatic portosystemic shunt (TIPS) for severe veno-occlusive disease of the liver following bone marrow transplantation. Bone Marrow Transplant 2000;25:987–992.

136. de la Rubia J, Carral A, Montes H, Urquijo JJ, Sanz GF, Sanz MA. Successful treatment of hepatic veno-occlusive disease in a peripheral blood progenitor cell transplant patient with a transjugular intrahepatic portosystemic stent-shunt (TIPS). Haematologica 1996;81:536–539.

137. Zenz T, Rossle M, Bertz H, Siegerstetter V, Ochs A, Finke J. Severe veno-occlusive disease after allogeneic bone marrow or peripheral stem cell transplantation—role of transjugular intrahepatic portosystemic shunt (TIPS). Liver 2001;21:31–36.

138. Rosen HR, Martin P, Schiller GJ, et al. Orthotopic liver transplantation for bone-marrow transplant-associated veno-occlusive disease and graft-versus-host disease of the liver. Liver Transplant Surg 1996;2:225–232.

139. Salat C, Holler E, Gohring P, et al. Protein C, protein S and antithrombin III levels in the course of bone marrow and subsequent liver transplantation due to veno-occlusive disease. Europ J Med Res 1996;1:571–574.

140. Kim ID, Egawa H, Marui Y, et al. A successful liver transplantation for refractory hepatic veno-occlusive disease originating from cord blood transplantation. Am J Transplant 2002;2:796–800.

27 Pulmonary Complications Associated with Portal Hypertension

Karen L. Swanson, DO
and Michael J. Krowka, MD

CONTENTS

DIAGNOSIS AND MANAGEMENT OF HEPATOPULMONARY SYNDROME
DIAGNOSIS AND MANAGEMENT OF PORTOPULMONARY HYPERTENSION
  (POPH)
DIAGNOSIS AND MANAGEMENT OF HEPATIC HYDROTHORAX
DIAGNOSIS AND MANAGEMENT OF CARDIAC COMPLICATIONS
  OF CIRRHOSIS
CONCLUSION
REFERENCES

DIAGNOSIS AND MANAGEMENT OF HEPATOPULMONARY SYNDROME

Definition

Hepatopulmonary syndrome (HPS) is a pulmonary vascular abnormality characterized by intrapulmonary vascular dilatations (IPVD) and arterial hypoxemia that occurs in the setting of either cirrhotic or noncirrhotic portal hypertension *(1–4)*. The clinical diagnostic triad is shown in Fig. 1. Prevalence rates for HPS in patients undergoing liver transplant evaluation have ranged from 5% to 29% *(5)*. HPS is not age-dependent and can be seen in children; it affects males and females equally. To date, no specific etiology of liver disease has been associated with HPS and the degree of HPS has not been correlated with the severity of liver disease using the Childs–Turcotte–Pugh classification or the model for end-stage liver disease scoring system (MELD) *(6)*.

An imbalance in vascular mediators may play a primary role in the vascular changes seen in HPS. Nitric oxide (a potent vasodilator) is thought to be an important mediator in the development of IPVD in HPS and, both inducible and constitutive nitric oxide synthase are upregulated in patients with cirrhosis *(7–9)*. Ironically, endothelin-1, which is a potent vasoconstrictor, may also be involved in the pathogenesis of HPS by stimulating the endothelin-B receptor in the pulmonary endothelium resulting in an increase in nitric

From: *Clinical Gastroenterology: Portal Hypertension*
Edited by: A. J. Sanyal and V. H. Shah © Humana Press Inc., Totowa, NJ

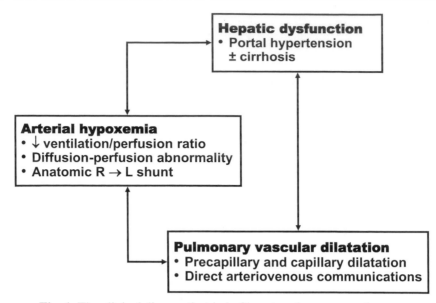

Fig. 1. The clinical diagnostic triad of hepatopulmonary syndrome.

oxide production *(10)*. Further defining the vascular biology in HPS will provide an increased understanding of the pathophysiologic mechanisms of this syndrome.

DIAGNOSIS

Arterial Hypoxemia

Arterial hypoxemia in HPS is documented by $PaO_2 < 70$ mmHg *(11–15)* or an alveolar–arterial oxygen difference $[P(A\text{-}a)O_2] > 20$ mmHg on room air assuming a respiratory quotient of 0.8 *(16)*. Orthodeoxia often occurs (a worsening of oxygenation in the upright position compared with the supine position) as a result of the predominance of vascular dilatations in the lung bases. Positional arterial blood gases (supine and upright) are used to document the degree of orthodeoxia (defined as a decrease in PaO_2 greater than 3 mmHg in the upright compared with supine position) *(2,16)*.

The multiple inert gas elimination technique has helped to define three mechanisms of hypoxemia in HPS *(2,5)*. The first is increased perfusion with normal ventilation due to the hyperdynamic circulatory state of these patients. This leads to a more rapid transit time through the pulmonary vascular bed influencing capillary oxygenation. The second mechanism relies on the diffusion–perfusion relationship. As the vascular dilatations increase in size, there is a further distance from the alveolus to the center of the capillary limiting the passive diffusion of oxygen. The third mechanism is that of direct right to left shunting through pulmonary arteriovenous malformations causing perfusion in the absence of ventilation.

IPVD

IPVD result in varying degrees of hypoxemia. Two types of vascular abnormalities have been described based on angiographic patterns and lung necropsy specimens *(17, 18)*. The type 1 pattern is that of diffuse precapillary and capillary dilatations causing ventilation/perfusion mismatching due to excessive perfusion. The type 2 pattern consists

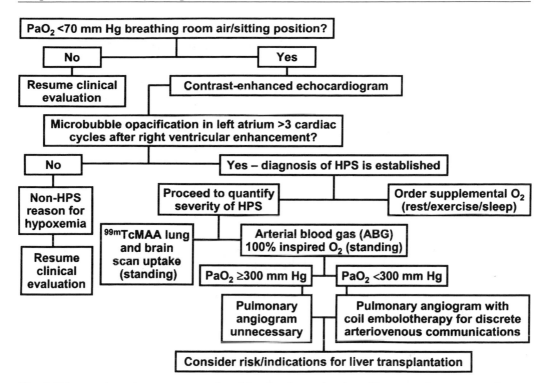

Fig. 2. Diagnostic and management algorithm for the evaluation of hepatopulmonary syndrome.

of distinct localized arteriovenous communications that cause perfusion in the absence of ventilation resulting in a true shunt. The response to 100% inspired oxygen can sometimes help to differentiate between the two types. In the presence of a true shunt, the response to 100% oxygen will be minimal. A useful guideline to follow is that if the PaO_2 is less than 300 mmHg in response to 100% oxygen, a pulmonary angiogram should be considered so that any distinct pulmonary arteriovenous communications can be considered for coil embolotherapy.

Contrast-enhanced transthoracic echocardiography is the most sensitive, qualitative screening test to detect the presence of IPVD (11). IPVD are present when microbubbles (agitated saline injected through a peripheral vein) are visualized in the left heart chambers four to six cardiac cycles after visualization in the right heart. This test may detect "subclinical" HPS however, as cirrhotic patients without hypoxemia may have positive contrast-enhanced echocardiograms (11).

Technetium labeled macroaggregated albumin (^{99m}TcMAA) lung perfusion scanning with brain uptake is a specific test that allows quantification of the degree of right to left shunting caused by IPVD (15,19). Abnormal uptake is defined as greater than 6% shunt. If positive in the setting of liver disease and arterial hypoxemia, the diagnosis of HPS is established. A diagnostic algorithm for HPS is shown in Fig. 2.

Management

Supplemental oxygen administration should be utilized in HPS patients although the response to oxygen therapy will vary depending on the degree of IPVD and will be less effective as IPVD increase in size. If the response to 100% oxygen is poor (<300 mmHg) a pulmonary angiogram is a reasonable next step. Pulmonary arteriovenous malformations that have "feeding" arteries larger than 3 mm can be effectively treated with coil embolotherapy *(20)*. Most commonly, however, the vascular abnormalities are of the diffuse type and are not amenable to treatment although a single case report has emerged documenting successful embolization therapy for diffusely dilated pulmonary vessels in a patient with HPS as palliative treatment prior to OLT *(21)*.

Multiple pharmacologic therapies have been used to treat HPS over the years; however, none thus far have been shown to be consistently effective *(17,22–25)*. There are no randomized controlled trials regarding pharmacologic therapies and most have been of short duration. A recent case report has provided encouraging data showing that inhibition of nitric oxide synthesis with nebulized N^G-nitro-L-arginine methyl ester (L-NAME) improved arterial oxygenation and 6-min walk distance in a patient with HPS *(7)*. This case report reiterates the delicate balance between vascular mediators and provides evidence that nitric oxide likely plays a role in the pathophysiology of HPS. Transjugular intrahepatic portosystemic shunting has been performed in HPS with variable results *(26,27)*. Rarely, HPS will spontaneously resolve.

Presently, the only effective treatment for HPS is orthotopic liver transplantation (OLT) with improvement or resolution of HPS in 61–91% of patients *(28–30)*. Survival in the absence of OLT in patients with HPS is poor compared to those undergoing OLT *(31,32)*. HPS can be severe even in the setting of stable hepatic dysfunction. Patients with PaO_2 < 50 mmHg appear to have a worse survival than those with PaO_2 > 50 mmHg *(31,32)*. As long as minimal listing criteria for transplantation are met, OLT remains an indication for the treatment of HPS. Oxygenation abnormalities resolve slowly after OLT (months). The lower the preoperative PaO_2, the longer the resolution of hypoxemia *(30)*. The current United Network for Organ Sharing policy recommends that HPS patients with PaO_2 < 60 mmHg be given additional MELD points so that they have a "reasonable probability of being transplanted within 3 mo" *(33)*.

DIAGNOSIS AND MANAGEMENT OF PORTOPULMONARY HYPERTENSION (POPH)

Definition

POPH results from a proliferative vascular process that occurs in the setting of liver disease, most commonly portal hypertension; and, is characterized by constrictive and obliterative changes in the pulmonary vascular bed that are indistinguishable from those seen in primary pulmonary hypertension *(34,35)*. The 3rd World Symposium on Pulmonary Arterial Hypertension in 2003 included POPH as a cause of pulmonary arterial hypertension *(36)*. Screening patients undergoing evaluation for liver transplantation is important because of the significant peri- and postoperative morbidity and mortality that can result from POPH. The prevalence of pulmonary hypertension in 1205 consecutive liver transplant patients has been shown to be 8.5% *(37)*. Other studies have determined the prevalence of POPH in liver transplant candidates to be 3.5 and 4%, respectively *(38,39)*. Males and females are affected equally and, neither the etiology nor the severity of hepatic dysfunction correlate with the degree of pulmonary hypertension.

The vasculopathy seen in POPH results from pulmonary endothelial proliferation leading to plexogenic arteriopathy and *in situ* thrombosis. These changes are pathologically similar to the findings in primary pulmonary hypertension.

Table 1
Variations in the Hemodynamic Profiles
That Can Be Seen in Patients with Liver Disease and Portal Hypertension

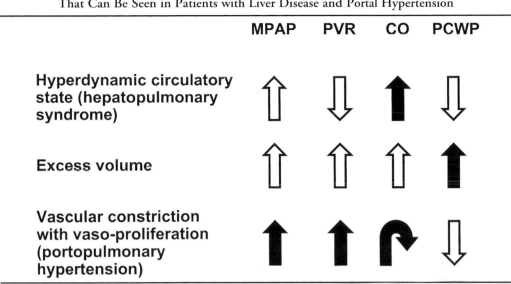

MPAP, mean pulmonary artery pressure; PVR, pulmonary vascular resistance; CO, cardiac output; PCWP, pulmonary capillary wedge pressure.

Diagnosis

The diagnosis of POPH relies on hemodynamic data obtained at right heart catheterization and includes a mean pulmonary artery pressure (MPAP) of > 25 mmHg at rest, a pulmonary vascular resistance (PVR) > 240 dynes.s.cm^{-5}, and a normal pulmonary capil-lary wedge pressure (PCWP) in patients with chronic liver disease (3,40). The PVR is cal-culated by [(MPAP–PCWP) ÷ cardiac output] × 80 (dynes.s.cm^{-5}). Including the PVR in the definition is important as many patients with liver disease can have moderate eleva-tions in MPAP largely in part because of high cardiac outputs from a hyperdynamic state. In these patients, however, the PVR should be close to normal. This is different from POPH where elevations in MPAP are a result of the changes in the pulmonary vascular bed often with reductions in cardiac output. Table 1 shows the variations in hemodynamic profiles that can exist in liver disease and portal hypertension.

Transthoracic echocardiography is a useful screening tool to estimate pulmonary artery systolic pressure (41). This pressure is estimated by using the tricuspid regurgitant flow velocity and the estimated right atrial pressure. Sensitivity and specificity of Doppler echocardiography for detecting POPH approaches 100% and 88% when using a systolic pulmonary arterial pressure of >40 mmHg or a pulmonary acceleration time of <100 ms (42). Echocardiography with Doppler assessment of the right ventricle should be performed in patients undergoing evaluation for liver transplantation with further testing if there is a suspicion of pulmonary hypertension. A diagnostic algorithm for the evaluation of POPH is shown in Fig. 3.

Management

Management of POPH consists of a multifaceted approach. Oxygen therapy should be considered once arterial saturations fall below 90% so that hypoxic vasoconstriction does not further compound the pulmonary hypertension. Symptomatic patients complaining

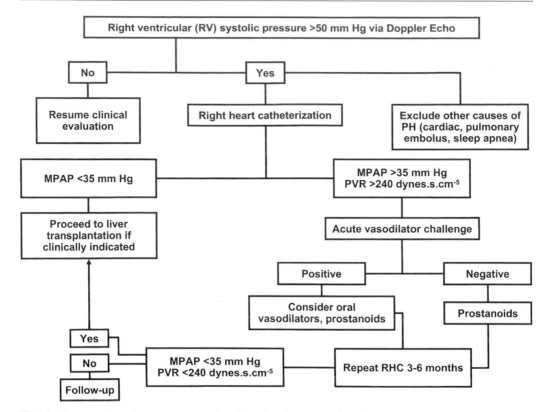

Fig. 3. Diagnostic and management algorithm for the evaluation of portopulmonary hypertension.

of shortness of breath often experience some symptom alleviation with oxygen therapy alone. Depending on the amount of edema that develops both from liver disease as well as from right heart dysfunction, diuretics and sodium restriction can be especially useful. Both loop diuretics and potassium-sparing diuretics are effective. B-type natriuretic peptide (BNP) is a cardiac neurohormone secreted from the ventricles *(43)*. Elevated BNP levels have been found to be a useful measure in patients with primary pulmonary hypertension and appear to have a strong independent association with mortality *(44)*. BNP may be helpful as a measure of right ventricular stress/strain in POPH.

The role of anticoagulation in POPH remains unclear. Hepatic dysfunction often results in an elevation of prothrombin time and, portal hypertension with resultant splenomegaly causes thrombocytopenia. Gastrointestinal bleeding from gastric and/or esophageal varices often complicates the situation as well. Anticoagulation may be considered in patients with stable hepatic dysfunction, reasonable platelet counts, and the lack of varices after discussion with the hepatologist or liver transplant surgeon.

Therapeutic agents available to specifically treat pulmonary hypertension include the prostanoids; intravenous (iv) epoprostenol (Flolan®) and subcutaneous (sc) treprostinil (Remodulin®) and, the oral nonspecific endothelin receptor antagonist bosentan (Tracleer®). More data are available regarding the use of iv epoprostenol in POPH. Epoprostenol is given as a continuous iv infusion through an indwelling, long-term central venous catheter. It is has been shown to decrease PVR and MPAP while increasing cardiac output, both acutely and long term in patients with POPH *(45)*. The overall goal is to improve pulmonary hemo-dynamics so that morbidity and mortality might be lessened and; to possibly facilitate OLT in specific instances. The degree of hemodynamic derangement influences survival after liver transplantation. In an evaluation of published liver transplantation outcomes in POPH, patients with MPAP >50 mmHg had 100% mortality, whereas patients with MPAP 35–50 mmHg and PVR >250 dynes.s.cm^{-5} showed a 50% mortality, and patients with MPAP <35 mmHg experienced no mortality (46,47).

To date, there are no published series regarding the use of subcutaneous treprostinil or oral bosentan in the treatment of POPH. A major side effect of bosentan treatment is that of hepatic dysfunction requiring monthly monitoring of liver enzymes, alkaline phosphatase, and bilirubin. The safe use of bosentan in patients with POPH has not been delineated.

DIAGNOSIS AND MANAGEMENT OF HEPATIC HYDROTHORAX

Definition

The definition of hepatic hydrothorax consists of a significant pleural effusion (generally greater than 500 mL) in a patient who has liver cirrhosis in the absence of primary cardiac or pulmonary disease (48,49). No particular etiology of liver disease is predictive for the development of hepatic hydrothorax. Prevalence rates of hepatic hydrothorax range from 4% to 10% of patients with advanced liver cirrhosis (50). The pleural fluid appears to develop owing to transfer of ascitic fluid through diaphragmatic fenestrations. Hepatic hydrothorax is most commonly located on the right side although can appear on the left as shown in Fig. 4 or, in some instances bilaterally.

Diagnosis

The diagnosis of hepatic hydrothorax relies on the documentation of a pleural effusion and the exclusion of any confounding cardiac or pulmonary disease (congestive heart failure, parapneumonic effusion, malignancy, and so on). The pleural fluid analysis of hepatic hydrothorax in general is transudative in nature. The cell count is usually <1000 cells/mm^3, the total protein concentration is <2.5 g/dL, and the pH ranges from 7.40 to 7.55 (49,51). Hepatic hydrothorax can occur in the absence of ascites and can be diagnosed with nuclear scanning techniques by injection of radioactive isotope (^{99m}Tc-sulfur colloid) into the peritoneal cavity and following the communication into the pleural space (50,52,53).

A careful history and physical examination are paramount in the evaluation of hepatic hydrothorax. Pleural fluid analysis via thoracentesis is important to define the fluid characteristics especially in patients with hemithorax pain or fever. Radiographic imaging including chest computed tomography scanning is important to evaluate the chest in its entirety to exclude significant mediastinal lymphadenopathy, as well as any gross pulmonary parenchymal or pleural lesions. Echocardiography is a helpful tool in assessing cardiac function as a potential etiology to pleural effusion.

Management

MEDICAL THERAPY

Patients who develop hepatic hydrothorax most often have advanced liver disease and may be candidates for OLT. The goal of therapy in hepatic hydrothorax is the relief of symptoms and the prevention of pulmonary complications such as compressive atelectasis and infection. Initial attempts at treating hepatic hydrothorax focus on strict sodium

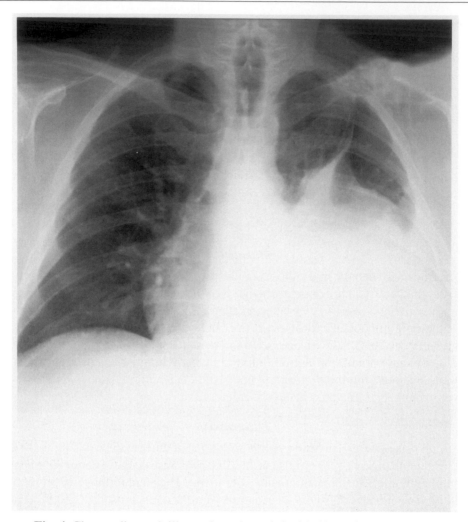

Fig. 4. Chest radiograph illustrating a large left-sided hepatic hydrothorax.

restriction and diuretic therapy. The effectiveness of these interventions relies on the patient's renal function and ability to excrete sodium. As glomerular filtration rates fall, diuretic therapy can result in rising BUN and creatinine values culminating in worsening encephalopathy. Occasionally, hepatic hydrothorax is controlled by these measures alone and the patient's symptoms are tolerable.

THORACENTESIS

Therapeutic thoracentesis is an effective procedure in eliminating pleural fluid and relieving symptomatology. Unfortunately, hepatic hydrothorax most commonly is a recurring process due to the unresolved hepatic dysfunction. Patients often require frequent thoracenteses for symptom relief. Complications of thoracentesis include postthoracentesis pulmonary edema, pneumothorax, and hemothorax. Hyponatremia and hypoalbuminemia can be significant problems in these patients because of recurrent large volume taps. Owing to the recurrent nature of hepatic hydrothorax other treatment options have been explored. To date, no consistent ideal treatment has been defined.

PLEURODESIS

Pleurodesis is a procedure whereby a sclerosing agent is instilled into the pleural space to eliminate the space where fluid accumulates. Unfortunately, pleurodesis has not been an effective treatment option in hepatic hydrothorax probably due to the large and recurrent volume of fluid that passes into the pleural space. Pleurodesis is generally effective only if the pleural space is able to be adequately drained prior to instillation of a sclerosing agent. This is usually not possible in hepatic hydrothorax. One study of talc pleurodesis found that the procedure was effective in 10 of 21 procedures with four recurrences *(54)*. Morbidity was seen in 57% and included fever, chest pain, empyema, wound infection, and persistent air leak. Thirty-nine percent of patients died within 30 d of the procedure.

DIAPHRAGMATIC REPAIR

Surgical repair of diaphragmatic defects has been performed in hepatic hydrothorax in attempts to decrease the passage of ascitic fluid into the pleural space. In one study of eight patients with ascites and hepatic hydrothorax, diaphragmatic defects were localized and repaired in six patients under surgical videothoracoscopy without recurrence of pleural effusion *(55)*. In the remaining two patients, no diaphragmatic defect was found and drainage persisted for 15–18 d. These patients were discharged with stable recurrent effusions occupying one-third of the hemithorax. This suggests that if obvious diaphragmatic defects can be localized and repaired, hepatic hydrothorax may be successfully treated by this method although ascitic burden may become more problematic.

SHUNT SYSTEMS

Pleurovenous shunting has emerged as a treatment consideration for hepatic hydrothorax. This involves the placement of a shunt system from the pleural cavity into the subclavian or jugular vein. Two types of shunt systems have been used. The LaVeen shunt system has largely been used in peritoneovenous shunting from the peritoneal cavity into the venous system. One disadvantage of this shunt system is that the pleural space has a lower pressure than both the peritoneal cavity and the venous system so that fluid may accumulate in the pleural space. Because of this problem, the Denver shunt was designed that has a unidirectional pump and, also allows for external manual compression so that fluid can be moved from an area of lower pressure (pleural space) to one of higher pressure (venous system). One study evaluated six patients with hepatic hydrothorax treated with pleurovenous shunting via the Denver shunt system and showed that hepatic hydrothorax related symptoms were reduced within a few days *(56)*. One patient died as a result of hepatic failure 4 wk after shunt implantation, however, the shunt was still functioning. This type of shunting may be an option for patients with symptomatic hepatic hydrothorax both for symptom control and, potentially as a bridge to liver transplantation.

TRANSJUGULAR INTRAHEPATIC PORTOSYSTEMIC SHUNT (TIPS)

Transjugular intrahepatic portosystemic shunt (TIPS) is an acceptable form of medical therapy for portal hypertension-related variceal bleeding, as well as intractable ascites. This procedure involves placing a stent between the portal and hepatic venous systems so that venous return bypasses the liver thereby reducing hepatic sinusoidal pressure. Early experience with TIPS in the treatment of hepatic hydrothorax in patients with and without ascites were encouraging *(57,58)*. More recently, 19 patients with hepatic hydrothorax treated with TIPS were evaluated to determine the safety and efficacy of TIPS *(59)*.

Complete clinical response was seen in 63% of patients, partial clinical response in 11%, and no clinical response in 26%. Radiographic response was deemed complete in 30%, partial in 50%, and none in 20%. The authors concluded that TIPS was a relatively safe and effective method of controlling hepatic hydrothorax, however, there was a variable reduction in the quantity of pleural fluid remaining after the procedure. Patients who did not respond to TIPS had a poor prognosis, with the majority dying within 30 d of the procedure. Complications of TIPS include worsening hepatic encephalopathy, shunt occlusion, and infection. Liver transplantation remains the only long-term effective treatment for refractory hepatic hydrothorax.

DIAGNOSIS AND MANAGEMENT OF CARDIAC COMPLICATIONS OF CIRRHOSIS

Definition

A variety of cardiac complications occur as a consequence of liver disease. Right heart failure associated with portopulmonary hypertension has already been discussed. Other cardiac complications, however, include cardiac compromise due to large pleural effusion, pericardial effusion in cirrhosis, and cirrhotic cardiomyopathy *(60–64)*. Patients with cirrhosis tend to have a hyperdynamic circulation characterized by a high cardiac output and low systemic vascular resistance. Many cirrhotic patients present with dyspnea, fluid retention, and diminished exercise capacity. A thorough cardiac and pulmonary evaluation is important in the assessment of these symptoms.

Diagnosis

CARDIAC EFFECTS OF LARGE PLEURAL EFFUSIONS

Large pleural effusions have the potential to transmit the resultant increase in intrapleural pressure to the pericardial space thereby diminishing right or left ventricular filling leading to hypotension and hypoperfusion (tamponade physiology) *(60,61)*. Physical examination findings include those of a large pleural effusion (diminished breath sounds, dullness to percussion, egophany) as well as evidence of cardiac tamponade (elevated jugular venous pressure, pulsus paradoxus, edema). Electrocardiography may show decreased voltage due to the tamponade physiology. Transthoracic echocardiography is the diagnostic tool of choice. Findings on echocardiography include right and/or left ventricular diastolic collapse, respiratory variation in flow velocities, and decreased left ventricular ejection fraction *(60)*. Pulmonary artery catheterization findings are consistent with cardiac tamponade showing equalization of pressures between the right atrium, right ventricle, pulmonary artery, and pulmonary capillary wedge pressure.

PERICARDIAL EFFUSION

The diagnosis of pericardial effusion in the setting of cirrhosis may be suspected by a patient's symptoms of dyspnea and physical examination findings of ascites and elevated jugular venous pressure. Chest radiography may be helpful if enlargement of the heart is seen. The diagnosis of pericardial effusion is established by transthoracic echocardiography, which can assess size of the effusion, as well as cardiac compromise or tamponade physiology. Pericardial effusion has been found in up to 63% of echocardiograms performed in patients with decompensated cirrhosis *(65)*.

CIRRHOTIC CARDIOMYOPATHY

Cirrhotic cardiomyopathy is the result of both structural and functional cardiac abnormalities. It is defined by a constellation of findings including myocardial hypertrophy, diastolic dysfunction, and inappropriate chronotropic and inotropic responses to stress or exercise *(62,63,66–69)*. An elevation in pulmonary capillary wedge pressure and pulmonary hypertension may be seen as a result of pulmonary venous excess. Transthoracic echocardiography is an important tool in the evaluation of cirrhotic cardiomyopathy. Diastolic dysfunction is suggested by an increased isovolumic relaxation time and reduced E/A ratio in the setting of a dilated left atrium *(66)*. Cardiopulmonary exercise testing can also be a useful tool to assess cardiac response to exercise if there is a suspicion of underlying cardiomyopathy.

BNP levels correlate with interventricular septal wall thickness, left ventricular diameter at the end of diastole, and deceleration time and, may be a useful marker in the screening of patients with cardiac complications of cirrhosis *(70)*. In patients with cirrhosis, circulating BNP has been shown to be related to severity of liver disease (Child score, serum albumin, hepatic venous pressure gradient) and to markers of cardiac dysfunction (QT interval, heart rate, plasma volume) but not to other measures of hyperdynamic circulation *(71)*. This tool deserves further evaluation in this patient population.

Management

CARDIAC EFFECTS OF LARGE PLEURAL EFFUSIONS

Sodium restriction and diuretics may be used in attempts to control the pleural effusion, however, in patients with cardiac compromise and tamponade physiology due to a large pleural effusion, thoracentesis is the treatment of choice to relieve cardiac compression and hemodynamic compromise. Following thoracentesis, other considerations for control of the pleural effusion include repair of diaphragmatic defects, TIPS, and OLT *(60,61)*.

PERICARDIAL EFFUSION

Pericardial effusions are related to the degree of fluid retention in decompensated cirrhosis and respond to the treatment and resolution of ascites *(64,65)*. A case report has also been published regarding resolution of a moderate sized pericardial effusion in a patient with primary biliary cirrhosis treated with colchicine and ursodeoxycholic acid *(72)*.

CIRRHOTIC CARDIOMYOPATHY

The management of cirrhotic cardiomyopathy focuses on sodium restriction and diuretic therapy. The diastolic dysfunction that occurs may be related to an increased plasma volume commonly seen in cirrhotic patients. Liver transplantation has been shown to improve exercise tolerance and cardiac function *(73)*.

CONCLUSION

A spectrum of both cardiac and pulmonary complications can occur in the setting of portal hypertension. This chapter has focused on hepatopulmonary syndrome, portopulmonary hypertension, hepatic hydrothorax, and cardiac complications of cirrhosis. It is important to systematically assess patients with cirrhosis especially in the presence of symptoms including dyspnea, edema, and reduced exercise tolerance. Useful studies to consider include chest radiography, pulmonary function testing, transthoracic echocardiography (with contrast enhancement and Doppler assessment of the right ventricle), arterial blood gases on room air, and potentially right and/or left heart catheterization. For patients undergoing liver transplantation evaluation, it is imperative to screen for hepatopulmonary syndrome and portopulmonary hypertension for reasons discussed herein.

REFERENCES

1. Kaymakoglu S, Kahraman T, Kudat H, et al. Hepatopulmonary syndrome in noncirrhotic portal hypertensive patients. Digest Dis Sci 2003;48:556–560.
2. Herve P, Lebrec D, Brenot F, et al. Pulmonary vascular disorders in portal hypertension. Eur Respir J 1998;11:1153–1166.
3. Krowka MJ. Hepatopulmonary syndromes. Gut 2000;40:1–4.
4. Lange PA, Stoller JK. The hepatopulmonary syndrome. Ann Intern Med 1995;122:521–529.
5. Rodriguez-Roisin R, Roca J. Hepatopulmonary syndrome: the paradigm of liver-induced hypoxaemia. Baillieres Clin Gastroenterol 1997;11:387–406.
6. Wiesner RH, Edwards E, Freeman R, et al. Model for end-stage liver disease (MELD) and allocation of donor livers. Gastroenterology 2003;124:91–96.
7. Brussino L, Bucca C, Morello M, Scappaticci E, Mauro M, Rolla G. Effect on dyspnoea and hypoxaemia of inhaled N^G-nitro-L-arginine methyl ester in hepatopulmonary syndrome. Lancet 2003;362: 43–44.
8. Rolla G, Brussino L, Colagrande P, et al. Exhaled nitric oxide and oxygenation abnormalities in hepatic cirrhosis. Hepatology 1997;26:842–847.
9. Rolla G, Brussino L, Colagrande P, et al. Exhaled nitric oxide and impaired oxygenation in cirrhotic patients before and after liver transplantation. Ann Intern Med 1998;129:375–378.
10. Fallon MB, Abrams GA. Pulmonary dysfunction in chronic liver disease. Hepatology 2000;32:859–865.
11. Abrams GA, Jaffe CC, Hoffer PB, et al. Diagnostic utility of contrast echocardiography and lung perfusion scan in patients with hepatopulmonary syndrome. Gastroenterology 1995;109:1283–1288.
12. Krowka MJ, Tajik AJ, Dickson E, et al. Intrapulmonary vascular dilatation in liver transplant candidates: screening by two-dimensional contrast enhanced echocardiography. Chest 1990;97:1165–1170.
13. Moller S, Hillingso J, Christensen E, Henriksen JH, et al. Arterial hypoxemia in cirrhosis: fact or fiction? Gut 1998;42:868–874.
14. Vachiery F, Moreau R, Hadengue A, et al. Hypoxemia in patients with cirrhosis: relationship with liver failure and hemodynamic alterations. J Hepatol 1997;27:492–495.
15. Abrams GA, Nanda NC, Dubovsky EV, Krowka MJ, Fallon MB. Use of macroaggregated albumin lung perfusion scan to diagnose hepatopulmonary syndrome: a new approach. Gastroenterology 1998; 114:305–310.
16. Castro M, Krowka MJ. Hepatopulmonary syndrome. A pulmonary vascular complication of liver disease. Clin Chest Med 1996;17:35–48.
17. Krowka MJ, Dickson E, Cortese D. Hepatopulmonary syndrome: clinical observations and lack of therapeutic response to somatostatin analogue. Chest 1993;104:515–521.
18. Rydell R, Hoffbauer FW. Multiple pulmonary arteriovenous fistulas in juvenile cirrhosis. Am J Med 1956;21:450–459.
19. Krowka MJ, Wiseman GA, Burnett OL, et al. Hepatopulmonary syndrome: a prospective study of relationships between severity of liver disease, PaO(2) response to 100% oxygen, and brain uptake after (99m)Tc MAA lung scanning. Chest 2000;118:615–624.
20. Gupta P, Mordin C, Curtis J, Hughes JMB, Shovlin CL, Jackson JE. Pulmonary arteriovenous malformations: effect of embolization on right-to-left shunt, hypoxemia, and exercise tolerance in 66 patients. Am J Radiol 2002;179:347–355.
21. Ryu JK, Oh JH. Hepatopulmonary syndrome: angiography and therapeutic embolization. J Clin Imag 2003;27:97–100.
22. Fallon MB. Methylene blue and cirrhosis: pathophysiologic insights, therapeutic dilemmas. Ann Intern Med 2000;133:738–740.
23. Groneberg DA, Fischer A. Methylene blue improves the hepatopulmonary syndrome. Ann Intern Med 2001;135:380,381.

24. Maniscalco M, Sofia M, Higenbottam T. Effects of an NO-synthase inhibitor L-NMMA in the hepato-pulmonary syndrome. Respiration 2001;68:226.

25. Schenk P, Madl C, Rezaie-Majd S, Lehr S, Muller C. Methylene blue improves the hepatopulmonary syndrome. Ann Intern Med 2000;133:701–706.

26. Paramesh AS, Husain SZ, Shneider B, et al. Improvement of hepatopulmonary syndrome after trans-jugular intrahepatic portasystemic shunting: case report and review of the literature. Pediat Transpl 2003;7:157–162.

27. Lasch HM, Fried MW, Zacks SL, et al. Use of transjugular intrahepatic portosystemic shunt as a bridge to liver transplantation in a patient with severe hepatopulmonary syndrome. Liver Transpl 2001;17: 147–149.

28. Egawa H, Kasahara M, Inomata Y, et al. Long-term outcome of living related liver transplantation for patients with intrapulmonary shunting and strategy for complications. Transplantation 1999;67:712–717.

29. Krowka M, Porayko M, Plevak D, et al. Hepatopulmonary syndrome with progressive hypoxemia as an indication for liver transplantation: case reports and review of the literature. Mayo Clinic Proc 1997; 72:44–53.

30. Taille C, Cadranel J, Bellocq A, et al. Liver transplantation for hepatopulmonary syndrome: a ten year experience in Paris, France. Transplantation 2003;75:1482–1489.

31. Swanson KL, Wiesner RH, Rosen CB, Krowka MJ. Pulmonary vascular complications of liver dis-ease: survival in 140 Mayo Clinic patients. Hepatology 2003;A250.

32. Schenk P, Schoniger-Hekele M, Fuhrmann V, Madl C, Silberhumer G, Muller C. Prognostic signifi-cance of the hepatopulmonary syndrome in patients with cirrhosis. Gastroenterology 2003;125:1042–1052.

33. (UNO3) UNOS.http//www.unos.org.

34. Edwards B, Weir K, Edwards WD, Ludwig J, Dykoski RK, Edwards JE. Coexistent pulmonary and portal hypertension: morphologic and clinical features. J Am Coll Cardiol 1987;10:1233–1238.

35. Krowka MJ. Hepatopulmonary syndromes. Gut 2000;46:1–4.

36. Third World Symp Pulmonary Arterial Hypertension, Venice, Italy; June 23–25, 2003.

37. Ramsay MAE, Simpson BR, Nguyen AT, Ramsay KJ, East C, Klintmalm GB. Severe pulmonary hyper-tension in liver transplant candidates. Liver Transpl Surg 1997;3:494–500.

38. Tamara P, Garcia-Valdecasas JC, Beltran J, et al. Moderate primary pulmonary hypertension in patients undergoing liver transplantation. Anaesth Analg 1996;83:675–680.

39. Castro M, Krowka MJ, Schroeder DR, et al. Frequency and clinical implications of increased pulmo-nary artery pressures in liver transplantation. Mayo Clinic Proc 1996;71:543–551.

40. Hoeper MM, Krowka MJ, Strassburg CP. Portopulmonary hypertension and hepatopulmonary syn-drome. Lancet 2004;363:1461–1468.

41. Kim WR, Krowka MJ, Plevak DJ, et al. Accuracy of doppler echocardiography in the assessment of pulmonary hypertension in liver transplant candidates. Liver Transpl 2000;6:453–458.

42. Torregrosa M, Genesca J, Gonzalez A, et al. Role of doppler echocardiography in the assessment of portopulmonary hypertension in liver transplantation candidates. Transplantation 2001;71:572–574.

43. Bhatia V, Nayyar P, Dhindsa S. Brain natriuretic peptide in diagnosis and treatment of heart failure. J Postgrad Med 2003;49:182–185.

44. Nagaya N, Nishikimi T, Uematsu M, et al. Plasma brain natriuretic peptide as a prognostic indicator in patients with primary pulmonary hypertension. Circulation 2000;102:865–970.

45. Krowka MJ, Frantz RP, McGoon MD, Severson C, Plevak DJ, Wiesner RH. Improvement in pulmo-nary hemodynamics during intravenous epoprostenol (prostacyclin): a study of 15 patients with mod-erate to severe portopulmonary hypertension. Hepatology 1999;30:641–648.

46. Kuo PC, Johnson LB, Plotkin JS, Howell CD, Bartlett ST, Rubin LJ. Continuous intravenous infusion of epoprostenol for the treatment of portopulmonary hypertension. Transplantation 1997;63:604–606.

47. Krowka MJ, Plevak DJ, Findlay JY, Rosen CB, Wiesner RH, Krom RA. Pulmonary hemodynamics and perioperative cardiopulmonary-related mortality in patients with portopulmonary hypertension undergoing liver transplantation. Liver Transpl 2000;6:443–450.

48. Morrow CS, Kantor M, Armen RN. Hepatic hydrothorax. Ann Int Med 1958;49:193–203.

49. Strauss RM, Boyer TD. Hepatic hydrothorax. Sem Liver Dis 1997;17:227–232.

50. Alberts WM, Salem AJ, Solomon DA, Boyce G. Hepatic hydrothorax: cause and management. Arch Int Med 1991;151:2383–2388.

51. Sahn SA. State of the art: the pleura. Am Rev Respirat Dis 1988;138:184–234.
52. Kinasewitz GT, Keddissi JI. Hepatic hydrothorax. Curr Opin Pulmon Med 2003;9:261–265.
53. Benet A, Vidal F, Toda R, et al. Diagnosis of hepatic hydrothorax in the absence of ascites by intraperitoneal injection of ^{99m}Tc-sulfur colloid. Postgrad Med J 1992;68:153.
54. Milenas de Campos JR, Filho LO, Campos Werebe E, et al. Thoracoscopy and talc poudrage in the management of hepatic hydrothorax. Chest 2000;118:13–17.
55. Mouroux J, Perrin C, Venissac N, Blaive B, Richelme H. Management of pleural effusion of cirrhotic origin. Chest 1996;109:1093–1096.
56. Artemiou O, Marta G, Klepetka W, Wolner E, Muller M. Pleurovenous shunting in the treatment of nonmalignant pleural effusion. Ann Thoracic Surg 2003;76:231–233.
57. Andrade RJ, Martin-Palance A, Faile JM, et al. Transjugular intrahepatic portosystemic shunt for the management of hepatic hydrothorax in the absence of ascites. J Clin Gastroenterol 1996;22:305–307.
58. Strauss RM, Martin LG, Kaufman SL, Boyer TD. Transjugular intrahepatic portal systemic shunt for the management of symptomatic cirrhotic hydrothorax. Am J Gastroenterol 1994;89:1520–1522.
59. Spencer EB, Cohen DT, Darcy MD. Safety and efficacy of transjugular intrahepatic portosystemic shunt creation for the treatment of hepatic hydrothorax. J Vasc Intl Radiol 2002;13:385–390.
60. Kaplan LM, Epstein SK, Schwartz SL, Cao QL, Pandian NG. Clinical, echocardiographic, and hemodynamic evidence of cardiac tamponade caused by large pleural effusions. Am J Respirat Crit Care Med 1995;151:904–908.
61. Van Thiel DH, Nadir A, Hassanein T, Wright HI. Simultaneous right-sided volume overload and left-sided hypovolemia in a man with massive ascites and a hydrothorax. Am J Gastroenterol 1995;90:478–481.
62. Wong F, Liu P, Lilly L, et al. The role of cardiac structural and functional abnormalities in the pathogenesis of hyperdynamic circulation and renal sodium retention in cirrhosis. Clin Sci 1999;97:259–267.
63. Pozzi M, Carugo S, Boari G, et al. Functional and structural cardiac abnormalities in cirrhotic patients with and without ascites. Hepatology 1997;26:1131–1137.
64. Naschitz JE, Slobodin G, Lewis RJ, Zuckerman E, Yeshurun D. Heart diseases affecting the liver and liver diseases affecting the heart. Am Heart J 2000;140:111–120.
65. Ahah A, Variyam E. Pericardial effusion and left ventricular dysfunction associated with ascites secondary to hepatic cirrhosis. Arch Int Med 1988;148:585–588.
66. Wong F, Girgrah N, Graba J, Allidina Y, Liu P, Blendis L. The cardiac response to exercise in cirrhosis. Gut 2001;49:268–275.
67. Finucci G, Desideri A, Sacerdoti D, et al. Left ventricular diastolic dysfunction in liver cirrhosis. Scand J Gastroenterol 1996;31:279–284.
68. Bernardi M, Rubboli A, Trevisani F, et al. Reduced cardiobascular responsiveness to exercise-induced sympathoadrenergic stimulation in patients with cirrhosis. J Hepatol 1991;12:207–216.
69. Grose RD, Nolan J, Dillon JF, et al. Exercise-induced left ventricular dysfunction in alcoholic and nonalcoholic cirrhosis. J Hepatol 1995;22:326–332.
70. Wong F, Siu S, Liu P, Blendis L. Brain natriuretic peptide: is it a predictor of cardiomyopathy in cirrhosis. Clin Sci 2001;101:621–628.
71. Henriksen JH, Gotze JP, Fuglsang S, Christensen E, Bendtsen F, Moller S. Increased circulating pro-brain natriuretic peptide (proBNP) and brain natriuretic peptide (BNP) in patients with cirrhosis: relation to cardiovascular dysfunction and severity of disease. Gut 2003;52:1511–1517.
72. Agraou B, Le Tourneau T, Agraou H, Leroy F, Asseman P, Dujardin JJ. Primary biliary cirrhosis associated with pericardial effusion. Ann Cardiol Angeiol (Paris) 1998;47:576–578.
73. Beyer N. Improved physical performance after orthotopic liver transplantation. Liver Transpl Surg 1999;5:301–309.

28 Health Status Assessment and Economic Analyses in Cirrhosis and Portal Hypertension

Jayant A. Talwalkar, MD, MPH
and W. Ray Kim, MD, MBA

CONTENTS

INTRODUCTION
HEALTH-RELATED QUALITY OF LIFE IN CIRRHOSIS
    AND PORTAL HYPERTENSION
ECONOMIC ANALYSES IN CIRRHOSIS AND PORTAL HYPERTENSION
REFERENCES

INTRODUCTION

Health status measurement in patients with cirrhosis and portal hypertension has received increasing attention from clinical investigators in recent times. This is based primarily on the continued absence of curative therapies for disease-related complications outside of liver transplantation. Patients with cirrhosis and portal hypertension have significant reductions in health status compared to general and select disease populations. Early detection and treatment of particular symptoms including muscle cramps and subclinical hepatic encephalopathy may afford the opportunity to improve quality of life in selected individuals. The use of health status as a study end point in controlled clinical trials requires further study on the responsiveness of existing liver disease-specific questionnaires. In conjunction with determining health status among patients with cirrhosis and portal hypertension, a number of investigations have sought to determine the cost effectiveness of clinical strategies for the prevention and treatment of disease-related complications. Further investigations of patient-based preferences for health states, however, are needed to fully understand the magnitude of net health benefits received from existing health care programs.

HEALTH-RELATED QUALITY OF LIFE IN CIRRHOSIS AND PORTAL HYPERTENSION

Purpose of Health Status Assessment

Health-related quality of life (or health status) is defined as a multidimensional construct consisting of domains which capture an individual's experience related to the presence or

From: *Clinical Gastroenterology: Portal Hypertension*
Edited by: A. J. Sanyal and V. H. Shah © Humana Press Inc., Totowa, NJ

absence of illness. The major domains involve physical, mental, and psychosocial factors. Identifying the extent of impairments in health status has allowed for an improved understanding of differences in clinical outcomes associated with similar chronic conditions (1,2). In recent years, the development of instruments using psychometric techniques has provided a more accurate representation of health status for an individual or population (3).

Health status measurement in patients with cirrhosis and portal hypertension has also received attention from clinical investigators. This is based primarily on the continued absence of curative therapies for disease-related complications. In addition, the impact of symptoms and toxicities of supportive therapy can be identified with health status measurement (1–3). Symptom severity, in particular, does not consistently correlate with pathophysiologic consequences of hepatic dysfunction described by existing summary measures of disease severity including the Child–Turcotte–Pugh (CTP) and Model for End-Stage Liver Disease (MELD) scores (4–6). In turn, the goal of health status measurement is to also identify a single number which captures the level of functional impairment resulting from cirrhosis.

SYSTEMIC EFFECTS OF CIRRHOSIS

The pathophysiologic processes associated with cirrhosis and portal hypertension are also responsible for systemic effects that contribute to overall disease status and health-related quality of life.

Fatigue is a common and potentially disabling symptom in patients with cirrhosis. As observed with many chronic diseases, the severity of fatigue is often independent of disease stage and underlying etiology (7). The absence of an objective index to quantify fatigue, however, has limited the understanding of its origin and subsequent development of potential therapies.

The estimated prevalence rate of depression in patients with cirrhosis (8) is 30% and similar to our experience among patients referred for liver transplant evaluation (unpublished). High-risk subgroups include those individuals with a prior history of depression and substance abuse. The psychosocial impact of disease progression and recurrent hospitalization for portal hypertensive complications has not been formally studied.

Sleep disorders are increasingly recognized but their frequency in association with cirrhosis remains underreported. When studied in a systematic fashion, an estimated 50% of patients without overt hepatic encephalopathy have evidence for poor sleep hygiene compared to healthy controls (9). Disruption of the circadian sleep–wake cycle rather than advanced liver disease or cognitive impairment is predictive of sleep disturbance in cirrhosis.

A number of investigations have documented increased prevalence rates for severe muscle cramps in patients with cirrhosis. Selected reports document frequencies between 52% and 88% (10–12). The underlying pathophysiology, however, remains unknown. The occurrence of muscle cramps is independent of the liver disease etiology, severity of cirrhosis, diuretic use, or serum electrolyte alterations. Reductions in effective arterial volume (6) may be the pathophysiologic alteration responsible for this troubling and underestimated symptom.

Health Status Questionnaires

Since the early 1980s, a number of standardized generic health status questionnaires have been developed for investigative use (13). The most common questionnaires used in studies of cirrhosis are the Short Form 36 (SF-36) Health Survey, Sickness Impact Profile, and Nottingham Health Profile. Based on concerns that generic questionnaires do not address unique problems experienced by patients with cirrhosis, several liver disease-specific questionnaires have been developed using psychometric *(14,15)* or module-based techniques *(16)*. For all questionnaires, however, the ability to make accurate health status assessments depends on their inherent reliability and validity.

RELIABILITY OF HEALTH STATUS INSTRUMENTS

Reliability is defined as the dependability of a questionnaire independent of its method of construction. Measures of reliability include internal consistency and test-retest reliability. *Internal consistency* is defined by how well items in a questionnaire are measuring health status. Cronbach's alpha is a statistical method which is based on the average correlation between items in a questionnaire (values range from 0 to 1). A Cronbach's alpha level of 0.7 or greater is associated with acceptable levels of reliability for health status questionnaires. *Test-retest reliability* is defined as the stability of a questionnaire in measuring health status on repeated occasions. Test-retest reliability coefficients between 0.80 and 0.90 are considered acceptable although values as low as 0.50 have also been recognized as satisfactory *(13,17)*.

VALIDITY OF HEALTH STATUS INSTRUMENTS

The two most important forms of validity are termed content and construct validity. *Content validity* measures the completeness of items within a questionnaire that captures the salient features of health status. *Construct validity* is defined by a questionnaire's ability to discriminate between different levels of impaired health status and between individuals. This is strengthened by documenting some degree of correlation to well-established clinical parameters of the disease under study. The *responsiveness* of a questionnaire is defined by its ability to detect changes in health status with disease progression and/or treatment effects over time. The inability to detect a negative change in health status when previously reported at its lowest level has been termed the "floor effect." Conversely, the inability to detect positive changes in health status from a previous maximum rating is termed the "ceiling effect" *(13,17)*. These effects can significantly limit the accuracy of health status assessment and occur more frequently with generic rather than disease-specific questionnaires.

The cross-sectional reliability and validity of selected generic and all disease-specific questionnaires in patients with cirrhosis has been demonstrated. None of the liver disease-specific instruments, however, has been shown to contain the ability for evaluating change in health status over time.

Results of Health Status Assessment in Cirrhosis and Portal Hypertension

The majority of cohort studies to date have used generic questionnaires for cross-sectional assessments of health status. When disease-specific questionnaires are used, they appear to have better discriminatory ability among patients with varying disease severity compared to generic instruments *(14–16,18)*. Nonetheless, a number of recurrent themes among published investigations have been observed. For the purposes of generalizability, the results that follow do not include studies focusing only on patients referred for liver transplantation.

The reported health status among patients with cirrhosis is markedly reduced compared to healthy or general populations. Reductions in physical function are the most dramatic when compared to mental function. In general, older individuals with cirrhosis report greater impairments in health status compared to younger patients. Overall health status, however, does not appear to be strongly influenced by sex, disease etiology, or duration of liver disease (19–23). Notably, the presence of muscle cramps has been most strongly associated with impairments of both physical and mental function. Interventions such as endoscopic sclerotherapy for prior variceal bleeding and nutritional supplementation have been associated with improved health status (19).

Impaired physical function is consistently the most common reason for reduced health status in patients with cirrhosis using generic (19–23) and disease-specific questionnaires (14–16,21). Decompensated liver disease with ascites and hepatic encephalopathy further reduce health status compared to compensated individuals (19–23). The need for hospitalization and medication use with β-blockers and oral diuretics are strongly correlated with reduced physical function (19). In some individuals with cirrhosis, reductions in health status may even be greater than impairments reported by selected individuals with congestive heart failure and chronic obstructive pulmonary disease (21).

Although increasing CTP classification is associated with greater reductions in physical function, the correlation between these variables is relatively weak (19–23). This is not surprising given that some patients with mild disease severity can report significant health status impairments based on symptoms (i.e., fatigue) rather than obvious clinical manifestations such as ascites. Decreased peripheral muscle strength (24) and reduced exercise capacity (25,26), both of which are associated with poor physical function, are also not captured by CTP or MELD scores. Notably, the presence of anxiety/depression (elicited by generic questionnaire) rather than cardiac structural abnormalities was associated with impaired health status in patients with cirrhotic cardiomyopathy (27).

Health status questionnaires have described only mild impairments in emotional and psychological function among patients with varying degrees of cirrhosis (14,15,18). The level of impairment does not decline with advancing liver disease as seen with physical function. From one investigation, the presence of sexual dysfunction and inability to work was strongly associated with reduced mental function among men with cirrhosis. Curtailments in social and home activities were of greatest concern to women (19).

Despite advances in the understanding of health status related to cirrhosis, several issues require further study. Information regarding the method of questionnaire administration, selection of patients, and handling of missing data has not been universally reported in all studies which raises concerns about selection bias. Similarly, the majority of studies involve referral-based populations whose self-reporting of health status is likely to differ from patients with milder disease who reside in the community. The majority of studies also do not systematically account for the effect of comorbid illness as a major contributor to impaired health status. The absence of greater emotional disturbance with increasing disease severity may reflect deficiencies with current disease-specific questionnaires based on their development using populations with milder disease severity.

Specific Hepatic Disease Etiologies

CHRONIC HEPATITIS C

Several investigations have documented significant reductions in health status among patients with chronic hepatitis C-related cirrhosis in comparison to general populations and patients with precirrhotic stage disease *(28–37)*. Unselected individuals report greater impairments in health status compared to study participants *(30)*. Comorbid illness may also further impair health status *(30,31)*. Of note, a history of substance abuse has not been shown to influence health status *(30)* although active psychiatric disease is an important determinant of poor function *(32,33)*. Among patients enrolled in registration trials for interferon-based therapy *(34–37)*, an improvement in health status following successful viral eradication compared to baseline values has been observed with compensated cirrhosis. For patients with advanced cirrhosis requiring liver transplantation, significant improvements in health status within the first year after surgery have also been observed *(38,39)*.

CHOLESTATIC LIVER DISEASE

Impaired health status from cirrhosis secondary to primary biliary cirrhosis (PBC) and primary sclerosing cholangitis (PSC) have been demonstrated when compared to healthy individuals and patients with precirrhotic stage *(16,40)*. Correlations between increasing Mayo risk score and reduced health status are better detected with disease-specific questionnaires for both conditions *(40)*. The importance of fatigue as a primary determinant of health status in PBC is recognized by several published investigations to date *(41–43)*. The effect of medical therapy with ursodeoxycholic acid on health status in PBC, however, remains unknown. Short-term improvements in health status following liver transplantation have also been observed in adults with cholestatic liver disease *(44)*.

Impact of Disease-Related Complications on Health Status

VARICEAL BLEEDING

Treatment approaches for acute variceal bleeding have resulted in greater survival rates over time *(45)*. Consequently, the impact of surviving a variceal bleed on health status may also be important in affected patients. Administration of the liver disease-specific NIDDK-QA questionnaire, however, did not reveal any significant differences in health status between patients with and without a prior history of variceal bleeding *(46)*. Study limitations including recall bias and the absence of specific questions about variceal bleeding may have contributed to this negative result. More importantly, there have been no published data examining health status in patients undergoing primary prophylaxis for esophageal variceal bleeding.

For patients with recurrent variceal bleeding, both short- and long-term (greater than 1 yr) gains in health status were initially reported following transjugular intrahepatic portosystemic shunt (TIPS) placement. Significant loss to follow-up from death and use of the Karnofsky scale (which measures physical activity alone) limit the external validity of these results *(47)*. In contrast, impaired emotional function from neuropsychologic dysfunction has been observed following TIPS placement for recurrent variceal bleeding *(48)*. Improvements in emotional function and fatigue subscale scores with the SF-36 Health Survey noted from a recent study are limited by retrospective methods of health status assessment and subsequent recall bias *(49)*. A prospective, randomized controlled trial showed no difference in health status among patients treated with medical therapy or TIPS to prevent recurrent variceal bleeding. Absence of a disease-specific questionnaire and the inability to detect minimal change with the Nottingham Health Profile may have been responsible for the observed results *(50)*.

ASCITES

In patients with mild to moderate ascites, the use of oral diuretics is responsible for reduced health status based primarily on adverse drug effects *(19)*. For the treatment of severe or refractory ascites, the majority of health status investigations have focused on the impact of TIPS placement. Significant gains in health status were initially reported in patients undergoing TIPS placement for refractory ascites. Significant losses to follow-up from death and retrospective methods of health status assessment, however, limit the validity of study results *(47,51)*. In 21 patients undergoing repeated large-volume paracentesis for at least 1 yr *(52)*, the greatest improvements in health status were reported among patients with a complete response following TIPS placement. The major absence of a control group limits the applicability of these findings. Recently, the use of medical therapy (including total paracentesis) versus medical therapy and TIPS was examined in a multicenter, randomized control trial. Despite improvements in control of ascites, there were no differences between groups in terms of survival or health-related quality of life measured by the SF-36 Health Survey *(53)*. Again, the use of liver disease-specific questionnaires may have provided further details about the experiences of patients in each treatment arm.

HEPATIC ENCEPHALOPATHY

Three studies have been published which examine the specific impact of hepatic encephalopathy on health status in patients with cirrhosis *(54–56)*. Individuals with subclinical hepatic encephalopathy have greater reductions in health status measured by the generic Sickness Impact Profile questionnaire compared to patients with cirrhosis alone. In this study, subclinical hepatic encephalopathy was independently related to a reduced Sickness Impact Profile score *(54)*. Similar results among patients eligible for liver transplantation in the United States with subclinical and overt hepatic encephalopathy have been reported using the SF-36 Health Survey *(55)*. With compensated cirrhosis, the presence of subclinical hepatic encephalopathy was associated with significant reductions in mental function scores alone. Among patients residing in Germany, the occurrence of premature workforce retirement owing to subclinical hepatic encephalopathy is strongly correlated with reduced health status independent of age or liver disease severity *(56)*.

HEPATOCELLULAR CARCINOMA

The most common risk factor for developing hepatocellular carcinoma (HCC) is cirrhosis *(57)*. Following operative resection of HCC in eligible patients, a reported increase in health status is observed when compared to individuals with unresectable disease undergoing transarterial chemoembolization *(58)*. Longitudinal declines in health status, however, are observed among surgically treated patients who experience recurrent HCC. From a subgroup analysis of a large cohort study, the presence of greater impairments in physical function, reported pain, and sleep was reported in patients with HCC vs controls with cirrhosis alone. For affected patients with HCC, health status was independent of tumor burden or hepatic disease severity, although disease-specific questionnaires were not administered *(59)*. Specific information about health status among patients with cirrhosis enrolled in screening and surveillance programs for HCC are not available.

NUTRITION

The importance of proper nutrition in the medical management of cirrhosis has received increasing attention *(60)*. Improved 1-yr survival, stabilization of liver disease, and reduced hospitalization rates have been reported following the use of branched-chain amino acids (BCAA) in controlled trial settings *(61)*. Compared to individuals given lactoalbumin or maltodextrin as nutritional supplements, patients with advanced cirrhosis receiving BCAA also reported statistically significant improvements in physical function compared to baseline values. The proportion of patients reporting poor health status decreased from 19% at baseline to 3% after 1 yr of BCAA therapy. Confirmatory studies examining the impact of nutrition on health status are awaited.

Health Status Assessment as a Clinical Trial End Point

Given the evidence in support of cross-sectional reliability and validity, the next challenge for health status questionnaires in patients with cirrhosis and portal hypertension is their use in clinical trial settings. Primary study end points including survival, time to treatment failure, or surrogate marker improvement are too insensitive for capturing important health effects. Information about the overall effects of novel treatment (compared to placebo or standard therapy) would be helpful for decision-making purposes to both clinicians and patients. The major limitation of longitudinal health status assessment in clinical trials is determining what represents a minimum clinically important difference (MCID) *(62)*. It has been suggested that the psychometric properties of health status questionnaires and correlations with global reports of change following treatment are required for determining the MCID. In clinical trials, however, the average response to a therapeutic intervention is often chosen as an end point. With reported health status as the end point, this approach may not reflect the actual distribution of individual responses found in a treatment group *(63)*. Further work in this area is necessary before firm conclusions about methodology can be reached.

Health State Utilities in Cirrhosis and Portal Hypertension

The majority of health status questionnaires allow respondents to rate their perceived health status with a quantitative value to allow for comparisons between other patient populations. Changes in an individual patient's health status can also be measured in terms of effects (i.e., life years gained from an intervention) or the values placed on health status *(64,65)*. The values place on health status have been termed health state preferences or utilities.

Health state utilities are determined by asking respondents about their threshold for risk in obtaining a desired outcome (e.g., the number of days given up for a current state of health to achieve 1 d of improved or perfect health). The elicited threshold is equivalent to the utility placed on an individual's current health state *(65,66)*. The basis of techniques to determine health state utility reside in economic theories of risk and utilitarianism. Fortunately, a number of assessment methods now exist which facilitate improved understanding for patients when utility values are being sought. The importance of health state utilities is underscored by formal recommendations to include these values for properly conducting economic analyses of health care programs *(66)*.

Two published investigations of health state preference in patients with cirrhosis are noted in refs. *67* and *68*. Results are varied depending on the techniques used. Overall, a relationship between declining health state utilities and worsening hepatic function is observed. Further investigations including the accuracy of longitudinal responses in clinical trial settings are eagerly awaited.

ECONOMIC ANALYSES IN CIRRHOSIS AND PORTAL HYPERTENSION

Background

Based on the recognition of limited resources, there is continued emphasis placed on identifying strategies or programs associated with optimal health care delivery. For economic evaluations of health care programs, a comparative analysis between alternate courses of action is required for decision-making at a policymaking level. The evaluation of a single program, which often results in a description of cost or outcome, is useful to estimate disease burden but is not considered an economic analysis based on the absence of a comparator program.

A number of methods have been developed for the economic evaluation of two or more competing strategies. Common to these designs is the determination of a ratio between consequences of health (outcomes) and the cost required to execute the program or strategy. For example, when outcomes of two or more alternative strategies are considered equivalent, the comparative study that is performed is called a *cost-minimization analysis*. In the medical literature, the most commonly employed technique is known as a *cost-effectiveness analysis*. The cost-effectiveness analysis defines that consequences of health are not valued by monetary indices but by metrics such as "quality of life years (QALY) gained." When comparing two or more strategies, the unit of measurement employed in these studies is called an incremental cost-effectiveness ratio (ICER). The recommended metric for ICER is "cost per QALY" as the description of health benefits appears to be most well described by this nomenclature *(69,70)*.

In the performance of economic analyses, a number of elements are required. These include: (1) a complete description of both costs and health outcomes; (2) the inclusion and complete description of a competing alternative strategy; (3) the identification of evidence to support previously established effectiveness; and (4) the appropriate valuation and inclusion of relevant costs. The importance of conducting evaluations with standardized methods is to allow for relevant comparisons between different programs to determine resource allocation priorities. Differences in resource availability, clinical practice patterns, and availability of alternate strategies may affect the results of economic evaluations *(69,70)*.

Specific Disease-Related Complications in Cirrhosis and Portal Hypertension

Acute Variceal Bleeding

The cost of managing acute variceal bleeding ranges between $15,000 and $50,000 (U.S.) per individual patient *(71–73)*. Severity of liver disease, duration of intensive care unit stay, and blood transfusion requirements are significant factors that increase cost *(71)*. In terms of cost per health benefit, there are no cost-effectiveness analyses reported that examine particular aspects in the management of variceal bleeding. However, the use of parenteral vasoconstrictors compared to strategies without these pharmacologic agents is associated with an additional cost of approx $26,000 (U.S.) per life saved *(73)*. Lower 2-yr costs per patient for endoscopic sclerotherapy compared to nonendoscopic therapies were reported from the 1980s before the advent of widespread band ligation *(74)*. A retrospective study of patients with acute gastric variceal bleeding demonstrated lower costs with N-butyl-2-cyanoacrylate (Histoacryl) glue therapy vs TIPS ($4138 vs $11,906 per patient treated) (75). In the absence of health state utility assessment, the overall effectiveness of either modality remains uncertain. From a controlled trial comparing endoscopic sclerotherapy with band ligation therapy where economic data were prospectively collected (76), the initial use of band ligation for acute variceal bleeding was associated with increased costs based on higher treatment failure rates. Effectiveness was measured, however, in terms of "life year saved" or "bleed prevented" without consideration of measured or estimated health state utilities.

PRIMARY PROPHYLAXIS FOR ESOPHAGEAL VARICEAL HEMORRHAGE

The cost-effectiveness of primary prophylaxis against esophageal variceal bleeding has been investigated in four published studies (77–80). Natural history simulation with Markov state-transition models was used in all instances. Strategies that were commonly examined included observation alone, screening for esophageal varices followed by treatment with β-blockers or band ligation, and universal β-blocker prophylaxis without screening. In three studies which included the costs of screening endoscopy, the most cost-effective strategy was universal prophylaxis with β-blockers which ranged between $1200 and $12,000 per life year saved (78–80). The widespread application of this strategy in clinical practice, however, remains questionable. Potential reasons include the absence of patient-elicited health state utilities accounting for clinical issues related to β-blocker use and diverging results about which subgroup would benefit the most from this strategy (CTP class A or CTP class B/C). Conflicting data also exist about the cost effectiveness of hepatic venous pressure gradient monitoring for primary prophylaxis with β blockers (81,82). Prospective study for definitive results will be required.

SECONDARY PROPHYLAXIS FOR ESOPHAGEAL VARICEAL HEMORRHAGE

A single cost-effectiveness analysis examining medical, endoscopic, and TIPS strategies for the prevention of recurrent variceal hemorrhage has been reported (83). In a 3-yr period, a combination of medical therapy with endoscopic band ligation was declared as the most cost-effective approach. The use of TIPS was favored only when patient adherence rates for competing strategies fell below 12%. Estimated patient preferences for medical therapy also influenced the model's results.

The majority of recent studies on TIPS for secondary prophylaxis, however, have focused on its economic impact alone. When compared to combination β-blocker and oral nitrate therapy, the use of TIPS was associated with greater costs despite higher recurrent bleeding rates with medical therapy (84). No difference in survival was observed between prophylaxis strategies. Secondary cost analyses from three investigations comparing the efficacy of TIPS with endoscopic therapy have been reported (85–87). When compared to endoscopic sclerotherapy, a greater long-term cost is associated with TIPS based on the development of shunt dysfunction and hepatic encephalopathy (85,86). A lower cost per patient, however, is observed with TIPS compared to band ligation therapy when only hospitalization costs are measured (87). From the only published economic analysis on this topic (88), the incremental cost-effectiveness ratio for TIPS vs sclerotherapy or band ligation over 1 yr ranged between $8800 and $12,660 per variceal bleed prevented. Increases in procedure-related costs and TIPS stenosis rates above 80% favored endoscopic therapy. Despite similar mortality rates for each strategy, the use of patient-based utilities for calculating quality-adjusted life-years was not performed.

For patients with CTP class A or B cirrhosis, the use of surgical shunt therapy is associated with fewer rebleeding episodes and reduced long-term costs compared with TIPS *(89,90)*. In a subsequent economic analysis, however, the incremental cost-effectiveness ratio for TIPS vs distal splenorenal shunt therapy was unfavorable at $147,340 per life year saved *(91)*.

ASCITES AND SPONTANEOUS BACTERIAL PERITONITIS

For the treatment of refractory or recividant ascites, the use of large volume paracentesis or TIPS is often used in clinical practice. Recent studies demonstrate no advantage in survival from TIPS although control of ascites is better compared to medical therapy *(53,92,93)*. Unfortunately, there is no cost-effectiveness analysis published to date which compares both strategies. However, a multicenter, randomized study of patients with refractory ascites from the United States and Spain reported cost increases between 44 and 103% for TIPS when compared to serial large volume paracentesis *(94)*. In both countries, the follow-up costs required for TIPS management exceeded the initial procedural costs.

Mortality rates from spontaneous bacterial peritonitis (SBP) have declined over the past two decades *(95)*. Three investigations have examined the cost effectiveness of antibiotic prophylaxis for SBP. For patients at high risk (ascitic fluid total protein concentrations ≤ 1 g/dL or a previous history of SBP), the use of either norfloxacin or trimethoprim-sulfamethoxazole (TMP-SMX) was associated with a decrease in total costs for SBP treatment between $4692 and $9251 per patient, respectively *(96,97)*. Smaller differences between antibiotic prophylaxis and no treatment are observed when lower inpatient treatment costs for SBP are assumed *(98)*. The cost per life-year saved in one study was estimated between $10,890 and $16,538 with antibiotic prophylaxis compared to no therapy *(99)*. However, the 20% annual probability rate for recurrent SBP assigned to TMP-SMX has not been demonstrated clinically *(99,100)*. In addition, the weekly administration of ciprofloxacin was not included as a potential strategy despite proven efficacy *(101)*. The assumption in all three studies that efficacy of antibiotic prophylaxis is stable over a 1-yr period requires prospective confirmation. No study incorporated measured or estimated health state utilities to determine the quality-adjusted life years gained from antibiotic prophylaxis.

HEPATOCELLULAR CARCINOMA

Despite objective evidence for the rising incidence of HCC in patients with cirrhosis, the cost effectiveness of early detection programs to improve survival and reduce morbidity remains controversial *(102–104)*. Three investigations focused on screening and surveillance for HCC in unselected populations have been published *(105–107)*. The majority of studies have compared serum α fetoprotein (AFP) with abdominal ultrasound at 6-mo intervals vs no screening. ICER of screening and surveillance, however, vary widely between $25,000 and $284,000 per life year saved. When all potential treatment options are considered (including ablative maneuvers, operative resection, and transplantation), the use of serum AFP with ultrasound every 6 mo is associated with an ICER of $112,993 per life year saved compared to no screening *(106)*. In this analysis, however, the use of charges rather than costs suggests that ICER values may actually be more favorable. Only one study *(107)* used elicited or assumed health state utility data for assessing benefit in terms of QALY. Notably, an estimated ICER between $25,000–$27,000 per

QALY with serum AFP plus ultrasound or computed tomography (CT) was reported in transplant-eligible patients with chronic hepatitis C. Notably, this is the only investigation where ICER values are below $50,000 per QALY which is generally considered an acceptable threshold for determining the value of medical surveillance programs in the United States. The failure to account for costs of recall procedures and therapeutic interventions for HCC was rarely observed in these studies (105).

A number of cost-effectiveness studies in selected populations with HCC have also been reported. Among patients eligible for either operative resection or liver transplantation (108), an ICER between $44,000 and $184,000 per additional year gained was observed if waiting time to transplant is less than 6–10 mo. When salvage liver transplantation is considered following initial operative resection vs primary liver transplantation (109), an ICER less than $50,000 per additional year gained is observed only for waiting times less than 12 mo. Similar results with operative resection as preadjuvant therapy in compensated liver transplant recipients are observed for waiting times beyond 12 mo (110). The cost-effectiveness of ablative therapy for HCC in patients waiting for liver transplantation is estimated between $50,000 and $100,000 per life-year saved (111). For patients with decompensated cirrhosis awaiting liver transplantation, the use of percutaneous ethanol injection therapy resulted in a cost effectiveness of $23,000 per life-year saved (111). Although many of these ICER values are considered cost ineffective, the assignment of elevated MELD scores for liver transplant recipients with HCC in the United States could improve the value of these strategies based on shorter waiting times. In areas where timely cadaveric liver transplantation remains problematic, the use of living donor liver transplantation appears cost effective (<$50,000 per QALY) when the waiting time exceeds 7 mo and high dropout rates from disease progression exist (112).

A single investigation of adjuvant interferon therapy after surgical resection for chronic hepatitis C-associated HCC was declared cost effective compared to observation alone (113). Assumptions in this study regarding the true incidence of recurrent HCC after interferon therapy, which are based on uncontrolled data, require prospective confirmation.

REFERENCES

1. Borgaonkar MR, Irvine EJ. Quality of life measurement in gastrointestinal and liver disorders. Gut 2000;47:444–454.
2. Glise H, Wiklund I. Health-related quality of life and gastrointestinal disease. J Gastroenterol Hepatol 2002;17(Supp 1):S72–S84.
3. Jones PA. Health status measurement in chronic obstructive pulmonary disease. Thorax 2001;56: 880–887.
4. Child CG III, Turcotte JG. Surgery and portal hypertension. In: Child CG III, ed. The Liver and Portal Hypertension. WB Saunders, Philadelphia, PA, 1964, pp. 49–50.
5. Pugh RN, Murray-Lyon IM, Dawson JL, Pietroni MC, Williams R. Transection of the oesophagus for bleeding oesophageal varices. Br J Surg 1973;60:646–649.
6. Kamath PS, Wiesner RH, Malinchoc M, et al. A model to predict survival in patients with end-stage liver disease. Hepatology 2001;33:464–470.
7. Swain MG. Fatigue in chronic disease. Clin Sci (Lond) 2000;99:1–8.
8. Singh N, Gayowski T, Wagener MM, Marino IR. Depression in patients with cirrhosis. Impact on outcome. Dig Dis Sci 1997;42:1421–1427.
9. Cordoba J, Cabrera J, Lataif L, Penev P, Zee P, Blei AT. High prevalence of sleep disturbance in cirrhosis. Hepatology 1998;27:339–345.
10. Konikoff F, Theodor E. Painful muscle cramps. A symptom of liver cirrhosis? J Clin Gastroenterol 1986;8(6):669–672.

11. Abrams GA, Concato J, Fallon MB. Muscle cramps in patients with cirrhosis. Am J Gastroenterol 1996;91(7):1363–1366.
12. Angeli P, Albino G, Carraro P, et al. Cirrhosis and muscle cramps: evidence of a causal relationship. Hepatology 1996;23(2):264–273.
13. Guyatt GH, Feeny DH, Patrick DL. Measuring health-related quality of life. Ann Intern Med 1993; 118:622–629.
14. Younossi ZM, Guyatt G, Kiwi M, Boparai N, King D. Development of a disease specific questionnaire to measure health related quality of life in patients with chronic liver disease. Gut 1999;45:295–300.
15. Gralnek IM, Hays RD, Kilbourne A, et al. Development and evaluation of the Liver Disease Quality of Life instrument in persons with advanced, chronic liver disease—the LDQOL 1.0. Am J Gastroenterol 2000;95:3552–3565.
16. Kim WR, Lindor KD, Malinchoc M, Petz JL, Jorgensen R, Dickson ER. Reliability and validity of the NIDDK-QA instrument in the assessment of quality of life in ambulatory patients with cholestatic liver disease. Hepatology 2000;32:924–929.
17. Younossi ZM, Guyatt G. Quality-of-life assessments and chronic liver disease. Am J Gastroenterol 1998;93:1037–1041.
18. Martin LM, Sheridan MJ, Younossi ZM. The impact of liver disease on health-related quality of life: a review of the literature. Curr Gastroenterol Rep 2002;4:79–83.
19. Marchesini G, Bianchi G, Amodio P, et al. Italian Study Group for quality of life in cirrhosis. Factors associated with poor health-related quality of life of patients with cirrhosis. Gastroenterology 2001; 120:170–178.
20. Lacevic N, Vanis N, Bratovic I. Reduced quality of life in liver cirrhosis. Med Arh 2000;54:93–96.
21. Younossi ZM, Boparai N, Price LL, Kiwi ML, McCormick M, Guyatt G. Health-related quality of life in chronic liver disease: the impact of type and severity of disease. Am J Gastroenterol 2001;96: 2199–2205.
22. Van Der Plas SM, Hansen BE, De Boer JB, et al. Generic and disease-specific health related quality of life in non-cirrhotic, cirrhotic and transplanted liver patients: a cross-sectional study. BMC Gastroenterol 2003;3:33.
23. Unal G, de Boer JB, Borsboom GJ, Brouwer JT, Essink-Bot M, de Man RA. A psychometric comparison of health-related quality of life measures in chronic liver disease. J Clin Epidemiol 2001;54: 587–596.
24. Panzak G, Tarter R, Murali S, et al. Isometric muscle strength in alcoholic and nonalcoholic liver-transplantation candidates. Am J Drug Alcohol Abuse 1998;24:499–512.
25. Wiesinger GF, Quittan M, Zimmermann K, et al. Physical performance and health-related quality of life in men on a liver transplantation waiting list. J Rehabil Med 2001;33:260–265.
26. Wong F, Girgrah N, Graba J, Allidina Y, Liu P, Blendis L. The cardiac response to exercise in cirrhosis. Gut 2001;49:268–275.
27. Girgrah N, Reid G, MacKenzie S, Wong F. Cirrhotic cardiomyopathy: does it contribute to chronic fatigue and decreased health-related quality of life in cirrhosis? Can J Gastroenterol 2003;17:545–551.
28. Bianchi G, Loguercio C, Sgarbi D, et al. Reduced quality of life in patients with chronic hepatitis C: effects of interferon treatment. Dig Liver Dis 2000;32:398–405.
29. Cordoba J, Flavia M, Jacas C, et al. Quality of life and cognitive function in hepatitis C at different stages of liver disease. J Hepatol 2003;39:231–238.
30. Hussain KB, Fontana RJ, Moyer CA, Su GL, Sneed-Pee N, Lok AS. Comorbid illness is an important determinant of health-related quality of life in patients with chronic hepatitis C. Am J Gastroenterol 2001;96:2737–2744.
31. Fontana RJ, Moyer CA, Sonnad S, et al. Comorbidities and quality of life in patients with interferon-refractory chronic hepatitis C. Am J Gastroenterol 2001;96:170–178.
32. Fontana RJ, Hussain KB, Schwartz SM, Moyer CA, Su GL, Lok AS. Emotional distress in chronic hepatitis C patients not receiving antiviral therapy. J Hepatol 2002;36:401–407.
33. Gallegos-Orozco JF, Fuentes AP, Gerardo Argueta J, et al. Health-related quality of life and depression in patients with chronic hepatitis C. Arch Med Res 2003;34:124–129.

34. McHutchison JG, Ware JE Jr, Bayliss MS, et al. Hepatitis Interventional Therapy Group. The effects of interferon alpha-2b in combination with ribavirin on health related quality of life and work productivity. J Hepatol 2001;34:140–147.

35. Ware JE Jr, Bayliss MS, Mannocchia M, Davis GL. Health-related quality of life in chronic hepatitis C: impact of disease and treatment response. The Interventional Therapy Group. Hepatology 1999;30: 550–555.

36. Bonkovsky HL, Woolley JM. Reduction of health-related quality of life in chronic hepatitis C and improvement with interferon therapy. The Consensus Interferon Study Group. Hepatology 1999;29: 264–270.

37. Bernstein D, Kleinman L, Barker CM, Revicki DA, Green J. Relationship of health-related quality of life to treatment adherence and sustained response in chronic hepatitis C patients. Hepatology 2002; 35:704–708.

38. Belle SH, Porayko MK, Hoofnagle JH, Lake JR, Zetterman RK. Changes in quality of life after liver transplantation among adults. National Institute of Diabetes and Digestive and Kidney Diseases (NIDDK) Liver Transplantation Database (LTD). Liver Transpl Surg 1997;3:93–104.

39. Younossi ZM, McCormick M, Price LL, et al. Impact of liver transplantation on health-related quality of life. Liver Transpl 2000;6:779–783.

40. Younossi ZM, Kiwi ML, Boparai N, Price LL, Guyatt G. Cholestatic liver diseases and health-related quality of life. Am J Gastroenterol 2000;95:497–502.

41. Cauch-Dudek K, Abbey S, Stewart DE, Heathcote EJ. Fatigue in primary biliary cirrhosis. Gut 1998; 43:705–710.

42. Huet PM, Deslauriers J, Tran A, Faucher C, Charbonneau J. Impact of fatigue on the quality of life of patients with primary biliary cirrhosis. Am J Gastroenterol 2000;95:760–767.

43. Prince MI, James OF, Holland NP, Jones DE. Validation of a fatigue impact score in primary biliary cirrhosis: towards a standard for clinical and trial use. J Hepatol 2000;32:368–373.

44. Gross CR, Malinchoc M, Kim WR, et al. Quality of life before and after liver transplantation for cholestatic liver disease. Hepatology 1999;29:356–364.

45. McCormick PA, O'Keefe C. Improving prognosis following a first variceal haemorrhage over four decades. Gut 2001;49:682–685.

46. Talwalkar JA, Kamath PS, Kim WR. Health-related quality of life assessment after variceal bleeding among patients with end-stage liver disease. Hepatology 2000;32(4 Pt 2):907A.

47 Nazarian GK, Ferral H, Bjarnason H, et al. Effect of transjugular intrahepatic portosystemic shunt on quality of life. AJR Am J Roentgenol 1996;167:963–969.

48. Jalan R, Gooday R, O'Carroll RE, Redhead DN, Elton RA, Hayes PC. A prospective evaluation of changes in neuropsychological and liver function tests following transjugular intrahepatic portosystemic stent-shunt. J Hepatol 1995;23:697–705.

49. Zhuang ZW, Teng GJ, Jeffery RF, Gemery JM, Janne d'Othee B, Bettmann MA. Long-term results and quality of life in patients treated with transjugular intrahepatic portosystemic shunts. AJR Am J Roentgenol 2002;179:1597–1603.

50. Escorsell A, Banares R, Garcia-Pagan JC, et al. TIPS versus drug therapy in preventing variceal rebleeding in advanced cirrhosis: a randomized controlled trial. Hepatology 2002;35:385–392.

51. Zhuang ZW, Teng GJ, Jeffery RF, Gemery JM, Janne d'Othee B, Bettmann MA. Long-term results and quality of life in patients treated with transjugular intrahepatic portosystemic shunts. AJR Am J Roentgenol 2002;179:1597–1603.

52. Gulberg V, Liss I, Bilzer M, Waggershauser T, Reiser M, Gerbes AL. Improved quality of life in patients with refractory or recidivant ascites after insertion of transjugular intrahepatic portosystemic shunts. Digestion 2002;66:127–130.

53. Sanyal AJ, Genning C, Reddy KR, et al. North American Study for the Treatment of Refractory Ascites Group. The North American study for the treatment of refractory ascites. Gastroenterology 2003;124: 634–641.

54. Groeneweg M, Quero JC, De Bruijn I, et al. Subclinical hepatic encephalopathy impairs daily functioning. Hepatology 1998;28:45–49.

55. Arguedas MR, DeLawrence TG, McGuire BM. Influence of hepatic encephalopathy on health-related quality of life in patients with cirrhosis. Dig Dis Sci 2003;48:1622–1626.

56. Schomerus H, Hamster W. Quality of life in cirrhotics with minimal hepatic encephalopathy. Metab Brain Dis 2001;16:37–41.

57. El-Serag HB. Hepatocellular carcinoma: an epidemiologic view. J Clin Gastroenterol 2002;35(5 Suppl 2):S72–S78.

58. Bianchi G, Loguercio C, Sgarbi D, et al. Reduced quality of life of patients with hepatocellular carcinoma. Dig Liver Dis 2003;35:46–54.

59. Poon RT, Fan ST, Yu WC, Lam BK, Chan FY, Wong J. A prospective longitudinal study of quality of life after resection of hepatocellular carcinoma. Arch Surg 2001;136:693–699.

60. Marchesini G, Bianchi G, Rossi B, Brizi M, Melchionda N. Nutritional treatment with branched-chain amino acids in advanced liver cirrhosis. J Gastroenterol 2000;35(Suppl 12):7–12.

61. Marchesini G, Bianchi G, Merli M, et al. Italian BCAA Study Group. Nutritional supplementation with branched-chain amino acids in advanced cirrhosis: a double-blind, randomized trial. Gastroenterology 2003;124:1792–1801.

62. Redelmeier DA, Guyatt GH, Goldstein RS. Assessing the minimal important difference in symptoms: a comparison of two techniques. J Clin Epidemiol 1996;49:1215–1219.

63. Guyatt GH, Osoba D, Wu AW, Wyrwich KW, Norman GR. Clinical Significance Consensus Meeting Group. Methods to explain the clinical significance of health status measures. Mayo Clin Proc 2002; 77:371–383.

64. Wright JC, Weinstein MC. Life years gained from a medical intervention. N Engl J Med 1998;339: 380–386.

65. Torrance GW. Utility approach to measuring health-related quality of life. J Chron Dis 1987;40:593–600.

66. Torrance GW. Measurement of health-state utilities for economic appraisal: a review. J Health Econom 1986;5:1–30.

67. Younossi ZM, Boparai N, McCormick M, Price LL, Guyatt G. Assessment of utilities and health-related quality of life in patients with chronic liver disease. Am J Gastroenterol 2001;96:579–583.

68. Chong CA, Gulamhussein A, Heathcote EJ, et al. Health-state utilities and quality of life in hepatitis C patients. Am J Gastroenterol 2003;98:630–638.

69. Drummond M. The role of health economics in clinical evaluation. J Eval Clin Pract 1995;1:71–75.

70. Weinstein MC, Siegel JE, Gold MR, Kamlet MS, Russell LB. Recommendations of the panel on cost-effectiveness in health and medicine. JAMA 1996;276:1253–1258.

71. Zaman A, Goldberg RJ, Pettit KG, et al. Cost of treating an episode of variceal bleeding in a VA setting. Am J Gastroenterol 2000;95:1323–1330.

72. O'Donnell TF Jr, Gembarowicz RM, Callow AD, Pauker SG, Kelly JJ, Deterling RA. The economic impact of acute variceal bleeding: cost-effectiveness implications for medical and surgical therapy. Surgery 1980;88:693–701.

73. McCormick PA, Greenslade L, Matheson LA, Matsaganis M, Bosanquet N, Burroughs AK. Vasoconstrictors in the management of bleeding from oesophageal varices. A clinico-economic appraisal in the UK. Scand J Gastroenterol 1995;30:377–383.

74. Chung R, Lewis JW. Cost of treatment of bleeding esophageal varices. Arch Surg 1983;118:482–485.

75. Mahadeva S, Bellamy MC, Kessel D, Davies MH, Millson CE. Cost-effectiveness of N-butyl-2-cyanoacrylate (histoacryl) glue injections versus transjugular intrahepatic portosystemic shunt in the management of acute gastric variceal bleeding. Am J Gastroenterol 2003;98:2688–2693.

76. Gralnek IM, Jensen DM, Kovacs TO, et al. The economic impact of esophageal variceal hemorrhage: cost-effectiveness implications of endoscopic therapy. Hepatology 1999;29:44–50.

77. Teran JC, Imperiale TF, Mullen KD, Tavill AS, McCullough AJ. Primary prophylaxis of variceal bleeding in cirrhosis: a cost-effectiveness analysis. Gastroenterology 1997;112:473–482.

78. Saab S, DeRosa V, Nieto J, Durazo F, Han S, Roth B. Costs and clinical outcomes of primary prophylaxis of variceal bleeding in patients with hepatic cirrhosis: a decision analytic model. Am J Gastroenterol 2003;98:763–770.

79. Arguedas MR, Heudebert GR, Eloubeidi MA, Abrams GA, Fallon MB. Cost-effectiveness of screening, surveillance, and primary prophylaxis strategies for esophageal varices. Am J Gastroenterol 2002; 97:2441–2452.

80. Spiegel BM, Targownik L, Dulai GS, Karsan HA, Gralnek IM. Endoscopic screening for esophageal varices in cirrhosis: is it ever cost effective? Hepatology 2003;37:366–377.
81. Hicken BL, Sharara AI, Abrams GA, Eloubeidi M, Fallon MB, Arguedas MR. Hepatic venous pressure gradient measurements to assess response to primary prophylaxis in patients with cirrhosis: a decision analytical study. Aliment Pharmacol Ther 2003;17:145–153.
82. Imperiale TF, Chalasani N, Klein RW. Measuring the hemodynamic response to primary pharmacoprophylaxis of variceal bleeding: a cost-effectiveness analysis. Am J Gastroenterol 2003;98:2742–2750.
83. Rubenstein JH, Eisen GM, Inadomi JM. A cost-utility analysis of secondary prophylaxis for variceal hemhorrage. Am J Gastroenterol 2004;99:274–288.
84. Escorsell A, Banares R, Garcia-Pagan JC, et al. TIPS versus drug therapy in preventing variceal rebleeding in advanced cirrhosis: a randomized controlled trial. Hepatology 2002;35:385–392.
85. Cello JP, Ring EJ, Olcott EW, et al. Endoscopic sclerotherapy compared with percutaneous transjugular intrahepatic portosystemic shunt after initial sclerotherapy in patients with acute variceal hemorrhage. A randomized, controlled trial. Ann Intern Med 1997;126:858–865.
86. Meddi P, Merli M, Lionetti R, et al. Cost analysis for the prevention of variceal rebleeding: a comparison between transjugular intrahepatic portosystemic shunt and endoscopic sclerotherapy in a selected group of Italian cirrhotic patients. Hepatology 1999;29:1074–1077.
87. Jalan R, Forrest EH, Stanley AJ, et al. A randomized trial comparing transjugular intrahepatic portosystemic stent-shunt with variceal band ligation in the prevention of rebleeding from esophageal varices. Hepatology 1997;26:1115–1122.
88. Russo MW, Zacks SL, Sandler RS, Brown RS. Cost-effectiveness analysis of transjugular intrahepatic portosystemic shunt (TIPS) versus endoscopic therapy for the prevention of recurrent esophageal variceal bleeding. Hepatology 2000;31:358–363.
89. Helton WS, Maves R, Wicks K, Johansen K. Transjugular intrahepatic portasystemic shunt vs surgical shunt in good-risk cirrhotic patients: a case-control comparison. Arch Surg 2001;136:17–20.
90. Rosemurgy AS 2nd, Bloomston M, Zervos EE, et al. Transjugular intrahepatic portosystemic shunt versus H-graft portacaval shunt in the management of bleeding varices: a cost-benefit analysis. Surgery 1997;122:794–799.
91. Zacks SL, Sandler RS, Biddle AK, Mauro MA, Brown RS Jr. Decision-analysis of transjugular intrahepatic portosystemic shunt versus distal splenorenal shunt for portal hypertension. Hepatology 1999;29:1399–1405.
92. Lebrec D, Giuily N, Hadengue A, et al. Transjugular intrahepatic portosystemic shunts: comparison with paracentesis in patients with cirrhosis and refractory ascites: a randomized trial. J Hepatol 1996;25:135–144.
93. Rossle M, Ochs A, Gulberg V, et al. A comparison of paracentesis and transjugular intrahepatic portosystemic shunting in patients with ascites. N Engl J Med 2000;342:1701–1707.
94. Gines P, Uriz J, Calahorra B, et al. Transjugular intrahepatic portosystemic shunting versus paracentesis plus albumin for refractory ascites in cirrhosis. Gastroenterology 2002;123:1839–1847.
95. Conn HO. Prevalence of spontaneous bacterial peritonitis. In: Conn HO, Rodes J, Navasa M, eds. Spontaneous Bacterial Peritonitis: The Disease, Pathogenesis, and Treatment. M. Dekker, New York, 2000, pp. 75–85.
96. Inadomi J, Sonnenberg A. Cost-analysis of prophylactic antibiotics in spontaneous bacterial peritonitis. Gastroenterology 1997;113:1289–1294.
97. Younossi ZM, McHutchison JG, Ganiats TG. An economic analysis of norfloxacin prophylaxis against spontaneous bacterial peritonitis. J Hepatol 1997;27:295–298.
98. Das A. A cost analysis of long term antibiotic prophylaxis for spontaneous bacterial peritonitis in cirrhosis. Am J Gastroenterol 1998;93:1895–1900.
99. Gines P, Rimola A, Planas R, et al. Norfloxacin prevents spontaneous bacterial peritonitis recurrence in cirrhosis: results of a double-blind, placebo-controlled trial. Hepatology 1990;12(4 Pt 1):716–724.
100. Singh N, Gayowski T, Yu VL, Wagener MM. Trimethoprim-sulfamethoxazole for the prevention of spontaneous bacterial peritonitis in cirrhosis: a randomized trial. Ann Intern Med 1995;122:595–598.
101. Rolachon A, Cordier L, Bacq Y, et al. Ciprofloxacin and long-term prevention of spontaneous bacterial peritonitis: results of a prospective controlled trial. Hepatology 1995;22(4 Pt 1):1171–1174.

102. Farinati F, Gianni S. Surveillance for hepatocellular carcinoma in cirrhosis: is it cost-effective? Eur J Cancer Prev 2001;10:111–115.
103. Bruix J, Llovet JM. Hepatocellular carcinoma: is surveillance cost effective? Gut 2001;48:149–150.
104. Wolf DC. Screening for hepatocellular carcinoma: is it cost-effective? Liver Transpl 2003;9:682,683.
105. Sarasin FP, Giostra E, Hadengue A. Cost-effectiveness of screening for detection of small hepatocellular carcinoma in western patients with Child-Pugh class A cirrhosis. Am J Med 1996;101:422–434.
106. Bolondi L, Sofia S, Siringo S, et al. Surveillance programme of cirrhotic patients for early diagnosis and treatment of hepatocellular carcinoma: a cost effectiveness analysis. Gut 2001;48:251–259.
107. Arguedas MR, Chen VK, Eloubeidi MA, Fallon MB. Screening for hepatocellular carcinoma in patients with hepatitis C cirrhosis: a cost-utility analysis. Am J Gastroenterol 2003;98:679–690.
108. Sarasin FP, Giostra E, Mentha G, Hadengue A. Partial hepatectomy or orthotopic liver transplantation for the treatment of resectable hepatocellular carcinoma? A cost-effectiveness perspective. Hepatology 1998;28:436–442.
109. Majno PE, Sarasin FP, Mentha G, Hadengue A. Primary liver resection and salvage transplantation or primary liver transplantation in patients with single, small hepatocellular carcinoma and preserved liver function: an outcome-oriented decision analysis. Hepatology 2000;31:899–906.
110. Saab S, Ly D, Nieto J, et al. Hepatocellular carcinoma screening in patients waiting for liver transplantation: a decision analytic model. Liver Transpl 2003;9:672–681.
111. Llovet JM, Mas X, Aponte JJ, et al. Cost effectiveness of adjuvant therapy for hepatocellular carcinoma during the waiting list for liver transplantation. Gut 2002;50:123–128.
112. Sarasin FP, Majno PE, Llovet JM, Bruix J, Mentha G, Hadengue A. Living donor liver transplantation for early hepatocellular carcinoma: a life-expectancy and cost-effectiveness perspective. Hepatology 2001;33:1073–1079.
113. Hoshida Y, Shiratori Y, Omata M. Cost-effectiveness of adjuvant interferon therapy after surgical resection of Hepatitis C-related hepatocellular carcinoma. Liver 2002;22:479–485.

29 Future Treatments

Antifibrotic Agents, Nitric Oxide Donors, and Gene Therapy in the Treatment of Portal Hypertension

Meena B. Bansal, MD
and Scott L. Friedman, MD

CONTENTS

INTRODUCTION
CELLULAR BASIS OF HEPATIC FIBROSIS AND PORTAL HYPERTENSION
ANTIFIBROTIC AGENTS
VASCULAR MEDIATORS IN THE INJURED LIVER
GENE THERAPY APPROACHES
SUMMARY
REFERENCES

INTRODUCTION

Increased resistance to portal blood flow leading to portal hypertension is the main cause of morbidity and mortality in patients with chronic liver disease, and reflects two parallel yet interrelated processes. First, the wound healing response to liver injury generates increased extracellular matrix (fibrosis) and the formation of regenerative nodules, which lead to architectural distortion that impedes intrahepatic blood flow. Second, dynamic sinusoidal changes caused by increased contractility of stellate cells in the perisinusoidal space also increase intrahepatic vascular resistance. The relative contribution of each of these components is difficult to quantify and may vary with the etiology and stage of fibrosis, but together they represent a key target for antifibrotic and vasoregulatory therapies. Clearly, the most effective therapy to treat hepatic fibrosis is to remove the causative agent. However, therapies that are able to retard or reverse the fibrotic response and/or inhibit stellate cell contraction could have a dramatic impact on the treatment of patients with chronic liver disease. This chapter reviews the cellular basis of hepatic fibrosis and increased intrahepatic vascular resistance, and how these insights are yielding novel approaches to the treatment of chronic liver disease.

From: *Clinical Gastroenterology: Portal Hypertension*
Edited by: A. J. Sanyal and V. H. Shah © Humana Press Inc., Totowa, NJ

CELLULAR BASIS OF HEPATIC FIBROSIS AND PORTAL HYPERTENSION

Cellular Basis of Hepatic Fibrosis

The hepatic stellate cell (previously called lipocyte, Ito, fat-storing, or perisinusoidal cell) is the primary source of the extracellular matrix in normal and fibrotic liver. Hepatic stellate cells are resident perisinusoidal cells in the subendothelial space between hepatocytes and sinusoidal endothelial cells. They are the primary site for storing retinoids and, therefore, can be recognized by their vitamin A autoflouresence in normal unfixed liver and following their isolation. In addition, their perisinusoidal orientation and expression of the cytoskeletal proteins desmin, glial acidic fibrillary protein and smooth muscle actin (in injured liver) facilitate their identification *in situ (1)*.

Studies in both animals and humans with progressive injury have defined a gradient of changes within stellate cells that collectively are termed *"activation"* (Fig. 1). Stellate cell activation refers to the transition from a quiescent vitamin A-rich cell to a highly fibrogenic cell type characterized morphologically by enlargement of rough endoplasmic reticulum, diminution of vitamin A droplets, ruffled nuclear membrane, appearance of contractile filaments, and proliferation. Proliferation of stellate cells generally occurs in regions of greatest injury, which is typically preceded by an influx of inflammatory cells and is associated with subsequent extracellular matrix accumulation.

Stellate cell activation, the central event in hepatic fibrosis, can be conceptualized as occurring in at least two stages: (1) *initiation* and (2) *perpetuation*. *Initiation* refers to early events encompassing rapid changes in gene expression and phenotype that render the cells responsive to cytokines and other stimuli. It results from paracrine stimulation caused by rapid, disruptive effects of liver injury on the homeostasis of neighboring cells and from early changes in ECM composition. *Perpetuation* incorporates those cellular events that amplify the activated phenotype through enhanced cytokine expression and responsiveness and involves at least seven discrete changes in cell behavior: (a) proliferation; (b) chemotaxis; (c) fibrogenesis; (d) contractility; (e) matrix degradation; (f) retinoid loss; (g) WBC chemoattractant and cytokine release. Either directly or indirectly, the net effect of these changes is accumulation of extracellular matrix, architectural distortion, and gradual increase in intrahepatic resistance ultimately leading to clinically significant portal hypertension.

The paradigm of stellate cell activation provides an important framework to define sites of antifibrotic therapy. These include: (a) Cure the primary disease to prevent injury. (b) Reduce inflammation or the host response to avoid stimulating stellate cell activation. (c) Directly downregulate stellate cell activation. (d) Neutralize proliferative, fibrogenic, contractile and/or proinflammatory responses of stellate cells. (e) Stimulate apoptosis of stellate cells. (f) Increase the degradation of scar matrix, either by stimulating cells which produce matrix proteases, downregulating their inhibitors, or by direct administration of matrix proteases.

Cellular Basis of Intrahepatic Portal Hypertension

Our understanding of the molecular basis of increased intrahepatic resistance in chronic liver disease is steadily expanding. A brief overview is provided here to set the stage for a review of therapies to treat intrahepatic portal hypertension. The microvascular unit of the liver, the sinusoid, is remarkably similar to peripheral capillary beds. Sinusoids are

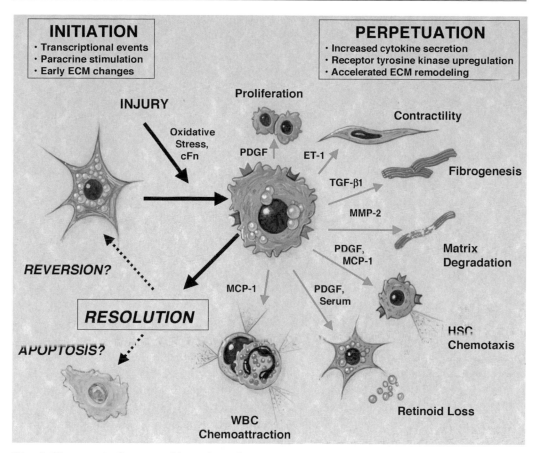

Fig. 1. Phenotypic features of hepatic stellate cell activation during liver injury and resolution. Following liver injury, hepatic stellate cells undergo "activation," which connotes a transition from quiescent vitamin A-rich cells into proliferative, fibrogenic, and contractile myofibroblasts. The major phenotypic changes after activation include proliferation, contractility, fibrogenesis, matrix degradation, chemotaxis, retinoid loss, and WBC chemoattraction. Key mediators underlying these effects are shown. The fate of activated stellate cells during resolution of liver injury is uncertain but may include reversion to a quiescent phenotype and/or selective clearance by apoptosis. Reprinted with permission from Friedman SL, Molecular regulation of hepatic fibrosis, an integrated cellular response to tissue injury. J Biol Chem 2000;275:2247–2250.

lined by endothelial cells, and on their basal surface are stellate cells within the space of Disse. Hepatic stellate cells resemble tissue pericytes, a cell population that has smooth muscle features and is thought to regulate blood flow by modulating pericapillary resistance *(2)*. During stellate cell activation, they increase their expression of the contractile protein α smooth muscle actin. Incubation of isolated human stellate cells with vasoconstrictors such as angiotensin II and thrombin, leads to phenotypic changes including cellular rounding, which are associated with increased intracellular calcium *(3)*. Furthermore, studies using in vivo microscopy to colocalize sinusoidal constriction with associated autoflourescence *(4–7)*, provide more direct evidence that stellate cells are contractile and can regulate intrahepatic blood flow. In summary, the contractile phenotype and perisinusoidal orientiation of stellate cells make them ideally positioned to regulate sinusoidal blood flow.

The increased intrahepatic vascular resistance characteristic of cirrhosis is thought to arise from an imbalance between vasodilator/vasoconstrictor forces that regulate hepatic vascular tone. Therefore, treatment strategies targeted to either inhibit contraction or stimulate relaxation of activated stellate cells and other vascular elements could decrease intrahepatic portal pressure, as reviewed below.

ANTIFIBROTIC AGENTS
Fibrosis Reversibility

A key issue in defining treatments for hepatic fibrosis is the point at which accumulation of matrix is no longer reversible. The exact moment at which fibrosis becomes irreversible is unknown, either in terms of a histologic marker or a specific change in the matrix composition or content. Dense cirrhosis with nodule formation, portal hypertension, and early liver failure is generally considered irreversible, but less advanced lesions can show remarkable reversibility when the underlying cause of the liver injury is controlled, or possibly by other therapeutic interventions. The ideal antifibrotic would be the one that could be easily delivered, is well tolerated, has high liver specificity, and promotes the resorption of excess interstitial matrix without abolishing the salutary effects of the normal hepatic ECM. The goal is not necessarily to abrogate fibrosis entirely, but rather to attenuate its development so that patients with chronic liver disease do not succumb to the end organ failure that it creates (e.g., portal hypertension, ascites, liver failure). Although no therapy yet meets these goals, the framework for developing such treatments is in place. As a general rule, the currently available antifibrotic therapies have been directed against suppressing hepatic inflammation rather than subduing fibrosis. In the future, targeting of stellate cells and fibrogenic mediators may be a mainstay of therapy. Points of therapeutic intervention may include efforts to remove the injurious stimuli, suppress hepatic inflammation, downregulate stellate cell activation, and promote matrix degradation (Fig. 2).

Remove Injurious Stimuli

Removing the underlying cause of liver injury is the most effective way to prevent fibrosis. This approach can be highly effective when instituted early. Examples include removal of excess iron or copper in genetic hemochromatosis or Wilson's disease, respectively, abstinence in alcoholic liver disease, antihelminthic therapy in schistosomiasis, clearance of HBV or HCV in chronic viral hepatitis, and biliary decompression in bile duct obstruction. In the future, identification of the pathogenetic mechanisms underlying primary biliary cirrhosis or sclerosing cholangitis may permit the elimination of bile duct injury and periductular fibrosis, possibly by improving bile flow through use of farnesoid X receptors or other choleretics *(8)*. Discontinuation of hepatotoxic drugs may prevent progression of drug-induced liver injury and fibrosis.

Because of the high worldwide prevalence of HBV or HCV, there are massive efforts underway to clear these viruses in chronically infected patients. Histologic improvement has been observed in patients responding to antiviral therapy with interferon/ribavirin for HCV and lamivudine for HBV. Beyond its antiviral effect, alpha interferon may have direct anti-fibrogenic activity *(9)*, which could explain the reports citing an antifibrotic effect of interferon/ribavirin, even in patients who fail to clear virus *(10)*.

Suppress Hepatic Inflammation

Inflammatory mediators may stimulate stellate cell activation in chronic liver diseases such as viral or autoimmune hepatitis and drug-induced liver injury. Thus, anti-inflamma-tory medications might be beneficial in preventing fibrosis in these conditions.

CORTICOSTEROIDS

Corticosteroids have been a mainstay of therapy for many inflammatory liver diseases. As an example, they can induce clinical remission and improve hepatic histopathology in patients with autoimmune hepatitis, even those with advanced histologic features. However, the incomplete suppression of fibrogenesis and undesirable side effects after prolonged administration limit its use.

COLCHICINE

Colchicine is an antiinflammatory drug but its value in treating chronic liver disease is minimal based on recent trials. In clinical trials of patients with primary biliary cirrhosis, colchicine improved laboratory values but mortality and transplantation rate were unaffected. In another trial, colchicine improved overall survival of patients with cirrhosis but did not reduce the mortality related specifically to liver disease *(11)*. Despite the lack of convincing data, colchicine is still being used by some physicians. One study suggests that its metabolite, colchiceine, may have better antifibrotic activity *(12)*.

URSODEOXYCHOLIC ACID (UDCA)

UDCA has clear efficacy in primary biliary cirrhosis *(13)*. Although no direct antifibrotic effect of UDCA is established, a putative effect has been reported in a rat model of bile duct ligation *(14)*. Moreover, recent studies using UDCA derivatives that release nitric oxide have shown promising effects on liver injury *(15,16)* (see below).

RECEPTOR ANTAGONISTS

Another antiinflammatory strategy is to neutralize inflammatory cytokines using specific receptor antagonists. As an example, a synthetic analog of Arg-Gly-Asp (RGD), which represents an integrin-binding motif shared by fibronectin and other ECM molecules, has been used in immune-mediated liver injury in mice induced by concanavalin A *(17, 18)*. In the same study, pretreatment of animals with soluble TNF-α receptor effectively reduced the serum elevation in liver enzymes and blocked TNF-α and interleukin-6 release. The reduced cytokine levels were accompanied by diminished necrosis and inflammation in tissue sections. No direct antifibrotic role of these compounds has been demonstrated, and their use in humans has not been reported.

IMMUNE MODULATION

Recent clinical studies suggest that immunosuppression may accelerate fibrosis progression, such as in patients with HCV and HIV co-infection, or in patients on immunosuppressives following liver transplantation. The role of immune phenotype in modulating the fibrogenic response is also supported by animal data in which the Th phenotype of mice significantly influences fibrogenesis after toxic liver injury *(19)*. Ongoing efforts are attempting to define the specific T-cell subsets responsible for these observations, which might ultimately yield new immunomodulatory approaches to dampening fibrosis in patients with ongoing liver injury.

A novel approach for treating schistosomiasis-induced fibrosis involves the coadministration of interleukin-12 and worm egg antigen to modulate the host immune response *(20)*. The inhibition of fibrosis in this model is accompanied by replacement of the Th2-dominated pattern of cytokine expression, which is characteristic of S. mansoni, by one dominated by Th1 cytokines, which has a more protective profile. This approach could have implications for other human liver diseases in which the host immune responses play a role in fibrogenesis, including viral hepatitis, primary biliary cirrhosis, and autoimmune hepatitis.

INTERLEUKIN 10

In a small uncontrolled trial in 24 patients with HCV infection and fibrosis, treatment with interleukin-10 was associated with dramatic antifibrogenic and antiinflammatory activity in some patients *(21)*. In a follow-up study, 30 patients with HCV-related advanced fibrosis who had failed antiviral therapy were enrolled in a 12-mo treatment regimen with SQ IL-10 given daily or three times a week. Thirty-nine percent of patients had a reduction in fibrosis score of at least one stage, but none who had a pretreatment Ishak score of 6 showed any improvement. In addition, long-term recombinant IL-10 therapy decreased disease activity but also was associated with increased HCV viral burden due to alterations in immunologic viral surveillance *(21)*. Studies in transgenic mice suggests that IL-10 exerts its antifibrotic effects by altering lymphoctye subpopulations and thus still may hold promise for specific liver diseases in which $CD8^+$ T cell-mediated injury is prominent *(22)*.

INHIBITION OF HEPATOCYTE APOPTOSIS

It has become increasingly clear that hepatocyte apoptosis contributes to inflammation and stellate cell activation *(23–25)*. Small interfering RNAs (siRNA) against *Fas* have been used to attenuate concavalin A–induced liver fibrosis *(26)*. In addition, inhibition of apoptosis by blocking caspases offers another potentially valuable approach *(24)*.

Downregulate Stellate Cell Activation

Suppression or reversal of stellate cell activation has inherent attractiveness as a therapeutic strategy because of the central role that stellate cells have in fibrogenesis.

INTERFERONS

The antifibrotic effects of the interferons may in part be related to downregulation of stellate cell activation, which may explain improvement in fibrosis that has been described in patients with HCV who do not have a virologic response to interferon-α *(27)*. Pegylated interferon given alone or in combination with ribavirin has been associated with improvement in fibrosis in HCV infected patients, including apparent reversal of early cirrhosis in some patients *(28)*. The precise mechanisms underlying these observations are incompletely understood. A contributing factor appears to be direct repression of collagen gene transcription *(9)*.

Interferon gamma is another interferon that has inhibitory effects on hepatic stellate cell activation *(29)*. It also reduces the expression of mRNAs of type I and IV collagen as well as fibronectin in activated hepatic stellate cells grown in tissue culture, inhibits stellate cell proliferation, and reduces smooth muscle actin expression *(30)*. Phase II controlled clinical trials, however, failed to show an antifibrotic effect in HCV-patients not responding to PEG/Ribavirin (see http://www.intermune.com, press releases).

ANTIOXIDANTS

Oxidative stress is an important stimulus to stellate cell activation, providing a rationale for the use of antioxidants such as vitamin E to suppress fibrogenesis. The issue is not whether antioxidants are rational, but whether they are sufficiently potent to impact on fibrosis progression. Limited data with vitamin E suggest efficacy in experimental conditions, although discordant data have also been reported *(31,32)*. Trials in humans are currently underway. Some studies have documented inhibition of stellate cell activation by other antioxidants such as resveratrol, quercetin, and N-acetylcysteine (NAC) *(33, 34)*. As will be discussed below, the antifibrotic properties of flavonoid compounds rely heavily upon their antioxidative effects.

SILYMARIN

Silymarin (silybum marianum) is a natural component of milk thistle, which has exhibited promising antifibrotic activity in experimental liver injury and is widely used as a nonprescription agent in patients with chronic liver disease, particularly those with HCV. Based upon its structure, silymarin belongs to a group of flavonoid compounds, the other members of which include quercetin, baicalin, and baicalein (see below). These flavonoids have drawn increasing attention because of their antifibrogenic properties. Silymarin functions as an antioxidant and may decrease hepatic injury via cytoprotection and inhibition of Kupffer cell function. Despite its theoretical benefit, a systematic review of 14 studies found no clear evidence of a reduction in mortality, improvement in liver histology, or biochemical markers of liver function in patients with chronic liver disease *(35)*. Similar conclusions were reached in an evidence report on the efficacy of milk thistle in liver disease performed through the Agency for Healthcare Research and Quality (http://www.ahrq.gov).

TGF-β ANTAGONISTS

TGF-β is a major fibrogenic cytokine; thus antagonists are under close investigation. Several TGF-β antagonists are being developed and tested, including soluble TGF-β type II receptor *(36)*, antisense oligonucleotides *(37)*, angiotensin II converting enzyme inhibitors *(38)*, and serine protease inhibitors (such as camostat mesilate) to inhibit proteolytic activation of latent TGF-β *(39)*. As an example, TGF-β type II receptor inhibits stellate cell activation and fibrogenesis in vivo when administered before or after the fibrogenic stimulus *(36)*. Other strategies to functionally block TGF-β are also being studied, including TGF-β-sequestering proteins such as decorin *(40)* or latency associated peptide (LAP) *(41)*. A concern related to TGF-β antagonists is the important role that TGF-β as a tumor suppressor gene, and its inhibition might theoretically increase the risk of HCC in patients with chronic liver disease.

ENDOTHELIN RECEPTOR ANTAGONISTS

Endothelin receptor antagonists have also been tested as antifibrotic agents and are among the most promising, because agents of this type are already undergoing clinical trials for hypertensive diseases *(42)*. One agent, bosentan, is antifibrotic and reduces stellate cell activation in experimental fibrosis *(43)*, but its safety in humans is not established yet. These agents are particularly attractive since they also have effects on inhibiting stellate cell contraction, an important component of increased intrahepatic vascular resistance as will be discussed in further detail below.

HEPATOCYTE GROWTH FACTOR (HGF)

HGF inhibits liver fibrosis and promotes liver regeneration in animal models of liver injury in part by increasing collagenase expression in hepatic stellate cells *(44,45)*. A deletion variant of HGF is effective in inhibiting stellate cell activation, downregulating the mRNA expression of procollagens and TGF-β-1, and stimulating liver regeneration *(46)*. Pretreatment with this deleted form of HGF also shows strong protective effects against some hepatotoxins *(47)*. Trials in humans are anticipated.

HALOFUGINONE

Halofuginone, a low-molecular-weight derivative of the anticoccidial quinoazolinone, has been studied as a potent inhibitor of type I collagen synthesis. It inhibits collagen I synthesis and extracellular matrix deposition in vitro and in vivo *(48,49)*. In dimethylnitrosamine or thioacetamide induced cirrhosis in rats, the dietary addition of halofuginone effectively prevented the occurrence of liver fibrosis and cirrhosis *(48,49)* and enhanced liver regeneration following partial hepatectomy *(50)*. Furthermore, the drug caused almost complete resolution of fibrosis in rats with established fibrosis *(51)*. Based upon the above data, this compound may become a promising candidate for future treatment of liver fibrosis.

RETINOIDS

In view of the export of retinoids during stellate cell activation, one might assume that restoration of cellular retinoid might reverse or downregulate activation. However, there is no evidence yet to support this idea, and studies even indicate that retinoids may exacerbate fibrosis in animal models *(52)*. There remain key gaps in our understanding of the interplay between retinoid metabolism and stellate cell activation and fibrogenesis.

HERBAL COMPOUNDS

In Asian countries such as China, herbal medicines have been used for centuries to treat liver diseases. Some studies have elucidated the cellular mechanisms of several herbal medicines, which have putative activity against liver fibrosis. Sho-saiko-to (Xiao-Chaihu-Tang), one of the most prominent herbal medicines, inhibits stellate cell activation and reduces fibrosis in vitro and in vivo *(53,54)*. Administration of Sho-saiko-to in experimental liver fibrosis reduced hepatic type I and III collagen expression and hydroxyproline content. It also decreased the number of α-smooth muscle actin positive stellate cells and increased retinoid concentration in injured liver. The antifibrotic mechanism of sho-saiko-to may include an antioxidative activity in which baicalin and baicalein are active components *(55)*.

Another herbal medicine under study is salvia miltiorrhiza (Dan-shen), which also inhibits fibrosis in animal model and downregulates mRNA expression of TGF-β-1, procollagen I and III *(56)*. Apart from the scientific insight they provide, these studies underscore the potential value of traditional medicine, a system which has been used for centuries in many parts of the world *(53)*. Traditional therapies could lead to innovative strategies for treating hepatic fibrosis and cirrhosis.

RAPAMYCIN

Rapamycin is an immunosuppressive drug used in liver transplantation. It inhibits stellate cell proliferation, which could attenuate the potential fibrotic response in patients with recurrent liver disease *(57)*. Use of rapamycin coated stents in coronary artery disease attests to its inhibitory effects on mesenchymal cell growth, however, recent concerns about its safety as an immunosuppressive immediately after liver transplantation have dampened enthusiasm. Still, other rapamycin-like drugs with good safety profiles could justify reassessment of these agents as antifibrotics.

PENTOXIFYLLINE

Pentoxifylline (a methylxanthine derivative that decreases tumor necrosis alpha synthesis) inhibits hepatic stellate cell proliferation and collagen synthesis in vitro and in a rat model of secondary biliary fibrosis *(58)*. It has been studied in the treatment of alcoholic hepatitis in humans where it appears to confer a survival advantage, possibly through a reduction in hepatorenal syndrome *(59)*.

Promote Matrix Degradation

The promotion of matrix degradation is of special clinical significance given the need to resorb matrix in patients with established fibrosis. Advances in understanding of matrix degradation in liver are likely to translate into new approaches to therapy *(60)*. As an example, preventing the upregulation of TIMP-1 and -2 during stellate cell activation might increase matrix degradation in vivo *(60)*. Strategies to increase the activity of matrix degrading enzymes or to introduce degrading enzymes with gene therapy are also of interest *(61)* and is discussed in further detail below ("Gene therapy approaches"). TGF-β antagonists can stimulate matrix degradation by downregulating TIMPs and increasing the net activity of interstitial collagenase.

Promote Stellate Cell Apoptosis

Promoting apoptosis of activated stellate cells is another potential strategy in theory, but is not yet feasible in practice. Obstacles to this approach include the need to target stellate cells and to titrate the apoptotic effect to avoid loss of normal cells. Furthermore, a coherent understanding of apoptosis in stellate cells is still developing *(24)*. Apoptosis can be induced by disruption of integrin-mediated adhesion *(62)* and administration of gliotoxin *(63)*.

Based upon the dramatic advances of the past decade, there is reason for optimism about the prospects for antifibrotic therapy. However, one major unanswered question is whether antifibrotics will result in a clinically significant reduction in portal pressures. Likely, the combination of antifibrotics and agents capable of reducing intrahepatic vascular resistance through modulation of stellate cell contractility carry the greatest promise (see below).

VASCULAR MEDIATORS IN THE INJURED LIVER

Recent work has elucidated the importance of numerous vasoactive agents in the development of increased intrahepatic vascular resistance *(64)* (Table 1). In general, abnormal vasoregulation in liver disease may arise as a result of abnormally elevated levels of contractile agents or reduced levels of vasodilatory/relaxation compounds. Therefore, potential therapies focus on either inhibition of stellate cell contraction or forced relaxation of activated stellate cells to decrease portal pressure (Fig. 2). Key agents regulating contraction and relaxation are reviewed below.

Table 1
Agents with Contractile
or Relaxing Effects on Hepatic Stellate Cells

Contraction	Relaxation
Endothelin(1,2,3)	Nitric oxide
Angiotensin II	Carbon monoxide
Thrombin	Prostaglandin E_2
Prostagland $F_{2\alpha}$	Adrenomedullin
Thromboxane A_2	
Vasopressin	
Substance P	
Serum	
Platelet activating factor	
Adenosine	

ENDOTHELIN

Endothelin is elevated in the serum of patients with advanced liver disease (65). Endothelins constitute a group of vasoconstrictors consisting of three members: ET-1, ET-2, ET-3. They are produced by endothelial and stellate cells, and exert autocrine and paracrine effects on adjacent stellate cells. Their major function appears to be in local control of vascular tone by inducing stellate cell contractility as well as proliferation (66,67). Stellate cells express both ET-A and ET-B receptors, both of which mediate endothelin's biological effects in this cell type. In addition, endothelin receptor expression is increased after injury (68) providing a rationale for therapeutically targeting these receptors in chronic liver injury and portal hypertension. In animal models of portal hypertension, ET-A receptor, ET-B receptor, and mixed ET-A/ET-B receptor antagonists can reduce portal pressures (69–71). In addition to its effects on stellate cell contractility, endothelin may provide a direct fibrogenic stimulus (see above).

NITRIC OXIDE (NO)

NO has emerged as an important regulator of vascular blood flow in many organ systems (72). In experimental models of liver injury and portal hypertension, NO production is reduced (73). Although the precise mechanism is unknown, endothelial cell NOS activity is reduced in cirrhosis. Furthermore, NO has important effects on stellate cells. Exogenous NO can antagonize endothelin-induced contraction and induce relaxation in precontracted cells (74) and endogenous NO produced by stellate cells in response to cytokines has relaxing effects (75).

As a result of these observations, multiple approaches have been employed to increase local NO production in the cirrhotic liver. Two especially promising approaches are the use of liver selective NO donors and gene therapy (see below).

LIVER-SELECTIVE NO DONORS

In addition to its role in vasodilatation, NO has hepatocyte cytoprotective effects against inflammation and tissue damage, and is directly cytotoxic toward invading micoorganisms and tumor cells (76). These features make NO a very attractive agent for the treatment of chronic liver disease. Because NO has a range of systemic activities including peripheral vasodilatation which could exacerbate the hypotension seen in cirrhotic patients, selective targeting to the liver is essential. V-PYYRO/NO is a newly synthesized stable diazeniumdiolate that can circulate freely in the body and is metabolized to nitric oxide by P450 enzymes in the liver *(77)*. It has been shown to reduce in situ hepatic vascular resistance without altering systolic blood pressure *(78)*. The systemic effects of V-PYRRO/NO appear to be minimal *(77,79)*. In animal models, V-PYRRO/NO can protect against acetominophen-induced hepatotoxicity in mice *(77,80)*, monocrotaline-induced hepatic sinusoid injury *(81)*, liver damage from ischemia reperfusion *(78)*, and D-galactosamine/endotoxin-induced hepatoxicity *(82)*, but only one preliminary study has reported an ability to reduce portal pressures and fibrosis in BDL-ligated rats *(83)*.

Recently, a NO-releasing derivative of ursodeoxycholic acid, NCX1000, has reportedly lowered portal pressures in rats *(15,16,84)*. In addition, this compound is hepatoprotective in multiple acute injury models, antifibrotic, and effective in reducing portal pressure. Thus, if safety is established in humans, the compound will certainly merit clinical trials. In addition, statins are thought to increase endothelial production of NO through a phosphatidylinositol 3-kinase dependent activation of Akt, leading to eNOS phosphorylation *(85)*. Recently, simvastatin was shown to increase hepatic nitric oxide production and decrease hepatic vascular tone in patients with cirrhosis and, thus, holds tremendous promise given its commercial availability and other beneficial effects *(86)*.

ANGIOTENSIN II

Angiotensin II can induce contraction and proliferation of human-activated hepatic stellate cells by acting through AT1 receptors *(87)*. Moreover, angiotensin II's effects on stellate cells are mediated by NAPDH oxidase, an enzyme that produces reactive oxygen species, further underscoring its potential use in the therapy of patients with chronic liver injury *(88)*. Because Angiotensin-II receptor antagonists are already FDA-approved for other indications, they are particularly attractive agents for study in patients with liver disease. Animal studies indicate that moderate doses of losartan decrease hepatic resistance in the fibrotic livers of BDL rats, but higher doses may have deleterious effects *(89)*. Trials in cirrhotic patients, however, have yielded mixed results. The major concern has been that these compounds decreased the glomerular filtration rate and led to systemic hypotension in cirrhotic patients *(90)*. In theory, liver-specific targeting, as has been achieved for NO-delivery, could overcome this limitation.

Prazosin: In cirrhotic patients, continuous α-adrenergic blockade with prazosin reduced portal pressure *(91,92)* but also reduced glomerular filtration rate and caused significant peripheral edema.

GENE THERAPY APPROACHES

General Considerations

Most simply, gene therapy involves the transfer of a gene into the body. The protein product of the transgene is expressed either locally or systemically, and functions to either replace a missing protein product or inhibit the functions of a deleterious protein. Over the past 30 yr, there have been over 23,000 publications on gene therapy with over 8000 in this past year. Ten percent of papers in the past year have described the use of gene therapy for the treatment of liver diseases. The ideal vector system is one that is regulable, highly cell-specific, efficient, nonimmunogenic, nonhepatotoxic, and capable of delivering large segments of DNA or RNA.

The issues that determine the ultimate efficacy of gene therapy include:

1. effectiveness of the specific vector system;
2. cellular targets of vector systems;
3. efficiency and longevity of cellular transduction;
4. deleterious side effects of genetic interventions.

Effectiveness of the Specific Vector System

Many vector systems have been used and each has specific advantages (for detailed review, see ref. *93*). In liver, the most commonly used delivery systems include:

ADENOVIRAL VECTORS

Adenoviral vectors have been the most popular because they result in high-level gene expression and have a significant tropism for hepatocytes, allowing for intravenous (iv) rather than portal vein administration. Significant drawbacks include the transient nature of transduction due to immune-mediated eradication of infected cells and decreased transduction in cirrhotic livers compared to uninjured livers *(94)*. In addition, mixed humoral and T-cell mediated immune response preclude its repeated administration. Lastly, high titers can result in hepatotoxicity which has been associated with death in humans *(95)*.

RETROVIRAL VECTORS

Unlike adenoviruses, these viruses integrate into the host genome and are passed onto progeny cells allowing for long-lasting gene expression. This advantage is also a disadvantage in that integration into the recipient genome may result in activation of latent oncogenes or inactivation of tumor-suppressor genes, as has been observed in pediatric patients in a handful of cases (see below). Tumor suppressor inactivation is less likely than oncogene activation, because loss of heterozygosity (inactivation of both alleles of the tumor suppressor gene) is required for tumorigenesis to proceed *(96)*. Until recently, retroviral insertion in the context of gene therapy has been considered a random event. In a recent clinical trial, 2 out of 10 patients receiving gene therapy for the treatment of X-linked severe combined immunodeficiency (SCID-X1) developed T-cell leukemia as a result of insertion of the retroviral vector in the same region near the promoter of the proto-oncogene LMO2. In addition, retroviruses only infect nondividing cells and, thus, in vivo gene therapy can only be utilized if liver cells are stimulated to regenerate. In principle, this might be accomplished by mitogen administration or treatment with thyroid hormone *(97)* but no clinical trials of this type have been undertaken to date.

LENTIVIRAL VECTORS

Unlike retroviruses, which cannot infect nondividing cells, lentiviruses are capable of infecting both dividing and nondividing cells *(98)*. They are, however, also subject to the problems that limit retroviruses, with possible activation of oncogenes due to integration into the host genome.

ADENOASSOCIATED VIRAL VECTORS

These viruses are a replication-defective parvovirus, that can integrate into a specific region on chromosome 19 *(99)*. Although wild-type viruses demonstrate this site-specific integration, recombinant viruses integrate more randomly. They can infect both dividing and nondividing cells and are noninfectious which make them particularly attractive for use in humans. They are more cumbersome to make and package and thus have been used less frequently to date.

Prospects for Gene Therapy in the Treatment of Fibrosis

Transforming Growth Factor-β (TGF-β)

TGF-β is a cytokine central to the fibrogenic process. Therefore, numerous approaches have been used to try to modulate this pathway. Adenoviral expression of a TGF-β1 antisense mRNA was effective in preventing liver fibrosis in bile-duct ligated rats *(100)*. In addition, overexpression of Smad7, an intracellular antagonist of TGF-β signaling, using an adenoviral vector resulted in a reduction in fibrosis in bile-duct ligated rats *(101)*.

Interferon-α

Several studies have suggested a potential anti-fibrotic effect of IFN-α. However, its systemic toxicity limits larger doses needed for this clinical end point. Therefore, adenoviral delivery to the liver is attractive in that high doses can be delivered to hepatocytes with very little systemic toxicity. In a rat model of dimethylnitrosamine-induced liver cirrhosis, an adenoviral vector expressing IFN-α prevented the progression of liver cirrhosis and improved survival in treated rats *(102)*. This same system was used to show that IFN-α gene transfer effectively inhibits HCV replication in hepatocytes *(103)*. This approach therefore could be of dual benefit in patients with HCV cirrhosis but it is uncertain if such approaches will yield sufficient advantage over current formulations to justify clinical trials.

Matrix Degrading Proteases

In cirrhosis, there is a gradual accumulation of interstitial collagens, type I and III. From a clinical standpoint patients generally present once scar is already established and, thus, one gene therapy approach is to express an interstitial collagenase to degrade the fibrotic scar. In humans, matrix metalloproteinase-1 is an important interstitial collagenase but its origin and importance in liver fibrosis are uncertain. In a model of established rat liver fibrosis, an adenoviral vector containing MMP-1 resulted in decreased fibrosis, decreased number of activated stellate cells, and hepatocyte proliferation *(61)*. Introduction of MMP-8, a neutrophil collagenase, in an adenoviral vector system also resulted in resorption of fibrosis in bile-duct ligated rats *(94)* and CCl$_4$-treated rats *(104)*. In both studies, adenoviral expression also resulted in mild liver injury as reflected by ALT levels, highlighting the potential hepatocellular toxicity which may be a significant concern in the cirrhotic patient if clinical trials are undertaken.

Gene Therapy in the Treatment of Portal Hypertension

Several issues must be addressed if gene therapy is to be effective in the treatment of portal hypertension. The first is which regulatory system should targeted. NO has received the most attention as a gene therapy to date. Second, the cellular target must be optimized. Endothelial and stellate cells may be ideal candidates given their roles in regulating vascular tone in the liver. One feature limiting clinical utility has been the short-lived nature of the transduction. For any significant impact on portal hypertension, achieving long-term transduction is a significant requirement.

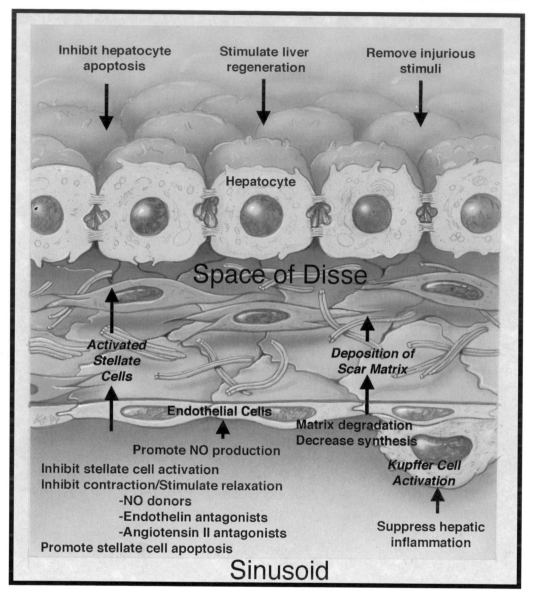

Fig. 2. Potential targets for antifibrotics and agents that modulate intrahepatic vascular resistance. Changes in the subendothelial Space of Disse and sinuoids as fibrosis develops in response to injury includes alterations in both cellular responses and extracellular matrix composition. Stellate cell activation leads to accumulation of scar. Kupffer cell activation accompanies liver injury and contributes to paracrine activation of stellate cells. Decrease in endothelial cell eNOS activity and nitric oxide and overall increase in stellate cell contractility leads to increased intrahepatic vascular resistance. Potential treatments at each of these sites of action are listed on the figure. Reprinted with modification from Friedman SL, Molecular regulation of hepatic fibrosis, an integrated cellular response to tissue injury. J Biol Chem 2000;275:2247–2250.

APPROACHES TO RESTORE HEPATIC SINUSOIDAL NO

In cirrhosis there is a relative deficiency of NO, likely secondary to decreased endothelial NO synthase. Therefore, direct delivery of either NO (see liver selective NO donors) or NO synthase are rational approaches. An adenoviral vector system was used to introduce neuronal NOS (nNOS) in both normal liver and liver injury models (bile duct ligation and CCl_4). Although transduction efficiency is slightly diminished in the injured liver, hepatocytes, endothelial cells, and stellate cells were efficiently transduced with nNOS resulting in decreased portal pressure in vivo and decrease in stellate cell contractility in vitro (105). Importantly, transduction of nNOS into injured liver reduced resting as well as flow-dependent portal pressure. The durability of this effect on portal pressures is not clear. Akt is a major activator of endothelial NO which may contribute to decreased NO production in cirrhosis, associated with portal hypertension. Adenoviral delivery of a constitutively active Akt restored Akt activation and NO production in the cirrhotic liver and resulted in normalization of portal pressures (106). Taken together, these data demonstrate the feasibility of transducing genes of interest into the liver's vascular compartment, even in the injured organ.

SUMMARY

In chronic liver injury there are two main factors contributing to increased hepatic resistance: (1) Mechanical factors secondary to fibrosis and regenerating nodules; and (2) interplay between sinusoidal endothelial cells and stellate cells resulting in stellate cell contraction. The relative contribution of these two elements is difficult to quantify. However, portal pressure can be reduced by 20–30% with pharmacologic agents that decrease intrahepatic resistance (6). It remains to be seen whether an effect of this magnitude is sufficient to reduce portal pressures enough to prevent the life-threatening sequelae of portal hypertension in cirrhotic patients. In addition, with so many cytokines and mediators converging on stellate cells, which ones are really important? It appears that antagonizing any given mediator in animal models is always antifibrotic, and the corresponding knock-out mice have attenuated fibrosis. Similarly, antagoinizing vasoconstrictive mediators or reconstituting vasodilatory mediators results in reduced stellate cell contractility and reduced portal pressures in animal models. Whether effective treatments in animal models will lead to successful treatments in human disease remains unknown. Compounds that have both antifibrotic and vasoregulatory properties, or combination therapies which can attack multiple pathways are most likely to succeed in the treatment of chronic liver injury.

REFERENCES

1. Geerts A. History and heterogeneity of stellate cells, and role in normal liver function. Semin Liver Dis 2001;21:311–336.
2. Sims D. Recent advances in pericyte biology and implications for health and disease. Can J Cardiol 1991;7:431–443.
3. Pinzani M, Failli P, Ruocco C, et al. Fat-storing cells as liver-specific pericytes. Spatial dynamics of agonist-stimulated intracellular calcium transients. J Clin Invest 1992;90:642–646.
4. Bauer M, Paquette N, Zhang J, et al. Chronic ethanol consumption increases hepatic sinusoidal contractile response to endothelin-1 in rat. Hepatology 1994;22:1565.
5. Bauer M, Zhang J, Bauer I, et al. ET-1 induced alterations of hepatic microcirculation: sinusoidal and extrasinusoidal sites of actions. Am J Physiol 1994;267:143–149.
6. Bhathal P, Grossman H. Reduction of the increased portal vascular resistance of the isolated perfused cirrhotic rat liver by vasodilators. J Hepatol 1985;1:325–337.
7. Okumura S, Takei Y, Kawano S. Vasoactive effect of endothelin-1 on rat liver in vivo. Hepatology 1994;19:155–161.
8. Liu Y, Binz J, Numerick M, et al. Hepatoprotection by the farsenoid X receptor agonist GW4064 in rat models of intra- and extrahepatic cholestasis. J Clin Invest 2003;112:1678–1687.

9. Inagaki Y, Nemoto T, Kushida M, et al. Interferon alfa down-regulates collagen gene transcription and suppresses experimental hepatic fibrosis in mice. Hepatology 2003;38:890–899.

10. Shiratori Y, Imazeki F, Moriyama M, et al. Histologic improvement of fibrosis in patients with hepatitis C who have sustained response to interferon therapy. Ann Intern Med 2000;132:517–524.

11. Kershenobich D, Vargas F, Garcia-Tsao G, Perez Tamayo R, Gent M, Rojkind M. Colchicine in the treatment of cirrhosis of the liver. N Engl J Med 1988;318:1709–1713.

12. Rodriguez L, Cerbon-Ambriz J, Munoz ML. Effects of colchicine and colchiceine in a biochemical model of liver injury and fibrosis. Arch Med Res 1998;29:109–116.

13. Poupon RE, Lindor KD, Cauch-Dudek K, Dickson ER, Poupon R, Heathcote EJ. Combined analysis of randomized controlled trials of ursodeoxycholic acid in primary biliary cirrhosis. Gastroenterology 1997;113:884–890.

14. Poo JL, Feldmann G, Erlinger S, et al. Ursodeoxycholic acid limits liver histologic alterations and portal hypertension induced by bile duct ligation in the rat. Gastroenterology 1992;102:1752–1759.

15. Fiorucci S, Antonelli E, Morelli A. Nitric oxide and portal hypertension: a nitric oxide-releasing derivative of ursodeoxycholic actd that selectively releases nitric oxide in the liver. Dig Liver Dis 2003; 35(Suppl):61–69.

16. Fiorucci S, Antonelli E, Morelli O, et al. NCX-1000, a NO-releasing derivative of ursodeoxycholic acid, selectively delivers NO to the liver and protects against development of portal hypertension. PNAS 2001;98:8897–8902.

17. Iwamoto H, Sakai H, Kotoh K, Nakamuta M, Nawata H. Soluble Arg-Gly-Asp peptides reduce collagen accumulation in cultured rat hepatic stellate cells. Dig Dis Sci 1999;44:1038–1045.

18. Bruck R, Hershkoviz R, Lider O, et al. Inhibition of experimentally-induced liver cirrhosis in rats by a nonpeptidic mimetic of the extracellular matrix-associated Arg-Gly-Asp epitope. J Hepatol 1996; 24:731–738.

19. Shi Z, Wakil AE, Rockey DC. Strain-specific differences in mouse hepatic wound healing are mediated by divergent T helper cytokine responses. Proc Natl Acad Sci USA 1997;94:10,663–10,668.

20. Sher A, Jankovic D, Cheever A, Wynn T. An IL-12-based vaccine approach for preventing immunopathology in schistosomiasis. Ann NY Acad Sci 1996;795:202–207.

21. Nelson DR, Lauwers GY, Lau JY, Davis GL. Interleukin 10 treatment reduces fibrosis in patients with chronic hepatitis C: a pilot trial of interferon nonresponders. Gastroenterology 2000;118:655–660.

22. Safadi S, Alvarez C, Cooreman M, Eng FJ, Friedman SL. Adoptive transfer of hepatic fibrosis by lymphocytes from mice with CCl_4 liver injury–implications for the role of the immune system in disease pathogenesis. Hepatology 2002;36:314A.

23. Canbay A, Higuchi H, Bronk SF, Taniai M, Sebo TJ, Gores GJ. Fas enhances fibrogenesis in the bile duct ligated mouse: a link between apoptosis and fibrosis. Gastroenterology 2002;123:1323–1330.

24. Canbay A, Friedman S, Gores G. Apoptosis: the nexus of liver injury and fibrosis. Hepatology 2004; 39:273–278.

25. Taimr P, Higuchi H, Kocova E, Rippe RA, Friedman S, Gores GJ. Activated stellate cells express the TRAIL receptor-2/death receptor-5 and undergo TRAIL-mediated apoptosis. Hepatology 2003;37: 87–95.

26. Song E, Lee SK, Wang J, et al. RNA interference targeting Fas protects mice from fulminant hepatitis. Nat Med 2003;9:347–351.

27. Shiratori Y, Imazeki F, Moriyama M, et al. Histologic improvement of fibrosis in patients with hepatitis C who have sustained response to interferon therapy. Ann Intern Med 2000;132:517–524.

28. Poynard T, McHutchison J, Manns M, et al. Impact of pegylated interferon alfa-2b and ribavirin on liver fibrosis in patients with chronic hepatitis C. Gastroenterology 2002;122:1303–1313.

29. Rockey DC, Maher JJ, Jarnagin WR, Gabbiani G, Friedman SL. Inhibition of rat hepatic lipocyte activation in culture by interferon-gamma. Hepatology 1992;16:776–784.

30. Rockey DC, Chung JJ. Interferon gamma inhibits lipocyte activation and extracellular matrix mRNA expression during experimental liver injury: implications for treatment of hepatic fibrosis. J Investig Med 1994;42:660–670.

31. Brown KE, Poulos JE, Li L, et al. Effect of vitamin E supplementation on hepatic fibrogenesis in chronic dietary iron overload. Am J Physiol 1997;272:G116–G123.

32. Houglum K, Venkataramani A, Lyche K, Chojkier M. A pilot study of the effects of d-alpha-tocopherol on hepatic stellate cell activation in chronic hepatitis C. Gastroenterology 1997;113:1069–1073.

33. Kawada N, Seki S, Inoue M, Kuroki T. Effect of antioxidants, resveratrol, quercetin, and N-acetylcysteine, on the functions of cultured rat hepatic stellate cells and Kupffer cells. Hepatology 1998; 27:1265–1274.

34. Stickel F, Brinkhaus B, Krahmer N, Seitz HK, Hahn EG, Schuppan D. Antifibrotic properties of botanicals in chronic liver disease. Hepatogastroenterology 2002;49:1102–1108.

35. Jacobs BP, Dennehy C, Ramirez G, Sapp J, Lawrence VA. Milk thistle for the treatment of liver disease: a systematic review and meta-analysis. Am J Med 2002;113:506–515.

36. George J, Roulot D, Koteliansky VE, Bissell DM. In vivo inhibition of rat stellate cell activation by soluble transforming growth factor beta type II receptor: a potential new therapy for hepatic fibrosis. Proc Natl Acad Sci USA 1999;96:12,719–12,724.

37. Spearman M, Taylor WR, Greenberg AH, Wright JA. Antisense oligodeoxyribonucleotide inhibition of TGF-beta 1 gene expression and alterations in the growth and malignant properties of mouse fibrosarcoma cells. Gene 1994;149:25–29.

38. Jonsson JR, Clouston AD, Ando Y, et al. Angiotensin-converting enzyme inhibition attenuates the progression of rat hepatic fibrosis. Gastroenterology 2001;121:148–155.

39. Okuno M, Akita K, Moriwaki H, et al. Prevention of rat hepatic fibrosis by the protease inhibitor, camostat mesilate, via reduced generation of active TGF-beta. Gastroenterology 2001;120:1784–1800.

40. Border WA, Okuda S, Languino LR, Sporn MB, Ruoslahti E. Suppression of experimental glomerulonephritis by antiserum against transforming growth factor beta 1. Nature 1990;346:371–374.

41. Roth S, Michel K, Gressner AM. (Latent) transforming growth factor beta in liver parenchymal cells, its injury-dependent release, and paracrine effects on rat hepatic stellate cells. Hepatology 1998;27: 1003–1012.

42. Luscher TF. Endothelin, endothelin receptors, and endothelin antagonists. Curr Opin Nephrol Hypertens 1994;3:92–98.

43. Rockey DC, Chung JJ. Endothelin antagonism in experimental hepatic fibrosis. Implications for endothelin in the pathogenesis of wound healing. J Clin Invest 1996;98:1381–1388.

44. Ueki T, Kaneda Y, Tsutsui H, et al. Hepatocyte growth factor gene therapy of liver cirrhosis in rats. Nat Med 1999;5:226–230.

45. Ozaki I, Zhao G, Mizuta T, et al. Hepatocyte growth factor induces collagenase (matrix metalloproteinase-1) via the transcription factor Ets-1 in human hepatic stellate cell line. J Hepatol 2002;36: 169–178.

46. Yasuda H, Imai E, Shiota A, Fujise N, Morinaga T, Higashio K. Antifibrogenic effect of a deletion variant of hepatocyte growth factor on liver fibrosis in rats. Hepatology 1996;24:636–642.

47. Masunaga H, Fujise N, Shiota A, et al. Preventive effects of the deleted form of hepatocyte growth factor against various liver injuries. Eur J Pharmacol 1998;342:267–279.

48. Pines M, Knopov V, Genina O, Lavelin I, Nagler A. Halofuginone, a specific inhibitor of collagen type I synthesis, prevents dimethylnitrosamine-induced liver cirrhosis. J Hepatol 1997;27:391–398.

49. Pines M, Nagler A. Halofuginone: a novel antifibrotic therapy. Gen Pharmacol 1998;30:445–450.

50. Spira G, Mawasi N, Paizi M, et al. Halofuginone, a collagen type I inhibitor improves liver regeneration in cirrhotic rats. J Hepatol 2002;37:331–339.

51. Bruck R, Genina O, Aeed H, et al. Halofuginone to prevent and treat thioacetamide-induced liver fibrosis in rats. Hepatology 2001;33:379–386.

52. Okuno M, Moriwaki H, Imai S, et al. Retinoids exacerbate rat liver fibrosis by inducing the activation of latent TGF-beta in liver stellate cells [see comments]. Hepatology 1997;26:913–921.

53. Geerts A, Rogiers V. Sho-saiko-To: the right blend of traditional Oriental medicine and liver cell biology [editorial; comment]. Hepatology 1999;29:282–284.

54. Sakaida I, Matsumura Y, Akiyama S, Hayashi K, Ishige A, Okita K. Herbal medicine Sho-saiko-to (TJ-9) prevents liver fibrosis and enzyme-altered lesions in rat liver cirrhosis induced by a choline-deficient L- amino acid-defined diet. J Hepatol 1998;28:298–306.

55. Shimizu I, Ma YR, Mizobuchi Y, et al. Effects of Sho-saiko-to, a Japanese herbal medicine, on hepatic fibrosis in rats [see comments]. Hepatology 1999;29:149–160.

56. Wasser S, Ho JM, Ang HK, Tan CE. Salvia miltiorrhiza reduces experimentally-induced hepatic fibrosis in rats [In Process Citation]. J Hepatol 1998;29:760-771 [MEDLINE record in process].

57. Zhu J, Wu J, Frizell E, et al. Rapamycin inhibits hepatic stellate cell proliferation in vitro and limits fibrogenesis in an in vivo model of liver fibrosis. Gastroenterology 1999;117:1198–1204.

58. Raetsch C, Jia JD, Boigk G, et al. Pentoxifylline downregulates profibrogenic cytokines and procollagen I expression in rat secondary biliary fibrosis. Gut 2002;50:241–247.

59. Akriviadis E, Botla R, Briggs W, Han S, Reynolds T, Shakil O. Pentoxifylline improves short-term survival in serve acute alcoholic hepatitis: a double-blind, placebo-controlled trial. Gastroenterology 2000;119:1637–1648.

60. Arthur MJ. Fibrosis and altered matrix degradation. Digestion 1998;59:376–380.

61. Iimuro Y, Nishio T, Morimoto T, et al. Delivery of matrix metalloproteinase-1 attenuates established liver fibrosis in the rat. Gastroenterology 2003;124:445–458.

62. Iwamoto H, Sakai H, Nawata H. Inhibition of integrin signaling with Arg-Gly-Asp motifs in rat hepatic stellate cells. J Hepatol 1998;29:752–759.

63. Wright MC, Issa R, Smart DE, et al. Gliotoxin stimulates the apoptosis of human and rat hepatic stellate cells and enhances the resolution of liver fibrosis in rats. Gastroenterology 2001;121:685–698.

64. Rockey DC. Vascular mediators in the injured liver. Hepatology 2003;37:4–12.

65. Moore K, Wendon J, Frazer M, et al. Plasma endothelin immunoreactivity in liver disease and the hepatorenal syndrome. N Engl J Med 1992;327:1774–1778.

66. Pinzani M, Milani S, De FR, et al. Endothelin 1 is overexpressed in human cirrhotic liver and exerts multiple effects on activated hepatic stellate cells. Gastroenterology 1996;110:534–548.

67. Rockey DC, Chung JJ. Reduced nitric oxide production by endothelial cells in cirrhotic rat liver: endothelial dysfunction in portal hypertension. Gastroenterology 1998;114:344–351.

68. Gandhi C, Behal R, Harvey S, et al. Increased hepatic endothelin-1 levels and endothelial receptor density in cirrhotic rats. Life Sci 1992;58:55–62.

69. Gandhi C, Nemoto E, Watkins S, et al. An endothelin-receptor antagonist TAK-044 ameliorates carbon tetrachloride-induced acute liver injury and portal hypertension in rats. Liver 1998;18:39–48.

70. Poo JL, Jimenez W, Maria Munoz R, et al. Chronic blockade of endothelin receptors in cirrhotic rats: hepatic and hemodynamic effects. Gastroenterology 1999;116:161–167.

71. Reichen J, Gerbes A, Steiner M, et al. The effect of endothelin and its antagonist Bosentan on hemodynamics and microvascular exchange in cirrhotic rat liver. J Hepatol 1998;28:1020–1030.

72. Michel T, Feron O. Nitric oxide synthases: which, where, how, and why? J Clin Invest 1997;100: 2146–2152.

73. Gupta TK, Toruner M, Groszmann RJ. Intrahepatic modulation of portal pressure and its role in portal hypertension. Role of nitric oxide. Digestion 1998;59:413–415.

74. Rockey DC, Chung JJ. Inducible nitric oxide synthase in rat hepatic lipocytes and the effect of nitric oxide on lipocyte contractility. J Clin Invest 1995;95:1199–1206.

75. Rockey DC. Characterization of endothelin receptors mediating rat hepatic stellate cell contraction. Biochem Biophys Res Commun 1995;207:725–731.

76. Suzuki H, Menegazzi M, Carcerero P, et al. Nitric oxide in the liver: physiopathological roles. Neuroimmunol 1995;5:379–410.

77. Saavedra J, Billiar T, Williams D. Targeting nitric oxide(NO) delivery in vivo. Design of a liver-selective NO prodrug that blocks TNF-α-induced apoptosis and toxicity in the liver. J Med Chem 1997; 40:1947–1954.

78. Ricciardi R, Foley D, Quarfordt S, et al. V-PYRRO/NO: an hepato-selective nitric oxide donor improves porcine hemodynamics and function after ischemia-reperfusion. Transplantation 2001:193–198.

79. Stinson S, House T, Bramhall C, et al. Plasma pharmokinetics of a liver-selective nitric oxide-donating diazeniumdiolate in the male C57BL/6. Xenobiotica 2002;32:339–347.

80. Kim Y, Kim T, Chung H, et al. Nitric oxide prevents tumor necrosis factor-α induced rat hepatocyte apoptosis by the interruption of mitochondrial apoptotic signaling through S-nitrosylation of caspase-8. Hepatology 2000;32:770–778.

81. Deleve L, Wang X, Kanel G, et al. Decreased hepatic nitric oxide production contributes to the development of rat sinusoidal obstruction syndrome. Hepatology 2003;38:900–908.

82. Liu J, Saveedra J, Lu T, et al. 02-vinyl 1-(pyrrolidin-1-yl) diazen-1-ium-1,2-diolate protection against D-galactosamine/endotoxin-induced hepatoxicity in mice: genomic analysis using microarrays. J Pharmacol Exp Ther 2002;300:18–25.

83. Moal F, Vuillemin E, Wang J, et al. Chronic antifibrotic and hemodynamic effects of a new liver specif NO donor(V-PYYRO/NO) in bile duct ligated(BDL) rats. Hepatology 2000;32(Suppl):94.

84. Fiorucci S, Antonelli E, Morelli O, et al. NCX-1000, a NO-releasing derivative of ursodeoxycholic acid, selectively delivers NO to the liver and protects against development of portal hypertension. Proc Natl Acad Sci USA 2001;98:8897–8902.

85. Kureishi Y, Luo Z, Shiojima I, et al. The HMG-CoA reductase inhibitor simvastatin activates the protein kinase Akt and promotes angiogenesis in normocholesterolemic animals. Nat Med 2000;6: 1004–1010.

86. Zafra C, Abraldes J, Turnes J. Simvastatin enhances hepatic nitric oxide production and decreases the hepatic vascular tone in patients with cirrhosis. Gastroenterology 2004;126:749–755.

87. Bataller R, Gines P, Nicolas JM, et al. Angiotensin II induces contraction and proliferation of human hepatic stellate cells. Gastroenterology 2000;118:1149–1156.

88. Bataller R, Sancho-Bru P, Gines P, et al. Activated human hepatic stellate cells express the renin-angiotensin system and synthesize angiotensin II. Gastroenterology 2003;125:117–125.

89. Croquet V, Moal F, Veal N, et al. Hemodynamic and antifibrotic effects of losartan in rats with liver fibrosis and/or portal hypertension. J Hepatol 2002;37:773–780.

90. Gonzalez-Abraldes J, Albillos A, Banares R, et al. Randomized comparison of long-term losartan versus propranolol in lowering portal pressures in cirrhosis. Gastroenterology 2001;121:382–388.

91. Albillos A, Lledo J, Rossi I, et al. Continuous prazosin administration in cirrhotic patients effects on portal hemodynamics and on liver and renal function. Gastroenterology 1995;109:1257–1265.

92. Lee W, Lin H, Yang Y. Hemodynamic effects of a combination of prazosin and terlipressin in patients with viral cirrhosis. Am J Gastroenterol 2001;96:1210–1216.

93. Kay M, Glorioso J, Naldini L. Viral vectors for gene therapy: the art of tuning infectious agents into vehicles of therapeutics. Nat Med 2001;7:33–40.

94. Garcia-Banuelos J, Siller-Lopez F, Miranda A, et al. Cirrhotic rat livers with extensive fibrosis can be safely transduced with clinical-grade adenoviral vectors. Evidence of cirrhosis reversion. Gene Ther 2002;9:127–134.

95. Shalala D. Protecting research subjects and what must be done. N Engl J Med 2000;343:808–810.

96. Williams DA, Baum C. Gene Therapy-new challenges ahead. Science 2003;302:400–410.

97. Oren R, Dabeva MD, Karnezis AN, et al. Role of thyroid hormone in stimulating liver repopulation in the rat by transplanted hepatocytes. Hepatology 1999;30:903–913.

98. Galimi F, Verma I. Opportunities for the use of lentiviral vectors in human gene therapy. Current Topics in Microbiol Immunol 2002;261:245–254.

99. Buning H, Nickin S, Perabo L, Hallek M, Baker A. AAV-based gene transfer. Curr Opin Mol Ther 2003;5:367–375.

100. Arias M, Sauer-Lehnen S, Treptau J, et al. Adenoviral expression of transforming growth factor-beta 1 antisense mRNA is effective in preventing liver fibrosis in bile-duct ligated rats. BMC Gastroenterology 2003;18:29.

101. Dooley D, Hamzavi J, Breitkopf K, et al. Smad7 prevents activation of hepatic stellate cells and liver fibrosis in rats. Gastroenterology 2003;125:178–191.

102. Suzuki K, Aoki K, Ohnami S, et al. Adenovirus-mediated gene transfer of interferon alpha improves dimethylnitrosamine-induced liver cirrhosis in rat model. Gene Ther 2003;10:765–773.

103. Suzuki K, Aoki K, Ohnami S. Adenovirus-mediated gene transfer of interferon alpha inhibits hepatitis C virus replication in hepatocytes. Biochem Biophys Res Commun 2003;307:814–819.

104. Siller-Lopez F, Sandoval A, Salgado S, et al. Treatment with human Metalloproteinase-8 gene delivery ameliorates experimental rat liver cirrhosis. Gastroenterology 2004;126:1122–1133.

105. Yu Q, Shao R, Qian HS, George SE, Rockey DC. Gene transfer of the neuronal NO synthase isoform to cirrhotic rat liver ameliorates portal hypertension. J Clin Invest 2000;105:741–748.

106. Morales-Ruiz M, Cejudo-Martin P, Fernandez-Varo G, et al. Transduction of the liver with activated Akt normalizes portal pressure in cirrhotic rats. Gastroenterology 2003;125:522–531.

Index